An Invitation to Health Brief

Health 11: Los Angeles City College

Dianne Hales

THOMSON

Australia · Canada · Mexico · Singapore · Spain · United Kingdom · United States

THOMSON

An Invitation to Health Brief
Dianne Hales

Executive Editors:
Michele Baird, Maureen Staudt &
Michael Stranz

Project Development Manager:
Linda deStefano

Sr. Marketing Coordinators:
Lindsay Annett and Sara Mercurio

Production/Manufacturing Manager:
Donna M. Brown

Pre-Media Services Supervisor:
Becki Walker

Rights and Permissions Specialist:
Kalina Ingham Hintz

Cover Image
Getty Images*

Printed in the
United States of America
1 2 3 4 5 6 7 10 09 08 07

For more information, please contact Thomson Custom Solutions, 5191 Natorp Boulevard, Mason, OH 45040. Or you can visit our Internet site at www.thomsoncustom.com

The Adaptable Courseware Program consists of products and additions to existing Thomson products that are produced from camera-ready copy. Peer review, class testing, and accuracy are primarily the responsibility of the author(s).

ISBN: 978-0-495-63479-9
ISBN: 0-495-63479-4

International Divisions List

Asia (Including India):
Thomson Learning
(a division of Thomson Asia Pte Ltd)
5 Shenton Way #01-01
UIC Building
Singapore 068808
Tel: (65) 6410-1200
Fax: (65) 6410-1208

Australia/New Zealand:
Thomson Learning Australia
102 Dodds Street
Southbank, Victoria 3006
Australia

Latin America:
Thomson Learning
Seneca 53
Colonia Polano
11560 Mexico, D.F., Mexico
Tel (525) 281-2906
Fax (525) 281-2656

Canada:
Thomson Nelson
1120 Birchmount Road
Toronto, Ontario
Canada M1K 5G4
Tel (416) 752-9100
Fax (416) 752-8102

UK/Europe/Middle East/Africa:
Thomson Learning
High Holborn House
50-51 Bedford Row
London, WC1R 4LS
United Kingdom
Tel 44 (020) 7067-2500
Fax 44 (020) 7067-2600

Spain (Includes Portugal):
Thomson Paraninfo
Calle Magallanes 25
28015 Madrid
España
Tel 34 (0)91 446-3350
Fax 34 (0)91 445-6218

CUSTOM CONTENTS

Attitude

The longer I live,
the more I realize the impact of attitude on life.
Attitude, to me, is more important than fact.
It is more important than the past,
than education, than money, than circumstances,
than failures, than successes, than what other people say or do.
It is more important than appearance, giftedness or skill.
It will make or break a company… a church… a home.
The remarkable thing is what have a choice everyday
regarding the attitude we will embrace for that day.
We can not change the past.
We can not change the inevitable.
The only thing we can do is play
on the one string we have, and that is attitude.
I am convinced that life is 10% what happens to me
and 90% how I react to it.
And so it is with you.
We are in charge of our attitudes.

-Charles Swindoll-

Welcome to Los Angeles City College

Department of Health and Physical Education

The Department of Health and Physical Education is dedicated to excellence in assisting students to understand not only the cognitive concepts in leading a healthy and productive life but also offers avenues of actual physical activities that alter the mind, body and spirit. Students will learn that the leading causes of death in the United States are, for the most part, directly related to the behaviors we choose each day. For example, 1 in 3 Americans are considered over fat or obese! This is frightening considering it is something that most of us have direct control over. Each day we wake up with a new opportunity to positively affect our lives and our health through the nutritional and exercise programs we choose to engage in. This is not an easy task and there is no "magic pill" for if there were, everyone would be thin and in shape. Many people want to be thinner but Americans keeps getting bigger and bigger. It's important for us to understand that we have locus of control over this area of our lives and that many of the problems we have in this area are the direct effect of our attitude towards it. Our nutritional choices are just one of the areas covered in this course. You will gain a wide body of knowledge to use each day if you choose to adopt the necessary behavior changes. Before going further let me digress and relate a quick story.

Several years ago a good friend of mine asked me what had gone wrong with her life. She was then in her fifties, and although she still retained a good deal of her youthful beauty she was now hugely over-fat and suffered from several degenerative ailments. Her sedentary life as a college professor in an academic field didn't allow for much exercise. She had grown up in an era when the idea of belonging to a health club was still novel. Her cultural background advocated the idea of suffering and penance as a means of attaining something akin to sainthood. She had been divorced five years previous to her bouts of what she waved off as "indigestion". One day, buckling under from pain that necessitated a trip to the hospital she realized that she needed to reassess her life. Now she had to ask the important questions, "What is life all about?' "What's the most important thing in my life?" "How much time do I have?" "What did I do wrong?"--- She had cancer.

It has been some years since my friend died, but I remember early on telling her "Health is first wealth". You may be the wealthiest person in town but if you're irreversibly sick and dying you'd give your millions away if you could just extend life for a year, a month, a week, a day,............a minute. So often at the end of our lives we want to barter for an extension to our lives. The wiser move is to invest in our lives near the beginning. We do this by understanding the demands the environment places on our physical bodies and minds, and the actions that have to be taken to promote a healthy, productive, happy and long life. This course contains the basics that will lead us in the right direction. Hopefully you won't have to ask at a premature end, "What did I do wrong?".

Our Health programs are the only ones on campus that comprehensively confront the issues of mental health, stress management, communication, nutrition, weight management, exercise, sexual behavior, family planning, alcohol, tobacco and drug addiction, degenerative and communicative diseases including STI's such as AIDS, self care, aging, consumerism, accident prevention, and of course understanding how our environment plays such a vital role in our health. Our health courses deal directly with your life and will give you some of the tools necessary to live not only a longer life but a QUALITY of life as well. Our faculty is at your disposal to help give you the knowledge necessary to avoid some of the pitfalls of life!

OUR FACULTY

Hayward Nishioka

Professor of Health and Physical Education, Pan American Games Gold Medallist in Judo, published author, SAG member, black belt in Judo and Karate, President of the Southern California Judo Federation, Assistant Instructor of Scuba (PADI)

Nancy Pierce M.S.

Professor of Health and Physical Education, Minor in Psychology, Bachelor of Science in Health Education and Masters of Science in Exercise Physiology from Cal State Northridge. Environmentalist, president of a consulting business, Motivational Speaker, L.A. Marathon finisher, specializes in volleyball, health, hiking, equestrian, and running.

Jan McEveety

Chairperson of Women's Physical Education, Professor of Health and Physical Education, swimming and volleyball coach, exercise physiologies, academic senator.

Tom Cano

Professor of Health and Physical Education, Former baseball, assistant football, basketball, and cross-country coach. Swimming and weight training specialist

Christine Tinberg,

Assistant Professor of Physical Education Fitness Center Coordinator, B.S. in Sports Medicine from Pepperdine University and a M.S. in Exercise Science from Arizona State University. Specializes in swimming, cycling, and exercise physiology.

John Erdhouse

Chairperson of Men's Physical Education, Professor of Physical Education, Former football coach, golf pro, weight training instructor

Daniel Cowgill

Associate Professor of Health and Physical Education, Former Baseball and Golf coach, Past Chairperson of Physical Education

Steve Rousey

Assistant Professor of Health and Physical Education, Head Baseball coach

Michael Miller

Assistant Professor of Physical Education, Athletic Director, Health Basketball coach

Adjunct Faculty

Lillian Yamaoka

Trisha San Martin

Robert McKinley

Beverly Russell

Robert Horowitz

Mark Kertinian

Jason Dietrich

George Vranau

Aykanush Gevenyan

LACC Health and Physical Education Courses

Take these courses to enrich your life and fulfill your AA requirement

Health

HEALTH 2
Health and Fitness
3 UNITS – (UC:CSU)
Course explores physical fitness as related to cardiovascular capacity, nutrition, stress, and addictive substances. The course involves laboratory assessment of each student's fitness status, lecture, and selected fitness activities. Based on these experiences students develop individualized fitness programs.

HEALTH 8
Women's Personal Health
3 UNITS – (UC:CSU)
Advisory: English 28/31 or equivalent.
The course examines the personal and social dimensions of women's health and the development of strategies for empowerment in decision making that impact changes and improvement in health welfare.

HEALTH 11
Principles of Healthful Living
3 UNITS – (UC:CSU)
The course offers health related concepts for today and the future as guidelines for a self-directed, responsible, satisfying, and productive life-style. Emphasis is on cognitive concepts and strategies of wellness for the individuals personal community, vocational, and leadership roles.

Physical Education

DANCE STUDIES 185
Directed Study - Dance
1 UNIT - (RPT 3) (UC:CSU)
Allows the student to pursue directed study in dance on a contract basis under the direction of a supervising instructor.

DANCE STUDIES 452
Introduction to Choreography
1 UNIT - (RPT 3) (UC:CSU)
This course introduces students to choreography with an emphasis on basic steps and combinations, creating dances, terminology, music, and appreciation of dance as a performing art form. Course may be taken four times.

DANCE SPECIALTIES 459
Flamenco and Spanish Dancing
1 UNIT - (RPT 3) (UC:CSU)
This course introduces the student to flamenco and Spanish dance with an emphasis on correct posture, individual steps, and arm movements. Terminology, various rhythms, basic step combinations and castanet technique will also be covered

DANCE STUDIOS 805

History and Appreciation of Dance
3 UNITS
Advisory: English 28
This course provides a historical perspective of dance from ritual to contemporary theatrical dance forms. It focuses on the ethnic, cultural and ritual forms of dance as it affected and reflected the world in which people lived. Primarily, this course will focus on how Dance reflects the times, historical, social and political climate of the day. The class will consider the impact of dance on the western world and how it has been affected by the different dance traditions world-wide.

DANCE TECHNIQUES 400
Stress Management Techniques Through Dance and Movement
1 UNIT - (RPT 3) (UC:CSU)
This course helps identify stressors and introduce techniques of dance and dance therapy. Movement mediations, authentic movement studies, breathing exercises, yoga, physical therapy and relaxation exercises are introduced. Multicultural rhythms and dance forms are used to enhance group experiences. May be taken 4 times.

DANCE TECHNIQUES 405
Yoga Conditioning for Dance
1 UNIT - (RPT 3) (UC:CSU)
This course introduces dance students to yoga skills that provide conditioning, flexibility and endurance to supplement dance technique. Course may be taken four times.

DANCE TECHNIQUES 406
Hatha Yoga Conditioning for Dancers
1 UNIT - (RPT 3) (UC:CSU)
Advisory: Dance 405.
This course provides dance students who have attained a basic level of yoga proficiency from Dance 405 (Yoga Conditioning for Dance) access to a more in-depth Hatha yoga practice that offer physical challenges beyond a beginning level and provides more advanced experiences in conditioning, flexibility and endurance to supplement dance technique. Course may be taken four times.

DANCE TECHNIQUES 408
Dance Movement for Instrumentalists and Vocalists
1 UNIT - (RPT 3) (UC:CSU)
This course will include different music and dance styles, tempo variations, and stage awareness to enhance a music student's movement on stage.

DANCE TECHNIQUES 410
Dance Aerobics
1 UNIT - (RPT 3) (UC:CSU)
Using the forms of dance aerobically, students will increase flexibility, strength, and cardiovascular endurance. Course may be taken four times.

DANCE TECHNIQUES 431
Modern Dance
1 UNIT - (RPT 3) (UC:CSU)
This course introduces students to modern dance with an emphasis on basic steps and combinations, terminology, music, and appreciation of dance as a performing art form. Course may be taken four times.

DANCE TECHNIQUES 434
Ballet

1 UNIT - (RPT 3) (UC:CSU)
This course introduces students to ballet with an emphasis on basic steps and combinations, terminology, music, and appreciation of dance as a performing art form. Course may be taken four times.

DANCE TECHNIQUES 437
Jazz Dance
1 UNIT - (RPT 3) (UC:CSU)
This course introduces students to jazz dance with an emphasis on basic steps and combinations, terminology, music, and appreciation of dance as a performing art form. Course may be taken four times.

DANCE TECHNIQUES 440
Social Dance
1 UNIT - (RPT 3) (UC:CSU)
In each dance form, special attention is paid to technique, terminology, history, style, and appreciation of related arts. Course may be taken four times.

DANCE TECHNIQUES 446
Tap Dance
1 UNIT - (RPT 3) (UC:CSU)
This course introduces students to tap dance with an emphasis on basic steps and combination, terminology, music, and appreciation of dance as a performing art form. Course may be taken four times.

DANCE TECHNIQUES 466
Ballet Combinations
1 UNIT - (RPT 3) (UC:CSU)
This course introduces students to ballet combinations with an emphasis on basic steps and combinations, terminology, music, and appreciation of dance as a performing art form. Course may be taken four times.

DANCE TECHNIQUES 467
Modern Dance Combinations
1 UNIT - (RPT 3) (UC:CSU)
This course introduces students to modern dance combinations with an emphasis on basic steps and combinations, terminology, music, and appreciation of dance as a performing art form. Course may be taken four times.

DANCE TECHNIQUES 468
Jazz Dance Combinations
1 UNIT - (RPT 3) (UC:CSU)
This course introduces students to jazz dance combinations with an emphasis on basic steps and combinations, terminology, music, and appreciation of dance as a performing art form. Course may be taken four times.

DANCE TECHNIQUES 469
Conditioning for Dance
1 UNIT - (RPT 3) (UC:CSU)
Students will learn dance and aerobic exercises to increase flexibility, strength, and endurance. Course may be taken four times.

PHYSICAL EDUCATION 401
International Folk Dance Skills
1 UNIT - (RPT 3) (UC:CSU)

PHYSICAL EDUCATION 480
Dances of Armenia and Greece
1 UNIT - (RPT 3) (UC:CSU)
Above courses acceptable for Dance 70 credits, UCLA.

PHYSICAL EDUCATION 101-142
Water Activities - Swimming
1 UNIT - (RPT 3) (UC:CSU)
Activity 2 hours.
Beginning, intermediate and advanced levels offered for all swim courses.

PHYSICAL EDUCATION 101
Water Activities - Non-Swimmer
1 UNIT - (RPT 3) (UC:CSU)

PHYSICAL EDUCATION 102
Water Activities - Swimming Skills
1 UNIT - (RPT 3) (UC:CSU)

PHYSICAL EDUCATION 110
Lap Swimming For Fitness
1 UNIT – (RPT 3) (UC:CSU)
For experienced swimmers who want to improve their speed, strength, and endurance. Students should be able to swim 50 yards without stopping in deep water using the freestyle stroke and rotary breathing. Class sessions consist of instructor directed, organized swimming workouts. At the first pool session, an assessment of swimming ability will be conducted to ensure minimum skills for participation.

PHYSICAL EDUCATION 122
Water Activities - Aqua Exercise
1 UNIT - (RPT 3) (UC:CSU)
Instruction includes progressive skills attainment.

PHYSICAL EDUCATION 128
Rock Climbing for Fitness
1 UNIT - (RPT 3) (UC:CSU)
This course was designed to provide exercise and fitness training for the beginning student who wants to learn more about equipment needs, new climbing areas, restrictions, and techniques for safe climbing. This class is created to accommodate first time climbers as well as those with some indoor rock climbing experience. The class is designed to be fun and challenging with the main emphasis on movement and self-esteem building. Students will develop muscular strength and endurance and improve their cardiovascular system.

PHYSICAL EDUCATION 170
Walking for Fitness
1 UNIT
This course focuses on achieving cardiovascular fitness and a healthy lifestyle through walking. Course topics include posture, gait, walking styles, strength and flexibility, proper clothing, nutrition and nutrirional aides, creating a walking program and fitness assessments.

PHYSICAL EDUCATION 185

see end of this section

PHYSICAL EDUCATION 203-299
Individual and Dual Activities
1 UNIT - (RPT 3) (UC:CSU)
Activity 2 hours.
In each sport or activity special attention is paid to techniques, strategy, etiquette, terminology, history, and rules.

PHYSICAL EDUCATION 203
Badminton Skills
1 UNIT - (RPT 3) (UC:CSU)

PHYSICAL EDUCATION 212
Tennis Skills
1 UNIT - (RPT 3) (UC:CSU)

PHYSICAL EDUCATION 216
Paddle Tennis Skills
1 UNIT - (RPT 3) (UC:CSU)

PHYSICAL EDUCATION 219
Table Tennis Skills
1 UNIT - (RPT 3) (UC:CSU)

PHYSICAL EDUCATION 225
Individual & Dual Activities - Yoga Skills
1 UNIT - (RPT 3) (UC:CSU)

PHYSICAL EDUCATION 228
Individual and Dual Activities Body Conditioning
1 UNIT - (RPT 3) (UC:CSU)
In each sport or activity, special attention is paid to techniques, strategy, etiquette, terminology, history, and rules. Individual courses may be taken four times.

PHYSICAL EDUCATION 229
Individual and Dual Activities: Body Dynamics
1 UNIT - (RPT 3) (UC:CSU)
In each sport or activity, special attention is paid to techniques, strategy, etiquette, terminology, history, and rules. Individual courses may be taken four times.

PHYSICAL EDUCATION 230
Weight Training
1 UNIT - (RPT 3) (UC:CSU)
In each sport or activity, special attention is paid to techniques, strategy, etiquette, terminology, history, and rules.

PHYSICAL EDUCATION 238
Self-Defense Skills
1 UNIT - (RPT 3) (UC:CSU)
In each sport or activity, special attention is paid to techniques, strategy, etiquette, terminology, history, and rules. Individual courses may be taken four times.

PHYSICAL EDUCATION 241
Judo Skills
1 UNIT - (RPT 3) (UC:CSU)

PHYSICAL EDUCATION 247
Gymnastics Skills
1 UNIT - (RPT 3) (UC:CSU)

PHYSICAL EDUCATION 259
Golf Skills
1 UNIT - (RPT 3) (UC:CSU)

PHYSICAL EDUCATION 262
Track and Field Skills
1 UNIT - (RPT 3) (UC:CSU)

PHYSICAL EDUCATION 299
Stress Management Techniques Through Movement and Dance
1 UNIT - (RPT 3) (UC:CSU)
This course helps us identify our stressors and introduces techniques such as breathing, yoga, relaxation exercises, movement, and dance as a means of coping with the stress in our lives.

PHYSICAL EDUCATION 300-399
Team Sports
1 UNIT - (RPT 3) (UC:CSU)
Activity 2 hours.
In each sport or activity, special attention is paid to techniques, strategy, etiquette, terminology, history, and rules.

PHYSICAL EDUCATION 301
Baseball Skills
1 UNIT - (RPT 3) (UC:CSU)

PHYSICAL EDUCATION 304
Basketball Skills
1 UNIT - (RPT 3) (UC:CSU)
In each sport or activity, special attention is paid to techniques, strategy, etiquette, terminology, history, and rules. Individual courses may be taken four times.

PHYSICAL EDUCATION 313
TEAM SPORTS - SOCCER SKILLS
1 UNIT - (RPT 3) (UC:CSU)

PHYSICAL EDUCATION 322
Volleyball Skills
1 UNIT - (RPT 3) (UC:CSU)

PHYSICAL EDUCATION 328
Softball Skills
1 UNIT - (RPT 3) (UC:CSU)

PHYSICAL EDUCATION 500-599
Intercollegiate Athletics Sports
2 UNITS - (RPT 1) (UC:CSU)
Activity 10 hours or more in the sports in season for the following courses.

PHYSICAL EDUCATION 500
Basketball Theory
3 UNITS - (RPT 1)
Prerequisite: Tryouts.
Co-requisite: Physical Education 504.

PHYSICAL EDUCATION 502
Badminton
2 UNITS - (RPT 1) (UC:CSU)

PHYSICAL EDUCATION 503
Baseball
2 UNITS - (RPT 1) (UC:CSU)

PHYSICAL EDUCATION 504
Basketball
2 UNITS - (RPT 1) (UC:CSU)
Prerequisite: Tryouts.

PHYSICAL EDUCATION 509
Intercollegiate Sports-Golf
2 UNITS - (RPT 1) (UC:CSU)
This course offers advanced instruction in the fundamental skills and techniques of golf and an opportunity for practical application in intercollegiate competition.

PHYSICAL EDUCATION 511
Soccer
2 UNITS - (RPT 1) (UC:CSU)
Prerequisite: Tryouts.

PHYSICAL EDUCATION 514
Intercollegiate Sports-Tennis
2 UNITS - (RPT 3) (UC:CSU)
Students with intermediate and advanced tennis skills need and opportunity to participate in higher levels of singles and doubles competition.

PHYSICAL EDUCATION 515
Track and Field
2 UNITS - (RPT 3) (UC:CSU)
This course offers men and women students with advanced track and field skills and opportunity to participate in intercollegiate track and field.

PHYSICAL EDUCATION 516
Volleyball
2 UNITS - (RPT 1) (UC:CSU)
Students with intermediate and advanced volleyball skills are given the opportunity to compete at the intercollegiate level.

PHYSICAL EDUCATION 552
Athletic Pre-season Conditioning
1 UNIT - (RPT 2) (UC:CSU)

PHYSICAL EDUCATION 630-810
FITNESS
0.5-2 UNITS - (RPT Varies) (UC:CSU)

Activity hours vary.

PHYSICAL EDUCATION 630
Aerobic Super Circuit Laboratory
1 UNIT - (RPT 3) (UC:CSU)
Using fundamentals of exercise physiology, each student will assess his/her level of physical fitness, develop a fitness profile, and design and implement a personalized exercise program.

PHYSICAL EDUCATION 635
Circuit Training
0.5 UNIT - (RPT 3) (UC:CSU)
An exercise program utilizing interval training to increase cardiovascular efficiency and muscular strength/endurance. Participants' transition, in timed intervals, from stationary bikes to strength training machines that condition all the major muscle groups in the body.

PHYSICAL EDUCATION 637
Spin Cycling Aerobic
0.5 UNIT - (RPT 3) (UC:CSU)
A vigorous cardiovascular workout using a stationary bicycle, energetic music and cycling drills. Drills include simulated hill climbs, sprints, and various cycling positions. Aerobic and anaerobic situations are created to condition the entire cardiovascular system.

PHYSICAL EDUCATION 639
Hatha Yoga
1 UNIT - (RPT 3) (UC:CSU)
Advisory: Physical Education Yoga Skills.
This class provides a more in-depth exposure and experience with Hatha Yoga. Special attention is paid to Hatha Yoga styles, terminology, history, and developing personal skill level. Individual course may be taken four times.

PHYSICAL EDUCATION 640
Beginning Lifelong Fitness Laboratory
1 UNIT - (RPT 3) (UC:CSU)
Advisory: Physical Education Yoga Skills.
In each sport activity, special attention is paid to techniques, strategy, etiquette, terminology, history and rules. Individuals' courses may be taken four times.

PHYSICAL EDUCATION 641
Introduction to Laboratory Techniques in Adapted Physical Education
2 UNITS – (RPT 3) (UC:CSU)
Advisory: Eligibility to enroll in English 28 or its equivalent.
Class provides an orientation to specific disabilities, methods, and techniques of working with the disabled. The arranged laboratory experience requires assisting a specialist with disabled students enrolled in adapted physical education activity classes. Valuable for students pursuing health/rehabilitative careers.

PHYSICAL EDUCATION 642
Adapted Fitness
1 UNIT – (RPT 3)
Course is designed to meet the needs of students with disabilities who require restricted or modified activities. Individualized exercise programs will be performed by students with instruction covering the basic elements of physical fitness and training principles.

PHYSICAL EDUCATION 643
Adapted Strength Training
1 Unit – (UC:CSU)

Course is designed to meet the needs of students with disabilities who require restricted or modified activities. Individualized exercise programs will be performed by students with instructional emphasis placed on strength training principles and techniques.

PHYSICAL EDUCATION 644
Adapted Swimming and Hydroexercise
1 UNIT – (RPT 3)
Course is designed to meet the needs of students with disabilities who require restricted or modified activities. Individualized exercise programs will focus on basic swimming and water safety skills. Hydroexercise programs will emphasize physical fitness, buoyancy, and hydrodynamic resistance principles.

PHYSICAL EDUCATION 645
Adapted Aerobics
1 UNIT – (RPT 3)
This course is designed for students with disabilities who need and individualized exercise program and can function independently. Students will develop cardiovascular and muscular endurance, strength, and flexibility while exercising with musical accompaniment.

PHYSICAL EDUCATION 646
Adapted Cardiovascular Fitness
1 Unit – (RPT 3) (UC:CSU)
Course is designed to meet the needs of students with disabilities who can benefit from individualized cardiovascular endurance training. Development of cardiovascular endurance through the use of bicycle ergometers with hand cranks will be the major class focus.

PHYSICAL EDUCATION 647
Adapted Aqua Aerobics
1 Unit – (RPT 3) (UC:CSU)
Course is designed to meet the needs of students with disabilities who require restricted or modified activities, and who can benefit from individualized non-impact aerobic exercises in the pool.

PHYSICAL EDUCATION 648
Adapted Exercise for Back Disorders
1 Unit – (RPT 3) (UC:CSU)
Course is designed for students with back and/or neck problems that can benefit from an individualized exercise program. Instruction and practice will be given in individualized exercises, including stretching, resistive exercises and cardiovascular fitness.

PHYSICAL EDUCATION 649
Adapted Sports and Games
1 Unit – (RPT 3) (UC: CSU)
Course is designed to develop students' gross motor skills and to facilitate their participation in life-long activities, enhancing improved fitness, self-esteem, and social interaction.

PHYSICAL EDUCATION 712
Introduction to Physical Education
3 UNITS – (RPT 3) (UC:CSU)
A study of the physical, mental, emotional, and social effects or organized physical education programs. Special emphasis is placed on the history, philosophy, professional qualifications, career opportunities, and current trends and curriculum development.

PHYSICAL EDUCATION 713
Introduction to Coaching Athletics
3 UNITS – (RPT 3) (UC:CSU)

A study of the physical, mental, emotional, and social effects or organized physical education programs. Special emphasis is placed on the history, philosophy, professional qualifications, career opportunities, and current trends and curriculum development.

PHYSICAL EDUCATION 714
Coaching Team Sports
3 UNITS – (RPT 3) (UC:CSU)
A comprehensive study of the physical, mental, emotional, and social aspect of coaching team sports. Special emphasis is placed on the history, philosophy, professional qualifications, career opportunities, and current trends and curriculum development in coaching. The theory and practice of team sports included in physical education and recreational programs. Basic skills, rules, regulations, and organization of activities are presented.

PHYSICAL EDUCATION 715
Coaching Individual Sports
3 UNITS – (UC:CSU)
The theory and practice of individual sports included in physical education and recreation. The student's skill in each sport is assessed; Basic skills, rules, regulations, and organization, of the activities are presented. Activities include Archery, Badminton, Handball, Golf, Tennis.

PHYSICAL EDUCATION 716
Games & Rhythms/Elementary School I
3 UNITS - (CSU)
A study of the physical, mental, emotional, and social effects of games and rhythms. Special emphasis is placed on the history, philosophy, professional qualifications, and current trends and curriculum development.

PHYSICAL EDUCATION 720
Theory and Practice of Olympic Sport Judo
3 UNITS - (RPT 3) (UC:CSU)
In each sport or activity, special attention is paid to techniques, strategy, etiquette, terminology, history, and rules. Individual courses may be taken four times.

PHYSICAL EDUCATION THEORY CLASSES
Physical Education Major
These classes do not meet credit for Physical Education activity. Required for Physical Education and Recreation majors and minors.

PHYSICAL EDUCATION 810
PE Folk Dance
2 UNITS - (UC:CSU)
This course offers an in depth study of folk dance, its history, characteristics, and music for students interested in teaching.

PHYSICAL EDUCATION 185
Directed Study — 1 UNIT (CSU)
PHYSICAL EDUCATION 285
Directed Study — 2 UNITS (CSU)
PHYSICAL EDUCATION 385
Directed Study — 3 UNITS (CSU)
Conference 1 hour per unit.
Allows students to pursue Directed Study on a contract basis under the direction of a supervising instructor. Refer to the "Directed Study" section of this catalog for additional information.
Credit Limit: A maximum of 3 units in Directed Study may be taken for credit.

An Invitation to Health Brief

FIFTH EDITION

1 An Invitation to Healthy Change

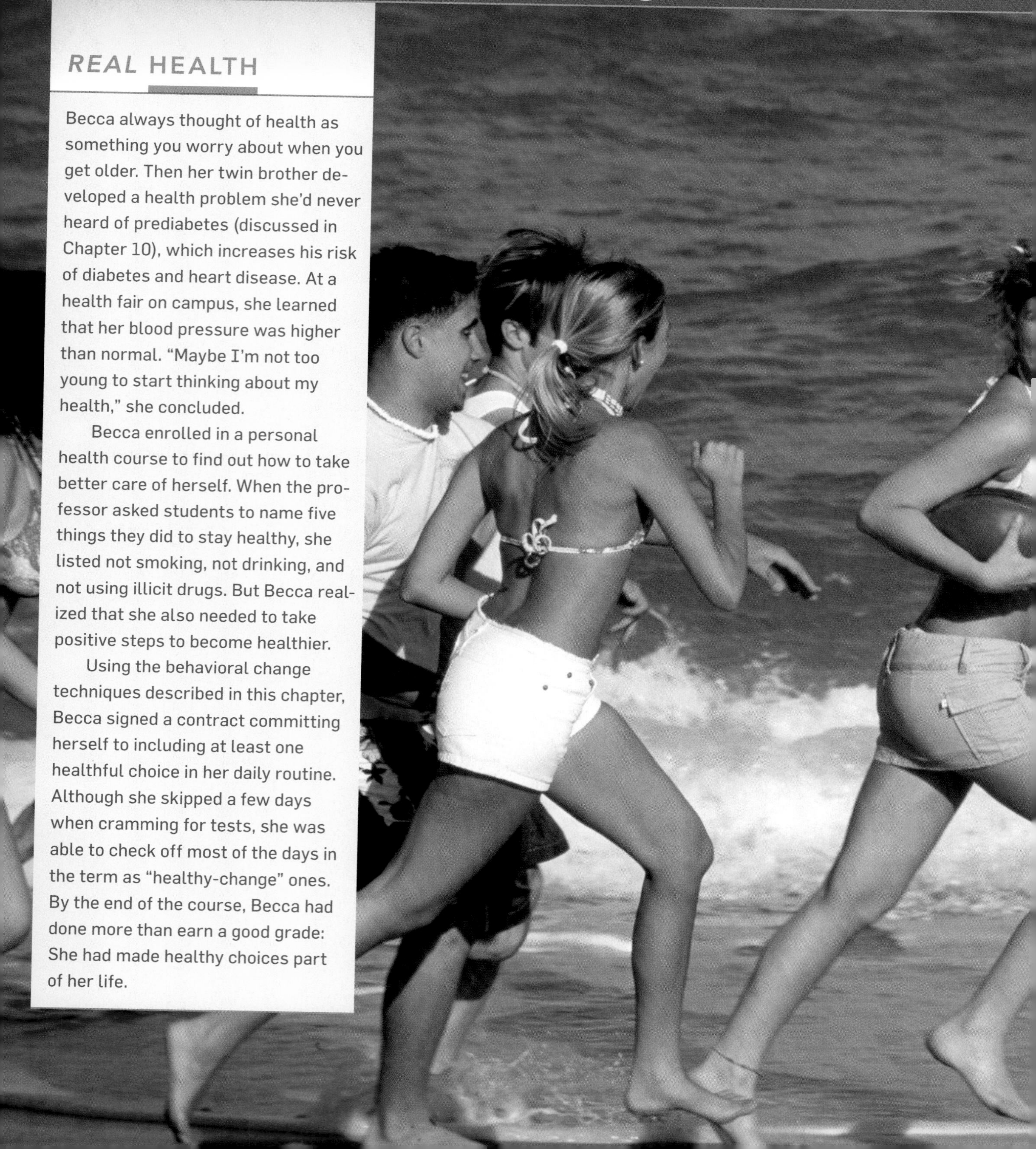

REAL HEALTH

Becca always thought of health as something you worry about when you get older. Then her twin brother developed a health problem she'd never heard of prediabetes (discussed in Chapter 10), which increases his risk of diabetes and heart disease. At a health fair on campus, she learned that her blood pressure was higher than normal. "Maybe I'm not too young to start thinking about my health," she concluded.

Becca enrolled in a personal health course to find out how to take better care of herself. When the professor asked students to name five things they did to stay healthy, she listed not smoking, not drinking, and not using illicit drugs. But Becca realized that she also needed to take positive steps to become healthier.

Using the behavioral change techniques described in this chapter, Becca signed a contract committing herself to including at least one healthful choice in her daily routine. Although she skipped a few days when cramming for tests, she was able to check off most of the days in the term as "healthy-change" ones. By the end of the course, Becca had done more than earn a good grade: She had made healthy choices part of her life.

© Roy Morsch/zefa/CORBIS

"How are you?" You may hear that question dozens of times each day. "Fine," you may answer. "Not bad." "Great." But how are you really doing?

How do you feel about yourself? Do you feel energetic and enthusiastic about your life? Do you have any health problems or limitations? Are you stressed? Do you eat well and exercise regularly? Do you have close friends? Do you drink, smoke, or use drugs? Do you get regular checkups? If you choose to be sexually active, do you take steps to prevent sexually transmitted infections and unwanted pregnancy? Do you try to avoid accidents and injuries? Are you making the most of the only life you'll ever get?

This book asks these questions and many more. It is a book about you: your mind and your body, your spirit and your social ties, your needs and your wants, your past and your potential. It will help you explore options, discover possibilities, and find new ways to make your life worthwhile. If you don't make the most of what you are, you risk never discovering what you might become.

Being healthy, as you'll learn in this chapter, means more than not being sick or in pain. Health is a personal choice that you make every day when you decide on everything from what to eat to whether to exercise to how to handle stress. Sometimes making the best choices demands making healthy changes in your life. This chapter will show you how.

This chapter also extends an invitation to live more fully, more happily, and more healthfully, It is an offer that you literally cannot afford to refuse. The quality of your life depends on it.

? FAQ Frequently Asked Questions

- How healthy are young Americans? *p. 7*
- Does gender matter? *p. 11*
- What are the stages of change? *p. 15*
- How can I change a bad health habit? *p. 18*

After studying the material in this chapter, you should be able to:

- **Define** health and wellness.
- **Name** the dimensions of health and **describe** how they relate to total wellness.
- **Define** the three factors that shape health behaviors.
- **Name** the three key components of the trans-theoretical model of change.
- **Describe** the stages of change and give an example of each.

ThomsonNOW™ Log on to ThomsonNOW at **www.thomsonedu.com/thomsonnow** to find your Behavior Change Planner and to explore self-assessments, interactive tutorials, and practice quizzes.

Health and Wellness

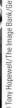

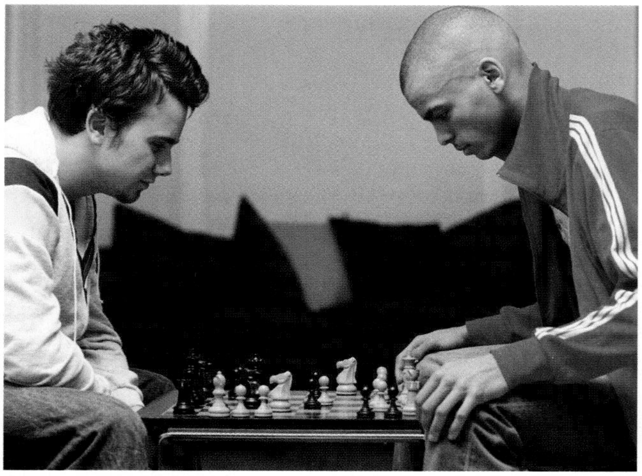

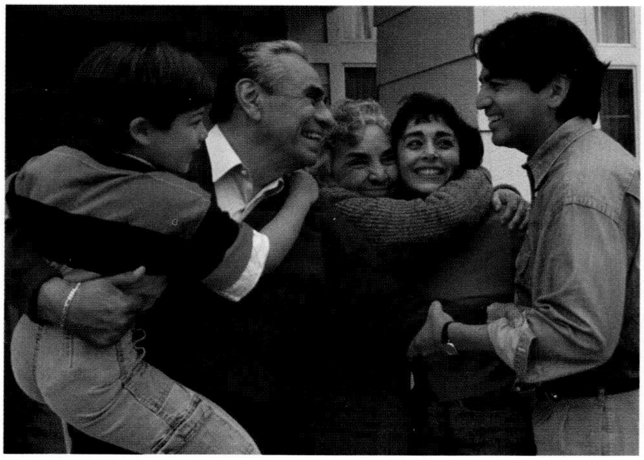

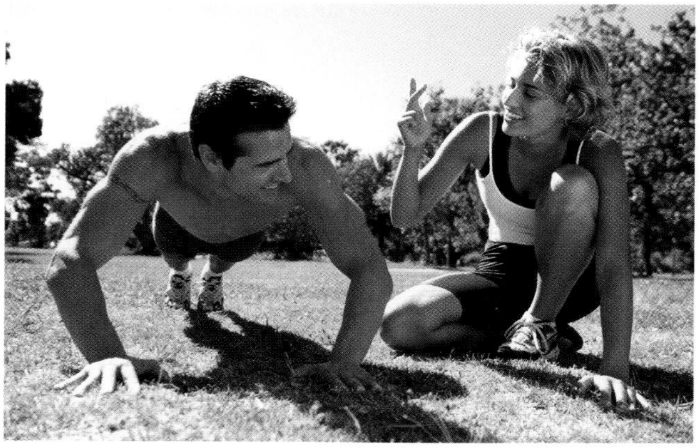

Health is the process of discovering, using, and protecting all the resources within our bodies, minds, spirits, families, communities, and environment.

By simplest definition, **health** means being sound in body, mind, and spirit. The World Health Organization defines health as "not merely the absence of disease or infirmity," but "a state of complete physical, mental, and social well-being."[1] Health is the process of discovering, using, and protecting all the resources within our bodies, minds, spirits, families, communities, and environment.

Health has many dimensions: physical, psychological, spiritual, social, intellectual, and environmental. This book takes a *holistic* approach, one that looks at health and the individual as a whole, rather than part by part. Your own definition of health may include different elements, but chances are you and your classmates agree that it includes at least some of the following:

- A positive, optimistic outlook.
- A sense of control over stress and worries; time to relax.
- Energy and vitality; freedom from pain or serious illness.
- Supportive friends and family and a nurturing intimate relationship with someone you love.
- A personally satisfying job.
- A clean environment.

Wellness can be defined as purposeful, enjoyable living or, more specifically, a deliberate lifestyle choice characterized by personal responsibility and optimal enhancement of physical, mental, and spiritual health. Health professionals use other definitions to encompass this broad, active meaning of wellness:

- As a decision you make to move toward optimal health.
- As a way of life you design to achieve your highest potential.
- As a process of developing awareness that health and happiness are possible in the present moment.
- As the integration of body, mind, and spirit.
- As the belief that everything you do, think, and feel has an impact on your state of health and the health of the world.[2]

"The 'well' person is not necessarily the strong, the brave, the successful, the young, the whole, or even the illness-free being," notes John Travis, M.D., author of *The Wellness Workbook*. "No matter what your current state of health, you can begin to appreciate yourself as a growing, changing person and allow yourself to move toward a happier life and positive health."

Dr. Travis, who created the Wellness Inventory (see The Self-Assessment Booklet) uses the analogy of an iceberg (Figure 1-1) to describe optimal health and wellness. Only about one-tenth of the mass of an iceberg is visible; the rest is submerged. Your current state of health is like the tip of the iceberg—the part that shows.

"To understand all that creates and supports your current state of health," says Dr. Travis, "you have to look 'underwater.'" The first hidden level—the "lifestyle/behavioral" level—consists of what you eat, how active you are, how you manage stress, and how you protect yourself from hazards. Below this dimension is the "cultural/psychological/motivational" level, the often invisible influences that lead us to choose a certain lifestyle. The foundation of the iceberg is the "spiritual/being/meaning" realm, which encompasses issues such as your reason for being, the meaning of your life, and your place in the universe. "Ultimately," says Dr. Travis, "this realm determines whether the tip of the iceberg, representing your state of health, is one of disease or wellness."[3]

In wellness, health, and sickness, there is considerable overlap of the functions of the mind, body, and spirit. As scientists have shown again and again in recent decades, psychological factors play a major role in enhancing physical well-being and preventing illness, but they also can trigger, worsen, or prolong physical symptoms. Similarly, almost every medical illness affects people psychologically as well as physically.

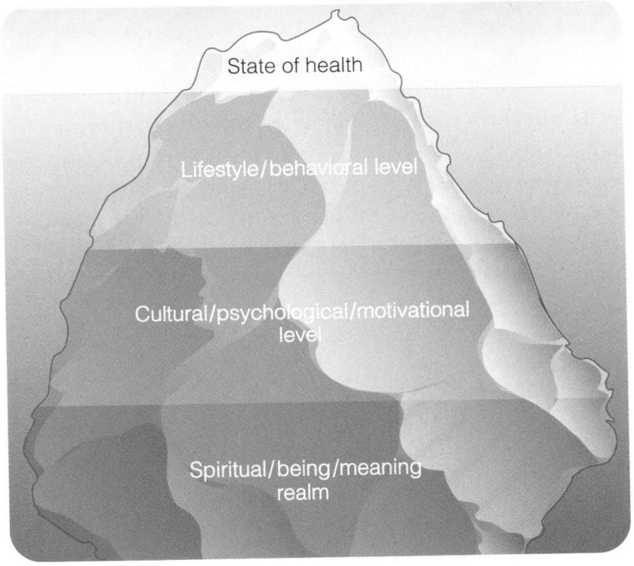

FIGURE 1-1 Iceberg Model of Wellness

Like an iceberg, only a small part of your total wellness is visible: your current state of health. Just as important are hidden dimensions, including lifestyle habits, cultural and psychological factors, and the realm of spiritual meaning and being.

Source: Reprinted with permission, *The Wellness Workbook*, 3rd edition, John W. Travis, MD, and Regina Sara Ryan, Celestial Arts, Berkeley, CA. © 1981, 1988, 2004 by John W. Travis. www.wellnessbook.com

The Dimensions of Health

By learning more about the six dimensions of health, you can explore the hidden levels of the iceberg.

Physical Health

The various states of health can be viewed as points on a continuum (Figure 1-2). At one end is early and needless death; at the other is optimal wellness, in which you feel and perform at your very best. In the middle, individuals are neither sick enough to need medical attention nor well enough to live each day with zest and vigor.

What matters even more than your place on the continuum is the direction in which you are moving: toward high-level wellness or toward premature death. Individuals in physical good health who are always worrying or not working to develop more fully may be on the right of the neutral point but facing left. Others who may be disabled or have a chronic health problem may have a positive outlook and a network of mutually supportive relationships that keeps them focused toward wellness.[4]

For the sake of optimal physical health, we must take positive steps away from illness and toward well-being. We must feed our bodies nutritiously, exercise them regularly, avoid harmful behaviors and substances, watch out for early signs of sickness, and protect ourselves from accidents.

health A state of complete well-being, including physical, psychological, spiritual, social, intellectual, and environmental dimensions.

wellness A deliberate lifestyle choice characterized by personal responsibility and optimal enhancement of physical, mental, and spiritual health.

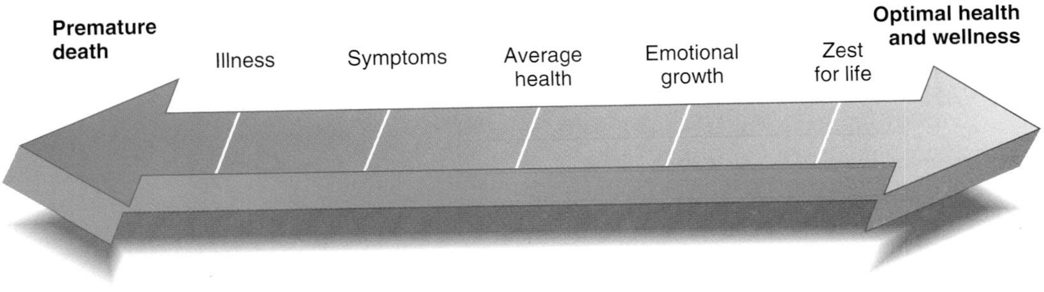

FIGURE 1-2 Wellness-Illness Continuum

Psychological Health

Like physical well-being, psychological health is more than the absence of problems or illness. Psychological health refers to both our emotional and mental states—that is, to our feelings and our thoughts. It involves awareness and acceptance of a wide range of feelings in oneself and others, the ability to express emotions, to function independently, and to cope with the challenges of daily stressors. (Chapter 2 provides more information on psychological health.)

Spiritual Health

Spiritually healthy individuals identify their own basic purpose in life; learn how to experience love, joy, peace, and fulfillment; and help themselves and others achieve their full potential. As they devote themselves to others' needs more than their own, their spiritual development produces a sense of greater meaning in their lives. (See Chapter 2 for an in-depth discussion of spirituality.)

Many studies have confirmed health benefits for individuals who pray, attend religious services, and engage in spiritual practices. However, the largest-ever study of "intercessory" prayer (praying for other individuals) found no benefits for coronary bypass patients. In fact, the patients who knew strangers were praying for them fared significantly worse than those who received no prayers.[5] These findings are "not an indictment of prayer or prayer's potential power," notes Dr. Mitchell Krucoff, a pioneer in spirituality research, but a call for more vigorous study and thinking about the complexity of the interactions between mind, body, and spirit.[6]

Social Health

Social health refers to the ability to interact effectively with other people and the social environment, to develop satisfying interpersonal relationships, and to fulfill social roles. It involves participating in and contributing to your community, living in harmony with fellow human beings, developing positive interdependent relationships (discussed in Chapter 7), and practicing healthy sexual behaviors.

In times of crisis, social connections provide comfort and support. Even in tranquil times, social isolation increases the risk of sickness and mortality. In a landmark study of 4,725 men and women in Alameda County, California, death rates were twice as high for loners as for those with strong social ties. In other studies, social isolation greatly increased the risk of dying of a heart attack. Heart attack patients have a better chance of long-term survival if they believe they have adequate help in performing daily tasks from family and friends. People with spouses, friends, and a rich social network may outlive isolated loners by as much as 30 years.

Health educators are placing greater emphasis on social health in its broadest sense as they expand the traditional individualistic concept of health to include the complex interrelationships between one person's health and the health of the community and environment. This change in perspective has given rise to a new emphasis on **health promotion,** which educators define as "any planned combination of educational, political, regulatory, and organizational supports for actions and conditions of living conducive to the health of individuals, groups, or communities." Examples on campus include smoke-free policies for all college buildings, residences, and dining areas, prohibiting tobacco advertising and sponsorship of campus social events, and banning tobacco sales on campus.

Intellectual Health

Your brain is the only one of your organs capable of self-awareness. Every day you use your mind to gather, process, and act on information; to think through your values; to make decisions, set goals, and figure out how to handle a problem or challenge. Intellectual health refers to your ability to think and learn from life experience, your openness to new ideas, and your capacity to question and evaluate information. Throughout your life, you'll use your critical thinking skills, including

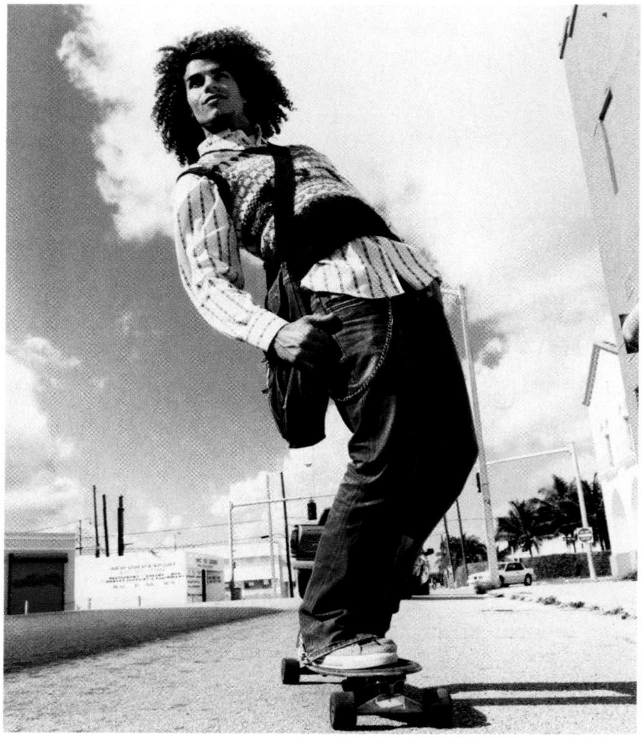

Where are you on the wellness-illness continuum? Which direction are you moving?

your ability to evaluate health information, to safeguard your well-being.

Environmental Health

You live in a physical and social setting that can affect every aspect of your health. Environmental health refers to the impact your world has on your well-being. It means protecting yourself from dangers in the air, water, and soil, and in products you use—and also working to preserve the environment itself. (Chapter 14 offers a thorough discussion of environmental health.)

The State of Our Health

Americans are living longer and healthier lives than ever before in history. Life expectancy has reached a new high of 77.9 years, increasing for both men and women and blacks and whites.[7] The gender gap between male and female life expectancies has narrowed to five years, but women are living longer than men across almost all the world.[8] The age-adjusted death rate has hit an all-time low of 801 deaths per 100,000 people, with declines in mortality from stroke, heart disease, cancer, and accidents.[9]

The top leading causes of preventable death are tobacco use and poor diet and inactivity. Others include alcohol and drug abuse, motor vehicle accidents, sexually transmitted infections (STIs), and firearms.[10]

Healthy People 2010

Healthy People 2010 is the prevention agenda for the nation. Every decade the federal government identifies the most significant preventable threats to health and creates leading indicators that assess the health of Americans. Its first goal is to help individuals of all ages increase life expectancy *and* improve their quality of life. Its second goal is to eliminate health disparities among different segments of the population.

Among the specific goals of *Healthy People 2010* are:

- **Reduce the prevalence of cigarette smoking** among adults to 12 percent from the current 21 percent.
- **Reduce the number of new cancer cases** as well as the illnesses, disabilities, and deaths caused by cancer.
- **Promote the health of people with disabilities,** prevent secondary conditions, and eliminate disparities between people with and without disabilities in the U.S. population.
- **Reduce foodborne illnesses.**
- **Reduce the proportion of obese children and adolescents** from 11 percent to 5 percent.
- **Reduce the number of adolescents and adults** using illegal substances.
- **Reduce the number of adults** engaging in binge drinking.[11]

Healthy Campus 2010

The American College Health Association has adapted the federal *Healthy People 2010* for college and universities. Its *Healthy Campus 2010* initiative has identified 28 focus areas (and 310 objectives) particularly relevant for students. Schools that participate in the program can compare data on their students to national norms and identify the key targets that would most improve health on their campuses.

As an example, the University of Southern California chose seven goals:

1. To improve access to comprehensive, high-quality health-care services by increasing the proportion of students with health insurance.
2. To decrease alcohol and drug use through increased access to information on preventing substance abuse.
3. To decrease unintentional pregnancies.
4. To improve health, fitness, and quality of life through daily physical activity.
5. To increase fruit and vegetable consumption in order to promote health and reduce chronic disease.
6. To decrease sexual assault, including rape, attempted rape, or sexual assault on campus.
7. To decrease depression through increased access to treatment.[12]

Find out if your school is participating in *Healthy Campus 2010.* If it is, what are the target objectives for your campus?

? FAQ How Healthy Are Young Americans?

According to the first longitudinal study that followed more than 10,000 young Americans, health risks increase significantly during the crucial transition from the teens into early adulthood. As they enter their twenties, men and women of every race and ethnic group are more likely to eat fast food, get no exercise, be obese, and smoke cigarettes. Many have no current health insurance, do not get regular physical or dental examinations, and do not receive health care when they need it. STIs and illicit drug use also become more common. Despite these realities, young men and women consider themselves in good health.[13]

health promotion An educational and informational process in which people are helped to change attitudes and behaviors in an effort to improve their health.

No single race or ethnic group leads or falters in health across all of the health indicators studied. White Americans, who have the best health in adolescence, experience the greatest decline in early adulthood. Native Americans face higher health risks both as teens and adults. Individuals in minority groups are most likely to need care but to be unable to pay for it.

None of these trends is inevitable. You—and only you—can reverse them by making healthy changes in the way you live. Regardless of your age, think back to your health habits when you were younger. Have they improved or deteriorated over time? Are you at risk of health problems now and in the future?

A Report Card on Student Health

According to the U.S. Department of Education, 16.6 million students—86 percent undergraduates—are enrolled in more than 4,000 colleges and universities.[14] Although various agencies survey students about their behaviors, the American College Health Association National College Health Assessment (ACHA-NCHA) provides the most comprehensive view of the state of student health. Among the key findings from its most recent report are:

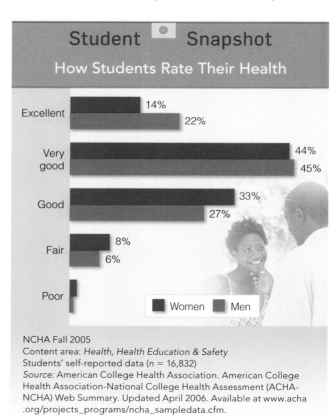

- More than nine in ten students describe their health as good, very good, or excellent (see Student Snapshot: "How Students Rate Their Health").
- About two-thirds of students—69 percent of women and 59 percent of men—are at healthy weights. One in five—17 percent of women and 29 percent of men—are overweight. Nine percent—8 percent of women and 11 percent of men—are obese.
- College women reported an average of 1.3 sex partners in the last year; college men, 1.8. Both sexes believed that other students were having sex with more partners.
- 40 percent of students who'd had vaginal intercourse relied on birth control pills for contraception; 39 percent on condoms; 14 percent on withdrawal (which, as discussed in Chapter 8, is not a reliable form of birth control).
- 61 percent of students have never smoked; 18 percent did not smoke in the last month.
- 61 percent of students have never used marijuana; 21 percent did not smoke pot in the previous month.
- About half of male students and a third of female students had had five or more alcoholic drinks at a single sitting in the previous three weeks. Men averaged 1.7 drinks per hour the last time they partied; women averaged 1.3 drinks.
- Asked about their perceptions of how other students behave, students generally overestimated the numbers engaging in risky behavior. For example, most students thought that only 10 percent of their peers had never smoked.[15]

Staying Healthy on Campus

Simply by acquiring more years of schooling, you increase your chance of a long and healthful life. Many risk factors for disease—including high blood pressure, elevated cholesterol, and cigarette smoking—decline steadily as education increases, regardless of how much money people make. Education may be good for the body as well as the mind by influencing lifestyle behaviors, problem-solving abilities, and values. People who earn college degrees acquire positive attitudes about the benefits of healthy living, learn how to gain access to preventive health services, join peer groups that promote healthy behavior, and develop higher self-esteem and greater control over their lives.

This course in itself may be good for your health. In studies on the impact of health and wellness courses, students reported that they not only learned about the many dimensions of health but made changes to improve their health. Many changed their diet and eating habits, began exercising at a campus gym, developed schedules for better time management, engaged in stress-releasing activities, or altered a dangerous habit, such as smoking or drinking.

Figure 1-3 shows the top ten physical and mental problems that students experienced in the last year.

Student Snapshot

How Students Rate Their Health

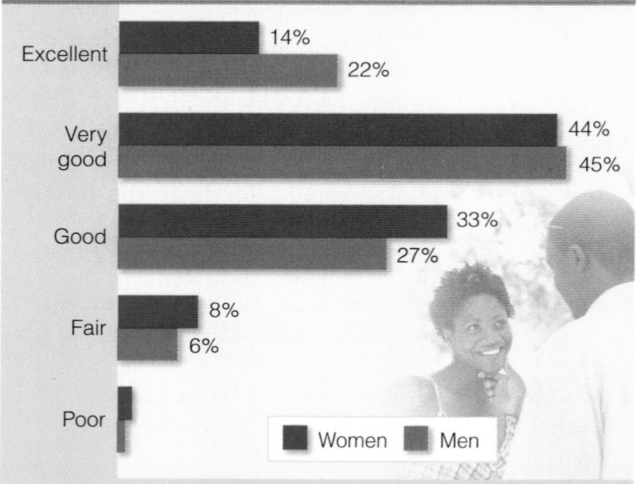

NCHA Fall 2005
Content area: *Health, Health Education & Safety*
Students' self-reported data (n = 16,832)
Source: American College Health Association. American College Health Association-National College Health Assessment (ACHA-NCHA) Web Summary. Updated April 2006. Available at www.acha.org/projects_programs/ncha_sampledata.cfm.

Strategies for Prevention — Smart Steps to Take Now

- To lower your risk of heart disease, get your blood pressure and cholesterol checked. Don't smoke. Stay at a healthy weight. Exercise regularly. (See Chapters 4, 6, and 10.)
- To lower your risks of major diseases, get regular checkups. Make sure you are immunized against infectious illnesses. (See Chapter 9.)
- To lower your risks of substance abuse and related illnesses and injuries, don't drink, or limit how much you drink. Avoid illegal drugs. (See Chapters 11 and 12.)
- To lower your risk of sexually transmitted infections (STIs) or unwanted pregnancy, abstain from sex. If you decide to engage in potentially risky sexual activities, protect yourself with contraceptives, condoms, and spermicides. (See Chapter 8.)
- To prevent car accidents, don't drive when road conditions are hazardous. When you drive, wear a seat belt, and use defensive driving techniques. (See Chapter 13.)

Some are occasional or one-time events (such as sinus and ear infections, or a broken bone), but the two most common—back pain and allergies—could be long-term health issues.

Preventing Health Problems

College students often think they are too young to worry about serious health conditions. Yet many chronic problems begin early in life. Two percent of college-age women already have osteoporosis, a bone-weakening disease; another 15 percent have osteopenia, low bone densities that put them at risk of osteoporosis. Many college students have several risk factors for heart disease, including high blood pressure and high cholesterol. Others increase their risk by eating a high-fat diet and not exercising regularly. The time to change is now.

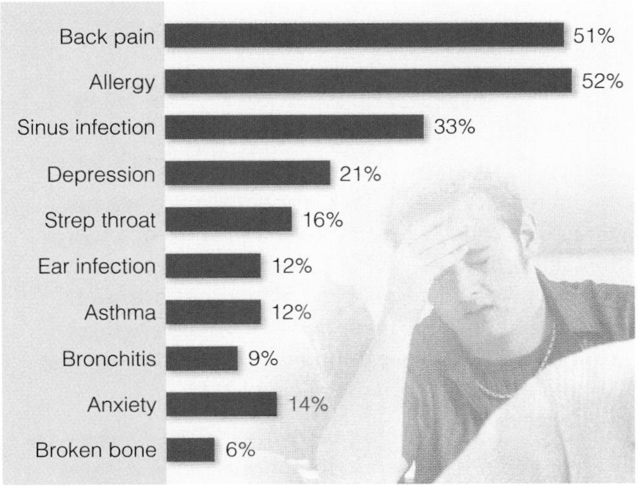

FIGURE 1-3 Top Ten Physical and Mental Problems on Campus (last 12 months)

Source: American College Health Association. American College Health Association-National College Health Assessment (ACHA-NCHA) Web Summary. Updated April 2006. www.acha.org/projects_programs/ncha_sampledata.cfm.

No medical treatment, however successful or sophisticated, can compare with the power of **prevention.** Two out of every three deaths and one in three hospitalizations in the United States could be prevented by changes in six main risk factors: tobacco use, alcohol abuse, accidents, high blood pressure, obesity, and gaps in screening and primary health care. Prevention remains the best weapon against cancer and heart disease.

Prevention can take many forms. Primary, or before-the-fact, prevention efforts might seek to reduce stressors and increase support to prevent problems in healthy people. Consumer education, for instance, provides guidance about how to change our lifestyles to prevent problems and enhance well-being. Other preventive programs identify people at risk and empower them with information and support so they can avoid potential problems. Prevention efforts may target an entire community and try to educate all of its members about the dangers of alcohol abuse or environmental hazards, or they may zero in on a particular group (for instance, seminars on safer sex practices offered to teens) or an individual (such as one-on-one counseling about substance abuse).

Protecting Yourself

There is a great deal of overlap between prevention and **protection.** Some people might think of immunizations (discussed in Chapter 9) as a way of preventing illness; others see them as a form of protection against dangerous diseases. In many ways, protection picks up where prevention leaves off. You can prevent STIs or unwanted pregnancy by abstaining from sex. But if you decide to engage in potentially risky sexual

prevention Information and support offered to help healthy people identify their health risks, reduce stressors, prevent potential medical problems, and enhance their well-being.

protection Measures that an individual can take when participating in risky behavior to prevent injury or unwanted risks.

activities, you can protect yourself with condoms and spermicides (discussed in Chapter 8). Similarly, you can prevent many automobile accidents by not driving when road conditions are hazardous. But if you do have to drive, you can protect yourself by wearing a seat belt and using defensive driving techniques (discussed in Chapter 13).

The very concept of protection implies some degree of risk—immediate and direct (for instance, the risk of intentional injury from an assailant or unintentional harm from a fire) or long-term and indirect (such as the risk of heart disease and cancer as a result of smoking). To know how best to protect yourself, you have to be able to realistically assess risks. (The information on risky behavior on page 11.)

Colleges and universities take varied steps to protect students' well-being. These range from requiring vaccination against meningitis to banning alcohol at athletic and social events. Find out what your school is doing to protect your health. Would you like to see more programs and policies to safeguard student well-being?

Informing Yourself

Reliable health information can help you take better care of yourself. In the ACHA-NCHA survey discussed in the previous section, 73 percent of students turned to parents for health-related information. However, parents may not have a realistic sense of the health risks their children face. In a recent study comparing parents' perceptions of their college student children's health and health risk behaviors with the students' own reports, parents tended to be overly optimistic. They rated their children's health higher than the students themselves and underestimated the frequency of their drinking, smoking, marijuana use, and sex-related behaviors. Parents were more accurate in assessing their children's nutrition, exercise, use of seatbelts and bicycle helmets, sun protection, and whether they would ride in a car with someone under the influence of alcohol.[16]

The second most common source of health information is the Internet, although only 22 percent consider it believable.[17] In a recent survey at two schools, three in four students reported getting health information online, and more than 40 percent frequently searched the Internet for health-related materials.[18] As discussed in Chapter 13, you can find reliable, reputable health advice online—if you know where to look and if you remain skeptical about news or breakthroughs that seem too good to be true (see Savvy Consumer: "Too Good to Be True?").

About half of students turn to health educators for information—and rank them as the most believable of sources. Health center medical staff rank almost equally as high. Although students regularly turn to flyers, pamphlets, magazines, and television for information, they are less likely to consider these as authoritative, believable sources.

Colleges and universities also provide health-related information to students. The most commonly covered

SAVVY CONSUMER

Too Good to Be True?

Almost every week you're likely to come across a commercial or an ad for a new health product that promises better sleep, more energy, clearer skin, firmer muscles, lower weight, brighter moods, longer life—or all of these combined. As the Savvy Consumer feature throughout this book points out, you can't believe every promise you read or hear. Keep these general guidelines in mind the next time you come across a health claim:

- If it sounds too good to be true, it probably is. If a magic pill could really trim off excess pounds or banish wrinkles, the world would be filled with thin people with unlined skin. Look around and you'll realize that's not the case.
- Look for objective evaluations. If you're watching an infomercial for a treatment or technique, you can be sure that the enthusiastic endorsements have been skillfully scripted and rehearsed. Even ads that claim to be presenting the science behind a new breakthrough are really sales pitches in disguise.
- Consider the sources. Research findings from carefully controlled scientific studies are reviewed by leading experts in the field and published in scholarly journals. Just because someone has conducted a study doesn't mean it was a valid scientific investigation.
- Check credentials. Anyone can claim to be a scientist or a health expert. Find out if advocates of any type of therapy have legitimate degrees from recognized institutions and are fully licensed in their fields.
- Do your own research. Check with your doctor or with the student health center. Go to the library or do some online research to gather as much information as you can.

topics are alcohol and drug use prevention, sexual assault/relationship violence prevention, sexually transmitted infections, physical activity and fitness, HIV/AIDS prevention, and nutrition and dietary behaviors.

Unhealthy Habits and Risky Behaviors

Often on their own for the first time, college students leave behind their family's ways of eating, sleeping, and relaxing and develop new habits and routines—usually not healthier ones. Many simply don't get enough sleep or keep irregular schedules that throw their sleep patterns off. Often it seems that there aren't enough hours in the day for all the things undergraduates need or want to do—study, socialize, pursue extracurricular activities, surf the Internet, work at part-time jobs, participate in community service. Sleeping less, juggling more, students can quickly end up exhausted—and at greater risk for colds, flus, digestive problems, and other maladies.

Students also become more sedentary in college, as they log more hours in classes and in front of computers. The combination of a high-fat diet and a sedentary lifestyle in college can set the stage for the development of health problems that include obesity, diabetes, metabolic syndrome, heart disease, and certain cancers.

College-age men are more likely than women to engage in risk-taking behaviors—to use drugs and alcohol; to engage in risky sexual behaviors, such as having sex while under the influence of alcohol; and to drive dangerously. Men also are more likely to be hospitalized for injuries and to commit suicide. Three-fourths of the deaths in the 15- to 24-year age range are men.

Drinking has long been part of college life and, despite the efforts across U.S. college campuses to curb alcohol abuse, two out of five students engage in binge drinking—consumption of five or more drinks at a single session for men, four for women. Heavy drinking increases the likelihood of other risky behaviors, such as smoking cigarettes, using drugs, or having multiple sexual partners.

Some behaviors are riskier than students realize. "Body art"—piercings and tattoos—may seem harmless, but health officials warn of hidden risks, including hepatitis B and C infection and transmission of HIV (see Chapter 9).

Personalizing Your Health Care

Thanks to advances in genomics (the study of the entire set of human genes), physicians are tailoring tests and treatments to individual patients. "Personalized" medicine can alert your doctor to potential threats that might be prevented, delayed, or detected at an earlier, more treatable stage and, if you do develop a disease, pinpoint the medications that will do the most good and cause the least harm.

But "personalizing" health care is also a personal responsibility. You can take charge of your own health by compiling a family health history and informing yourself about risks related to your gender, race, and ethnicity.

Your Family Health History

Someday a DNA scan from a single drop of blood may tell you the diseases you're most likely to develop. A family history can do the same—now.

Mapping your family medical history can help identify health risks you may face in the future. One way of charting your health history is to draw a medical family "tree" that includes your parents and siblings (who share half your genes), as well as grandparents, uncles, aunts, and cousins. Depending on how much information you're able to obtain for each relative, your medical family tree can include health issues each family member has faced, including illnesses with a hereditary component, such as high blood pressure, diabetes, some cancers, and certain psychiatric disorders. Although having a relative with a certain disease may increase your risk, your likelihood of ending up with the same condition also depends on your health habits, such as diet and exercise. Knowing now that you're at risk can motivate you to change any unhealthy behaviors. Realizing that you have a relative with, say, colon cancer could mean that you should start screening tests ten years before others because you're at risk of developing a tumor at an earlier age.

For guidance on creating a family history, check these websites: **www.mayoclinic.com** or **www.ashg.org/genetics/ashg/educ/007.shtml.**

? FAQ Does Gender Matter?

"Sex does matter. It matters in ways that we did not expect. Undoubtedly, it also matters in ways that we have not begun to imagine." This was the conclusion of the Institute of Medicine Committee on Understanding the Biology of Sex and Gender Differences in the first significant review of the status of sex and gender differences in biomedical research.

Sex, the committee stated, is "a classification, generally as male or female, according to the reproductive organs and functions that derive from the chromosomal complement." *Gender* refers to "a person's self-representation as male or female or how that person is responded to by social institutions on the basis of the individual's gender presentation." Rooted in biology, gender is shaped by environment and experience.

The experience of being male or female in a particular culture and society can and does have an effect on physical and psychological well-being. In fact, sex and gender may have a greater impact than any other variable on how our bodies function, how long we live, and the symptoms, course, and treatment of the diseases that strike us.

This realization is both new and revolutionary. For centuries, scientists based biological theories solely on a male model and viewed women as shorter, smaller, and rounder versions of men. Even modern medicine is based on the assumption that, except for their reproductive organs, both sexes are biologically interchangeable. We now know that this simply isn't so (Figure 1-4). Sex begins in the womb, but sex and gender differences affect behavior, perception, and health throughout life.

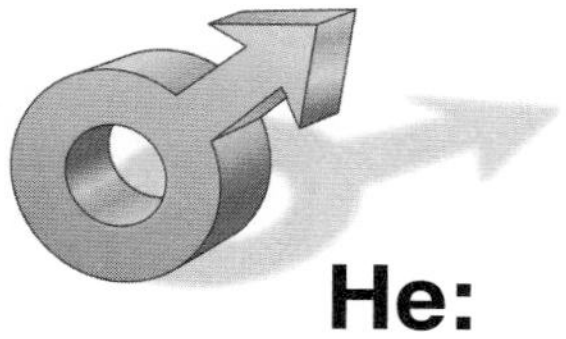

He:

- averages 12 breaths a minute
- has lower core body temperature
- has a slower heart rate
- has more oxygen-rich hemoglobin in his blood
- is more sensitive to sound
- produces twice as much saliva
- has a 10 percent larger brain
- is 10 times more likely to have attention deficit disorder
- as a teen, has an attention span of 5 minutes
- is more likely to be physically active
- is more prone to lethal diseases, including heart attacks, cancer, and liver failure
- is five times more likely to become an alcoholic
- has a life expectancy of 75.2 years

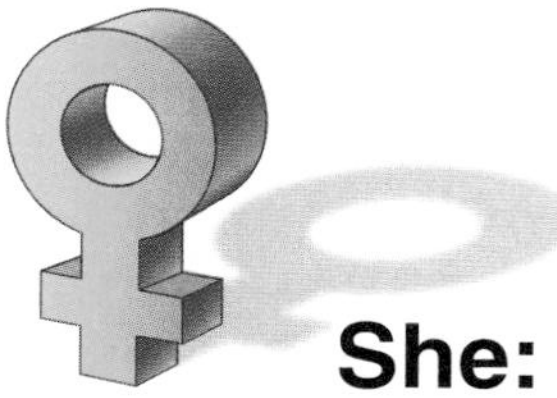

She:

- averages 9 breaths a minute
- has higher core body temperature
- has a faster heart rate
- has higher levels of protective immunoglobulin in her blood
- is more sensitive to light
- takes twice as long to process food
- has more neurons in certain brain regions
- is twice as likely to have an eating disorder
- as a teen, has an attention span of 20 minutes
- is more likely to be overweight
- is more vulnerable to chronic diseases, like arthritis and autoimmune disorders, and age-related conditions like osteoporosis
- is twice as likely to develop depression
- has a life expectancy of 80.4 years

FIGURE 1-4 Men and women *are* different in many ways.

Recognition of these gender differences is transforming medical research and practice. *Gender-specific medicine* is replacing one-size-fits-all health care with new definitions of what is normal in both men and women, more complex concepts of disease, more precise diagnostic tests, and more effective treatments.

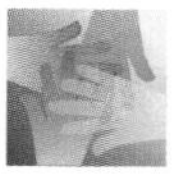

Diversity and Health

We live in the most diverse nation on Earth, one that is becoming increasingly diverse. For society, this variety can be both enriching and divisive. Tolerance and acceptance of others have always been part of the American creed. By working together, Americans have created a country that remains, to those outside our borders, a symbol of opportunity. Yet members of different ethnic groups still have to struggle against discrimination.

Black Americans lose substantially more years of potential life to homicide (nine times as many), stroke (three times as many), and diabetes (three times as many) as whites.[19] Hispanics suffer more fatal injuries, chronic liver disease, and cirrhosis of the liver.

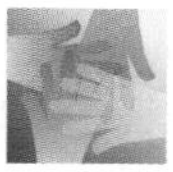

How Race Affects Health

Race and ethnicity affect the health of various minority groups in the United States in many ways.

- The infant mortality rate for African-American babies remains higher than for white babies.
- Life expectancy for African Americans, though increasing, is five years lower than for whites.
- African Americans have higher rates of high blood pressure (hypertension), develop this problem earlier in life, suffer more severe hypertension, and have higher rates of stroke.
- African Americans have higher rates of glaucoma, systemic lupus erythematosus, liver disease, and kidney failure than whites. They also have less access to kidney transplants.[20]
- Overall, black Americans are more likely to develop cancer than persons of any other racial or ethnic group. Black women have higher rates of colon, pancreatic, and stomach cancer. Black men have higher rates of prostate, colon, and stomach cancer.[21]
- African Americans have the highest death rates for lung cancer of any racial or ethnic group in the United States. Medical scientists have debated whether the reason might be that treatments are less effective in blacks or whether many are not diagnosed early enough nor treated rigorously enough.[22] A recent study of men with lung cancer has shown that equal treatment leads to equal outcomes. African-American patients who received the same treatments as whites were just as likely to survive.[23]
- Fewer African-American and Hispanic children are given prescriptions. White children receive more pain medication than black children treated for the

same conditions in emergency centers. Fewer psychiatric medications are provided to African-American youths.[24]

- Latinos living in the United States have high rates of eye disease and visual impairment, particularly of diabetic retinopathy, an eye complication of diabetes, and open-angle glaucoma, a disease that damages the optic nerve.[25]
- Women of Filipino, Hawaiian, Indian, Pakistani, Mexican, South and Central American, and Puerto Rican descent are 20 to 260 percent more likely to be diagnosed with late-stage breast cancer than white women.
- Caucasians are prone to osteoporosis (progressive weakening of bone tissue); cystic fibrosis; skin cancer; and phenylketonuria (PKU), a metabolic disorder that can lead to mental retardation.
- Asians and Asian Americans metabolize some medications faster than whites and thus require much smaller doses.
- Native Americans have the highest rate of diabetes in the world. Among the Pima Indians, half of all adults have diabetes.
- Native Hawaiian women have a higher rate of breast cancer than women from other racial and ethnic groups.
- Native Americans, including those indigenous to Alaska, are more likely to die young than the population as a whole, primarily as a result of accidental injuries, cirrhosis of the liver, homicide, pneumonia, and the complications of diabetes.
- The suicide rate among American Indians and Alaska Natives is 50 percent higher than the national rate. The rates of co-occurring mental illness and substance abuse (especially alcohol) are also higher among Native American youth and adults.
- American Indians and Alaska Natives have the poorest survival rates from all cancers combined, when compared with all other racial and ethnic groups.[26]

Are these increased susceptibilities the result of genetics, an unhealthy lifestyle, lack of access to health services, poverty, or the stress of living with discrimination? It is hard to say precisely. Certainly, poverty presents a major barrier to seeking preventive care and getting timely and effective treatment.

In some cases, both genetic and environmental factors may play a role. Take, for example, the high rates of diabetes among the Pima Indians. Until 50 years ago, these Native Americans were not notably obese or prone to diabetes. After World War II, the tribe started trading handmade baskets for lard and flour. Their lifestyle became more sedentary and their diet higher in fats. In addition, researchers have discovered that many Pima Indians have an inherited resistance to insulin that increases their susceptibility to diabetes. The combination of a hereditary predisposition and environmental factors may explain why the Pimas now have epidemic levels of diabetes.

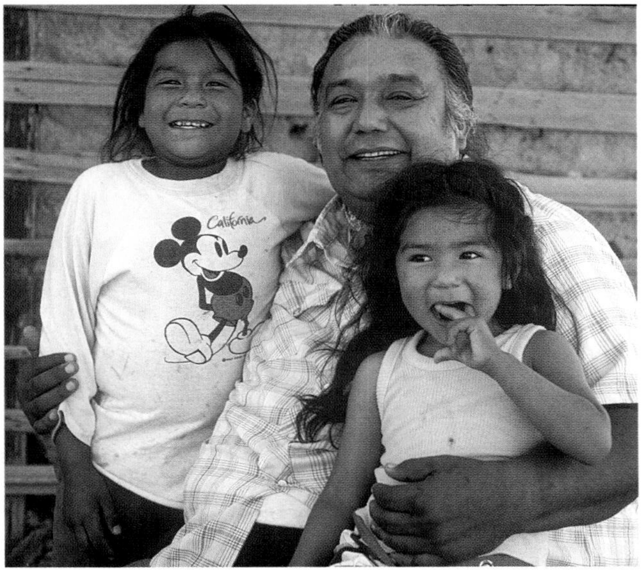

Steven Trimble Photography

Both genetic and environmental factors have contributed to the increase in diabetes among the Pima tribe. Half of all Pima adults have diabetes.

Ending Health Disparities

In the words of a National Institutes of Health report, minorities have carried "an unequal burden with respect to disease and disability, resulting in a lower life expectancy." Each year minorities in the United States—African Americans, Hispanics, Asian Americans, Pacific Islanders, Native Americans, and other groups—experience as many as 75,000 more deaths than they would if they lived under the same health conditions as the white population.

But race itself isn't the primary reason for the health problems faced by minorities in the United States. Poverty is. Without adequate insurance or the ability to pay, many cannot afford the tests and treatments that could prevent illness or overcome it at the earliest possible stages. One in three Hispanics under age 65 has no health insurance. According to public health experts, low income may account for one-third of the racial differences in death rates for middle-aged African-American adults. High blood pressure, high cholesterol, obesity, diabetes, and smoking are responsible for another third. The final third has been blamed on "unexplained factors," which may well include poor access to health care and the stress of living in a society in which skin color remains a major barrier to equality.

The racial gap in health care may be closing. A national survey monitored whether more than 6,700 patients received the highest standard of treatment for hundreds of conditions, ranging from routine care such as blood sugar testing for diabetes to specific procedures such as kidney dialysis or heart bypass surgery. Young people under age 31, blacks, and Hispanics had the highest percentage of those receiving top-quality health care (58 percent, compared with 54 percent of whites and 52 percent of those age 65 or older). However, many poor people and minorities do not see doctors in the first place or receive any care at all.[27]

Making Healthy Changes

Nothing is certain in life except change. Every day ushers in changes large and small, but the changes that matter most are those we make ourselves. In recent decades behavioral scientists have dissected the process of how people change, mapping the stages of change and identifying the components of successful change. The following sections describe some of the steps that can help you make changes for the better.

Understanding Health Behavior

Your choices and behaviors affect how long and how well you live. Nearly half of all deaths in the United States are linked to behaviors such as tobacco use, improper diet, abuse of alcohol and other drugs, use of firearms, motor vehicle accidents, risky sexual practices, and lack of exercise.

If you would like to improve your health behavior, you have to realize that change isn't easy. Between 40 and 80 percent of those who try to kick bad health habits lapse back into their unhealthy ways within six weeks. To make lasting beneficial changes, you have to understand the three types of influences that shape behavior: predisposing, enabling, and reinforcing factors (Figure 1-5).

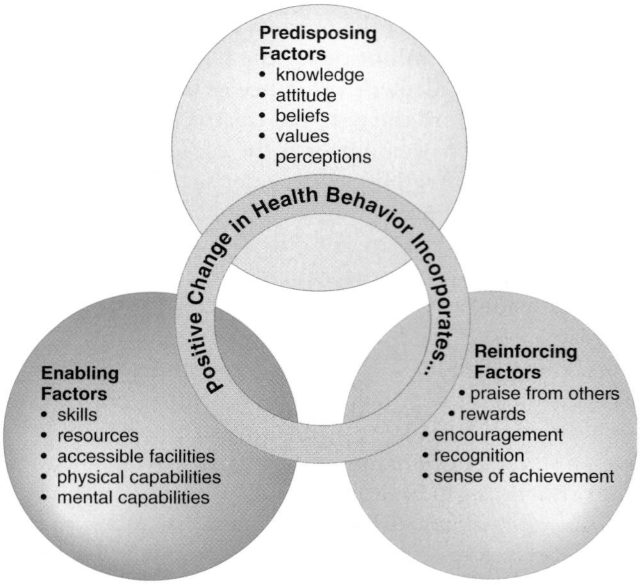

FIGURE 1-5 Factors that Shape Positive Behavior

Predisposing Factors

Predisposing factors include knowledge, attitudes, beliefs, values, and perceptions. Unfortunately, knowledge isn't enough to cause most people to change their behavior; for example, people fully aware of the grim consequences of smoking often continue to puff away. Nor is attitude—one's likes and dislikes—sufficient; an individual may dislike the smell and taste of cigarettes but continue to smoke regardless.

Beliefs are more powerful than knowledge and attitudes, and researchers report that people are most likely to change health behavior if they hold three beliefs:

- **Susceptibility.** They acknowledge that they are at risk for the negative consequences of their behavior.
- **Severity.** They believe that they may pay a very high price if they don't make a change.
- **Benefits.** They believe that the proposed change will be advantageous to their health.

There can be a gap between stated and actual beliefs, however. Young adults may say they recognize the very real dangers of casual, careless sex in this day and age. Yet, rather than act in accordance with these statements, they may impulsively engage in unprotected sex with individuals whose health status and histories they do not know. The reason: Like young people everywhere and in every time, they feel invulnerable, that nothing bad can or will happen to them, that if there were a real

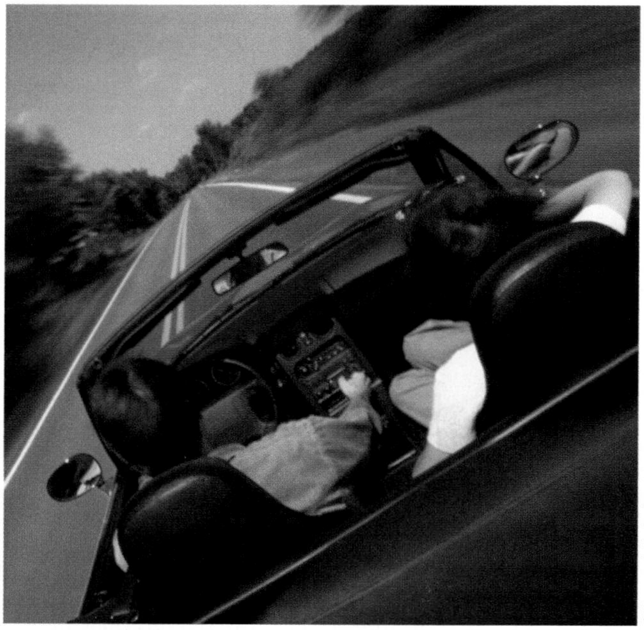

Your *stated* knowledge-based belief may be that unsafe driving can cause accidents. Your *actual* belief is that it won't happen to you.

danger, they would somehow know it. Often it's not until something happens—a former lover may admit to having a sexually transmitted infection—that their behaviors become consistent with their stated beliefs.

Enabling Factors

Enabling factors include skills, resources, accessible facilities, and physical and mental capacities. Before you initiate a change, assess the means available to reach your goal. No matter how motivated you are, you'll become frustrated if you keep encountering obstacles. That's why breaking a task or goal down into step-by-step strategies is so important in behavioral change.

Reinforcing Factors

Reinforcing factors may be praise from family and friends, rewards from teachers or parents, or encouragement and recognition for meeting a goal. Although these help a great deal in the short run, lasting change depends not on external rewards but on an internal commitment and sense of achievement. To make a difference, reinforcement must come from within.

A decision to change a health behavior should stem from a permanent, personal goal, not from a desire to please or impress someone else. If you lose weight for the homecoming dance, you're almost sure to regain pounds afterward. But if you shed extra pounds because you want to feel better about yourself or get into shape, you're far more likely to keep off the weight.

> *Some instructors offer extra credit to students who commit to and follow through on a healthy change, for example, exercising regularly or quitting smoking. Can this sort of incentive lead to permanent behavioral change? Or will students go back to their unhealthy habits as soon as the term ends?*
>
> You Decide

Models of Behavioral Change

Change can simply happen. You get older. You put on or lose weight. You have an accident. Intentional change is different: A person consciously, deliberately sets out either to change a negative behavior, such as chronic procrastination, or to initiate a healthy behavior, such as daily exercise. For decades psychologists have studied how people intentionally change and have developed various models that reveal the anatomy of change.

In the moral model, you take responsibility for a problem (such as smoking) and its solution; success depends on adequate motivation, while failure is seen as a sign of character weakness. In the enlightenment model, you submit to strict discipline to correct a problem; this is the approach used in Alcoholics Anonymous. The behavioral model involves rewarding yourself when you make positive changes. The medical model sees the behavior as caused by forces beyond your control (a genetic predisposition to being overweight, for example) and employs an expert to provide advice or treatment. For many people, the most effective approach is the compensatory model, which doesn't assign blame but puts responsibility on individuals to acquire whatever skills or power they need to overcome their problems.

The Transtheoretical Model

This theoretical model of behavioral change, developed by psychologist James Prochaska and his colleagues, focuses on the individual's decision making rather than on social or biological influences on behavior.[28] It is the foundation of programs for smoking cessation, exercise, healthy food choices, alcohol abuse, weight control, condom use, drug abuse, mammography screening, and stress management. However, conclusive scientific evidence for its usefulness in lifestyle change remains limited.

These key components of the **transtheoretical model of change** are described in the following sections:

- **Stages of Change.**
- **Processes of Change**—cognitive and behavioral activities that facilitate change.
- **Self-efficacy**—the confidence people have in their ability to cope with challenge.

> **predisposing factors** The beliefs, values, attitudes, knowledge, and perceptions that influence our behavior.
>
> **enabling factors** The skills, resources, and physical and mental capabilities that shape our behavior.
>
> **reinforcing factors** Rewards, encouragement, and recognition that influence our behavior in the short run.
>
> **transtheoretical model of change** A model of behavioral change that focuses on the individual's decision making; it states that an individual progresses through a sequence of six stages as he or she makes a change in behavior.

? FAQ What Are the Stages of Change?

According to the transtheoretical model of change, individuals progress through a sequence of stages as they make a change (Figure 1-6). No one stage is more important than another, and people often move back and forth between them. Most "spiral" from stage to stage, slipping from maintenance to contemplation or from action to precontemplation before moving forward again.

People usually cycle and recycle through the stages several times. Smokers, for instance, report making three or four serious efforts to quit before they succeed.

The six stages of change are:

1. **Precontemplation.** Whether or not they're aware of a problem behavior, people in this stage have no intention of making a change in the next six months. Busy college students in good health, for instance, might never think about getting more exercise.
2. **Contemplation.** Individuals in this stage are aware they have a problem behavior and are considering changing it within the next six months. However, they may be torn between the positives of the new behavior and the amount of energy, time, and other resources required to change. Students in a health course, for instance, may start thinking about exercising but struggle to balance potential benefits with the effort of getting up early to jog or go to the gym.
3. **Preparation.** People in this stage intend to change a problem behavior within the next month. Some focus on a master plan. For instance, they might look into fitness classes, gyms, or other options for working out. Others might start by making small changes, such as walking to classes rather than taking a campus shuttle bus.
4. **Action.** People in this stage are modifying their behavior according to their plan. For instance, they might be jogging or working out at the gym three times a week.
5. **Maintenance.** In this stage, individuals have continued to work at changing their behavior and have avoided relapse for at least six months. New exercisers are likely to stop during the first three to six months. One reason that researchers have identified: the temptation not to exercise. However, follow-up, whether by mail, e-mail, or phone calls from supportive friends, family, or a counselor, can help maintain physical activity levels.
6. **Termination.** While it may take two to five years, a behavior becomes so deeply ingrained that a person can't imagine abandoning it. More than eight in ten college seniors who exercised regularly remain as active, or even more active, after graduation.

As research on college students has shown, attitudes and feelings are related to stages of change. Smokers who believe that continuing to smoke would have only a minor or no impact on their health remain in the precontemplation stage; those with respiratory symptoms move on to contemplation and preparation. In a study at Ohio State University, researchers classified student heavy drinkers according to the stages of change: Nearly two-thirds of the "precontemplators" continued to drink heavily and had no intention of changing their behavior. In the maintenance stage, students drank an average of one alcoholic drink a month even though they felt that heavy drinking was the norm on their campus.[29]

The Processes of Change

Anything you do to modify your thinking, feeling, or behavior can be called a change process. The nine included in the transtheoretical model are shown in Figure 1-6 in their corresponding stages:

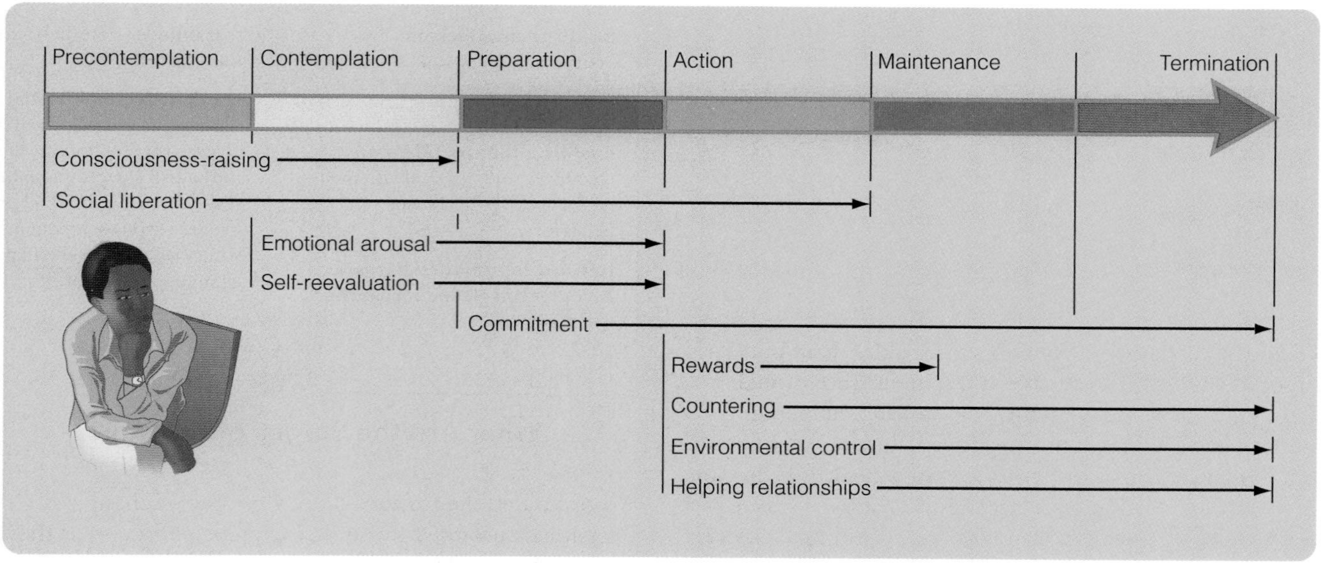

FIGURE 1-6 The Stages of Change and Some Change Processes
These change processes can help you progress through the stages of change. Each may be most useful at particular stages.

Consciousness-raising The most widely used change process involves increasing knowledge about yourself or the nature of your problem. As you learn more, you gain understanding and feedback about your behavior.

Example: Reading Chapter 5 on making healthy food choices.

Social liberation This process takes advantage of alternatives in the external environment that can help you begin or continue your efforts to change.

Example: Spending as much time as possible in nonsmoking areas.

Emotional arousal This process, also known as dramatic relief, works on a deeper level than consciousness-raising and is equally important in the early stages of change. Emotional arousal means experiencing and expressing feelings about a problem behavior and its potential solutions.

Example: Resolving never to drink and drive after the death of a friend in a car accident.

Self-reevaluation This process requires a thoughtful reappraisal of your problem, including an assessment of the person you might be once you have changed the behavior.

Example: Recognizing that you have a gambling problem and imagining yourself as a nongambler.

Commitment This process acknowledges—first privately and then publicly—that you are responsible for your behavior and the only one who can change it.

Example: Joining a self-help or support group.

Countering Countering, or counterconditioning, substitutes healthy behaviors for unhealthy ones.

Example: Chewing gum rather than smoking.

Environmental control This action-oriented process restructures your environment so you are less likely to engage in a problem behavior.

Example: Getting rid of your stash of sweets.

Rewards This process reinforces positive behavioral changes with self-praise or small gifts.

Example: Getting a massage after a month of consistent exercise.

Helping relationships This process recruits individuals—family, friends, therapist, coach—to provide support, caring, understanding, and acceptance.

Example: Finding an exercise buddy.

Self-Efficacy and Locus of Control

Do you see yourself as master of your fate, asserting control over your destiny? Or do so many things happen in your life that you just hang on and hope for the best? The answers to these questions reveal two important characteristics that affect your health: your sense of **self-efficacy** (the belief in your ability to change and to reach a goal) and your **locus of control** (the sense of being in control of your life).

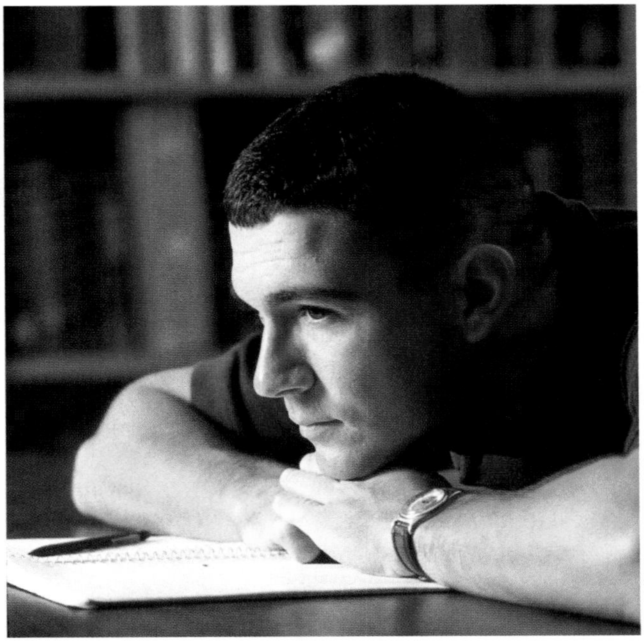

Do you picture yourself as master of your own destiny? You are more likely to achieve your health goals if you do.

Your confidence in your ability to cope with challenge can determine whether you can and will succeed in making a change. In his research on self-efficacy, psychologist Albert Bandura of Stanford University found that the individuals most likely to reach a goal are those who believe that they can. The stronger their faith in themselves, the more energy and persistence they put into making a change. The opposite is also true, especially for health behaviors. Among people who begin an exercise program, those with lower self-efficacy are more likely to drop out.

If you believe that your actions will make a difference in your health, your locus of control is internal. If you believe that external forces or factors play a greater role, your locus of control is external. Hundreds of studies have compared people who have these different perceptions of control. "Internals," who believe that their actions largely determine what happens to them, act more independently, enjoy better health, and are more optimistic about their future. "Externals," who perceive that chance or outside forces determine their fate, find it harder to cope with stress and feel increasingly helpless over time. When it comes to

self-efficacy Belief in one's ability to accomplish a goal or change a behavior.

locus of control An individual's belief about the sources of power and influence over his or her life.

Strategies for Change — Use the Language of Change

Pay attention both to what you say when you talk or think about a health behavior change and how you say it. Then consciously edit the words in your mind and as you say them.

- **Watch out for weasel words.** Are you "planning" to quit smoking? "Hoping" to lose weight? When you use linguistic loopholes like "trying" or "hoping," you give yourself permission to settle for whatever happens. When you speak of goals, use definitive, unequivocal language.
- **Trade tenses.** When thinking or talking about bad health habits, switch to the past tense. Instead of saying, "I'm too lazy to exercise," tell yourself, "I used to be too lazy to exercise." This reminds you that you have changed, are changing, or at the least are capable of change.
- **Not "if" but "when."** Instead of saying, "If I could exercise more," say to yourself, "When I start exercising more." This simple switch sets the stage for believing that you will be able to change your lifestyle.
- **Just "because."** According to social psychology research, using the word "because" when making a request or seeking agreement can boost your compliance as high as 80 to 90 percent. For instance, you might tell yourself: "I won't buy doughnuts *because* I don't want to be tempted."
- **Guard against demeaning words and phrases.** When a derogatory statement about yourself forms in your brain, say firmly, "Stop!" or "Delete!"
- **Don't focus on what you can't do.** Remind yourself of your strengths every day. Say to yourself, "I can go another five minutes on the treadmill" or "I can stand another half hour without a cigarette."

weight, for instance, they see themselves as destined to be fat.

The Health Belief Model

Psychologists developed the **health belief model (HBM)** about 50 years ago to explain and predict health behaviors by focusing on the attitudes and beliefs of individuals. (Remember that your attitudes and beliefs are predisposing influences on your capacity for change.) According to this model, people will take a health-related action (e.g., use condoms) if they:

- **Feel that they can avoid a negative consequence,** such as a sexually transmitted infection (STI).
- **Expect a positive outcome** if they take the recommended advice, for instance, that condoms will protect them from STIs.
- **Believe that they can successfully take action,** for example, use condoms comfortably and confidently.

Readiness to act on health beliefs, in this model, depends on how vulnerable individuals feel, how severe they perceive the danger to be, the benefits they expect to gain, and the barriers they think they will encounter. Another key factor, discussed earlier in this chapter, is self-efficacy, their confidence in their ability to take action.

Over the years the health belief model has been used to help people change unhealthy behaviors, such as smoking, overeating, and inactivity, or to encourage them to take positive health actions, such as using condoms and getting needed vaccinations and medical checkups.

? FAQ How Can I Change a Bad Health Habit?

Change is never easy—even if it's done for the best possible reasons. When you decide to change a behavior, you have to give up something familiar and easy for something new and challenging. Change always involves risk—and the prospect of rewards.

Before they reach the stage where they can and do take action to change, most people go through a process comparable to religious conversion. First, they reach a level of accumulated unhappiness that makes them ready for change. Then they have a moment of truth that makes them want to change. One pregnant woman, for instance, felt her unborn baby quiver when she drank a beer and swore never to drink again. As people change their behavior, they change their lifestyles and identities as well. Ex-smokers, for instance, may start an aggressive exercise program, make new friends at the track or gym, and participate in new types of activities, like racquetball games or fun runs.

Think about the behavior you want to change. Now think about which of the six stages of change you are in with regard to that behavior. Table 1-1 lists some appropriate change goals for each stage. Set your goal and go for it! The next section provides more keys on how to make this change successful, and then Your Life Coach talks about goal-setting.

TABLE 1-1 Stages of Lifestyle Change

Stage of Change	Appropriate Change Goal
1. **Precontemplation:** You are not truly convinced about the importance of the lifestyle goal.	Get more information about the value of the lifestyle change goal.
2. **Contemplation:** You have no definite plan for when to begin but would like to change.	Set a date for making the change.
3. **Preparation:** You have set a date to begin the new behavior and are planning the best strategy to carry out the change.	Develop a plan and tell others about the change.
4. **Action:** You are engaged in making changes.	Adjust to new lifestyle and manage unexpected emotional and physical reactions.
5. **Maintenance:** You are working to integrate the lifestyle change into normal day-to-day life.	Continue to pay attention to the behavior and work through any relapse. Help others achieve similar lifestyle goals.
6. **Termination/Moving On:** You have maintained the change for six months to a year and are ready to move on to other lifestyle interests.	Set new health-enhancing goals. Move on from support systems that are focused exclusively on the prior lifestyle goal.

Source: Human Resources Institute, www.healthyculture.com/Articles/mentorarticle.html. Reprinted with permission.

How You Change

Awareness of a negative behavior is always the first step toward changing it. Once you identify what you'd like to change, keep a diary for one or two weeks, noting what you do, when, where, and what you're feeling at the time. If you'd like, enlist the help of friends or family to call attention to your behavior. Sometimes self-observation in itself proves therapeutic: Just the act of keeping a diary can be enough to help you lose weight or kick the smoking habit.

In making a change, you have to weigh its potential pluses and minuses. **Decisional balance** involves consideration of the consequences of change to yourself and others and the reactions of both yourself and others as a result of change. These can be both positive and negative.

For instance, if your target health behavior goal is to stop smoking, you will definitely benefit in many ways, such as breathing more easily and lowering your risk of heart disease and cancer. But you may gain a few pounds or miss the camaraderie of hanging out with fellow smokers. You are more likely to make—and maintain—a health change if you see the pros of the change outweighing the cons.

Once you've identified the situations, moods, thoughts, or people that act as cues for a behavior, identify the most powerful ones and develop a plan to avoid them. For instance, if you snack continuously when studying in your room, try working in the library, where food is forbidden.

Some people find it helpful to sign a "contract," a written agreement in which they make a commitment to change, with their partner, parent, or health educator. Spelling out what they intend to do, and why, underscores the seriousness of what they're trying to accomplish (see the sample contract in the Self-Assessment Booklet).

Social and cultural **norms**—behaviors that are expected, accepted, or supported by a group—can work against a person's best intentions. You may resolve to eat less, for instance, yet your mother may keep offering you home-made fudge and brownies because your family's norm is to show love by making and offering delicious treats. Or you might decide to drink less, yet your friends' norm may be to equate drinking with having a good time.

In a recent study at a large public university in the Northeast, students overestimated how many of their peers drank heavily, used drugs, and engaged in sex. These misperceptions had a small to moderate effect on the students' own drinking, drug use, and sexual activities.[30] Providing correct information about students' actual behavior, the authors concluded, might be particularly helpful in targeting high-risk groups, such as heavy drinkers.

Your **self-talk**—the messages you send yourself—also can play a role. In recent decades, mental health professionals have recognized the conscious use of positive self-talk as a powerful force for changing the way individuals think, feel, and behave. "We have a choice about how we think," explains psychologist Martin Seligman, Ph.D., author of *Learned Optimism*. As he notes, by learning to challenge automatic negative thoughts that enter our brains and asserting our own statements of self-worth, we can transform ourselves into optimists who see what's right rather than pessimists forever focusing on what's wrong.[31]

Reinforcements—either positive (a reward) or negative (a punishment)—also can play a role. Plan a pleasant reward as an incentive for every week you stick to your new behavior—sleeping in on a Saturday morn-

health belief model (HBM) A model of behavioral change that focuses on the individual's attitudes and beliefs.

decisional balance Weighing the positive and negative consequences of change to yourself and to others.

norms The unwritten rules regarding behavior and conduct expected or accepted by a group.

self-talk Repetition of positive messages about one's self-worth to learn more optimistic patterns of thought, feeling, and behavior.

reinforcement Reward or punishment for a behavior that will increase or decrease one's likelihood of repeating the behavior.

Strategies for Change — Is Your Goal S.M.A.R.T.?

Many professional coaches use the following questions to help clients set effective goals:

- **Specific?** Identifying exactly what you want to accomplish helps you plan the steps that lead to your goal.
- **Measurable?** Your goal should be concrete enough so that both you and others can see the progress you're making.
- **Attainable?** Set goals that are slightly out of your immediate grasp but not so far that there is no hope of achieving them.
- **Realistic?** Maybe you dream of being an Olympian, but a realistic goal might be to try out for the rowing team.
- **Targeted?** A clear objective, such as quitting smoking, encourages laserlike focus.

ing, going out with some friends, or spending a sunny afternoon outdoors. Small, regular rewards are more effective in keeping up motivation than one big reward that won't come for many months.

YOUR LIFE COACH

Going for Your Goals

Think of goals as road maps that give you both a destination and a planned itinerary for getting there. "To set goals means to set a course for your life," says psychologist James Fadiman, author of *Unlimit Your Life: Setting and Getting Goals.* "Without goals, you remain what you were. With goals, you become what you wish." As studies of performance in students, athletes, and employees have shown, the one single characteristic that separates high- and low-achievers is having a clear, specific goal. The following sections describe the most effective strategies for using goals to map your way to the life you want.

Set Your Sights on a Destination or Target

The more vividly that you can see, feel, touch, and taste what you want, the more likely you are to achieve it. The reason, explains psychologist Kenneth W. Christian, author of *Your Own Worst Enemy,* is that a destination goal transforms your brain into a satellite dish picking up the signals that are most relevant to your quest. "You begin to see possibilities that pull you closer to your goal. You meet people who can help you. It can seem magical, but it's not. Your unconscious mind is working on your goal while you go on with your life."[32]

Take a Step and a Stretch

With your target goal in sight, set "step-and-stretch" goals. Think of them like stair steps that lift you out of your comfort zone and keep you moving forward. It doesn't matter how many there are. In some instances, it may be six; in others, sixty. Every goal should be a reach from where you are that will bring you to the next level.

Break down each step goal into projects and every project into tasks. Ask yourself the following questions, and write down the answers.

- What skills do I need to achieve this?
- What information and knowledge must I acquire?
- What help, assistance, or resources do I need?
- What can block my progress? (For each potential barrier, list solutions.)
- Whom can I turn to for support?

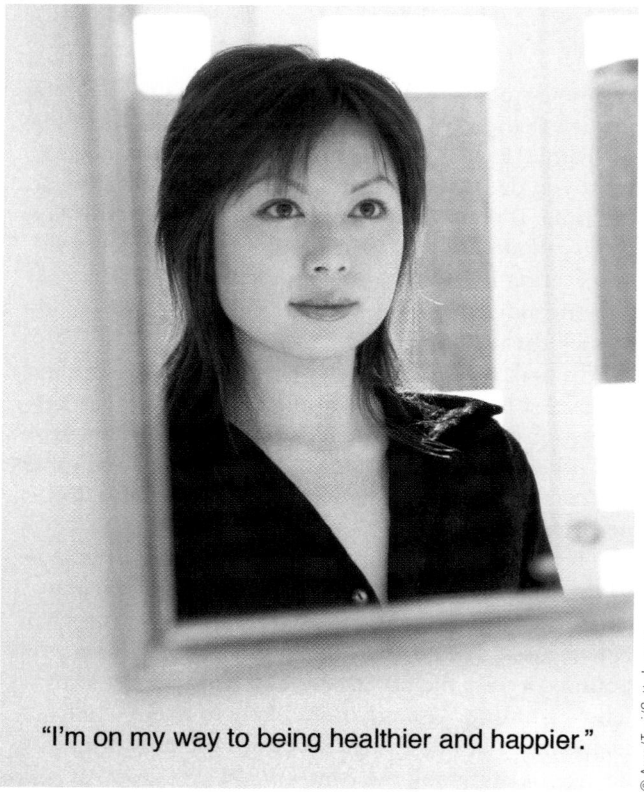

"I'm on my way to being healthier and happier."

An affirmation is a powerful tool to help you make a change.

- Who or what is likely to get in my way?
- How am I most likely to sabotage myself?

Use an Affirmation

Once you've pictured your goal in detail, express it in an **affirmation,** a single positive sentence. As decades of psychological research have shown, affirmations serve as powerful tools for behavioral change. Make sure to use the present tense. For example, tell yourself "I am not a smoker" daily—even though you may still light up occasionally.

Once you've polished your affirmation, put it on paper. By putting it in writing, you become more committed to making your words come true. Some people post their affirmations on their computers and night stands or carry them in their wallets. Wherever you jot yours, look at your affirmation often—ideally at least once a day.

Go All the Way

Despite good intentions and considerable progress, many people give up their goals just before the rainbow's end—and congratulate themselves for getting that far. "Would you ever board a plane for Chicago and say, 'Well, we got three-quarters of the way there!' as if that were good?" asks psychologist Christian, who urges goal-seekers to persist, persevere, and "not settle for almost-there." If you stall on the final stretch, do a quick reality check. Maybe you need to add some smaller-step goals, seek more support, or simply allow yourself more time.

Whenever you achieve a goal, acknowledge it, tell a friend, or just raise your hands above your head like a runner crossing the finish line. This is what builds your sense of, "I can do it. I AM doing it. Look how far I've come!"

Recovering from a Relapse

Once you are ready to change, getting started is not the greatest challenge you'll face. That usually comes weeks or months later, when your progress hits a wall or you return to your old, unhealthy habits. Rather than looking for someone or something to help you get back on track, try the following:

- **Gather data.** Keep a detailed log of your behavior for a week, including a weekend. If your goal is to get into better shape, keep track of how much time you spend on sedentary pursuits, what derails your plans to exercise, the types of activities you most enjoy, and so forth.
- **Reassess your goals.** Are your expectations too high? Is your timetable unrealistic? Have you been derailed by finals, stress, the flu, a family crisis?
- **Check with your doctor.** Various medical conditions, such as infections, depression, diabetes, and medications (including corticosteroids and hormones) can undermine your energy and ability to pursue your wellness goals.
- **Autopsy setbacks.** If you blow your diet or slide back into couch-potato habits, analyze what went wrong and why. Start with the following questions:
  - What blindsided, distracted, demoralized, or otherwise derailed you?
  - What excuses did you use?
  - Who were the saboteurs who undermined your efforts?
  - How did they sidetrack you?

  Now focus on the future.
  - What potential pitfalls do you anticipate?
  - How will you overcome them?
  - What are your back-up plans in case something or someone unexpectedly tries to sabotage your current efforts to change a health behavior?

affirmation A single positive sentence used as a tool for behavior change.

LEARN IT / LIVE IT

Making Healthy Changes

Ultimately you have more control over your health than anyone else. Use this course as an opportunity to zero in on at least one less-than-healthful behavior and improve it. Here are some suggestions for small steps that can have a big payoff:

- **Use seat belts.** In the last decade, seat belts have saved more than 40,000 lives and prevented millions of injuries.
- **Eat an extra fruit or vegetable every day.** Adding more fruit and vegetables to your diet can improve your digestion and lower your risk of several cancers.
- **Get enough sleep.** A good night's rest provides the energy you need to make it through the following day.
- **Take regular stress breaks.** A few quiet minutes spent stretching, looking out the window, or simply letting yourself unwind are good for body and soul.
- **Lose a pound.** If you're overweight, you may not think a pound will make a difference, but it's a step in the right direction.

(Continued)

- **If you're a woman, examine your breasts regularly.** Get in the habit of performing a breast self-examination every month after your period (when breasts are least swollen or tender).
- **If you're a man, examine your testicles regularly.** These simple self-exams can spot the early signs of cancer when they're most likely to be cured.
- **Get physical.** Just a little exercise will do some good. A regular workout schedule will be good for your heart, lungs, muscles, bones—even your mood.
- **Drink more water.** Eight glasses a day are what you need to replenish lost fluids, prevent constipation, and keep your digestive system working efficiently.
- **Do a good deed.** Caring for others is a wonderful way to care for your own soul and connect with others.

1 Making This Chapter Work for You

Review Questions

1. Which of the following statements about the dimensions of health are true?
   a. Spirituality provides solace and comfort for those who are severely ill, but it has no health benefits.
   b. The people who reflect the highest levels of social health are usually among the most popular individuals in a group and are often thought of as the life of the party.
   c. Intellectual health refers to one's academic abilities.
   d. Optimal physical health requires a nutritious diet, regular exercise, avoidance of harmful behaviors and substances, and self-protection from accidents.
2. The goals of the *Healthy People 2010* initiative include all of the following *except*
   a. Reduce the proportion of obese children and adolescents in the population.
   b. Decrease the number of teens using illegal substances.
   c. Increase the number of adults engaging in daily, vigorous, physical activity for 30 minutes per occasion.
   d. Reduce the percentage of teens and adults who report smoking cigarettes.
3. Which statement about today's college students is *not* true?
   a. A majority of students are at a healthy weight.
   b. Fewer than 25 percent of students had five or more alcoholic drinks at a single sitting in the past three weeks.
   c. More than 60 percent of students have never smoked.
   d. Almost 80 percent of students who'd had vaginal intercourse used birth control pills or condoms.
4. A group of students is discussing the differences between the sexes. Whose statement is *incorrect?*
   a. Matt: "Men breathe faster but have a slower heart rate—and have a larger brain."
   b. Elena: "But women have more neurons in certain brain regions."
   c. Kristin: "And women are less likely to get arthritis."
   d. Rick: "Got me there—Men *are* more likely to have heart attacks and to get cancer."
5. Health risks faced by different ethnic and racial groups include all of the following *except*
   a. Whites have higher rates of hypertension, lupus, liver disease, and kidney failure than African Americans.
   b. Native Americans have a higher rate of diabetes than other racial and ethnic groups.
   c. Infant mortality is higher for African-American babies than for white babies.
   d. Latinos living in the United States have high rates of eye disease.
6. The development of health behaviors is influenced by all of the following *except*
   a. reinforcing factors, which involve external recognition for achieving a goal.
   b. preexisting health factors, which take into account the individual's current position on the wellness continuum.
   c. predisposing factors, which include knowledge, attitudes, and beliefs.
   d. enabling factors, which are related to an individual's skills and capabilities to make behavioral changes.
7. Change processes, cognitive and behavioral activities that facilitate change, include all of these *except*
   a. consciousness-raising
   b. countering
   c. health awareness
   d. helping relationships
8. According to the stages of change in the transtheoretical model of change, which statement is *incorrect?*
   a. In the maintenance stage, individuals have avoided relapse for six months.
   b. In the contemplation stage, individuals are considering changing a problem behavior in the next six months.
   c. In the action stage, individuals are actually modifying their behavior according to their plan.
   d. In the preparation stage, individuals intend to change a problem behavior in the next six months.
9. If you want to change unhealthy behavior, which of the following strategies is *least* likely to promote success?
   a. Believe that you can make the change.
   b. Reward yourself regularly.
   c. During self-talks, remind yourself about all your faults.
   d. Accept that you are in control of your health.

LACC Extra Credit Assignment

1. List and discuss three of the most important issues in this chapter.

10. Relapses are common (you're human, aren't you?), but don't let them keep you from your goal. Which of these strategies might help you recover from a relapse?
    a. Have a hot fudge sundae.
    b. Decide to think about it after finals.
    c. Analyze what went wrong and why.
    d. Put yourself back into contemplation stage.

Answers to these questions can be found on page 422.

Critical Thinking

1. Where are you on the wellness–illness continuum? What variables might affect your place on the scale? What do you consider your optimum state of health to be?
2. Talk to classmates from different racial or ethnic backgrounds than yours about their culture's health attitudes. Ask them what is considered healthy behavior in their cultures. For example, is having a good appetite a sign of health? What kinds of self-care practices did their parents and grandparents use to treat colds, fevers, rashes, and other health problems? What are their attitudes about the health-care system?
3. Think about a behavioral change you have made in your life in the past three years in any of the dimensions of health (physical, psychological, spiritual, social, intellectual, environmental). Can you remember going through each of the six stages of the transtheoretical model of change?
4. In what ways would you like to change your present lifestyle? What steps could you take to make those changes?

Media Menu

ThomsonNOW™ Go to the ThomsonNOW website at **http://www.thomsonedu.com** that will:

- Help you evaluate your knowledge of the material.
- Allow you to take an exam-prep quiz.
- Provide a Personalized Learning Plan targeting resources that address areas you should study.
- Coach you through identifying target goals for behavioral change and creating and monitoring your personal change plan throughout the semester.

INTERNET CONNECTIONS

Go Ask Alice
www.goaskalice.columbia.edu/index.html

Sponsored by Columbia University, this site offers questions and answers as well as an interactive service on a wide variety of health-related topics.

Lifescan Health Risk Appraisal
http://wellness.uwsp.edu/Other/lifescan

This site, created by Bill Hettler, M.D., of the National Wellness Institute, helps you identify specific lifestyle factors that can impair your health and longevity. Take the health questionnaire to determine your personal lifestyle risks. Your results provide a score for general results, nutrition results, and height/weight results. Your ranking among the top ten causes of death is provided, as well as suggestions on how to improve.

Transtheoretical Model—Cancer Prevention Research Center
www.uri.edu/research/cprc/TTM/detailedoverview.htm

This site describes the transtheoretical model of change, including descriptions of effective interventions to promote health behavior change, focusing on the individual's decision-making strategies.

InfoTrac College Edition Activities Log on, insert **self-efficacy** into the Keyword search box, and limit your search to the past year. When you get the results, Mark articles to review, then Select one to read. Summarize three or four key points from the article.

You can find additional readings related to personal health with InfoTrac College Edition, an online library of more than 900 journals and publications. Follow the instructions for accessing InfoTrac College Edition that were packaged with your textbook; then search for articles using a keyword search.

For additional links, resources, and suggested readings on the InfoTrac College Edition, visit our Health and Wellness Resource Center at http://health.wadsworth.com.

Key Terms

The terms listed are used on the page indicated. Definitions of the terms are in the Glossary at the end of this book.

affirmation 21
decisional balance 19
enabling factors 15
health 4
health belief model (HBM) 18
health promotion 6
locus of control 17
norms 19
predisposing factors 14
prevention 9
protection 9
reinforcement 19
reinforcing factors 15
self-efficacy 17
self-talk 19
transtheoretical model of change 15
wellness 4

2 Psychological Health

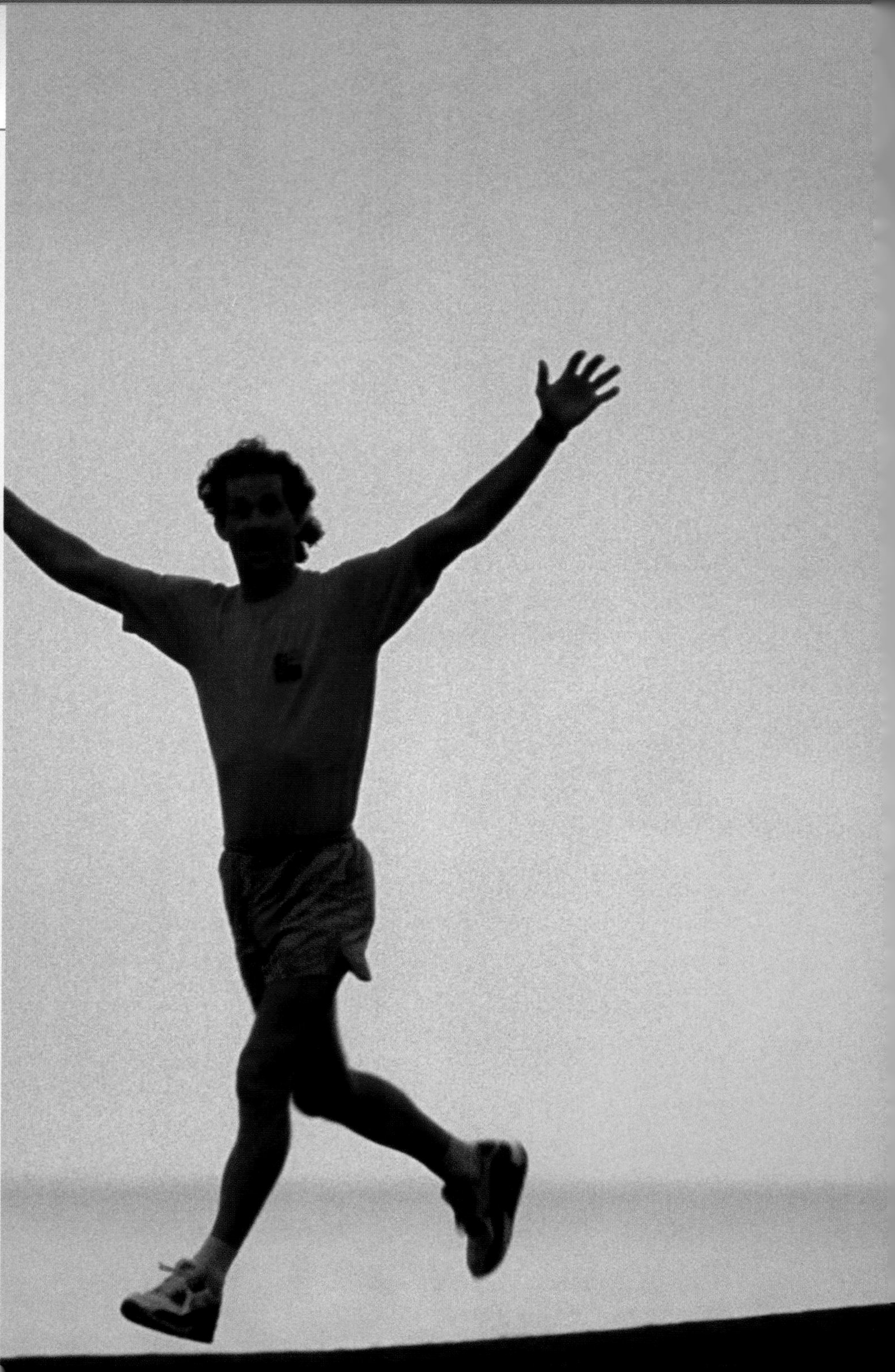

REAL HEALTH

In the middle of his freshman year, Travis once again began to sink into a major depression. At first he blamed his unhappiness on the difficulties of adapting to a new life as a college student. Even though he tossed and turned at night, he couldn't muster the energy to get out of bed for his 8:00 a.m. classes. His mood turned darker, especially when he drank. Travis began to fantasize about ways he could just let go of his troubles—and his life.

Walking across the main quad, Travis spotted a poster from a student organization promoting awareness of psychological problems. He looked at the photograph of a sullen young man with lifeless eyes and thought, That could be me. The next day he met with a therapist at the campus health center.

"I thought college was supposed to be the happiest time of your life," Travis said. "What went wrong?" As the counselor explained, no one is immune to psychological problems, and depression is common among college students. Rather than blaming himself, Travis began a combination of regular psychotherapy and psychiatric medication. "I was smart—or lucky," he says. "I got help before I went over the brink and tried to harm myself."

Although youth can seem a golden time, when body and mind glow with potential, the process of becoming an adult is a challenging one in every culture and country. Psychological health can make the difference between facing this challenge with optimism and confidence or feeling overwhelmed by expectations and responsibilities.

This isn't always easy. At some point in life almost half of Americans develop an emotional disorder.[1] Young adulthood—the years from the late teens to the midtwenties—is a time when many serious disorders, including bipolar illness (manic depression) and schizophrenia, often develop. The saddest fact is not that so many feel so bad, but that so few realize they can feel better. In the course of a year, 60 percent of those with a mental disorder receive no treatment at all.[2] Yet 80 to 90 percent of those treated for psychological problems recover, most within a few months.

By learning about psychological disorders, you may be able to recognize early warning signals in yourself or your loved ones so that you can deal with potential difficulties or seek professional help for more serious problems.

? FAQ Frequently Asked Questions

- How can I get out of a bad mood? *p. 29*
- Can prayer keep us healthy? *p. 32*
- How much sleep do I need? *p. 36*
- Why are so many young people depressed? *p. 39*
- Are antidepressants dangerous? *p. 42*
- What leads to suicide? *p. 46*

After studying the material in this chapter, you should be able to:

- **Identify** the characteristics of emotional, mental, and spiritual health.
- **Describe** the values and other self-esteem components of psychological health.
- **Discuss** ways of enhancing spirituality in your daily life.
- **Explain** the differences between mental health and mental illness.
- **Name** the characteristic symptoms of depression.
- **Discuss** some of the factors that may lead to suicide, as well as strategies for prevention.
- **Describe** the treatment options available for those with psychological problems.

ThomsonNOW™ Log on to ThomsonNOW at **www.thomsonedu.com/thomsonnow** to find your Behavior Change Planner and to explore self-assessments, interactive tutorials, and practice quizzes.

What Is Psychological Health?

Unlike physical health, psychological well-being cannot be measured, tested, X-rayed, or dissected. Yet psychologically healthy men and women generally share certain characteristics: They value themselves and strive toward happiness and fulfillment. They establish and maintain close relationships with others. They accept the limitations as well as the possibilities that life has to offer. And they feel a sense of meaning and purpose that makes the gestures of living worth the effort required.

Psychological health encompasses both our emotional and mental states—that is, our feelings and our thoughts. **Emotional health** generally refers to feelings and moods, both of which are discussed later in this chapter. Characteristics of emotionally healthy people include the following:

- Determination and effort to be healthy.
- Flexibility and adaptability to a variety of circumstances.
- Development of a sense of meaning and affirmation of life.
- An understanding that the self is not the center of the universe.
- Compassion for others.
- The ability to be unselfish in serving or relating to others.
- Increased depth and satisfaction in intimate relationships.
- A sense of control over the mind and body that enables the person to make health-enhancing choices and decisions.

Mental health describes our ability to perceive reality as it is, to respond to its challenges, and to develop rational strategies for living. The mentally healthy person doesn't try to avoid conflicts and distress but can cope with life's transitions, traumas, and losses in a way that allows for emotional stability and growth. The characteristics of mental health include:

- The ability to function and carry out responsibilities.
- The ability to form relationships.
- Realistic perceptions of the motivations of others.
- Rational, logical thought processes.
- The ability to adapt to change and to cope with adversity.

There is considerable overlap between psychological and **spiritual health,** which involves our ability to identify our basic purpose in life and to experience the fulfillment of achieving our full potential. In one study, more than half of individuals with mental disorders, including depression, turned to spiritual readings or practices to increase calmness, find inner strength and meaning, improve self-awareness, and increase their sense of well-being. Religious support has also been shown to help lower depression and increase life

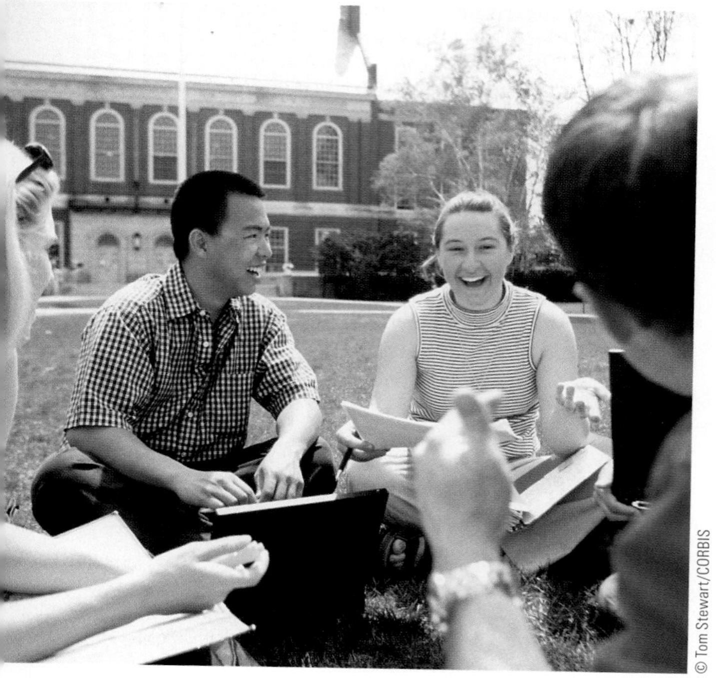

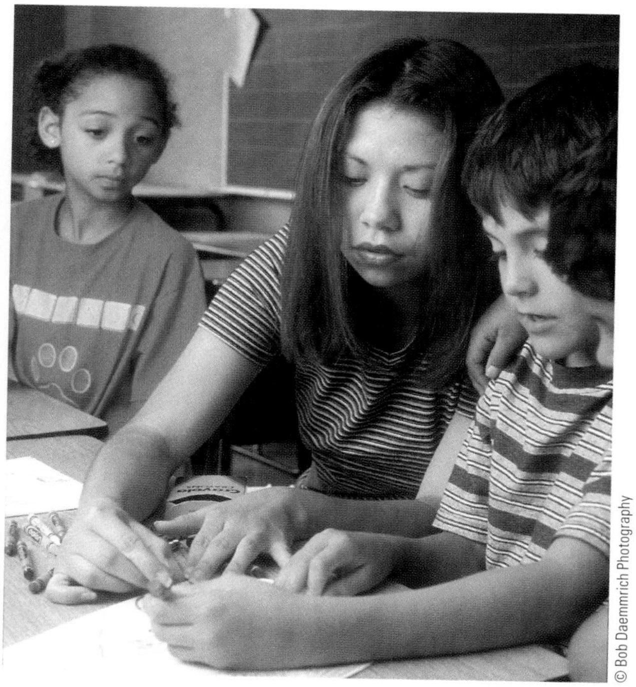

Psychologically healthy people have compassion for others and form strong and deep relationships. They adapt to a variety of circumstances, overcome challenges, and strive to achieve their full potential.

satisfaction beyond the benefits of social support from friends and family.

In addition, **culture** helps to define psychological health. In one culture, men and women may express feelings with great intensity, shouting in joy or wailing in grief, while in another culture such behavior might be considered abnormal or unhealthy. In our diverse society, many cultural influences affect Americans' sense of who they are, where they came from, and what they believe. Cultural rituals help bring people together, strengthen their bonds, reinforce the values and beliefs they share, and provide a sense of belonging, meaning, and purpose.

Emotional Intelligence

A person's "IQ"—or intelligence quotient—was once considered the leading predictor of achievement. However, psychologists have determined that another "way of knowing," dubbed **emotional intelligence,** makes an even greater difference in a person's personal and professional success.

"EQ" (for emotional quotient) is the ability to monitor and use emotions to guide thinking and actions. As more than a decade of research has shown, people with high EQ are more productive at work and happier at home. They're also less prone to stress, depression, and anxiety and bounce back quicker from serious illnesses.

Spiritual Intelligence

Mental health professionals have recognized the power of **spiritual intelligence,** which some define as "the capacity to sense, understand, and tap into the highest parts of ourselves, others, and the world around us." Spiritual intelligence, unlike spirituality, does not center on the worship of a God above, but on the discovery of a wisdom within. All of us are born with the potential to develop spiritual intelligence, but relatively few do. (Spirituality is discussed in depth on page 30.)

While we're all born with this capacity, most of us aren't even aware of it—and do little or nothing to nurture it. Part of the reason is that we confuse spiritual intelligence with religion, dogma, or old-fashioned morality. "You don't have to go to church to be spiritually intelligent; you don't even have to believe in God," say Reverend Paul Edwards, a retired Episcopalian minister and therapist in Fullerton, California. "It is a scientific fact that when you are feeling secure, at peace, loved, and happy, you see, hear, and act differently than when you're feeling insecure, unhappy, and unloved. Spiritual intelligence allows you to use the wisdom you have when you're in a state of inner peace. And you get there by changing the way you think, basically by listening less to what's in your head and more to what's in your heart."[3]

The Lessons of Positive Psychology

Psychology, a field that traditionally concentrated on what goes wrong in our lives and in our minds, has shifted its focus to the study of human strengths, virtues, and positive emotions. The three pillars of positive psychology are the study of positive emotions, such as hope and trust; positive traits, such as wisdom and courage; and positive institutions, such as strong families and democracy.

According to psychologist Martin Seligman, Ph.D., the "father" of positive psychology, everyone, regardless of genes or fate, can achieve a happy, gratifying, meaningful life. The goal is not simply to feel good momentarily or to avoid bad experiences, but to build positive strengths and virtues that enable us to find meaning and purpose in life.[4]

"Psychology is not just the study of weakness and damage," Seligman argues, "it is also the study of strength and virtue. Treatment is not just fixing what is broken, it is nurturing what is best within ourselves." The traits that may well protect us from physical and mental illness include courage, optimism, hope, interpersonal skills, a work ethic, responsibility, future-mindedness, honesty, and perseverance.

Knowing Your Needs

Newborns are unable to survive on their own. They depend on others for the satisfaction of their physical needs for food, shelter, warmth, and protection, as well as their less tangible emotional needs. In growing to maturity, children take on more responsibility and become more independent. No one, however, becomes totally self-sufficient. As adults, we easily recognize our basic physical needs, but we often fail to acknowledge

emotional health The ability to express and acknowledge one's feelings and moods and exhibit adaptability and compassion for others.

mental health The ability to perceive reality as it is, respond to its challenges, and develop rational strategies for living.

spiritual health The ability to identify one's basic purpose in life and achieve one's full potential; the sense of connectedness to a greater power.

culture The set of shared attitudes, values, goals, and practices of a group that are internalized by an individual within the group.

emotional intelligence A term used by some psychologists to evaluate the capacity of people to understand themselves and relate well with others.

spiritual intelligence The capacity to sense, understand, and tap into ourselves, others, and the world around us.

our emotional needs. Yet they, too, must be met if we are to be as fulfilled as possible.

The humanist theorist Abraham Maslow believed that human needs are the motivating factors in personality development. First, we must satisfy basic physiological needs, such as those for food, shelter, and sleep. Only then can we pursue fulfillment of our higher needs—for safety and security, love and affection, and self-esteem. Few individuals reach the state of **self-actualization,** in which one functions at the highest possible level and derives the greatest possible satisfaction from life (Figure 2-1).

The Power of Self-Esteem

Each of us wants and needs to feel significant as a human being with unique talents, abilities, and roles in life. A sense of **self-esteem,** of belief or pride in ourselves, gives us confidence to dare to attempt to achieve at school or work and to reach out to others to form friendships and close relationships. Self-esteem is the little voice that whispers, "You're worth it. You can do it. You're okay."

Self-esteem is based, not on external factors like wealth or beauty, but on what you believe about yourself. It's not something you're born with; self-esteem develops over time. It's also not something anyone else can give to you, although those around you can either help boost or diminish your self-esteem.

The seeds of self-esteem are planted in childhood when parents provide the assurance and appreciation youngsters need to push themselves toward new accomplishments: crawling, walking, forming words and sentences, learning control over their bladder and bowels.

Adults, too, must consider themselves worthy of love, friendship, and success if they are to be loved, to make friends, and to achieve their goals. Low self-esteem is more common in people who have been abused as children and in those with psychiatric disorders, including depression, anxiety, alcoholism, and drug dependence. Feeling a lack of love and encouragement as a child can also lead to poor self-esteem. Adults with poor self-esteem may unconsciously enter relationships that reinforce their self-perceptions and may prefer and even seek out people who think poorly of them.

Self-esteem has proved to be one of the best predictors of college adjustment. Students with high self-esteem report better personal, emotional, social, and academic adjustment.

The Pursuit of Happiness

Just like physical health, psychological well-being involves more than an absence of problems. By developing your inner strengths and resources, you become the

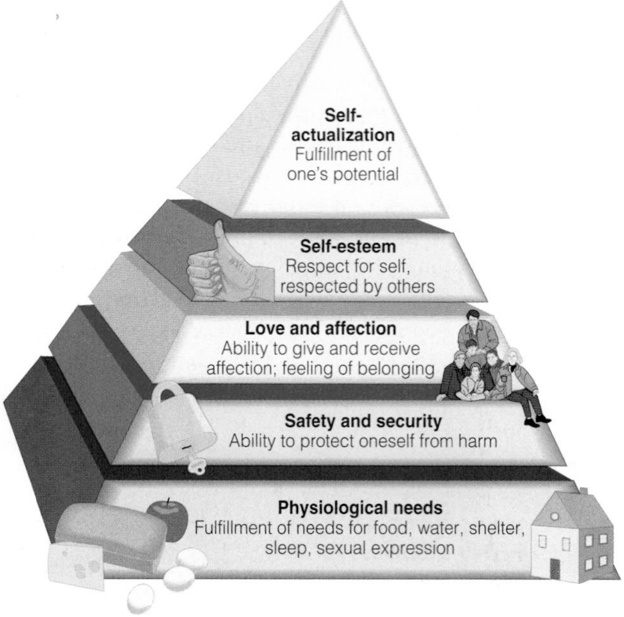

FIGURE 2-1 The Maslow Pyramid

To attain the highest level of psychological health, you must first satisfy your needs for safety and security, love and affection, and self-esteem.

Source: Maslow, A. *Motivation and Personality,* 3rd ed., © 1997. Reprinted by permission of Pearson Education, Inc.

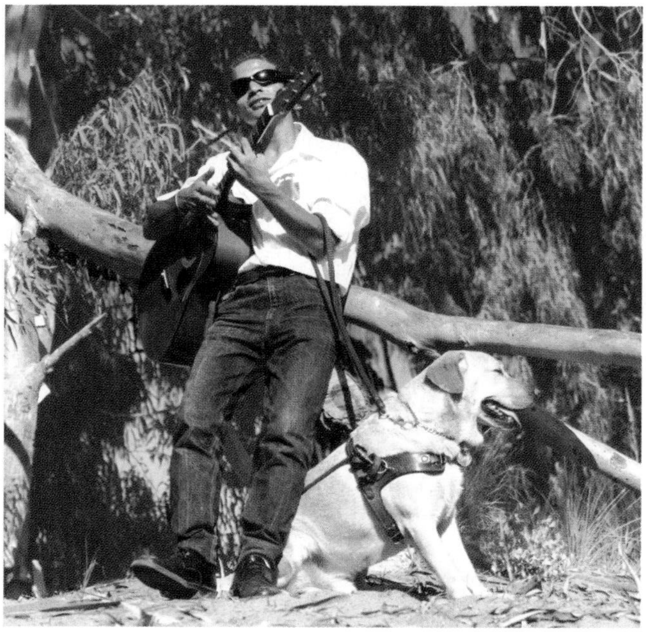

© Eldad Rafaeli/CORBIS.

Health and wealth don't equal happiness. People with disabilities show almost the same level of life satisfaction as people without disabilities.

Strategies for Change — How to be Happy

- Make time for yourself. It's impossible to meet the needs of others without recognizing and fulfilling your own.
- Invest yourself in closeness. Give your loved ones the gift of your time and caring.
- Work hard at what you like. Search for challenges that satisfy your need to do something meaningful.
- Be upbeat. If you always look for what's wrong about yourself or your life, you'll find it—and feel even worse.
- Organize but stay loose. Be ready to seize an unexpected opportunity to try something different.

author of your life, capable of confronting challenges and learning from them. As positive psychologists have discovered, you have greater control over how happy, optimistic, upbeat, and lovable you are than anyone or anything else. But only by consciously taking charge of your life can you find happiness and fulfillment.

A joke, a chocolate, a compliment, or a back rub can make us happy—briefly. The more such happy moments we experience, the more pleasant life feels. But happiness researchers distinguish between short-lived pleasures and long-term joy and satisfaction. Enduring happiness comes from attention, awareness, emotional balance, compassion, commitment, and altruism (discussed later in this chapter), giving your talents, time, and energy in the service of some larger purpose.[5]

Wealth and health have different and often surprising effects on happiness. Rich people are, on average, only slightly happier than poor ones. Good health is not a prerequisite for happiness. Even seriously ill cancer patients and individuals with serious disabilities differ only slightly from healthier people in life satisfaction. Life satisfaction goes up slightly with age, and emotions become less intense and more stable.

Education, intelligence, gender, and race do not matter much for happiness. African Americans and Hispanics have lower rates of depression than white Americans, but they do not report greater happiness. Neither gender is clearly happier, but in different studies women are both happier and sadder than men.

Relationships are key to happiness among undergraduates. In a survey of 222 college students, psychologists found that the "happiest" 10 percent, as determined by six different rating scales, shared one distinctive characteristic: a rich and fulfilling social life. Almost all were involved in a romantic relationship as well as in rewarding friendships. The happiest students spent the least time alone, and their friends rated them as highest on good relationships.[6]

If you're older than the traditional college student, take heart: You're probably happier. Young people naturally pay more attention to the negative, which may be a way of alerting them to dangers as they encounter novel experiences. Over time, we are increasingly drawn to the familiar, like close friends and relatives. When researchers ask people of different ages if they'd rather have lunch with their favorite author or a close friend, younger people choose the former while older ones opt for the company of someone near and dear.[7]

? FAQ How Can I Get Out of a Bad Mood?

Feelings come and go within minutes. A **mood** is a more sustained emotional state that colors our view of the world for hours or days. According to surveys by psychologist Randy Larsen of the University of Michigan, bad moods descend upon us an average of three out of every ten days. "A few people—about 2 percent—are happy just about every day," he says. "About 5 percent report bad moods four out of every five days."[8]

There are gender differences in mood management: Men typically try to distract themselves (a partially successful strategy) or use alcohol or drugs (an ineffective tactic). Women are more likely to talk to someone (which can help) or to ruminate on why they feel bad (which doesn't help). Learning effective mood-boosting, mood-regulating strategies can help both men and women pull themselves up and out of an emotional slump.

The most effective way to banish a sad or bad mood is by changing what caused it in the first place—if you can figure out what made you upset and why. "Most bad moods are caused by loss or failure in work or intimate relationships," says

self-actualization A state of wellness and fulfillment that can be achieved once certain human needs are satisfied; living to one's full potential.

self-esteem Confidence and satisfaction in oneself.

mood A sustained emotional state that colors one's view of the world for hours or days.

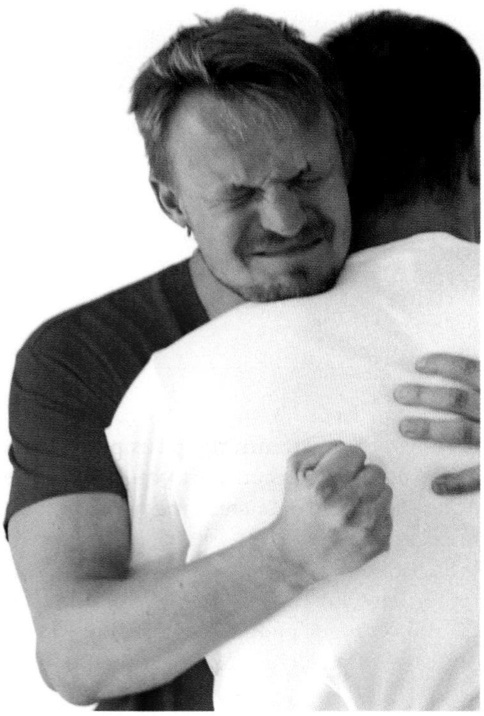

© Eva Mueller/Nonstock/Jupiter Images

Giving and getting support from others is fundamental to good psychological health.

Larsen. "The questions to ask are What can I do to fix the failure? What can I do to remedy the loss? Is there anything under my control that I can change? If there is, take action and solve it." Rewrite the report. Ask to take a makeup exam. Apologize to the friend whose feelings you hurt. Tell your parents you feel bad about the argument you had.

If there's nothing you can do, accept what happened and focus on doing things differently next time. "In our studies, resolving to try harder actually was as effective in improving mood as taking action in the present," says Larsen. You also can try to think about what happened in a different way and put a positive spin on it. This technique, known as *cognitive reappraisal,* or *reframing,* helps you look at a setback in a new light: What lessons did it teach you? What would you have done differently? Could there be a silver lining or hidden benefit?

If you can't identify or resolve the problem responsible for your emotional funk, the next-best solution is to concentrate on altering your negative feelings. For example, try setting a quick, achievable goal that can boost your spirits with a small success. Clean out a drawer; sort through the piles of paper on your desk; send an e-mail or instant message to an old friend.

Another good option is to get moving. In studies of mood regulation, exercise consistently ranks as the single most effective strategy for banishing bad feelings. Numerous studies have confirmed that aerobic workouts, such as walking or jogging, significantly improve mood. Even nonaerobic exercise, such as weight lifting, can boost spirits; improve sleep and appetite; reduce anxiety, irritability, and anger; and produce feelings of mastery and accomplishment.

Spirituality

Whatever your faith, whether or not you belong to any formal religion, you are more than a body of a certain height and weight occupying space on the planet. You have a mind that equips you to learn and question. And you have a spirit that animates everything you say and do. Spiritual health refers to this breath of life.

Spirituality is a belief in what some call a higher power, in someone or something that transcends the boundaries of self. It gives rise to a strong sense of purpose, values, morals, and ethics. Throughout life you make choices and decide to behave in one way rather than another because your spirituality serves as both a compass and a guide.

The term *religiosity* refers to various spiritual practices. That definition may seem vague, but one thing is clear. According to thousands of studies on the relationship between religious beliefs and practices and health, religious individuals are less depressed, less anxious, and better able to cope with crises such as illness or divorce than nonreligious ones. The more that a believer incorporates spiritual practices, such as prayer, meditation, or attending services, into daily life, the greater their sense of satisfaction with life.

Even when age, health, habits, demographics, and other factors are considered, individuals who pray regularly and attend religious services stay healthier and live longer than those who rarely or never do. In studies at several medical centers, prayer and faith speeded recovery from alcoholism, hip surgery, drug addiction, stroke, rheumatoid arthritis, heart attacks, and bypass surgery.

In one study, researchers assessed religiosity and symptoms of depression in 104 intercollegiate athletes at a public university in the Southeast. The greater the athletes' intrinsic religiosity, the less likely they were to suffer depressive symptoms. "Perhaps intrinsic religious beliefs provide a sense of hope and security that protect against distressing events," the researchers speculated. "It may also be that unconditional love by one's God provides a stable sense of self worth" that buffers against stress.[9]

Clarifying Your Values

Your **values** are the criteria by which you evaluate things, people, events, and yourself; they represent what's most important to you. In a world of almost

Strategies for Change — Being True to Yourself

- Take the tombstone test: What would you like to have written on your tombstone? In other words, how would you like to be remembered? Your honest answer should tell you, very succinctly, what you value most.
- Describe yourself, as you are today, in a brief sentence. Ask friends or family members for their descriptions of you. How would you have to change to become the person you want to be remembered as?
- Try the adjective test: Choose three adjectives that you'd like to see associated with your reputation. Then list what you've done or can do to earn such descriptions.

dizzying complexity, values can provide guidelines for making decisions that are right for you. If understood and applied, they help give life meaning and structure.

There can be a large discrepancy between what people say they value and what their actions indicate about their values. That's why it's important to clarify your own values, making sure you understand what you believe so that you can live in accordance with your beliefs.

When you confront a situation in which you must choose different paths or behaviors, follow these steps:

1. Carefully consider the consequences of each choice.
2. Choose freely from among all the options.
3. Publicly affirm your values by sharing them with others.
4. Act out your values.

Values clarification is not a once-in-a-lifetime task, but an ongoing process of sorting out what matters most to you. If you believe in protecting the environment, do you shut off lights, or walk rather than drive, in order to conserve energy? Do you vote for political candidates who support environmental protection? Do you recycle newspapers, bottles, and cans? Values are more than ideals we'd like to attain; they should be reflected in the way we live day by day.

YOUR LIFE COACH

Enriching Your Spiritual Life

Do you attend religious services? Pray or meditate on a weekly basis? In a national survey, a majority of the members of the Class of 2009 answered yes: Eight in ten went to religious services frequently or occasionally, while a third prayed or meditated every week. These percentages are somewhat lower than in the past, but a growing number of students report frequent discussions of religion.[10]

Whatever role religion plays in your life, you have the capacity for deep, meaningful spiritual experiences that can add great meaning to everyday existence. You don't need to enroll in theology classes or commit to a certain religious preference. The following simple steps can start you on an inner journey to a new level of understanding:

- **Sit quietly.** The process of cultivating spiritual intelligence begins in solitude and silence. "There is an inner wisdom," says Dr. Dean Ornish, the pioneering cardiologist who incorporates spiritual health into his mind-body therapies, "but it speaks very, very softly." To tune into its whisper, you have to turn down the volume in your busy, noisy, complicated life and force yourself to do nothing at all. This may sound easy; it's anything but.

  Start small: Create islands of silence in your day. Don't reach for the radio dial as soon as you get in the car. Leave your earpods on as you walk across campus but turn off the music. Shut the door to your room, take a few huge deep breaths, and let them out very, very slowly. Don't worry if you're too busy to carve out half an hour for quiet contemplation. Even ten minutes every day can make a difference.
- **Step outside.** For many people, nature sets their spirit free. Being outdoors, walking by the ocean, or looking at the hills gives us a sense of timelessness and puts the little hassles of daily living into perspective. As you wait for the bus or for a traffic light to change, let your gaze linger on silvery ice glazing a branch or an azalea bush in wild bloom. Follow the flight of a bird; watch clouds float overhead. Gaze into the night sky and think of the stars as holes in the darkness letting heaven shine through.
- **Use activity to tune into your spirit.** Spirituality exists in every cell of the body, not just in the brain. As a student, mental labor takes up much of your day. To tap into your spirit, try a less cerebral activity, such as singing, chanting, dancing, or drumming. Alternative ways of quieting your mind and tuning into your spirit include gardening,

values The criteria by which one makes choices about one's thoughts, actions, goals, and ideals.

walking, arranging flowers, listening to music that touches your soul, or immersing yourself in a simple process like preparing a meal.

- **Ask questions of yourself.** Some people use their contemplative time to focus on a line of scripture or poetry. Others ask open-ended questions, such as What am I feeling? What are my choices? Where am I heading? Dr. Ornish ends his own daily meditations by asking, "What am I not paying attention to that's important?"

  In her meditations, one minister often paints a lush scene with a golden meadow, a shade tree, and a gentle brook and invites the divine spirit to enter. "Rarely do I get an immediate answer or solution, but later that day something may happen—often just a random conversation—and I suddenly find myself thinking about a problem from a perspective I never considered before."
- **Trust your spirit.** While most of us rely on gut feelings to alert us to danger, our inner spirit usually nudges us, not away from, but toward some action that will somehow lead to a greater good—even if we can't see it at the time. You may suddenly feel the urge to call or e-mail a friend you've lost touch with—only to discover that he just lost a loved one and needed the comfort of your caring. If you ignore such silent signals, you may look back and regret the consequences. Pay a little more attention the next time you feel an unexpected need to say or do something for someone.
- **Develop a spiritual practice.**
  - **If you are religious:** Deepen your spiritual commitment through prayer, more frequent church attendance, or joining a prayer group.
  - **If you are not religious:** Keep an open mind about the value of religion or spirituality. Consider visiting a church or synagogue. Read the writings of inspired people of deep faith, such as Rabbi Harold Kushner and Rev. Martin Luther King, Jr.
  - **If you are not ready to consider religion:** Try nonreligious meditation or relaxation training. In decades of research, Dr. Herbert Benson of Harvard University has shown that focusing the mind on a single sound or image can slow heart rate, respiration, and brain waves; relax muscles; and lower stress-related hormones—responses similar to those induced by prayer.

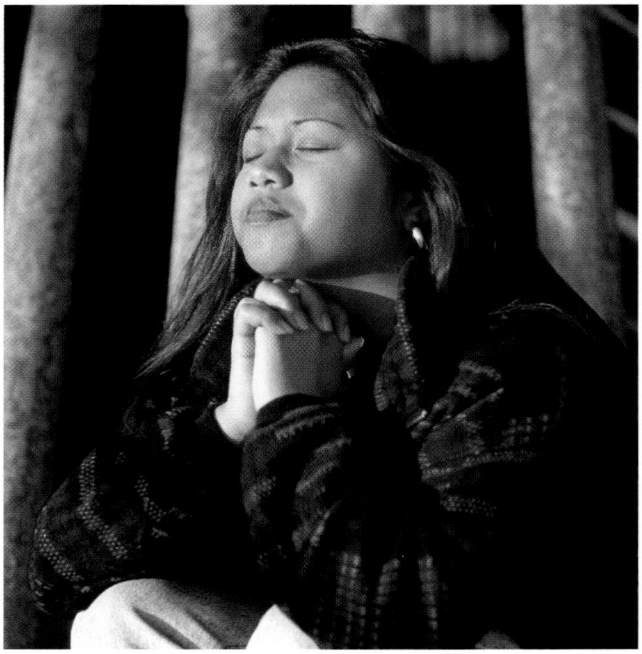

Prayer enhances physical health as well as spiritual and psychological well-being.

? FAQ Can Prayer Keep Us Healthy?

Prayer, a spiritual practice of millions, is the most commonly used form of complementary and alternative medicine. However, only in recent years has science launched rigorous investigations of the healing power of prayer.

Petitionary prayer—praying directly to a higher power—affects both the quality and quantity of life, says Dr. Harold Koenig, director of Duke University's Center for the Study of Religion/Spirituality and Health. "It boosts morale, lowers agitation, loneliness, and life dissatisfaction and enhances ability to cope in men, women, the elderly, the young, the healthy, and the sick."[11]

Some scientists speculate that prayer may foster a state of peace and calm that could lead to beneficial changes in the cardiovascular and immune systems. Sophisticated brain imaging techniques have shown that prayer and meditation cause changes in blood flow in particular regions of the brain that may lead to lower blood pressure, slower heart rate, decreased anxiety, and an enhanced sense of well-being. Membership in a faith community provides an identity as well as support, although individuals vary in their religious practices and observances.

Expressing Gratitude

A grateful spirit brightens mood, boosts energy, and infuses daily living with a sense of glad abundance. Although giving thanks is an ancient virtue, only recently have researchers focused on the "trait" of gratitude—appreciation, not just for a special gift, but for everything that makes life a bit better.[12]

Since gratitude is not just a feeling but a mental outlook, we can consciously become more grateful—with practice. "Volunteers on college campuses who are asked to list things they're grateful for every day report more positive feelings," says psychologist Michael McCullough of Southern Methodist University, a pioneer in gratitude research. "They have more energy. They sleep better. They feel richer, regardless of how much money they have. Even their families notice visible, positive changes."[13]

How can you help your gratitude grow? Here are some suggestions:

- Write a "gratitude letter," a belated thank you to someone in your life whom you're never properly thanked for a kindness.
- Build a time for thankfulness into your day. Some people write nightly in a gratitude journal or log.
- Develop a "good" memory, one that stores the kindnesses and comforts that have come your way.
- Pass on simple kindnesses. Open the door for a student juggling a backpack and an umbrella. Flash a smile at a server in the cafeteria. Pitch in on a beach or park cleanup. Give others a reason to savor a moment of gratitude.

Doing Good

Altruism—helping or giving to others—enhances self-esteem, relieves physical and mental stress, and protects psychological well-being. Hans Selye, the father of stress research, described cooperation with others for the self's sake as altruistic egotism, whereby we satisfy our own needs while helping others satisfy theirs. This concept is essentially an updated version of the golden rule: Do unto others as you would have them do unto you. The important difference is that you earn your neighbor's love and help by offering them love and help.

Volunteerism helps those who give as well as those who receive. People involved in community organizations, for instance, consistently report a surge of well-being called *helper's high,* which they describe as a unique sense of calmness, warmth, and enhanced self-worth. College students who provided community service as part of a semester-long course reported changes in attitude (including a decreased tendency to blame people for their misfortunes), self-esteem (primarily a belief that they can make a difference), and behavior (a greater commitment to do more volunteer work).

The options for giving of yourself are limitless: Volunteer to serve a meal at a homeless shelter. Collect donations for a charity auction. Teach in an illiteracy program. Perform the simplest act of charity: Pray for others.

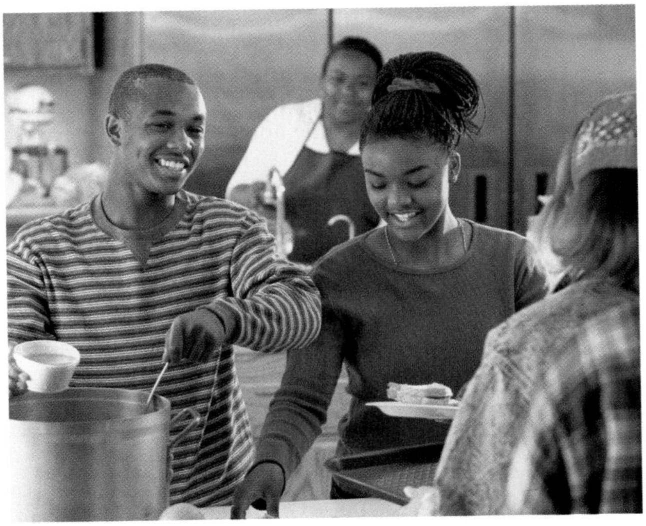

Helping others makes us feel better about ourselves.

Feeling in Control

Although no one has absolute control over destiny, we can do a great deal to control how we think, feel, and behave. By assessing our life situations realistically, we can make plans and preparations that allow us to make the most of our circumstances. By doing so, we gain a sense of mastery. In nationwide surveys, Americans who feel in control of their lives report greater psychological well-being than those who do not, as well as extraordinarily positive feelings of happiness.

Developing Autonomy

One goal that many people strive for is **autonomy,** or independence. Both family and society influence our ability to grow toward independence. Autonomous individuals are true to themselves. As they weigh the pros and cons of any decision, whether it's using or refusing drugs or choosing a major or career, they base their judgment on their own values, not those of others. Their ability to draw on internal resources and cope with challenges has a positive impact on both their psychological well-being and their physical health, including recovery from illness.

Those who've achieved autonomy may seek the opinions of others, but they do not allow their decisions to be dictated by external

altruism Acts of helping or giving to others without thought of self-benefit.

autonomy The ability to draw on internal resources; independence from familial and societal influences.

Strategies for Change — How to Assert Yourself

- Use "I" statements to explain your feelings. This allows you to take ownership of your opinions and feelings without putting down others for how they feel and think.
- Listen to and acknowledge what the other person says. After you speak, find out if the other person understands your position. Ask how he or she feels about what you've said.
- Be direct and specific. Describe the problem as you see it, using neutral language rather than assigning blame. Also suggest a specific solution, but make it clear that you'd like the lines of communication and negotiation to remain open.
- Don't think you have to be obnoxious in order to be assertive. It's most effective to state your needs and preferences without any sarcasm or hostility.

influences. For autonomous individuals, their **locus of control**—that is, where they view control as originating—is *internal* (from within themselves) rather than *external* (from others).

Asserting Yourself

Being **assertive** means recognizing your feelings and making your needs and desires clear to others. Unlike aggression, a far less healthy means of expression, assertiveness usually works. You can change a situation you don't like by communicating your feelings and thoughts in nonprovocative words, by focusing on specifics, and by making sure you're talking with the person who is directly responsible.

Becoming assertive isn't always easy. Many people have learned to cope by being passive and not communicating their feelings or opinions. Sooner or later they become so irritated, frustrated, or overwhelmed that they explode in an outburst—which they think of as being assertive. However, such behavior is so distasteful to them that they'd rather be passive. But assertiveness doesn't mean screaming or telling someone off. You can communicate your wishes calmly and clearly. Assertiveness is a behavior that respects your rights and the rights of other people even when you disagree.

Even at its mildest, assertiveness can make you feel better about yourself and your life. The reason: When you speak up or take action, you're in the pilot seat. And that's always much less stressful than taking a back seat and trying to hang on for dear life.

Connecting with Others

At every age, people who feel connected to others tend to be healthier physically and psychologically. This is as, if not more, true in college when young adults, often living independently for the first time, need to form new relationships.

In a recent study at a large midwestern university, the students—particularly the women—who felt the greatest sense of belonging reported fewer physical symptoms than those who had not forged close friendships.

The research also revealed a gender difference: Female students seek out, forge, and maintain more supportive ties than men, rely on friends more in times of stress, and provide more support than men.[14]

The opposite of *connectedness* is **social isolation,** a major risk factor for illness and early death. Individuals with few social contacts face two to four times the mortality rate of others. The reason may be that their social isolation weakens the body's ability to ward off disease. Medical students with higher-than-average scores on a loneliness scale had lower levels of protective immune cells. The end of a long-term relationship—through separation, divorce, or death—also dampens immunity.

It is part of our nature as mammals and as human beings to crave relationships. But invariably we end up alone at times. Solitude is not without its own quiet joys—time for introspection, self-assessment, learning from the past, and looking toward the future. Each of us can cultivate the joy of our own company, of being alone without crossing the line and becoming lonely.

Overcoming Loneliness

More so than many other countries, we are a nation of loners. Recent trends—longer work hours, busy family schedules, frequent moves, high divorce rates—have created even more lonely people. Only 23 percent of Americans say they're never lonely. Loneliest of all are those who are divorced, separated, or widowed and those who live alone or solely with children. Among single adults who have never been married, 42 percent feel lonely at least sometimes. However, loneliness is most likely to cause emotional distress when it is chronic rather than episodic.

To combat loneliness, people may join groups, fling themselves into projects and activities, or surround themselves with superficial acquaintances. Others avoid the effort of trying to connect, sometimes limiting most of their personal interactions to chat groups on the Internet.

The true keys to overcoming loneliness are developing resources to fulfill our own potential and learning to reach out to others. In this way, loneliness can become a means to personal growth and discovery.

Facing Shyness and Social Anxiety

Many people are uncomfortable meeting strangers or speaking or performing in public. In some surveys, as many as 40 percent of people describe themselves as shy or socially anxious. Some shy people—an estimated 10 to 15 percent of children—are born with a predisposition to shyness. Others become shy because they don't learn proper social responses or because they experience rejection or shame.

Some people are "fearfully" shy; that is, they withdraw and avoid contact with others and experience a high degree of anxiety and fear in social situations. Others are "self-consciously" shy. They enjoy the company of others but become highly self-aware and anxious in social situations.

In one study of college students, men reported somewhat more shyness than women. African Americans were less shy than either Asian Americans or Caucasians.[15] Students may develop symptoms of shyness or social anxiety when they go to a party or are called on in class. Some experience symptoms when they try to perform any sort of action in the presence of others, even such everyday activities as eating in public, using a public restroom, or writing a check.

About 7 percent of the population could be diagnosed with a severe form of social anxiety, called **social phobia,** in which individuals typically fear and avoid various social situations. Adolescents and young adults with severe social anxiety are at increased risk of major depression. Phobias are discussed later in this chapter. The key difference between these problems and normal shyness and self-consciousness is the degree of distress and impairment that individuals experience.

If you're shy, you can overcome much of your social apprehensiveness on your own, in much the same way as you might set out to stop smoking or lose weight. For example, you can improve your social skills by pushing yourself to introduce yourself to a stranger at a party or to chat about the weather or the food selections with the person next to you in a cafeteria line. Gradually, you'll acquire a sense of social timing and a verbal ease that will take the worry out of close encounters with others. Those with more disabling social anxiety may do best with psychotherapy and medication, which have proved highly effective.

Sleepless in America—And on Campus

You stay up late cramming for a final. You drive through the night to visit a friend at another campus. You get up for an early class during the week but stay in bed until noon on weekends. And you wonder: "Why am I so tired?" The answer: You're not getting enough sleep.

You're hardly alone. According to a recent report by the Institute of Medicine, 50 to 70 million Americans have chronic sleep problems that jeopardize their ability to function at their best as well as their health and longevity. The cumulative long-term effects of sleep loss and sleep disorders include an increased risk of hypertension, diabetes, obesity, depression, heart attack, and stroke. Drowsy drivers are responsible for almost 20 percent of all serious car crash injuries.[16]

Sleep problems start young. Nearly one-half of adolescents sleep less than eight hours on school nights; more than half report feeling sleepy during the day.[17] College students are notorious for staying up late to study and socialize during the week and sleeping in on weekends. In recent studies only 11 percent of college students reported good quality sleep, while 30 percent suffered chronic sleep difficulties.[18]

College students can learn to sleep better. In an experiment with introductory psychology students—mostly freshmen—those who learned basic sleep skills (including the Strategies for Change on page 36) significantly improved their overall sleep quality compared with students who did not receive such training. They took fewer naps, went to bed hungry less frequently, and consumed less caffeine. Over time they fell asleep more quickly and woke less often in the night.[19]

Why Sleep Matters

Sleep problems, as medical scientists now recognize, are hazardous to health. Breathing-related sleep disorders, such as chronic snoring and obstructive sleep apnea, increase the risk of high blood pressure, heart attacks, and stroke. Individuals with insomnia, the most

locus of control An individual's belief about the source of power and influence over his or her life.

assertive Behaving in a confident manner to make your needs and desires clear to others in a nonhostile way.

social isolation A feeling of unconnectedness with others caused by and reinforced by infrequency of social contacts.

social phobia A severe form of social anxiety marked by extreme fears and avoidance of social situations.

Strategies for Change — How to Sleep Like a Baby

- Keep regular hours for going to bed and getting up in the morning. Stay as close as possible to this schedule on weekends as well as weekdays.
- Develop a sleep ritual—such as stretching, meditation, yoga, prayer, or reading a not-too-thrilling novel— to ease the transition from wakefulness to sleep.
- Don't drink coffee late in the day. The effects of caffeine can linger for up to eight hours. And don't smoke. Nicotine is an even more powerful stimulant—and sleep saboteur—than caffeine.
- Don't rely on alcohol to get to sleep. Alcohol disrupts normal sleep stages, so you won't sleep as deeply or as restfully as you normally would.
- Don't nap during the day if you're having problems sleeping through the night.

common sleep complaint, become irritable and depressed, get into more traffic accidents, develop memory problems, and have difficulties concentrating and doing their jobs.

According to recent research, inadequate sleep affects growth hormone secretion, increasing the likelihood of obesity, and impairs the body's ability to use insulin, which can lead to diabetes.[20] Sleeping less than six hours per night more than doubles the risk of developing hypertension.[21] Individuals chronically deprived of enough sleep may become more susceptible to certain illnesses, and researchers speculate that disturbed sleep may be the reason why individuals under stress—such as students taking exams or grieving widows and widowers—may have lower levels of certain infection-fighting cells than normal.

Sleep-deprived university students experience more feelings of tension, anger, depression, fatigue, and confusion. They find it harder to concentrate and memorize new material. They score lower on life-satisfaction scales. Students who get eight hours of sleep but shift their sleep schedules by as little as two hours suffer more depressive symptoms, lower sociability, and more frequent attention and concentration problems. They're even likely to get lower grades.[22]

Are you sleep deprived? Take the "BEARS" quiz in Table 2-1 to see if you have a sleep problem.

? FAQ How Much Sleep Do I Need?

Over the last century, we have cut our average nightly sleep time by 20 percent. More than half of us try to get by with less than seven hours of shut-eye a night.

College students are no exception. In a study of 212 undergraduates, their average sleep time was slightly less than seven hours, with little difference between men and women.

No formula can say how long a good night's sleep should be. Normal sleep times range from five to ten hours; the average is seven and a half. About one or two people in a hundred can get by with just five hours; another small minority needs twice that amount.[23] Each of us seems to have an innate sleep *appetite* that is as much a part of our genetic programming as hair color and skin tone.

To figure out your sleep needs, keep your wake-up time the same every morning and vary your bedtime. Are you groggy after six hours of shut-eye? Does an extra hour give you more stamina? What about an extra two hours? Since too much sleep can make you feel sluggish, don't assume that more is always better. Listen to your body's signals, and adjust your sleep schedule to suit them.

Are you better off pulling an all-nighter before a big test or closing the books and getting a good night's sleep? According to researchers, that depends on the nature of the exam. If it's a test of facts—Civil War battles, for instance—cramming all night works. However, if you will have to write analytical essays in which you compare, contrast, and make connections, you need to

TABLE 2-1 "BEARS": How Well Do You Sleep?

B = Bedtime problems: Do you have any problems falling asleep at bedtime?

E = Excessive daytime sleepiness: Do you feel sleepy a lot during the day? In school? While driving?

A = Awakenings during the night: Do you wake up a lot at night?

R = Regularity and duration of sleep: What time do you usually go to bed on school nights? Weekends? How much sleep do you usually get?

S = Sleep-disordered breathing: Has anyone ever told you that you snore loudly at night?

Your answers to this self-assessment, developed by sleep specialists, may reveal a sleep problem that can interfere with your daytime functioning. If it persists, discuss it with a doctor.

Source: Millman, Richard, et al. "Excessive Sleepiness in Adolescents and Young Adults: Causes, Consequences, and Treatment Strategies." *Pediatrics,* Vol. 115, No. 6, June 2005, p. 1774.

sleep in order to make the most of your reasoning abilities.

Understanding Mental Health

Mentally healthy individuals value themselves, perceive reality as it is, accept their limitations and possibilities, carry out their responsibilities, establish and maintain close relationships, pursue work that suits their talent and training, and feel a sense of fulfillment that makes the efforts of daily living worthwhile (Figure 2-2).

According to a national report by the Centers for Disease Control (CDC), American adults spend an average of three days a month feeling "sad, blue, or depressed." Individuals who spend more time down in the dumps are more likely to report unhealthy behaviors such as cigarette smoking and physical inactivity. College-age young adults (18 to 24 years old) report the most days with depressive symptoms. Women had more gloomy days than men (3.5 compared to 2.4). College graduates and those earning more than $50,000 reported half as many sad, bad days as those without a high school diploma or earning less than $15,000. Regular exercisers had 1.3 fewer days with symptoms of depression than those who did not work out regularly. Those who smoked a pack or more of cigarettes a day had more down days than those who never smoked.[24]

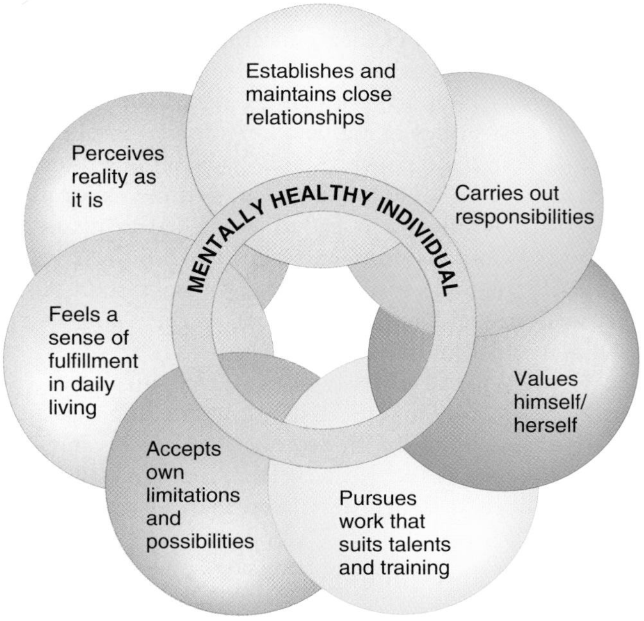

FIGURE 2-2 The Mentally Healthy Individual
Mental well-being is a combination of many factors.

What Is a Mental Disorder?

While lay people may speak of "nervous breakdowns" or "insanity," these are not scientific terms. The U.S. government's official definition states that a serious mental illness is "a diagnosable mental, behavioral, or emotional disorder that interferes with one or more major activities in life, like dressing, eating, or working."

The mental health profession's standard for diagnosing a mental disorder is the pattern of symptoms, or diagnostic criteria, spelled out for the almost 300 disorders in the American Psychiatric Association's *Diagnostic and Statistical Manual,* 4th edition (DSM-IV). Psychiatrists define a **mental disorder** as "a clinically significant behavioral or psychological syndrome or pattern that occurs in an individual and that is associated with present distress (a painful symptom) or disability (impairment in one or more important areas of functioning) or with a significantly increased risk of suffering death, pain, disability, or an important loss of freedom."[25]

Mental Health on Campus

The emotional difficulties of college students have become more complex and more severe than in the past. In one national survey, more than 80 percent of directors of counseling centers reported an increase in the number of students with serious psychological disorders. However, studies that tested students seeking help at counseling centers show that they are not more disturbed and do not have more or more serious psychiatric problems than in the past.[26] (Eating disorders, which are common among college students, are discussed in Chapter 6.)

About one in eight undergraduates seeks counseling during college. In the past students were most likely to have trouble with dating and other relationships. More recently stress

mental disorder Behavioral or psychological syndrome associated with distress or disability or with a significantly increased risk of suffering death, pain, disability, or loss of freedom.

TABLE 2-2 Mental Disorders in the United States

Disorder	18- to 29-Year-Olds	All Adults
Any mental disorder	52%	46%
Anxiety disorders	30%	29%
Impulse control disorders	27%	25%
Mood disorders	21%	21%
Substance abuse disorders	17%	15%

Source: Kessler, Ronald, et al. "Lifetime Prevalence and Age-of-Onset Distributions of *DSM-IV* Disorders in the National Comorbidity Survey Replication." *Archives of General Psychiatry,* Vol. 62, No. 6, June 2005, p. 593.

TABLE 2-3 Mental Disorders on Campus

Type of Problem	Percentage of Diagnoses at a College Counseling Center
Adjustment disorder	16.7%
Major depression and bipolar disorder	16.4%
Dysthymic disorder	15.6%
Anxiety and phobic disorders	8.0%

Source: Schwartz, Allan. "Are College Students More Disturbed Today? Stability in the Acuity and Qualitative Character of Psychopathology of College Counseling Center Clients: 1992–1993 through 2001–2002." *American Journal of College Health*, Vol. 54, No. 6, May–June 2006, pp. 327–337.

and anxiety have become more common reasons for seeking help.

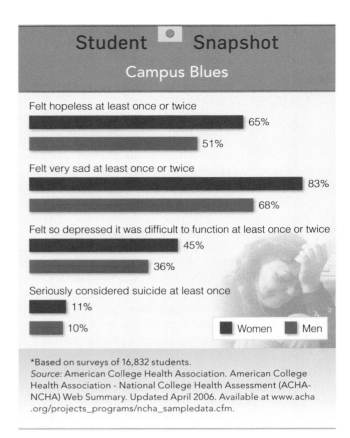

Many college students experience a broad range of psychological symptoms and disorders. The most common are adjustment disorders (the abnormal persistence of otherwise normal emotional or behavioral symptoms) and various forms of **depression,** which are discussed later in this chapter[27] (Table 2-3). According to the most recent findings from the American College Health Association-National College Health Assessment, more than 50 percent of men and 65 percent of women felt hopeless at least once or twice during the academic year; a higher percentage reported episodes of sadness. About 45 percent of college women and 36 percent of college men found it difficult to function because they were so depressed.[28] (See Student Snapshot: "Campus Blues.") One in ten has seriously considered suicide, the second-leading cause of death among college students.[29]

Researchers at the University of Michigan have identified three key contributors to depression in college students; stress, substance abuse, and sleep loss. As they adjust to campus life, undergraduates face the ongoing stress of forging a new identity and finding a place for themselves in various social hierarchies. This triggers the release of the so-called stress harmones (discussed in Chapter 3), which can change brain activity. Drugs and alcohol, widely used on campus, also affect the brain in ways that make stress even harder to manage. Too little sleep adds another ingredient to this dangerous brew. Computers, the Internet, around-the-clock cable television, and the college tradition of pulling all-nighters can conspire to sabotage rest and increase vulnerability to depression.[30] Among the most vulnerable students are those being treated for mental disorders.

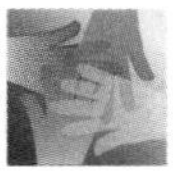

The few studies that have looked into ethnic differences in psychological health have yielded conflicting or inconclusive results: Some found no differences; others suggested higher rates of depression among Korean and South Asian students.

Some colleges offer seminars, movies, and 24-hour hot lines that students can call to talk about everything from stress to substance abuse. A few schools have redesigned dormitories to decrease isolation and foster more interaction.

Student Snapshot

Campus Blues

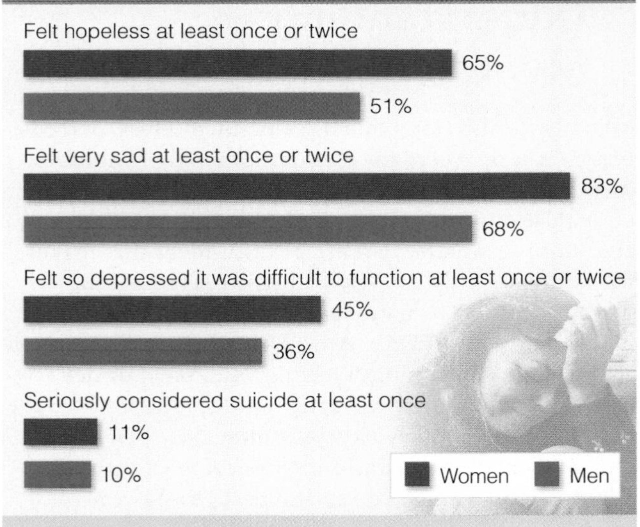

*Based on surveys of 16,832 students.
Source: American College Health Association. American College Health Association - National College Health Assessment (ACHA-NCHA) Web Summary. Updated April 2006. Available at www.acha.org/projects_programs/ncha_sampledata.cfm.

The Mind-Body Connection

According to a growing number of studies, mental attitude may be just as important a risk factor for certain diseases as age, race, gender, education, habits, and health history.[31] Positive states like happiness and optimism have been linked with longer lifespans as well as lower risk of cardiovascular and lung disease, stroke, diabetes, colds, and upper respiratory infections. Mental disorders, on the other hand, can undermine physical well-being. **Anxiety** can lead to intensified asthmatic reactions, skin conditions, and digestive disorders. Stress can play a role in hypertension, heart attacks, sudden cardiac death, and immune disorders in the young as well as in older individuals.

Depression has increasingly been recognized as a serious risk factor for physical illness. According to large-scale studies on depression, depressed individuals are up to four times more likely to develop heart problems. In still unknown ways, depression may increase risk factors for heart disease, such as high blood pressure, and for premature death. Together, depression and heart disease worsen a patient's prognosis more than either condition alone. One in five patients hospitalized for a heart attack suffers from major depression, and they are three times more likely to die from a future heart problem.[32]

Major depression is associated with lower bone density in young men, but not in women. A history of depression increases the risk of physical problems such as headache and shoulder and neck pain in women as they reach middle age.

The Mind-Exercise Connection

Imagine a drug so powerful it can alter brain chemistry, so versatile it can help prevent or treat many common mental disorders, so safe that moderate doses cause few, if any, side effects, and so inexpensive that anyone can afford it. This wonder drug, proved in years of research, is exercise.

In addition to its head-to-toe physical benefits, discussed in Chapter 4, exercise may be, as one therapist puts it, the single most effective way to lift a person's spirits and to restore feelings of potency about all aspects of life. People who exercise regularly report a more cheerful mood, higher self-esteem, and less stress. Their sleep and appetite also tend to improve. In clinical studies, exercise has proved effective as a treatment for depression and anxiety disorders.[33] But remember: Although exercise can help prevent and ease problems for many people, it's no substitute for professional treatment of serious psychiatric disorders.

Depressive Disorders

Depression, the world's most common mental ailment, affects the brain, the mind, and the body in complex ways. An estimated 16.2 percent of adults experience depression at some point in their lives, according to a recent national survey. After a single episode, the risk of a recurrence, or second episode, is about 50 percent. After a third, the risk of a fourth is about 90 percent. Stress-related events may trigger half of all depressive episodes; great trauma in childhood can increase vulnerability to depression later in life.

In a study of young adults ages 18 to 23, those who'd experienced the most adversity were at greatest risk of depression or an anxiety disorder.[34] An estimated 15 to 40 percent of college-age men and women (18- to 24-year-olds) may develop depression. Over a four-year period, depression increased 4.6 percent among college students.[35] Medical students also have higher rates of depression than the general population, but only about a quarter receive treatment.[36]

? FAQ Why Are So Many Young People Depressed?

Once young people were considered immune to sadness. Now mental health professionals know better. An estimated 5 to 10 percent of American teenagers suffer from a serious depressive disorder; girls are twice as susceptible as boys. Prior to puberty, girls and boys are equally likely to develop depression.

According to a survey of more than 2,000 young women ages 16 to 23, white girls become less depressed as they age while black girls continue feeling the same. The reason may be that Caucasian girls tend to be unhappy with their bodies in their teens and may develop symptoms of depression as a result. Over time they become more satisfied with their shapes and sizes and less depressed. African-American girls tend to accept their bodies from early adolescence into adulthood.[37]

The risks of depression in the young are high. Four in ten depressed adolescents think about killing themselves; two in ten actually try to do so. Every year an estimated 11 to 13 in every 100,000 teens take their own lives, twice as many as the number who die from all natural causes combined.

"Depression is the most common emotional problem in adolescence and the single greatest risk factor for teen suicide," says child psychiatrist Peter Jensen, M.D., director for the Center for the Advancement of Children's Mental Health at Columbia University, who notes that depression rates have been rising over the last half century.[38]

No one knows the reason for this steady surge in sadness, but experts point to the breakdown of families, the pressures of the information age, and increased isolation. A family history of depression greatly increases a young person's vulnerability. A mother's anxiety and depression during early childhood can increase the risk that adolescents will develop symptoms of anxiety and depression.

However, the strongest predictor of depression is cigarette smoking. Depressed teens may smoke because they think smoking will make them feel better, but nicotine alters brain chemistry and actually worsens symptoms of depression.

The link between tobacco and depression continues during college. Students who had been diagnosed with or treated for depression were 7.5 times as likely as other students to use tobacco, possibly because of nicotine's stimulating effects.[39] Young women with symptoms of depression and those who do not feel connected with a peer group are more likely to smoke. Individuals with other mental illnesses also are more likely to smoke. Nicotine may have a beneficial effect on their brains, which makes it more difficult for them to quit.[40]

Depression can be hard to recognize in the young, who may not look or act sad. Rather than crying, they may snap grouchily at par-

depression In general, feelings of unhappiness and despair; as a mental illness, also characterized by an inability to function normally.

anxiety A feeling of apprehension and dread, with or without a known cause; may range from mild to severe and may be accompanied by physical symptoms.

ents or burst into angry tirades. Some turn to alcohol or drugs in hopes of feeling better; others become depressed after they start abusing these substances. As they drop out of activities and pull away from friends, depressed teens spend more time alone. Their schoolwork suffers, and many are labeled as underachievers. Those whose anger explodes in public are branded as troublemakers.

Only in the last decade have researchers in mental health specifically studied treatments for teen depression. They now know that 60 to 75 percent of teenagers—the same percentage as adults—respond to treatment with the medications called SSRIs (a group of antidepressants that includes Prozac and Paxil). The use of these antidepressants in children and teenagers has increased three- to fivefold in recent years, but there is controversy over a potential increase in the risk of suicide (discussed later in this chapter).

According to a landmark study of therapies for depression in adolescents, the most effective treatment is a combination of antidepressant medication and cognitive-behavioral therapy (CBT), which teaches problem-solving skills and ways to change negative thinking (discussed later in this chapter).

Gender and Depression

Female Depression

Depression is twice as common in women as men, a gender gap found through most of the world. Some have argued that women are simply more willing than men to admit to being depressed or more likely to seek help. But even when these factors are accounted for, the sex difference persists. Others contend that men in distress drown their problems in alcohol rather than becoming sad, tearful, and hopeless. In studies of the Amish, who prohibit alcohol use, and of Jewish Americans, who also drink less than other groups, women and men are equally likely to develop depression. Yet these data do not mean that fewer women among teetotalers become depressed but that more men do.

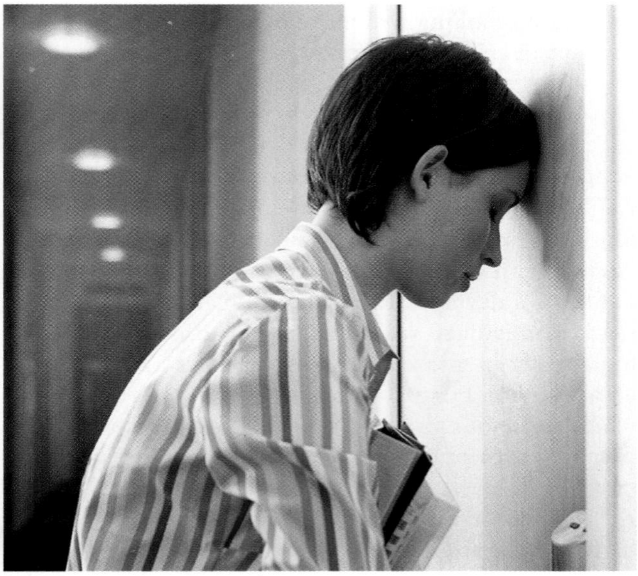

Factors that can contribute to the development of depression in college include stressful events, poor academic performance, loneliness, and relationship problems.

Genes may make both men and women more vulnerable to depression. Brain chemistry and sex hormones also may play a role. Women produce less of certain metabolites of serotonin, a messenger chemical that helps regulate mood. Their brains also register sadness much more intensely than men's, and they are more sensitive to changes in light and temperature. Women are at least four times more likely than men to develop seasonal affective disorder (SAD) and to become depressed in the dark winter months.

Some women also seem more sensitive to their own hormones or to the changes in them that occur at puberty, during the menstrual cycle, after childbirth, or during perimenopause and menopause. Pregnancy, contrary to what many people assume, does not "protect" a woman from depression, and women who discontinue treatment when they become pregnant are at risk of a relapse.[41] Women and their psychiatrists must carefully weigh the risks and benefits of psychiatric medications during pregnancy.[42]

Childhood abuse also contributes to female vulnerability. In epidemiological studies, 60 percent of women diagnosed with depression—compared with 39 percent of men—were abused as children. In adulthood, relationships may protect women from depression, while a lack of social support increases vulnerability to depression.[43] Women with at least one "confiding relationship," as researchers put it, are physically and psychologically more resilient.

Male Depression

More than six million men in the United States—one in every 14—suffer from this insidious disorder, many without recognizing what's wrong. Experts describe male depression as an "under" disease: underdiscussed, underrecognized, underdiagnosed, and undertreated.

Depression "looks" different in men than women. Rather than becoming sad, men may be irritable or tremendously fatigued. They feel a sense of being dead inside, of worthlessness, hopelessness, helplessness, of losing their life force. Physical symptoms, such as headaches, pain, and insomnia, are common, as are attempts to "self-medicate" with alcohol or drugs.

Genes may make some men more vulnerable, but chronic stress of any sort plays a major role in male depression, possibly by raising levels of cortisol, a stress hormone, and lowering testosterone. Men also are more likely than women to become depressed following divorce, job loss, or a career setback. Whatever its roots, depression alters brain chemistry in potentially deadly ways. Four times as many men as women kill themselves; depressed men are two to four times more likely to take their own lives than depressed women.

Minor Depression

Minor depression is a common disorder that is often unrecognized and untreated, affecting about 7.5 percent of Americans during their lifetime. Its symptoms are the same as those of major depression, but less severe and fewer in number. They include either a depressed mood most of the day, nearly every day, or diminished interest or pleasure in daily activities.

Psychotherapy is remarkably effective for mild depression. In more serious cases, antidepressant medication can lead to dramatic improvement in 40 to 80 percent of depressed patients. Exercise also works—several studies have shown that exercise effectively lifts mild to moderate depression.

Dysthymic Disorder

Dysthymia is a depressive disorder characterized by a chronically depressed mood. Symptoms include feelings of inadequacy, hopelessness, and guilt; low self-esteem; low energy; fatigue; indecisiveness; and an inability to enjoy pleasurable activities.

Major Depression

The simplest definition of **major depression** is sadness that does not end. The incidence of major depression has soared over the last two decades, especially among young adults. Major depression can destroy a person's joy for living. Food, friends, sex, or any form of pleasure no longer appeals. It is impossible to concentrate on work and responsibilities. Unable to escape a sense of utter hopelessness, depressed individuals may fight back tears throughout the day and toss and turn through long, empty nights. Thoughts of death or suicide may push into their minds.

The characteristic symptoms of major depression include:

- **Feeling depressed,** sad, empty, discouraged, tearful.
- **Loss of interest** or pleasure in once-enjoyable activities.
- **Eating more or less** than usual and either gaining or losing weight.
- **Having trouble sleeping** or sleeping much more than usual.
- **Feeling slowed down** or restless and unable to sit still.
- **Lack of energy.**
- **Feeling helpless,** hopeless, worthless, inadequate.
- **Difficulty concentrating,** forgetfulness.
- **Difficulty thinking clearly** or making decisions.
- **Persistent thoughts of death** or suicide.
- **Withdrawal from others,** lack of interest in sex.
- **Physical symptoms** (headaches, digestive problems, aches and pains).

As many as half of major depressive episodes are not recognized because the symptoms are "masked." Rather than feeling sad or depressed, individuals may experience low energy, insomnia, difficulty concentrating, and physical symptoms. An episode of major depression can trigger a relapse in individuals with substance abuse problems.

Treating Depression

Treatment with psychotherapy, medication, or both relieves depression for 80 percent of sufferers—yet only half of those with depression seek help and only 10 to 15 percent get optimal care.

Psychotherapy helps individuals pinpoint the life problems that contribute to their depression, identify negative or distorted thinking patterns, explore behaviors that contribute to depression, and regain a sense of control and pleasure in life. Two specific psychotherapies—cognitive-behavioral therapy and interpersonal therapy (described later in this chapter)—have proved as helpful as antidepressant drugs, although they take longer than medication to achieve results.

Antidepressants help about 70 percent of individuals feel better within six to ten weeks. According to long-term studies, treatment should continue for at least nine months after a single acute episode of depression, longer for chronic or recurrent depression.

When either medication or psychotherapy fails to lift depression, switching from one to the other or adding a second antidepressant can be highly effective.[44] Medications have proved effective for patients who did not recover with psychotherapy alone, and psychotherapy can help those who do not benefit from medication alone.[45]

Exercise also has proved beneficial in both the short- and long-term for both men and women. Although walking and jogging have been studied most extensively, all forms of exercise decrease depression to some degree. The greater the length of the exercise program and the larger the total number of sessions, the greater the decrease in depression.

For individuals who cannot take antidepressant medications because of medical problems, or who do not improve with

dysthymia Frequent, prolonged mild depression.

major depression Sadness that does not end; ongoing feelings of utter hopelessness.

psychotherapy or drugs, *electroconvulsive therapy* (ECT)—the administration of a controlled electrical current through electrodes attached to the scalp—remains the safest and most effective treatment. About 50 percent of depressed individuals who do not get better with antidepressant medication and psychotherapy improve after ECT. Experimental new techniques are using electrical and magnetic stimulation to treat depression.[46]

Even without treatment, depression generally lifts after six to nine months. However, in more than 80 percent of people, it recurs, with each episode lasting longer and becoming more severe and difficult to treat. "All the while the depression goes untreated, it is causing ongoing damage that shrivels important regions of the brain" says John Greden, M.D., director of the University of Michigan Depression Center. "The exciting news is that, as brain scans show, treatment turns the destructive process around and stops depression in its tracks."[47]

If a loved one is depressed:

- **Express your concern,** but don't nag. You might say: "I'm concerned about you. You are struggling right now. We need to find some help."
- **Don't be distracted** by behaviors like drinking or gambling, which can disguise depression in men.
- **Encourage the individual to remain in treatment** until symptoms begin to lift (which takes several weeks).
- **Provide emotional support.** Listen carefully. Offer hope and reassurance that with time and treatment, things will get better.
- **Do not ignore remarks about suicide.** Report them to his or her doctor or, in an emergency, call 911.

? FAQ Are Antidepressants Dangerous?

Millions of individuals have benefited from the category of **antidepressant** drugs called selective serotonin reuptake inhibitors (SSRIs) over the last two decades. However, like all drugs, they can cause side effects that range from temporary physical symptoms, such as stomach upset and headaches, to more persistent problems, such as sexual dysfunction. The most serious—and controversial—risk is suicide.

Although studies have showed varying results, they generally indicate that, compared with a placebo, all antidepressants, including the SSRIs, seem to double the risk of suicidal thinking, from 1 to 2 percent to 2 to 4 percent in both children and adults.[48] The FDA has issued a "black box" warning about the risk of suicidal thoughts, hostility, and aggression in both children and adults. The danger is greatest just after pill use begins, before depression is really alleviated but when some patients experience more energy and agitation and may be more likely to act on suicidal tendencies.

The debate continues, however, because of the complexity of the problem. Depression itself can be fatal: The lifetime suicide rate for people with major depression is 15 percent, and depression increases the risk of heart disease and other serious illnesses. While the use of SSRIs in adolescents soared in the 1990s, the suicide rate declined. Only 20 percent of teenagers who take their own lives have ever taken an antidepressant.

A recent review of more than 80,000 cases of antidepressant use found that the risk of suicide for both children and adults was higher in the month *before* starting treatment and gradually declined after taking newer antidepressant drugs. The risk of suicide while taking an antidepressant is about 1 in 3,000; the risk of a serious attempt is 1 in 1,000.[49]

In every case, physicians have to weigh the potential benefits of antidepressant medication against the possible risks. Both adults and children taking antidepressants should be watched closely for a worsening of depression or an increase in suicidal thoughts, particularly when medications are started for the first time or the dose is changed.

Bipolar Disorder (Manic Depression)

Bipolar disorder, or manic depression, consists of mood swings that may take individuals from *manic* states of feeling euphoric and energetic to depressive states of utter despair. In episodes of full mania, they may become so impulsive and out of touch with reality that they endanger their careers, relationships, health, or even survival.[50] One percent of the population—about 2 million American adults—suffer from this serious but treatable disorder. Men tend to develop bipolar disorder earlier in life (between ages 16 to 25), but women have higher rates overall.[51] About 50 percent of patients with bipolar illness have a family history of the disorder.

The characteristic symptoms of bipolar disorder include:

- **Mood swings** (from happy to miserable, optimistic to despairing, and so on).
- **Changes in thinking** (thoughts speeding through one's mind, unrealistic self-confidence, difficulty concentrating, delusions, hallucinations).
- **Changes in behavior** (sudden immersion in plans and projects, talking very rapidly and much more than usual, excessive spending, impaired judgment, impulsive sexual involvement).
- **Changes in physical condition** (less need for sleep, increased energy, fewer health complaints than usual).

During "manic" periods, individuals may make grandiose plans or take dangerous risks. But they often plunge from this highest of highs to a horrible, low depressive episode, in which they may feel sad, hopeless, and helpless and develop other symptoms of major depression. The risk of suicide is very real.

Professional therapy is essential in treating bipolar disorders. Mood-stabilizing medications are the keystone of treatment, although psychotherapy plays a critical role in helping individuals understand their illness and rebuild their lives. Most individuals continue taking medication indefinitely after remission of their symptoms because the risk of recurrence is high.

Anxiety Disorders

Anxiety disorders may involve inordinate fears of certain objects or situations (**phobias**), episodes of sudden, inexplicable terror (**panic attacks**), chronic distress (**generalized anxiety disorder,** or **GAD**), or persistent, disturbing thoughts and behaviors (**obsessive-compulsive disorder,** or **OCD**). These disorders can increase the risk of developing depression. Over a lifetime, as many as one in four Americans may experience an anxiety disorder. Only one of every four of these individuals is ever correctly diagnosed and treated. Yet most who do get treatment, even for severe and disabling problems, improve dramatically.

Phobias

Phobias—the most prevalent type of anxiety disorder—are out-of-the-ordinary, irrational, intense, persistent fears of certain objects or situations. About two million Americans develop such acute terror that they go to extremes to avoid whatever it is that they fear, even though they realize that these feelings are excessive or unreasonable. The most common phobias involve animals, particularly dogs, snakes, insects, and mice; the sight of blood; closed spaces (*claustrophobia*); heights (*acrophobia*); air travel and being in open or public places or situations from which one perceives it would be difficult or embarrassing to escape (*agoraphobia*).

Although various medications have been tried, none is effective by itself in relieving phobias. The best approach is behavioral therapy, which consists of gradual, systematic exposure to the feared object (a process called *systematic desensitization*). Numerous studies have proved that exposure—especially in vivo exposure, in which individuals are exposed to the actual source of their fear rather than simply imagining it—is highly effective. Medical hypnosis—the use of induction of an altered state of consciousness—also can help.

Panic Attacks and Panic Disorder

Individuals who have had panic attacks describe them as the most frightening experiences of their lives. Without reason or warning, their hearts race wildly. They may become light-headed or dizzy. Because they can't catch their breath, they may start breathing rapidly and hyperventilate. Parts of their bodies, such as their fingers or toes, may tingle or feel numb. Worst of all is the terrible sense that something horrible is about to happen: that they will die, lose their minds, or have a heart attack. Most attacks reach peak intensity within ten minutes. Afterward, individuals live in dread of another one. In the course of a lifetime, your risk of having a single panic attack is 7.2 percent.

Panic disorder develops when attacks recur or apprehension about them becomes so intense that

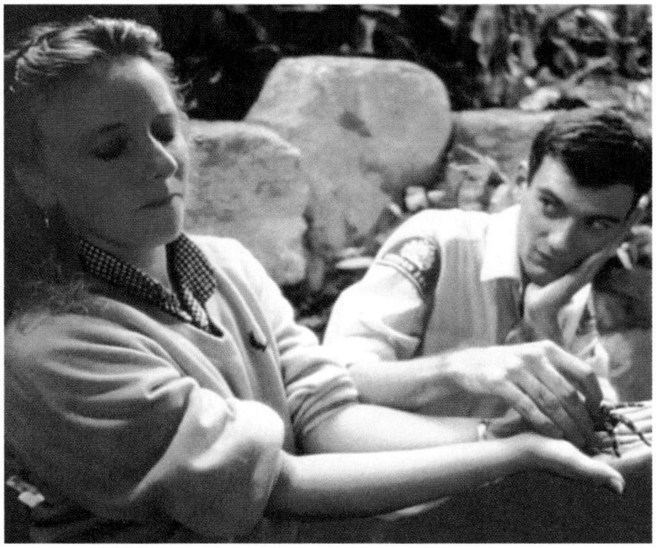

Systematic decensitization is one of the behavioral therapies used in the treatment of phobias.

antidepressant A drug used primarily to treat symptoms of depression.

bipolar disorder Severe depression alternating with periods of manic activity and elation.

anxiety disorders A group of psychological disorders involving episodes of apprehension, tension, or uneasiness, stemming from the anticipation of danger and sometimes accompanied by physical symptoms, which cause significant distress and impairment to an individual.

phobia An anxiety disorder marked by an inordinate fear of an object, a class of objects, or a situation, resulting in extreme avoidance behaviors.

panic attack A short episode characterized by physical sensations of light-headedness, dizziness, hyperventilation, and numbness of extremities, accompanied by an inexplicable terror, usually of a physical disaster such as death.

generalized anxiety disorder (GAD) An anxiety disorder characterized as chronic distress.

obsessive-compulsive disorder (OCD) An anxiety disorder characterized by obsessions and/or compulsions that impair one's ability to function and form relationships.

panic disorder An anxiety disorder in which the apprehension or experience of recurring panic attacks is so intense that normal functioning is impaired.

individuals cannot function normally. Full-blown panic disorder occurs in about 1.6 percent of all adults in the course of a lifetime and usually develops before age 30. Women are more than twice as likely as men to experience panic attacks, although no one knows why. Parents, siblings, and children of individuals with panic disorders also are more likely to develop them than are others.

The two primary treatments for panic disorder are (1) cognitive-behavioral therapy, which teaches specific strategies for coping with symptoms like rapid breathing, and (2) medication. Treatment helps as many as 90 percent of those with panic disorder either improve significantly or recover completely, usually within six to eight weeks. Individuals who receive cognitive-behavioral therapy as well as medication are less likely to suffer relapses than those taking medication alone and often can learn to control their symptoms without drugs.

Generalized Anxiety Disorder

About 10 million adults in the United States suffer from a generalized anxiety disorder (GAD), excessive or unrealistic apprehension that causes physical symptoms and lasts for six months or longer. It usually starts when people are in their twenties. Unlike fear, which helps us recognize and avoid real danger, GAD is an irrational or unwarranted response to harmless objects or situations of exaggerated danger. The most common symptoms are faster heart rate, sweating, increased blood pressure, muscle aches, intestinal pains, irritability, sleep problems, and difficulty concentrating.

Chronically anxious individuals worry—not just some of the time, and not just about the stresses and strains of ordinary life—but constantly, about almost everything: their health, families, finances, marriages, potential dangers. Treatment for GAD may consist of a combination of psychotherapy, behavioral therapy, and antianxiety drugs.

Obsessive-Compulsive Disorder

As many as 1 in 40 Americans has a type of anxiety called obsessive-compulsive disorder (OCD). Some of these individuals suffer only from an *obsession,* a recurring idea, thought, or image that they realize, at least initially, is senseless. The most common obsessions are repetitive thoughts of violence (for example, killing a child), contamination (becoming infected by shaking hands), and doubt (wondering whether one has performed some act, such as having hurt someone in a traffic accident). Most people with OCD also suffer from a compulsion, repetitive behavior performed according to certain rules or in a stereotyped fashion. The most common compulsions involve handwashing, cleaning, hoarding useless items, counting, or checking (for example, making sure dozens of times that a door is locked).

Individuals with OCD realize that their thoughts or behaviors are bizarre, but they cannot resist or control them. Eventually, the obsessions or compulsions consume a great deal of time and significantly interfere with normal routines, job functioning, or usual social activities or relationships with others. A young woman who must follow a very rigid dressing routine may always be late for class, for example; a student who must count each letter of the alphabet as he types may not be able to complete a term paper.

Treatment may consist of cognitive therapy to correct irrational assumptions, behavioral techniques such as progressively limiting the amount of time someone obsessed with cleanliness can spend washing and scrubbing, and medication. About 70 to 80 percent of those with OCD improve with treatment.

Attention Disorders

Attention-deficit/hyperactivity disorder (ADHD) is the most common mental disorder in childhood. About 10 percent of boys and 5 percent of girls between ages 5 to 18 suffer from ADHD. Contrary to previous beliefs, most children do not outgrow it. For as many as 65 percent of youngsters, ADHD persists into adolescence and young adulthood. Among adults, 4 to 5 percent may have ADHD.

ADHD looks and feels different in adults. Hyperactivity is more subtle, an internal fidgety feeling rather than a physical restlessness. As youngsters with ADHD mature, academic difficulties become much more of a problem. Students with ADHD may find it hard to concentrate, read, make decisions, complete complex projects, and meet deadlines. Relationships with peers also can become more challenging. Young people with ADHD may become frustrated easily, have a short fuse, and erupt into angry outbursts. Some become more argumentative, negative, and defiant than most other teens. Sleep problems, including sleeping much more or less than normal, are common. The likelihood of developing other emotional problems, including depression and anxiety disorders, is higher. As many as 20 percent of those diagnosed with depression, anxiety, or substance abuse also have ADHD.

The risk of substance use disorders for individuals with ADHD is twice that of the general population. According to several reports, between 15 and 25 percent of adults with substance use disorders have ADHD. In addition, individuals with ADHD start smoking at a younger age and have higher rates of smoking and drinking. (The use of stimulant medication to treat ADHD does not increase the risk of substance abuse.)

The medications most often used for this disorder are stimulants (such as Ritalin), which improve behavior and cognition for about 70 percent of adolescents.

Thanks to extended-release preparations (including a skin patch), which are longer acting, individuals do not have to take these medications as often as in the past. As discussed in Chapter 11, abuse of prescription stimulants by students without ADHD is a growing problem on college campuses. In one report, 8 percent of students reported using prescription stimulants in their lifetime, 5 percent in the last year. Their primary motivations were to stay awake or feel more energetic or to get high.[52]

An alternative nonstimulant treatment is Strattera (atomoxetine), which treats ADHD and co-existing problems such as depression and anxiety. Its effects are more gradual, and it does not seem to have any known potential for abuse. Adverse effects include drowsiness, loss of appetite, nausea, vomiting, and headaches. Its long-term effects are not known.

An estimated 1 percent of college students have an attention disorder that can have a significant impact on their academic performance and personal lives. Pediatricians caution undergraduates with ADHD that they are at higher risk of becoming smokers, abusing alcohol and drugs, and having automobile accidents. The normal challenges of college, including navigating the complexities of scheduling, course planning, and acquiring study skills, also may be especially daunting. If you have ADHD, check with your student health or counseling center to see if any special services are available.

Suicide

Suicide is not in itself a psychiatric disorder, but it is often the tragic consequence of emotional and psychological problems. Every year 30,000 Americans—among them many young people who seem to have "everything to live for"—commit suicide. An estimated 752,000 attempt to take their own lives; there may be 4.5 million suicide "survivors" in the United States.

The suicide rate for African-American and Caucasian men peaks between ages 20 and 40. It rises again after age 65 among white men and after age 75 among blacks. In general, whites are at highest risk for suicide, followed by Native Americans, African Americans, Hispanic Americans, and Asian Americans. Internationally, suicide rates are highest in Germany, Scandinavia, Eastern Europe, and Japan, average in the United States, Canada, and Great Britain, and low in Italy, Spain, and Ireland.

At all ages, men *commit* suicide three to four times more frequently than women, but women *attempt* suicide much more often than men (Table 2-4). Elderly men are ten times more likely to take their own lives than older women.[53]

TABLE 2-4 Suicide Risk

	Who attempts suicide?	Who completes suicide?
Sex	Female	Male
Age	Under 35	Under 20 or over 60
Means	Less deadly, such as wrist slashing	More deadly, such as a gun
Circumstances	High chance of rescue	Low chance of rescue

Suicide in the Young

Although rates have declined in the last decade, suicide remains the third-leading cause of death among children and adolescents 10 to 19 years old in the United States. An estimated 500,000 U.S. teens attempt suicide every year. About 1,500 die.[54]

Suicide is the second-leading cause of death among students at American colleges and universities. Although many people believe that suicide rates are increasing, the suicide rate for young adults has been stable or declining since 1976. Among college-aged women, the rate is the lowest it has been in the last 100 years. More young men than women take their own lives, but the suicide rate for college-aged men has declined 20 percent in the past ten years.[55] The suicide rate among college students is about 6.5 per 100,000, half the rate of the U.S. population in general.[56]

One-half of the adolescents who take their own lives suffer from major depression. "In psychological interviews after a teen suicide, we see that the warning signs were there," notes child psychiatrist Madelyn Gould, M.D., of Columbia University, "but no one realized the underlying problem was depression."[57]

Native American communities have especially high rates of suicide among both young men and women. Young African-American men, historically at low suicide risk, are narrowing the gap with their white peers, while suicide by Hispanic young men has declined. The lowest rates are for Asian Pacific males and African-American females.[58]

Firearms and suffocation (mainly by hanging) are the most common methods of suicide among young people. In recent years, deaths with firearms have decreased, in part because of laws restricting access to guns by youngsters. However, deaths by hanging have increased, particularly among younger teens.[59]

Researchers also have identified factors that protect young people from suicide. Number one for both boys and girls was feeling connected to their

attention deficit/hyperactivity disorder (ADHD) A spectrum of difficulties in controlling motion and sustaining attention, including hyperactivity, impulsivity, and distractibility.

parents and family. For girls, emotional well-being was also protective; grade point average was an additional protective factor for boys. High parental expectations for their child's school achievement, more people living in the household, and religiosity were protective for some of the boys, but not for the girls. Availability of counseling services at school and parental presence at key times during the day were protective for some of the girls, but not for the boys.

Suicide is not inevitable. Appropriate treatment can help as many as 70 to 80 percent of those at risk for suicide. Among young people, early recognition and treatment for depressive disorders and alcohol and drug use could save thousands of lives each year.

? FAQ What Leads to Suicide?

Researchers have looked for explanations for suicide by studying everything from phases of the moon to seasons (suicides peak in the spring and early summer) to birth order in the family. They have found no conclusive answers. A constellation of influences—mental disorders, personality traits, biologic and genetic vulnerability, medical illness, and psychosocial stressors—may combine in ways that lower an individual's threshold of vulnerability. The risk of suicide is higher in people who live in cities, are single, have a low income, or are unemployed. No one factor in itself may ever explain fully why a person chooses death.

Mental Disorders More than 95 percent of those who commit suicide have a mental disorder. Two in particular—depression and alcoholism—account for two-thirds of all suicides. Suicide also is a risk for those with other disorders, including schizophrenia, posttraumatic stress disorder, and personality disorders.

Antidepressant Medications As the FDA has warned, antidepressants can increase the risk of suicidal thoughts and attempts. Recent studies have confirmed an increase in suicide attempts in some individuals, including adolescents, during the first four weeks of treatment, especially the first nine days, with various antidepressants, including Prozac and Paxil.[60] Because depression itself increases the danger of suicide, psychiatrists contend that the benefits of treatment outweigh the risk but call for increased monitoring for increased agitation or suicidal thoughts.[61]

Substance Abuse Many of those who commit suicide drink beforehand, and their use of alcohol may lower their inhibitions. Since alcohol itself is a depressant, it can intensify the despondency suicidal individuals are already feeling. Alcoholics who attempt suicide often have other risk factors, including major depression, poor social support, serious medical illness, and unemployment. Drugs of abuse also can alter thinking and lower inhibitions against suicide.

Hopelessness The sense of utter hopelessness and helplessness may be the most common contributing factor in suicide. When hope dies, individuals view every experience in negative terms and come to expect the worst possible outcomes for their problems. Given this way of thinking, suicide often seems a reasonable response to a life seen as not worth living.

Family History One of every four people who attempt suicide has a family member who also tried to commit suicide. While a family history of suicide is not in itself considered a predictor of suicide, two mental disorders that can lead to suicide—depression and bipolar disorder (manic depression)—do run in families.

Physical Illness People who commit suicide are likely to be ill or to believe that they are. About 5 percent actually have a serious physical disorder, such as AIDS or cancer. While suicide may seem to be a decision rationally arrived at in persons with serious or fatal illness, this may not be the case. Depression, not uncommon in such instances, can warp judgment. When the depression is treated, the person may no longer have suicidal intentions.

Brain Chemistry Investigators have found abnormalities in the brain chemistry of individuals who complete suicide, especially low levels of a metabolite of the neurotransmitter serotonin. There are indications that individuals with a deficiency in this substance may have as much as a ten times greater risk of committing suicide than those with higher levels.

Access to Guns For individuals already facing a combination of predisposing factors, access to a means of committing suicide, particularly to guns, can add to the risk. Unlike other methods of suicide, guns almost always work. States with stricter gun-control laws have much lower rates of suicide than states with more lenient laws. Health professionals are urging parents whose children undergo psychological treatment or assessment to remove all weapons from their homes and to make sure their youngsters do not have access to potentially lethal medications or to alcohol.

Other Factors Individuals who kill themselves often have gone through more major life crises—job changes, births, financial reversals, divorce, retirement—in the previous six months, compared with others. Long-standing, intense conflict with family members or other important people may add to the danger. In some cases, suicide may be an act of revenge that offers the person a sense of control—however temporary or illusory. For example, a husband whose wife has had an affair may rationalize that he can get back at her, and have the final word, by killing himself. Others may feel that, by rejecting life, they are rejecting a partner or parent who abandoned or betrayed them.

Suicide Prevention

If someone you know has talked about suicide, behaved unpredictably, or suddenly emerged from a severe depression into a calm, settled state of mind, don't rule out the possibility that he or she may attempt suicide.

- **Encourage your friend to talk.** Ask concerned questions. Listen attentively. Show that you take the person's feelings seriously and truly care.
- **Don't offer trite reassurances.** List reasons to go on living, try to analyze the person's motives, or try to shock or challenge him or her.
- **Suggest solutions or alternatives to problems.** Make plans. Encourage positive action, such as getting away for a while to gain a better perspective on a problem.
- **Don't be afraid to ask** whether your friend has considered suicide. The opportunity to talk about thoughts of suicide may be an enormous relief and—contrary to a long-standing myth—will not fix the idea of suicide more firmly in a person's mind.
- **Don't think that people who talk** about killing themselves never carry out their threat. Most individuals who commit suicide give definite indications of their intent to die.

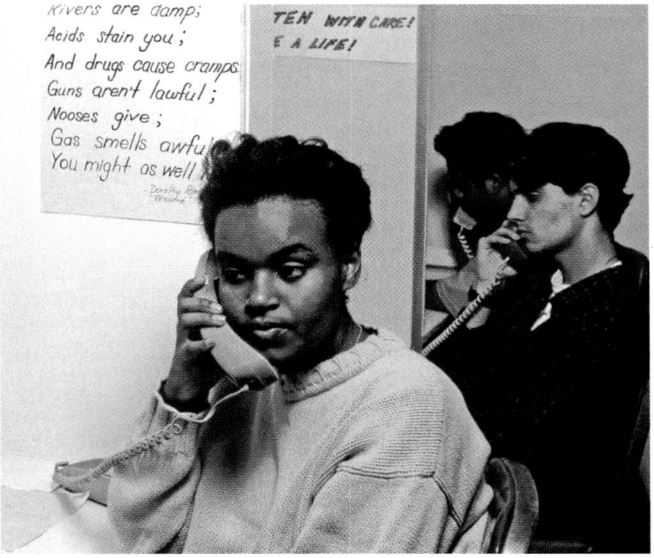

© Mary Kate Denny/PhotoEdit

About 20 percent of teenagers seriously consider suicide; a much smaller number actually attempt to take their own lives. Talking to a counselor at a suicide hot line may help a young person deal with feelings of despondency.

When her brother committed suicide in college, a sophomore at the University of Pennsylvania formed a student group to raise awareness and change attitudes toward mental illness. Should undergraduates speak out and take action to make sure that troubled students get the help they need? Or is it the responsibility of colleges and universities to provide programs to enhance the mental health of their students?

You Decide

Strategies for Prevention — *If You Start Thinking About Suicide*

At some point, the thought of ending it all—the disappointments, problems, bad feelings—may cross your mind. This experience isn't unusual. But if the idea of taking your life persists or intensifies, you should respond as you would to other warnings of potential threats to your health—by getting the help you need:

- Talk to a mental health professional. If you have a therapist, call immediately. If not, call a suicide hot line.
- Find someone you can trust and talk honestly about what you're feeling. If you suffer from depression or another mental disorder, educate trusted friends or relatives about your condition so they are prepared if called upon to help.
- Write down your more uplifting thoughts. Even if you are despondent, you can help yourself by taking the time to retrieve some more positive thoughts or memories. A simple record of your hopes for the future and the people you value in your life can remind you of why your own life is worth continuing.
- Avoid drugs and alcohol. Most suicides are the result of sudden, uncontrolled impulses, and drugs and alcohol can make it harder to resist these destructive urges.
- Go to the hospital. Hospitalization can sometimes be the best way to protect your health and safety.

Overcoming Problems of the Mind

Mental illness costs our society an estimated $150 billion a year in lost work time and productivity, employee turnover, disability payments, and death. Yet many Americans do not have access to mental health services, nor do they have insurance for such services. Despite the fact that treatments for mental disorders have a higher success rate than those for many other diseases, employers often restrict mental health benefits. HMOs and health insurance plans are much more likely to limit psychotherapy visits and psychiatric hospitalizations than treatments for medical illnesses.

Even when cost is not a barrier, many people do not seek treatment because they see psychological problems as a sign of weakness rather than illness. They also may not realize that scientifically proven therapies can bring relief, often in a matter of weeks or months.

Where Can I Turn for Help?

As a student, your best contact for identifying local services may be your health education instructor or department. The health instructors can tell you about general and mental health counseling available on campus, school-based support groups, community-based programs, and special emergency services. On campus, you can also turn to the student health services or the office of the dean of student services or student affairs.

Within the community, you may be able to get help through the city or county health department and neighborhood health centers. Local hospitals often have special clinics and services; and there are usually local branches of national service organizations, such as United Way or Alcoholics Anonymous, other 12-step programs, and various support groups. You can call the psychiatric or psychological association in your city or state for the names of licensed professionals. (Check the telephone directory for listings.) Your primary physician may also be able to help.

The telephone book and the Internet are also good resources for special programs, found either by the nature of the service, by the name of the neighborhood or city, or by the name of the sponsoring group. In some places, the city's name may precede a listing: the New York City Suicide Hot Line, for instance. In addition to suicide-prevention programs, look for crisis intervention, violence prevention, and child-abuse prevention programs; drug-treatment information; shelters for battered women; senior citizen centers; and self-help and counseling services. Many services have special hot lines for coping with emergencies. Others provide information as well as counseling over the phone.

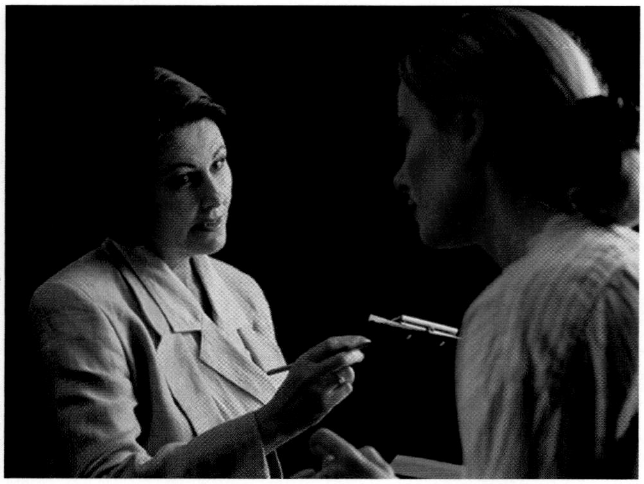

© Tony Latham/Stone/Getty Images

When choosing a therapist, you should always consider the individual's education, title, and qualifications. Also important are qualities such as compassion and caring.

Types of Therapy

The term **psychotherapy** refers to any type of counseling based on the exchange of words in the context of the unique relationship that develops between a mental health professional and a person seeking help. The process of talking and listening can lead to new insight, relief from distressing psychological symptoms, changes in unhealthy or maladaptive behaviors, and more effective ways of dealing with the world.

Most mental health professionals today are trained in a variety of psychotherapeutic techniques and tailor their approach to the problem, personality, and needs of each person seeking their help. Because skilled therapists may combine different techniques in the course of therapy, the lines between the various approaches often blur.

Because insurance companies and health-care plans often limit the duration of psychotherapy, many mental health professionals are adopting a *time-limited* format in order to make the most of every session, regardless of the length of treatment. Brief or short-term psychotherapy typically focuses on a central theme, problem, or topic and may continue for several weeks to several months. The individuals most likely to benefit are those who are interested in solving immediate problems rather than changing their characters, who can think in psychological terms, and who are motivated to change.

Psychodynamic Psychotherapy

For the most part, today's mental health professionals base their assessment of individuals on a **psychodynamic** understanding that takes into account the role of early experiences and unconscious influences in *actively* shaping behavior. (This is the *dynamic* in psychodynamic.) Psychodynamic treatments work toward the goal of providing greater insight into problems and bringing about behavioral change. Therapy may be brief, consisting of 12 to 25 sessions, or may continue for several years. According to current thinking, psychotherapy can actually rewire the network of neurons within the brain in ways that ease distress and improve functioning in many areas of daily life.

Cognitive-Behavioral Therapy (CBT)

Cognitive-behavioral therapy (CBT) focuses on inappropriate or inaccurate thoughts or beliefs to help individuals break out of a distorted way of thinking. The techniques of **cognitive therapy** include identification of an individual's beliefs and attitudes, recognition of negative thought patterns, and education in alternative ways of thinking. Individuals with major depression or anxiety disorders are most likely to benefit, usually in 15 to 25 sessions. However, many of the positive messages used in cognitive therapy can help anyone improve a bad mood or negative outlook.

Behavioral therapy strives to substitute healthier ways of behaving for maladaptive patterns used in the past. Its premise is that distressing psychological symptoms, like all behaviors, are learned responses that can be modified or unlearned. Some therapists believe that changing behavior also changes how people think and feel. As they put it, "Change the behavior, and the feelings will follow." Behavior therapies work best for disorders characterized by specific, abnormal patterns of acting—such as alcohol and drug abuse, anxiety disorders, and phobias—and for individuals who want to change bad habits.

Interpersonal Therapy (IPT)

Interpersonal therapy (IPT), originally developed for research into the treatment of major depression, focuses on relationships in order to help individuals deal with unrecognized feelings and needs and improve their communication skills. IPT does not deal with the psychological origins of symptoms but rather concentrates on current problems of getting along with others. The supportive, empathic relationship that is developed with the therapist, who takes an even more active role than in psychodynamic psychotherapy, is the most crucial component of this therapy. The emphasis is on the here and now and on interpersonal—rather than intrapsychic—issues. Individuals with major depression, chronic difficulties developing relationships, chronic mild depression, or bulimia (see Chapter 6 on eating disorders) are most likely to benefit. IPT usually consists of 12 to 16 sessions.

Psychiatric Drugs

Medications that alter brain chemistry and relieve psychiatric symptoms have brought great hope and help to millions of people. Thanks to the recent development of a new generation of more precise and effective **psychiatric drugs,** success rates for treating many common and disabling disorders—depression, panic disorder, schizophrenia, and others—have soared. Often used in conjunction with psychotherapy, sometimes used as the primary treatment, these medications have revolutionized mental health care.

At some point in their lives, about half of all Americans will take a psychiatric drug. The reason may be depression, anxiety, a sleep difficulty, an eating disorder, alcohol or drug dependence, impaired memory, or another disorder that disrupts the intricate chemistry of the brain. (See Savvy Consumer: "What You Need to Know About Mind-Mood Medications.")

Psychiatric drugs are now among the most widely prescribed drugs in the United States. Serotonin-boosting medications (SSRIs), have become the drugs of choice in treating depression. They also are effective in treating obsessive compulsive disorder, panic disorder, social phobia, posttraumatic stress disorder, premenstrual dysphoric disorder, and generalized anxiety disorder. In patients who don't respond, psychiatrists may add another drug to boost the efficacy of the treatment.

According to various studies, 5 to 7 percent of college students take antidepressant medications. Direct-to-consumer advertisements for antidepressant drugs can influence students' perceptions of what is wrong with them. In one study, college women were more likely to rate themselves as having mild-to-moderate depression as a result of reading pharmaceutical company information for popular antidepressants. The researchers cautioned that students

psychotherapy Treatment designed to produce a response by psychological rather than physical means, such as suggestion, persuasion, reassurance, and support.

psychodynamic Interpreting behaviors in terms of early experiences and unconscious influences.

cognitive therapy A technique used to identify an individual's beliefs and attitudes, recognize negative thought patterns, and educate in alternative ways of thinking.

behavioral therapy Psychotherapy that emphasizes application of the principles of learning to substitute desirable responses and behavior patterns for undesirable ones.

interpersonal therapy (IPT) A technique used to develop communication skills and relationships.

psychiatric drugs Medications that regulate a person's mental, emotional, and physical functions to facilitate normal functioning.

SAVVY CONSUMER

What You Need to Know About Mind-Mood Medications

Before taking any "psychoactive" drug (one that affects the brain), talk to a qualified health professional. Here are some points to raise:

- What can this medication do for me? What specific symptoms will it relieve? Are there other possible benefits?
- When will I notice a difference? How long does it take for the medicine to have an effect?
- Are there any risks? What about side effects? Do I have to take it before or after eating? Will it affect my ability to study, work, drive, or operate machinery?
- Is there a risk of increased aggression or suicide? What should I do if I start thinking about taking my own life or of harming others?
- How will I be able to tell if the medication is working? What are the odds that it will help me?
- How long will I have to take medication? Is there any danger that I'll become addicted?
- What if it doesn't help?
- Is there an herbal or natural alternative? If so, has it been studied? What do you know about its possible risks and side effects?

should try alternative treatments for mild depression, including simple changes such as reduced class load, increased exercise, and more sleep, before starting medication.[62]

Alternative Mind-Mood Products

People with serious mental illnesses, including depression and bipolar disorder, often use at least one alternative health-care practice, such as yoga or meditation. They also are trying "natural" products, such as herbs and enzymes, that claim to have psychological effects. However, because they are not classified as drugs, these products have not undergone the rigorous scientific testing required of psychiatric medications, and little is known about their safety or efficacy. "Natural" doesn't mean risk-free. Opium and cocaine are "natural" substances that have dramatic and potentially deadly effects on the mind.

St. John's wort has been used to treat anxiety and depression in Europe for many years. Data from clinical studies in the United States do not support the efficacy of St. John's wort for moderate to severe depression. In two carefully controlled studies, the herb did not prove more effective than a placebo. However, more than two-dozen studies have found that St. John's wort was similar in efficacy to standard antidepressants. Side effects include dizziness, abdominal pain and bloating, constipation, nausea, fatigue, and dry mouth. St. John's wort should not be taken in combination with other prescription antidepressants. St. John's wort can lower the efficacy of oral contraceptives and increase the risk of an unwanted pregnancy.

LEARN IT / LIVE IT

Surviving and Thriving

Feeling good does not depend on money, success, recognition, or status. At any age, at any level of education and achievement, regardless of disability or disease, it is possible to find happiness and fulfillment in life. Achieving the highest possible level of psychological well-being, like achieving peak physical well-being, depends primarily on assuming responsibility for yourself.

Like physical health, psychological well-being is not a fixed state of being, but a process. The way you live every day affects how you feel about yourself and your world. Here are some basic guidelines that you can rely on to make the most of the process of living:

- **Accept yourself.** As a human being, you are, by definition, imperfect. Come to terms with the fact that you are a worthwhile person despite your mistakes.
- **Respect yourself.** Recognize your abilities and talents. Acknowledge your competence and achievements, and take pride in them.
- **Trust yourself.** Learn to listen to the voice within you, and let your intuition be your guide.
- **Love yourself.** Be happy to spend time by yourself. Learn to appreciate your own company and to be glad you're you.

- **Stretch yourself.** Be willing to change and grow, to try something new, and dare to be vulnerable.
- **Look at challenges as opportunities for personal growth.** "Every problem brings the possibility of a widening of consciousness," psychologist Carl Jung once noted. Put his words to the test.
- **Think of not only where but also who you want to be a decade from now.** The goals you set, the decisions you make, the values you adopt now will determine how you feel about yourself and your life in the future.

2 Making This Chapter Work for You

Review Questions

1. Psychological health is influenced by all of the following *except*
   a. spiritual health.
   b. physical agility.
   c. culture.
   d. a firm grasp on reality.
2. Emotional intelligence encompasses which of the following components?
   a. creativity, sense of humor, scholastic achievement
   b. integrity, honesty, and perseverance
   c. piety, tolerance, and self-esteem
   d. empathy, self-awareness, and altruism
3. Which of the following activities can contribute to a lasting sense of personal fulfillment?
   a. becoming a Big Sister or Big Brother to a child from an inner city, single-parent home
   b. volunteering at a local soup kitchen on Thanksgiving
   c. being a regular participant in an Internet chat room
   d. going on a shopping spree
4. Individuals who have developed a sense of mastery over their lives are
   a. skilled at controlling the actions of others.
   b. usually passive and silent when faced with a situation they don't like.
   c. aware that their locus of control is internal, not external.
   d. aware that their locus of control is external, not internal.
5. People who pray regularly
   a. are able to quit smoking more easily.
   b. never get sick.
   c. recover from heart attacks more quickly.
   d. get better grades.
6. A mental disorder can be described as
   a. a condition associated with migraine headaches and narcolepsy.
   b. a condition that is usually caused by severe trauma to the brain.
   c. a behavioral or psychological disorder that impairs an individual's ability to conduct one or more important activities of daily life.
   d. a psychological disorder that is easily controlled with medication and a change in diet.
7. Some characteristic symptoms of major depression are
   a. difficulty concentrating, lack of energy, and changes in eating habits.
   b. exaggerated sense of euphoria and energy.
   c. palpitations, sweating, numbness, and tingling sensations.
   d. talking in rambling ways, inability to think in a logical manner, and delusions.
8. Which of the following statements about anxiety disorders is true?
   a. Anxiety disorders are the least prevalent type of mental illness.
   b. An individual suffering from a panic attack may mistake her symptoms for a heart attack.
   c. The primary symptom of obsessive-compulsive disorder is irrational, intense, and persistent fear of a specific object or situation.
   d. Generalized anxiety disorders respond to systematic desensitization behavioral therapy.
9. A person may be at higher risk of committing suicide if
   a. he is taking blood pressure medication.
   b. he lives in a rural environment and is married.
   c. he has been diagnosed with hyperactivity disorder.
   d. he has lost his job because of alcoholism.
10. Which of the following statements is true?
    a. Individuals with phobias are most likely to benefit from psychiatric medications.
    b. Antidepressant medications now require a warning label about the increased risk of suicidal thoughts.
    c. Only children have attention disorders.
    d. Interpersonal therapy focuses on the role of early experiences and unconscious influences in shaping patterns of behavior, such as repeated failed relationships.

Answers to these questions can be found on page 422.

Critical Thinking

1. Would you say that you view life positively or negatively? Would your friends and family agree with your assessment? Ask two of your closest friends for feedback about what they perceive are your typical responses to a problematic situation. Are these indicative of positive

attitudes? If not, what could you do to become more psychologically positive?

2. Paula went to a therapist when she was feeling depressed and was given a prescription for an antidepressant called fluoxetine (trade name Prozac). Her therapist recommended the drug because it causes fewer side effects than other medications. However, Paula later read in a news magazine that some patients, claiming that Prozac had made them violent or suicidal, had sued the drug's manufacturers. Their suits didn't win in court, but Paula was less certain about taking the prescribed medication. What do you think she should do? How would you weigh the risks and benefits of taking a psychiatric drug?
3. Research has indicated that many homeless men and women are in need of outpatient psychiatric care, often because they suffer from chronic mental illnesses or alcoholism. Yet government funding for the mentally ill is inadequate, and homelessness itself can make it difficult, if not impossible, for people to gain access to the care they need. How do you feel when you pass homeless individuals who seem disoriented or out of touch with reality? Who should take responsibility for their welfare? Should they be forced to undergo treatment at psychiatric institutions?

Media Menu

ThomsonNOW™ Go to the ThomsonNOW website at **http://www.thomsonedu.com** that will:

- Help you evaluate your knowledge of the material.
- Allow you to take an exam-prep quiz.
- Provide a Personalized Learning Plan targeting resources that address areas you should study.
- Coach you through identifying target goals for behavioral change and creating and monitoring your personal change plan throughout the semester.

INTERNET CONNECTIONS

SAVE: Suicide Awareness Voices of Education
www.save.org

This site (formerly American Foundation for Suicide Prevention) offers research, facts, survivor support, and more.

National Institute of Mental Health
www.nimh.nih.gov

The National Institute of Mental Health is a federally sponsored organization that provides useful information on a variety of mental health topics including current mental health research.

Spirituality and Health
www.spiritualityhealth.com

Developed by the Publishing Group of Trinity Church, Wall Street in New York City, this website offers self-tests, guidance on spiritual practices, resources for people on spiritual journeys, and subscriptions to a bimonthly print magazine.

www.spirituality.org

Spirituality for Today is an interactive monthly magazine dedicated to current themes and questions concerning faith in this postmodern age.

www.spiritweb.org

Combination of New Age and ancient teachings for those interested in exploring alternative views of spirituality.

www.newvision-psychic.com/bookshelf

A comprehensive list of books dealing with women and spirituality.

www.beliefnet.com

An eclectic, informative guide to different forms of religion and spirituality.

American Psychological Association
www.apa.org

The APA is the scientific and professional organization for psychology in the United States. Its website provides up-to-date information on psychological issues and disorders.

National Mental Health Association
www.nmha.org

This site features fact sheets on a variety of mental health topics, including depression screening, college initiative, substance abuse prevention, and information for families. Also available are current mental health articles, an e-mail newsletter, and a bookstore.

InfoTrac College Edition Activities Log on, insert **psychological depression** into the Keyword search box, and limit your search to the past year. When you get the results, Mark articles to review, then Select one to read. Summarize three or four key points from the article.

You can find additional readings related to personal health with InfoTrac College Edition, an online library of more than 900 journals and publications. Follow the instructions for accessing InfoTrac College Edition that were packaged with your textbook; then search for articles using a keyword search.

For additional links, resources, and suggested readings on the InfoTrac College Edition, visit our Health and Wellness Resource Center at **http://health.wadsworth.com.**

Key Terms

The terms listed are used on the page indicated. Definitions of the terms are in the Glossary at the end of this book.

altruism 33
antidepressant 42
anxiety 38
anxiety disorders 43
assertive 34

LACC Extra Credit Assignment

2. Your friend may be suffering from one of the following disorders. Discuss at least one option for each: A. Major Depression, B. Dementia, C. Bipolar disorder, D. Phobia, E. Schizophrenia.

attention deficit/hyperactivity disorder (ADHD) 44
autonomy 33
behavioral therapy 49
bipolar disorder 42
cognitive therapy 49
culture 27
depression 38
dysthymia 41
emotional health 26
emotional intelligence 27
generalized anxiety disorder (GAD) 43
interpersonal therapy (IPT) 49
locus of control 34
major depression 41
mental disorder 37
mental health 26
mood 29
obsessive-compulsive disorder (OCD) 43
panic attack 43
panic disorder 43
phobia 43
psychiatric drugs 49
psychodynamic 48
psychotherapy 48
self-actualization 28
self-esteem 28
social isolation 34
social phobia 35
spiritual health 26
spiritual intelligence 27
values 30

3 Personal Stress Management

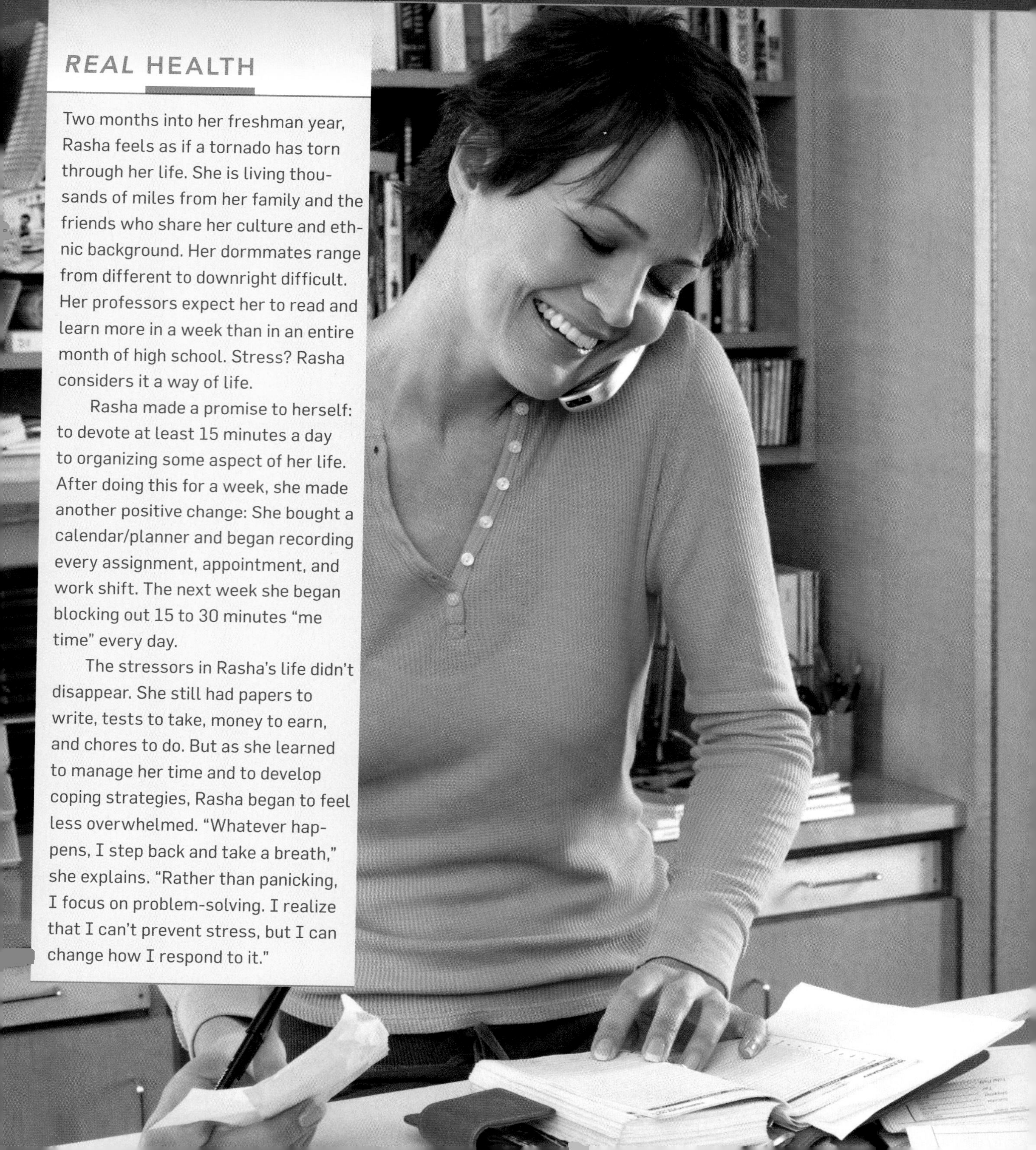

REAL HEALTH

Two months into her freshman year, Rasha feels as if a tornado has torn through her life. She is living thousands of miles from her family and the friends who share her culture and ethnic background. Her dormmates range from different to downright difficult. Her professors expect her to read and learn more in a week than in an entire month of high school. Stress? Rasha considers it a way of life.

Rasha made a promise to herself: to devote at least 15 minutes a day to organizing some aspect of her life. After doing this for a week, she made another positive change: She bought a calendar/planner and began recording every assignment, appointment, and work shift. The next week she began blocking out 15 to 30 minutes "me time" every day.

The stressors in Rasha's life didn't disappear. She still had papers to write, tests to take, money to earn, and chores to do. But as she learned to manage her time and to develop coping strategies, Rasha began to feel less overwhelmed. "Whatever happens, I step back and take a breath," she explains. "Rather than panicking, I focus on problem-solving. I realize that I can't prevent stress, but I can change how I respond to it."

You know about stress. You live with it every day, whether you're studying for exams, meeting people, facing new experiences, or figuring out how to live on a budget. You're not alone. Everyone, regardless of age, gender, race, or income, has to deal with stress—as an individual and as a member of society.

As researchers have demonstrated time and again, stress has profound effects, both immediate and long-term, on our bodies and minds. While stress alone doesn't cause disease, it triggers molecular changes throughout the body that make us more susceptible to many illnesses. Its impact on the mind is no less significant. The burden of chronic stress can undermine one's ability to cope with day-to-day hassles and can exacerbate psychological problems like depression and anxiety disorders.

Yet stress in itself isn't necessarily bad. What matters most is not the stressful situation itself, but an individual's response to it. By learning to anticipate stressful events, to manage day-to-day hassles, and to prevent stress overload, you can find alternatives to running endlessly on a treadmill of alarm, panic, and exhaustion. As you organize your schedule, find ways to release tension, and build up coping skills, you will begin to experience the sense of control and confidence that makes stress a challenge rather than an ordeal.

? FAQ Frequently Asked Questions

After studying the material in this chapter, you should be able to:

- **Define** stress and stressors and **describe** how the body responds to stress according to the general adaptation syndrome theory.
- **List** the physical changes associated with frequent or severe stress and **discuss** how stress can affect the cardiovascular, immune, and digestive systems.
- **Describe** some personal causes of stress, especially those experienced by students, and **discuss** how their effects can be prevented or minimized.
- **Describe** some techniques to help manage stress.
- **Explain** how stressful events can affect psychological health and **describe** the factors contributing to posttraumatic stress disorder.
- **Identify** ways of managing time more efficiently.

ThomsonNOW Log on to ThomsonNOW at **www.thomsonedu.com/thomsonnow** to find your Behavior Change Planner and to explore self-assessments, interactive tutorials, and practice quizzes.

What Is Stress?

People use the word *stress* in different ways: as an external force that causes a person to become tense or upset, as the internal state of arousal, and as the physical response of the body to various demands. Dr. Hans Selye, a pioneer in studying physiological responses to challenge, defined **stress** as "the nonspecific response of the body to any demand made upon it." In other words, the body reacts to **stressors**—the things that upset or excite us—in the same way, regardless of whether they are positive or negative.

Based on nearly 300 studies over four decades, researchers have distinguished five categories of stressors:

- **Acute time-limited stressors** include anxiety-provoking situations such as having to give a talk in public or work out a math problem, such as calculating a tip or dividing a bill, under pressure.
- **Brief naturalistic stressors** are more serious challenges such as taking SATs or meeting a deadline for a big project.
- **Stressful event sequences** are the difficult consequences of a natural disaster or another traumatic occurrence, such as the death of a spouse. The individuals involved recognize that these difficulties will end at some point in the future.
- **Chronic stressors** are ongoing demands caused by life-changing circumstances, such as permanent disability following an accident or caregiving for a parent with dementia, that do not have any clear end point.
- **Distant stressors** are traumatic experiences that occurred long ago, such as child abuse or combat, yet continue to have an emotional and psychological impact.

Not all stressors are negative. Some of life's happiest moments—births, reunions, weddings—are enormously stressful. We weep with the stress of frustration or loss; we weep, too, with the stress of love and joy. Selye coined the term **eustress** for positive stress in our lives (*eu* is a Greek prefix meaning "good"). Eustress challenges us to grow, adapt, and find creative solutions in our lives. **Distress** refers to the negative effects of stress that can deplete or even destroy life energy. Ideally, the level of stress in our lives should be just high enough to motivate us to satisfy our needs and not so high that it interferes with our ability to reach our fullest potential.

What Causes Stress?

Of the many biological theories of stress, the best known may be the **general adaptation syndrome (GAS),** developed by Hans Selye. He postulated that our bodies constantly strive to maintain a stable and consistent physiological state, called **homeostasis.** Stressors, whether in the form of physical illness or a demanding job, disturb this state and trigger a nonspecific physiological response. The body attempts to restore homeostasis by means of an **adaptive response.**

Selye's general adaptation syndrome, which describes the body's response to a stressor—whether threatening or exhilarating—consists of three distinct stages:

1. **Alarm.** When a stressor first occurs, the body responds with changes that temporarily lower resistance. Levels of certain hormones may rise; blood pressure may increase (Figure 3-1). The body quickly makes internal adjustments to cope with the stressor and return to normal activity.
2. **Resistance.** If the stressor continues, the body mobilizes its internal resources to try to sustain homeostasis. For example, if a loved one is seriously hurt in an accident, we initially respond intensely and feel great anxiety. During the subsequent stressful period of recuperation, we struggle to carry on as normally as possible, but this requires considerable effort.
3. **Exhaustion.** If the stress continues long enough, we cannot keep up our normal functioning. Even a small amount of additional stress at this point can cause a breakdown.

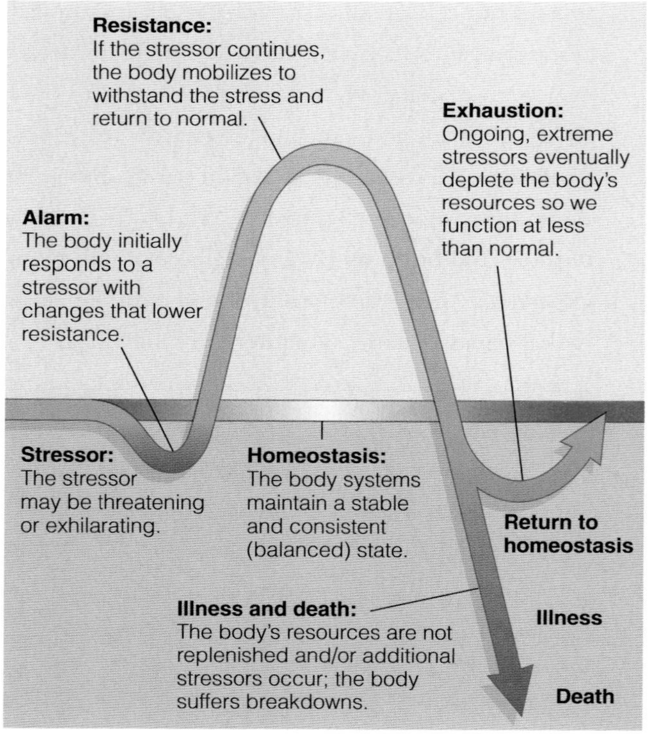

Resistance:
If the stressor continues, the body mobilizes to withstand the stress and return to normal.
Exhaustion:
Ongoing, extreme stressors eventually deplete the body's resources so we function at less than normal.
Alarm:
The body initially responds to a stressor with changes that lower resistance.
Stressor:
The stressor may be threatening or exhilarating.
Homeostasis:
The body systems maintain a stable and consistent (balanced) state.
Return to homeostasis
Illness and death:
The body's resources are not replenished and/or additional stressors occur; the body suffers breakdowns.
Illness
Death

FIGURE 3-1 General Adaptation Syndrome (GAS)
The three stages of Hans Selye's GAS are alarm, resistance, exhaustion.

Among the nonbiological theories is the cognitive-transactional model of stress, developed by Richard Lazarus, which looks at the relation between stress and health. As he sees it, stress can have a powerful impact on health. Conversely, health can affect a person's resistance or coping ability. Stress, according to Lazarus, is "neither an environmental stimulus, a characteristic of the person, nor a response, but a relationship between demands and the power to deal with them without unreasonable or destructive costs."[1] Thus, an event may be stressful for one person but not for another, or it may seem stressful on one occasion but not on another. For instance, one student may think of speaking in front of the class as extremely stressful, while another relishes the chance to do so—except on days when he's not well prepared.

"Perceived" stress—an individual's view of how challenging life is—undermines a sense of well-being in people of all ages and circumstances. However, good self-esteem, social support, and internal resources buffer the impact of perceived stress.

Stress experts Thomas Holmes, M.D., and Richard Rahe, M.D., devised a scale to evaluate individual levels of stress and potential for coping, based on *life-change units* that estimate each change's impact. The death of a partner or parent ranks high on the list, but even changing apartments is considered a stressor. People who accumulate more than 300 life-change units in a year are more likely to suffer serious health problems. Scores on the scale, however, represent "potential stress"; the actual impact of the life change depends on the individual's response. (See Self Survey: "Student Stress Scale" in the Self-Assessment Booklet.)

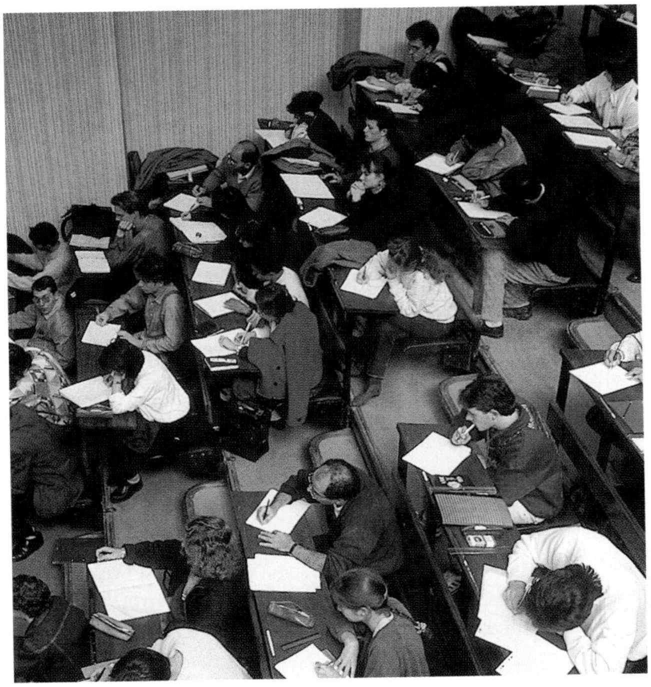

© Ulrike Welsch

Tests are acute time-limited stressors that provoke your body's adaptive stress response.

? FAQ Is Stress Hazardous to Physical Health?

These days we've grown accustomed to warning lables advising us of the health risks of substances like alcohol and cigarettes. Medical researchers speculate that another component of twenty-first-century living also warrants a warning: stress. In recent years, an ever-growing number of studies has implicated stress as a culprit in a range of medical problems. While stress itself may not kill, it clearly undermines our ability to stay well.

While stress alone doesn't cause disease, it triggers molecular changes throughout the body that make us more susceptible to many illnesses. Severe emotional distress—whether caused by a divorce, the loss of a job, or caring for an ill child or parent—can have such a powerful effect on the DNA in body cells that it speeds up aging, adding the equivalent of a decade to biological age. This occurs because of a shortening of structures called telomeres in the chromosomes of cells. An enzyme called telomerase maintains these structures but declines with age. Every time a cell divides, which is a continuous process, the telomeres shorten. The shorter your telomeres, the more likely you are to die.

Stress also triggers complex changes in the body's endocrine, or hormone-secreting, system. When you confront a stressor, the adrenal glands, two triangle-shaped glands that sit atop the kidneys, respond by producing stress hormones, including catecholamines, cortisol (hydrocortisone), and epinephrine (adrenaline), that speed up heart rate and raise blood pressure and prepare the body to deal with the threat. This "fight-or-flight" response prepares you for quick action: Your heart works harder to pump more blood to your legs and arms. Your muscles tense, your breathing quickens, and

stress The nonspecific response of the body to any demands made upon it; may be characterized by muscle tension and acute anxiety, or may be a positive force for action.

stressor Specific or nonspecific agents or situations that cause the stress response in a body.

eustress Positive stress, which stimulates a person to function properly.

distress A negative stress that may result in illness.

general adaptation syndrome (GAS) The sequenced physiological response to a stressful situation; consists of three stages: alarm, resistance, and exhaustion.

homeostasis The body's natural state of balance or stability.

adaptive response The body's attempt to reestablish homeostasis or stability.

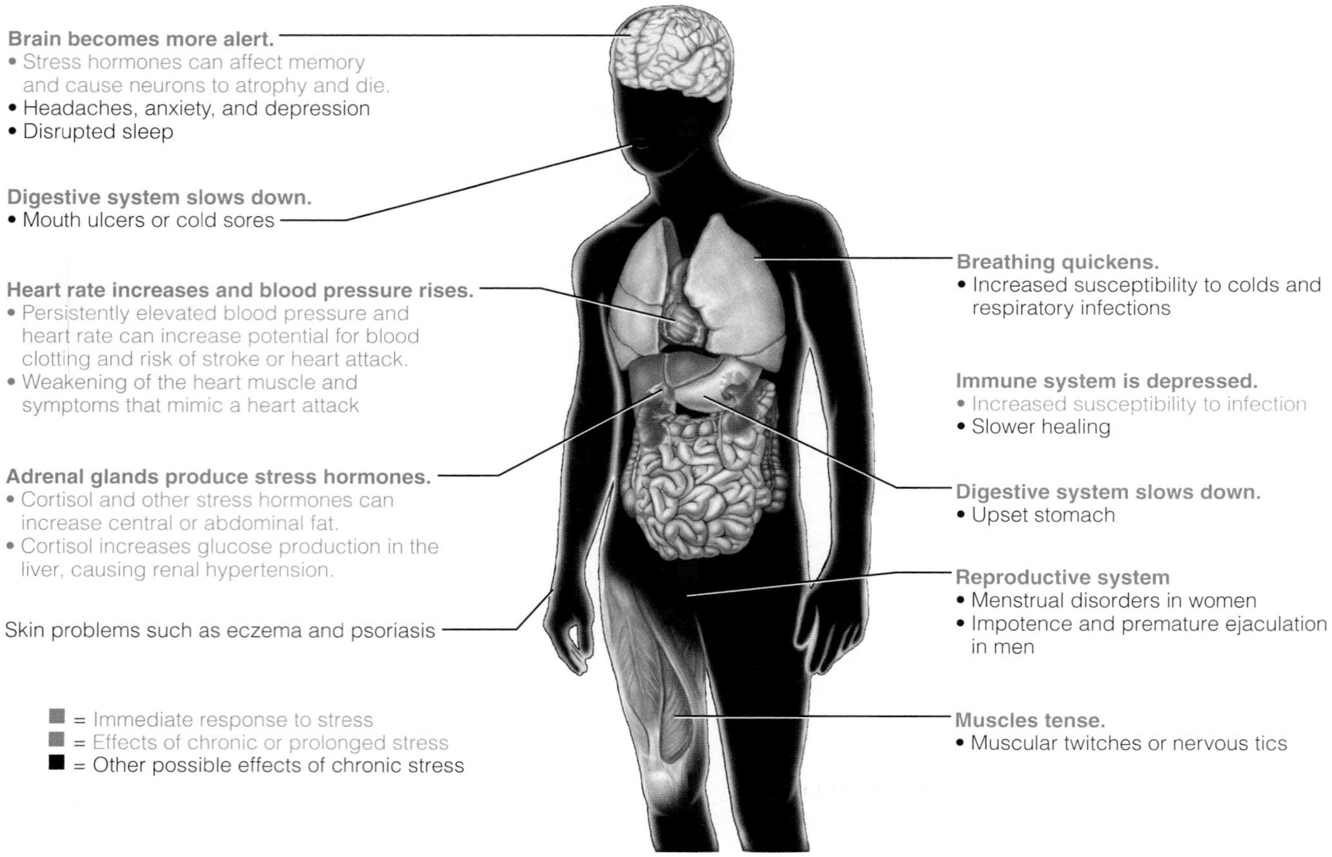
Brain becomes more alert.
• Stress hormones can affect memory and cause neurons to atrophy and die.
• Headaches, anxiety, and depression
• Disrupted sleep
Digestive system slows down.
• Mouth ulcers or cold sores
Heart rate increases and blood pressure rises.
• Persistently elevated blood pressure and heart rate can increase potential for blood clotting and risk of stroke or heart attack.
• Weakening of the heart muscle and symptoms that mimic a heart attack
Adrenal glands produce stress hormones.
• Cortisol and other stress hormones can increase central or abdominal fat.
• Cortisol increases glucose production in the liver, causing renal hypertension.
Skin problems such as eczema and psoriasis
■ = Immediate response to stress
■ = Effects of chronic or prolonged stress
■ = Other possible effects of chronic stress
Breathing quickens.
• Increased susceptibility to colds and respiratory infections
Immune system is depressed.
• Increased susceptibility to infection
• Slower healing
Digestive system slows down.
• Upset stomach
Reproductive system
• Menstrual disorders in women
• Impotence and premature ejaculation in men
Muscles tense.
• Muscular twitches or nervous tics

FIGURE 3-2 The Effects of Stress on the Body

your brain becomes extra alert. Because it's nonessential in a crisis, your digestive system practically shuts down (Figure 3-2).

Cortisol speeds the conversion of proteins and fats into carbohydrates, the body's basic fuel, so we have the energy to fight or flee from a threat. However, stress increases the amount of time required to clear triglycerides, a type of fat linked to heart disease, from the bloodstream.

Cortisol can cause excessive central or abdominal fat, which heightens the risk of diseases such as diabetes, high blood pressure, and stroke. Even slender, premenopausal women faced with increased stress and lacking good coping skills are more likely to accumulate excess weight around their waists, thereby increasing their risk of heart disease and other health problems.

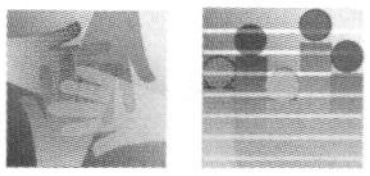

In one study, African-American college students who scored low in coping skills had higher levels of cortisol than those better equipped to cope with stress.[2] Challenges that seem uncontrollable or unpredictable have a greater impact on cortisol than others.

Figure 3-2 illustrates how persistent or repeated increases in the stress hormones can be hazardous throughout the body. In the brain, stress hormones linked to powerful emotions may help create long-lasting memories of events such as Hurricane Katrina, But very prolonged or severe stress can damage the brain's ability to remember and can actually cause brain cells, or neurons, to atrophy and die.

Stress and the Heart

Stress may be the most significant inherited risk factor in people who develop heart disease at a young age. According to behavioral researchers, family transmission of emotional and psychosocial stress, specifically anger in males, greatly increases the likelihood of early heart disease. Young adults whose blood pressure spikes in response to stress may be at risk of hypertension as they get older.

In the 1970s, cardiologists Meyer Friedman, M.D., and Ray Rosenman, M.D., compared their patients to individuals of the same age with healthy hearts and developed two general categories of personality: Type A and Type B. Hardworking, aggressive, and competitive, Type As never have time for all they want to accomplish, even though they usually try to do several tasks at once. Type Bs are more relaxed, though not necessarily less ambitious or successful.

The degree of danger associated with Type-A behavior remains controversial. Of all the personality traits linked with Type-A behavior, the most sinister are anger and chronic hostility. People who are always mistrustful, cynical, and suspicious are twice as likely to suffer blockages of their coronary arteries. Social isolation, depression, and stress may be even stronger risk factors for men.

Stress and Immunity

The immune system is the network of organs, tissues, and white blood cells that defend against disease. Impaired immunity makes the body more susceptible to many diseases, including infections (from the common cold to tuberculosis) and disorders of the immune system itself.

A recent "meta-analysis"—a study of studies in peer-reviewed scientific journals—confirmed earlier findings that stress alters immunity, but the effects differ between short-term and long-term stress. In short-term, stress "revs up" the immune system, a way of preparing for injury or infection. Acute time-limited stressors, the type that produce a "fight-or-flight" response, prompt the immune system to ready itself for the possibility of infections resulting from bites, punctures, or other wounds.

However, long-term, or chronic, stress creates excessive wear and tear, and the system breaks down. Chronic stressors, so profound and persistent that they seem endless and beyond a person's control, suppress immune responses the most. The longer the stress, the more the immune system shifts from potentially adaptive changes to potentially harmful ones, first in cellular immunity and then in broader immune function. Traumatic stress, such as losing a loved one through death or divorce, can impair immunity for as long as a year.

Minor hassles that aren't related to trauma do take a toll. Under exam stress, students experience a dip in immune function and a higher rate of infections. Ohio State University researchers found that during exam periods, there is a significant drop in the immune cells that normally ward off infection and cancer in medical students.

Age and overall health also affect immune response. The immune systems of individuals who are elderly or ill are more vulnerable to acute and chronic stressors, possibly because their bodies find it more difficult to regulate their reactions.

Stress and Digestion

Do you ever get butterflies in your stomach before giving a speech in class or before a big game? The digestive system is, as one psychologist quips, "an important stop on the tension trail." No studies have ever demonstrated that stress alone causes ulcers, but it may make people more vulnerable to infection with *Helicobacter pylori* bacteria, a known culprit in many cases.[3] To avoid problems, pay attention to how you eat. Eating on the run, gulping food, or overeating results in poorly chewed foods, an overworked stomach, and increased abdominal pressure.

Some simple strategies can help you avoid stress-related stomachaches. Many people experience dry mouth or sweat more under stress. By drinking plenty of water, you replenish lost fluids and prevent dehydration. Fiber-rich foods counteract common stress-related problems, such as cramps and constipation. Do not skip meals. If you do, you're more likely to feel fatigued and irritable.

Be wary of overeating under stress. Some people eat more because they scarf down meals too quickly. Others reach for snacks to calm their nerves or comfort themselves.

In a study of college women, higher stress increased the risk of binge eating.[4] Watch out for caffeine. Coffee, tea, and cola drinks can make your strained nerves jangle even more. Also avoid sugary snacks. They'll send your blood sugar levels on a roller coaster ride—up one minute, down the next.

Other Stress Symptoms

The first signs of stress include muscle tightness, tension headaches, backaches, upset stomach, and sleep disruptions (caused by stress-altered brain-wave activity). Some people feel fatigued, their hearts may race or beat faster than usual at rest, and they may feel tense all the time, easily frustrated and often irritable. Others feel sad; lose their energy, appetite, or sex drive; and develop psychological problems, including depression anxiety and panic attacks (Chapter 2).

Hundreds of studies over the last 20 years have shown that stress contributes to approximately 80 percent of all major illnesses: cardiovascular disease, cancer, endocrine and metabolic disease, skin rashes, ulcers, ulcerative colitis, emotional disorders, musculoskeletal disease, infectious ailments, premenstrual syndrome (PMS), uterine fibroid cysts, and breast cysts. As many as 75 to 90 percent of visits to physicians are related to stress.

Stress on Campus

Being a student—full-time or part-time, in your late teens, early twenties, or later in life—can be extremely stressful. You may feel pressure to perform well to qualify for a good job or graduate school. To meet steep tuition payments, you may have to juggle part-time work and coursework. You may feel stressed about choosing a major, getting along with a difficult roommate, passing a particularly hard course, or living up to your parents' and teachers' expectations. If you're an older student, you may have children, housework, and

Student Snapshot
Stressed Out on Campus

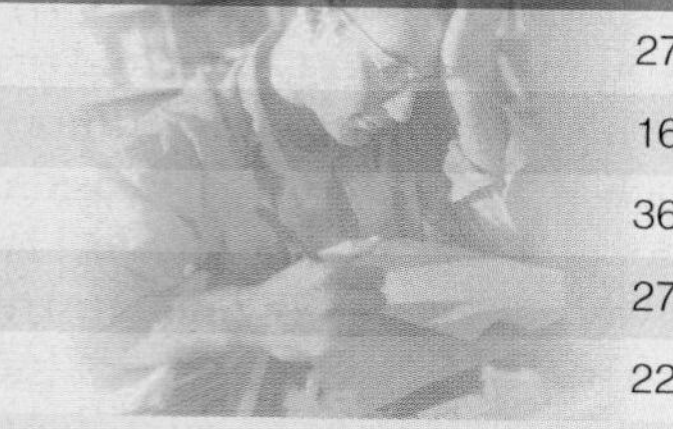

© Purestock/Alamy

Have You Felt Overwhelmed by All You Had to Do?	Percentage of Students
All undergraduates	27%
Men	16%
Women	36%
Four-year colleges	27%
Two-year colleges	22%

Source: Pryor, John, et al. *The American Freshman: National Norms for Fall 2005.* Los Angeles: University of California, Los Angeles Higher Education Research Institute, 2005.

homework to balance. Your days may seem so busy and your life so full that you worry about coming apart at the seams. One thing is for certain: You're not alone. (See Student Snapshot: "Stressed Out on Campus.") According to surveys of students at colleges and universities around the country and the world, stressors are remarkably similar. Among the most common are:

- **Test pressures.**
- **Financial problems.**
- **Frustrations,** such as delays in reaching goals.
- **Problems in friendships** and dating relationships.
- **Daily hassles.**
- **Academic failure.**
- **Pressures** as a result of competition, deadlines, and the like.
- **Changes,** which may be unpleasant, disruptive, or too frequent.
- **Losses,** whether caused by the breakup of a relationship or the death of a loved one.

Many students bring complex psychological problems with them to campus, including learning disabilities and mood disorders like depression and anxiety. "Students arrive with the underpinnings of problems that are brought out by the stress of campus life," says one counselor. Some have grown up in broken homes and bear the scars of family troubles. Others fall into the same patterns of alcohol abuse that they observed for years in their families or suffer lingering emotional scars from childhood physical or sexual abuse.

Students Under Stress

More than a quarter of freshmen feel overwhelmed by all they have to do at the beginning of the academic year; by the year's end, 44 percent feel overwhelmed. In research at three universities, underclassmen were most vulnerable to negative life events, perhaps because they lacked experience in coping with stressful situations. Freshmen had the highest levels of depression; sophomores had the most anger and hostility. Seniors may handle life's challenges better because they have developed better coping mechanisms. In the study, more seniors reported that they faced problems squarely and took action to resolve them, while younger students were more likely to respond passively, for instance, by trying not to let things bother them.

First-generation college students—those whose parents never experienced at least one full year of college—encounter more difficulties with social adjustment than freshmen whose parents attended college. Second-generation students may have several advantages: more knowledge of college life, greater social support, more preparation for college in high school, a greater focus on college activities, and more financial resources.

The percentage of students seeking psychological help because of stress or anxiety has risen dramatically in the last 15 years. Students say they react to stress in various ways: physiologically (by sweating, stuttering, trembling, or developing physical symptoms); emotionally (by becoming anxious, fearful, angry, guilty, or depressed); behaviorally (by crying, eating, smoking, being irritable or abusive); or cognitively (by thinking about and analyzing stressful situations and strategies that might be useful in dealing with them).

A supportive network of friends and family makes a difference. Undergraduates with higher levels of social support and self-efficacy reported feeling less stressed and more satisfied with life than others.

Does stress increase drinking among college students? Many assume so, since life stress is a recognized risk for alcohol use, particularly for people with a family history of alcoholism.[5] The relationship between drinking and stress is more complex. For some, drinking occasions are times to discuss problems with friends, regardless of the day's stress. Students tend to drink more on days when they are feeling good—possibly because of what the researchers call the "celebratory and social" nature of college drinking. Drinking—and positive emotions—peak on weekends. (See Chapter 12 for more on student drinking.)

Campuses are providing more frontline services than they have in the past, including career-guidance workshops, telephone hot lines, and special social programs for lonely, homesick freshmen. Undergraduates, who learn relaxation and stress-reduction techniques report less stress, anxiety, and psychological distress than other students.

? FAQ How Can I Cope with Test Stress?

For many students, midterms and final exams are the most stressful times of the year. Studies at various colleges and universities found that

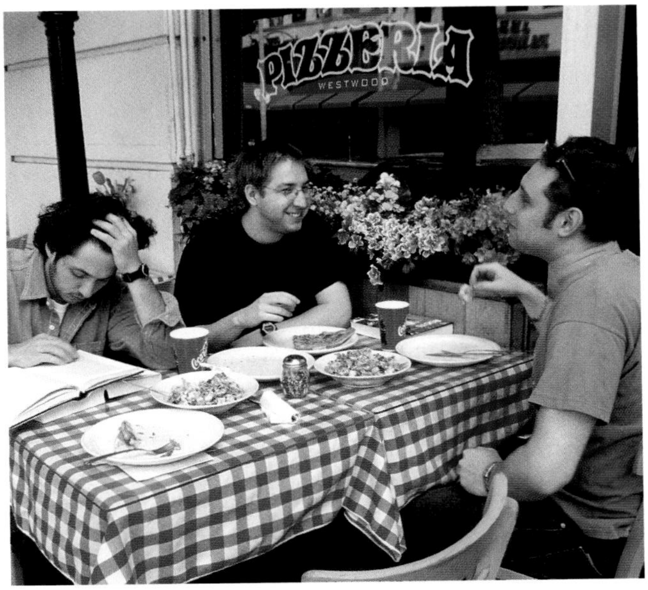

© Bill Aron/PhotoEdit

The first year of college can be overwhelming as you learn your way around the campus, meet new people, and strive to succeed.

the incidence of colds and flu soared during finals. Some students feel the impact of test stress in other ways—headaches, upset stomachs, skin flare-ups, or insomnia.

Because of stress's impact on memory, students with advanced skills may perform worse under exam pressure than their less skilled peers. Sometimes students become so preoccupied with the possibility of failing that they can't concentrate on studying. Others, including many of the best and brightest students, freeze up during tests and can't comprehend multiple-choice questions or write essay answers, even if they know the material.

The students most susceptible to exam stress are those who believe they'll do poorly and who see tests as extremely threatening. Unfortunately, such negative thoughts often become a self-fulfilling prophecy. As they study, these students keep wondering: What good will studying do? I never do well on tests. As their fear increases, they try harder, pulling all-nighters. Fueled by caffeine, munching on sugary snacks, they become edgy and find it harder and harder to concentrate. By the time of the test, they're nervous wrecks, scarcely able to sit still and focus on the exam.

Can you do anything to reduce test stress and feel more in control? Absolutely. One way is to defuse stress through relaxation. Students taught relaxation techniques—such as controlled breathing, meditation, progressive relaxation, and guided imagery (visualization)—a month before finals tend to have higher levels of immune cells during the exam period and feel in better control during their tests.

Minorities Under Stress

Regardless of your race or ethnic background, college may bring culture shock. You may never have encountered such a degree of diversity in one setting. You probably will meet students with different values, unfamiliar customs, entirely new ways of looking at the world—experiences you may find both stimulating and stressful.

Mental health professionals have long assumed that minority students may feel a double burden of stress. Many undergraduates experience emotional difficulties (see Chapter 2), and researchers have theorized that students from a racial or ethnic minority would be especially likely to develop psychological symptoms, such as anger, anxiety, and depression, as a result of increased stress.

Strategies for Prevention — Defusing Test Stress

- **Plan ahead.** A month before finals, map out a study schedule for each course. Set aside a small amount of time every day or every other day to review the course materials.
- **Be positive.** Picture yourself taking your final exam. Imagine yourself walking into the exam room feeling confident, opening up the test booklet, and seeing questions for which you know the answers.
- **Take regular breaks.** Get up from your desk, breathe deeply, stretch, and visualize a pleasant scene. You'll feel more refreshed than you would if you chugged another cup of coffee.
- **Practice.** Some teachers are willing to give practice finals to prepare students for test situations, or you and your friends can test each other.
- **Talk to other students.** Chances are that many of them share your fears about test taking and may have discovered some helpful techniques of their own. Sometimes talking to your adviser or a counselor can also help.
- **Be satisfied with doing your best.** You can't expect to ace every test; all you can and should expect is your best effort. Once you've completed the exam, allow yourself the sweet pleasure of relief that it's over.

Racism has indeed been shown to be a source of stress that can affect health and well-being. In the past, some African-American students have described predominately white campuses as hostile, alienating, and socially isolating and have reported greater estrangement from the campus community and heightened estrangement in interactions with faculty and peers. However, the generalization that all minority students are more stressed may not be valid.

"Diversity, in and of itself, is unlikely to be related to higher levels of reported psychological symptoms on campus," researchers concluded in one study, theorizing that minority students "may have developed strengths while growing up within their particular cultures, subcommunities, and families that have often gone unrecognized or unnoted. And some coping mechanisms, especially spirituality, can buffer the negative effects of racism.

All minority students do share some common stressors. In one study of minority freshmen entering a large, competitive university, Asian, Filipino, African-American, and Native American students all felt more sensitive and vulnerable to the college social climate, to interpersonal tensions between themselves and nonminority students and faculty, to experiences of actual or perceived racism, and to racist attitudes and discrimination (discussed later in this chapter). Despite scoring above the national average on the SAT, the minority students in this study did not feel accepted as legitimate students and sensed that others viewed them as unworthy beneficiaries of affirmative action initiatives. While most said that overt racism was rare and relatively easy to deal with, they reported subtle pressures that undermined their academic confidence and their ability to bond with the university. Balancing these stressors, however, was a strong sense of ethnic identity, which helped buffer some stressful effects.

Hispanic students have identified three major types of stressors in their college experiences: academic (related to exam preparation and faculty interaction, social (related to ethnicity and interpersonal competence), and financial (related to their economic situation). Some Asian students who recently immigrated to the United States report feeling ostracized by students of similar ancestry who are second- or third-generation Americans. While they take pride in being truly bicultural and bilingual, the newcomers feel ambivalent about mainstream American culture. "My parents stress the importance of traditions; my friends tell me to get with it and act like an American," says one Asian-born student who has spent five years in the United States. "I feel trapped between cultures."

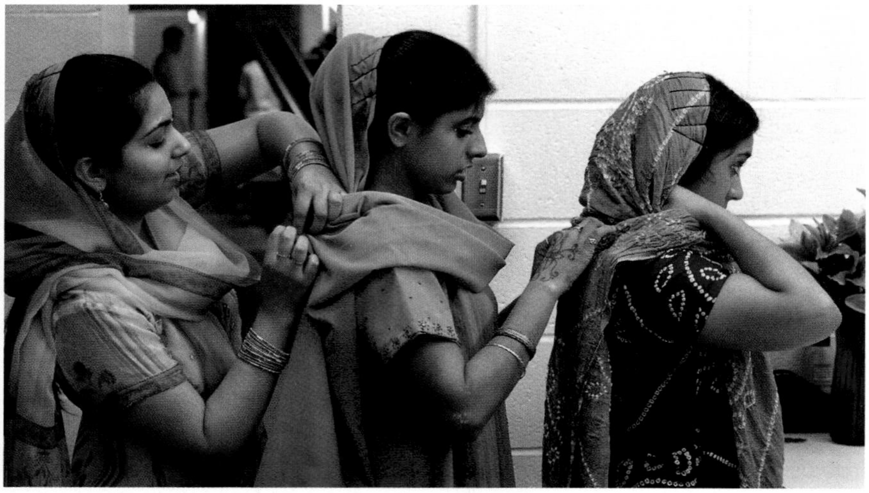

Campus clubs and organizations provide an opportunity for individuals from different ethnic backgrounds to celebrate their culture and educate others about it. These undergraduates are preparing to perform an Indian dance at a special evening sponsored by Asian Students in America.

Men, Women, and Stress

Women, who make up 56 percent of today's college students, also shoulder the majority of the stress load. In a nationwide survey of students in the class of 2009, more women (36 percent) described themselves as "overwhelmed by all I have to do," compared with just 16 percent of men. More women than men reported feeling depressed, insecure about their physical and mental health, and worried about paying for college. More men than women considered themselves above average or in the top 10 percent of people their age in terms of emotional health.[6]

The immune and hormonal systems of men and women may respond differently to stressors.[7] Gender differences in lifestyle also explain why women feel so stressed. College men, the survey revealed, spend significantly more time doing things that are fun and relaxing: exercising, partying, watching TV, and playing video games. Women, on the other hand, tend to study more, do more volunteer work, and handle more household and childcare chores.

Where can stressed-out college women turn for support? The best source, according to University of California research, is other women. In general, the social support women offer their friends and relatives seems more effective in reducing the blood-pressure response to stress than that provided by men.

At all ages, women and men tend to respond to stress differently. While males (human and those of other species) react with the classic fight-or-flight response, females under attack try to protect their children and seek help from other females—a strategy dubbed *tend and befriend*. When exposed to experimental stress (such as a loud, harsh noise), women show more affection for friends and relatives; men show less. When working mothers studied by psychologists had a bad day, they coped by concentrating on their children when they got home. Stressed-out fathers were more likely to withdraw.

Other Personal Stressors

At every stage of life, you will encounter challenges and stressors. Among the most common are those related to anger, work, and illness.

? FAQ Why is Everyone So Angry?

In recent years, violent aggressive driving—which some dub *road rage*—has exploded. Sideline rage at amateur and professional sporting events has become so widespread that a Pennsylvania midget football game ended in a brawl involving more than 100 coaches, players, parents, and fans.

No one seems immune. Women fly off the handle just as often as men, although they're less likely to get physical. The young and the infamous, including several rappers and musicians sentenced to anger management classes for violent outbursts, may seem more volatile. However, ordinary senior citizens have erupted into "line rage" and pushed ahead of others simply because they feel they've "waited long enough" in their lives.

"Everyone everywhere seems to be hotter under the collar these days," observes Sybil Evans, a conflict resolution expert who singles out three primary culprits: time, technology, and tension. "Americans are working longer hours than anyone else in the world. The cell phones and pagers that were supposed to make our lives easier have put us on call 24–7–365. Since we're always running, we're tense and low on patience, and the less patience we have, the less we monitor what we say to people and how we treat them."[8]

Job Stress

More so than ever, many people find that they are working more and enjoying it less. Many people, including working parents, spend 55 to 60 hours a week on the job. More people are caught up in an exhausting cycle of overwork, which causes stress, which makes work harder, which leads to more stress. Even the workplace itself can contribute to stress. A noisy, open-office environment can increase levels of stress without workers realizing it.

Yet work in itself is not hazardous to health. Attitudes about work and habits related to how we work are the true threats. In fact, a job—stressful or not, enjoyable or not—can be therapeutic.

Illness and Disability

Just as the mind can have profound effects on the body, the body can have an enormous impact on our emotions. Whenever we come down with the flu or pull a muscle, we feel under par. When the problem is more serious or persistent—a chronic disease like diabetes, for

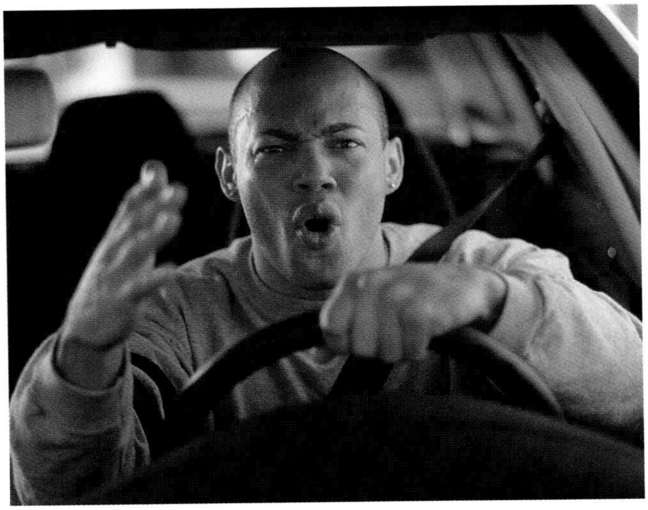

© Anthony Redpath/CORBIS

How you manage your anger has consequences for your health and for your interactions with others.

Strategies for Change — How to Deal with an Angry Person

- **Become an impartial observer.** Act as if you were watching someone else's two-year-old have a temper tantrum at the supermarket.
- **Stay calm.** Letting your emotions loose only adds fuel to fury. Talk quietly and slowly; let the person know you understand that he or she is angry.
- **Refuse to engage.** Step back to avoid invading his or her space. Retreat farther if need be until the person is back in control.
- **Find something to agree with.** Look for common ground, if only to acknowledge that you're both in a difficult situation.

instance, or a lifelong hearing impairment—the emotional stress of constantly coping with it is even greater.

A common source of stress for college students is a learning disability, which may affect one of every ten Americans. Most learning-disabled students have average or above-average intelligence, but they rarely live up to their ability in school. Some have only one area of difficulty, such as reading or math. Others have problems with attention, writing, communicating, reasoning, coordination, and social skills.

Not all students with learning disabilities experience greater stress. In one in-depth study comparing undergraduates with and without learning disabilities, the learning-disabled (LD) students reported significantly fewer college stressors and demonstrated a higher need for achievement. The LD students also scored significantly higher in resiliency and initiative in solving problems and working toward goals.

Societal Stressors

Centuries ago the poet John Donne observed that no man is an island. Today, on an increasingly crowded and troubled planet, these words seem truer than ever. Problems such as discrimination and terrorism can no longer be viewed only as economic or political issues. Directly or indirectly, they affect the well-being of all who inhabit the Earth—now and in the future.

The deliberate use of physical force to abuse or injure is a leading killer of young people in the United States—and a potential source of stress in all our lives. Even a single childhood trauma increases the likelihood that college students may engage in risky behaviors.[9] If you or someone you know has been a victim of a violent crime, a sense of vulnerability may add to the stress of daily living.

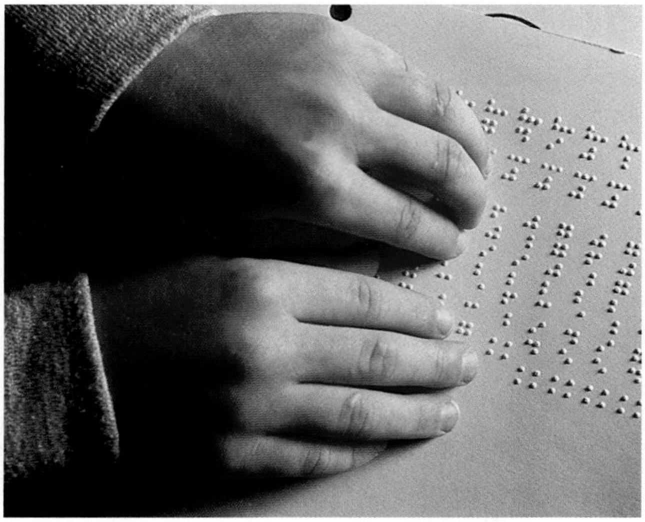

A blind college student has unique challenges and stressors that sighted students do not.

Americans often deal with stress in ways that can damage their physical and mental health, according to a recent survey conducted by the American Psychological Association. One in four turns to food for comfort. Individuals who describe themselves as "very concerned" about stress also are more likely to smoke and not exercise.[10]

Discrimination

Discrimination can take many forms—some as subtle as not being included in a conversation or joke, some as blatant as threats scrawled on a wall, some as violent as brutal beatings and other hate crimes. Because it can be hard to deal with individually, discrimination is a particularly sinister form of stress. By banding together, however, those who experience discrimination can take action to protect themselves, challenge the ignorance and hateful assumptions that fuel bigotry, and promote a healthier environment for all.

In the last decade, there have been reports of increased intolerance among young people and greater tolerance of expressions and acts of hate on college campuses. To counteract this trend, many schools have set up programs and classes to educate students about each other's backgrounds and to acknowledge and celebrate the richness diversity brings to campus life. Educators have called on universities to make campuses less alienating and more culturally and emotionally accessible, with programs and policies targeted not only at minority students but also at the university as a whole.

YOUR LIFE COACH

Coping with Stress

The key to coping with stress is realizing that your *perception* of and *response* to a stressor are crucial. Changing the way you interpret events or situations—a skill called *reframing*—makes all the difference. An event, such as a move to a new city, is not stressful in itself. A move becomes stressful if you see it as a traumatic upheaval rather than an exciting beginning of a new chapter in your life.

In times of stress, the following simple exercises can stop the stress buildup inside your body and help you regain a sense of calm and control.

- **Breathing.** Deep breathing relaxes the body and quiets the mind. Draw air deeply into your lungs, allowing your chest to fill with air and your belly to rise and fall. You will feel the muscle tension and stress begin to melt away. When you're feeling extremely stressed, try this calming breath: Sit or lie with your back straight and place the tip of your tongue on the roof of your mouth behind your teeth. Exhale completely through the mouth, then inhale through the nose for 4 seconds. Hold the breath for 7 seconds, then exhale audibly through the mouth for 8 seconds. Repeat four times.

- **Refocusing.** Thinking about a situation you can't change or control only increases the stress you feel. Force your mind to focus on other subjects. If you're stuck in a long line, distract yourself. Check out what other people are buying or imagine what they do for a living. Imagine that you're in a hot shower and a wave of relaxation is washing your stress down the drain.
- **Serenity breaks.** Build moments of tranquility into your day. For instance, while waiting for your computer to start up or a file to download, look at a photograph of someone you love or a poster of a tropical island. If none is available, close your eyes and visualize a soothing scene, such as walking in a meadow or along a beach.
- **Stress signals.** Learn to recognize the first signs that your stress load is getting out of hand: Is your back bothering you? Do you have a headache? Do you find yourself speeding or misplacing things? Whenever you spot these early warnings, force yourself to stop and say, I'm under stress. I need to do something about it.
- **Reality checks.** To put things into proper perspective, ask yourself: Will I remember what's made me so upset a month from now? If I had to rank this problem on a scale of 1 to 10, with worldwide catastrophe as 10, where would it rate?
- **Stress inoculation.** Rehearse everyday situations that you find stressful, such as speaking in class. Think of how you might make the situation less tense, for instance, by breathing deeply before you talk or jotting down notes beforehand. Think of these small "doses" of stress as the psychological equivalent of allergy shots: They immunize you so you feel less stressed when bigger challenges come along.
- **Rx: Laughter.** Humor counters stress by focusing on comic aspects of difficult situations and may, as various studies have shown, lessen harmful effects on the immune system and overall health. However, humor may have different effects on stress in men and women.

  In a study of undergraduates, humor buffered stress-related physical symptoms in men and women. However, it reduced stress-linked anxiety only in men. The researchers theorized that men may prefer humor as a more appropriate way of expressing emotions such as anxiety, whereas women are more likely to use self-disclosure, that is, to confide in friends.
- **Spiritual coping.** Saying a prayer under stress is one of the oldest and most effective ways of calming yourself. Other forms of spiritual coping, such as putting trust in God and doing for others (for instance, by volunteering at a shelter for battered women) also can provide a different perspective on daily hassles and stresses.
- **Sublimation.** This term refers to the redirection of any drives considered unacceptable into socially acceptable channels. Outdoor activity is one of the best ways to reduce stress through sublimation. For instance, if you're furious with a friend who betrayed your trust or frustrated because your boss rejects all of your proposals, you might go for a long run or hike to sublimate your anger.

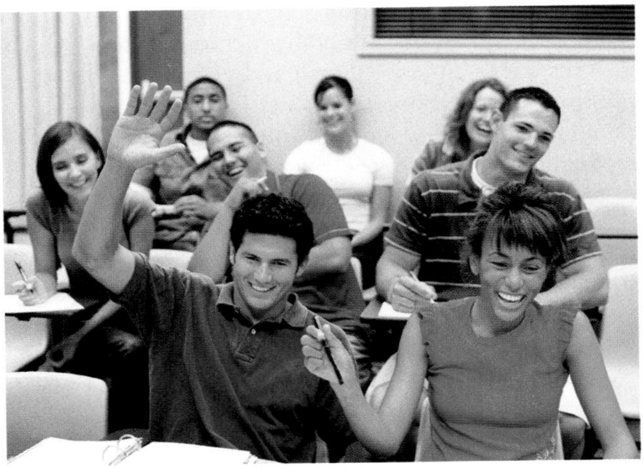

© BananaStock/Alamy

Shared laughter is a powerful antidote to stress.

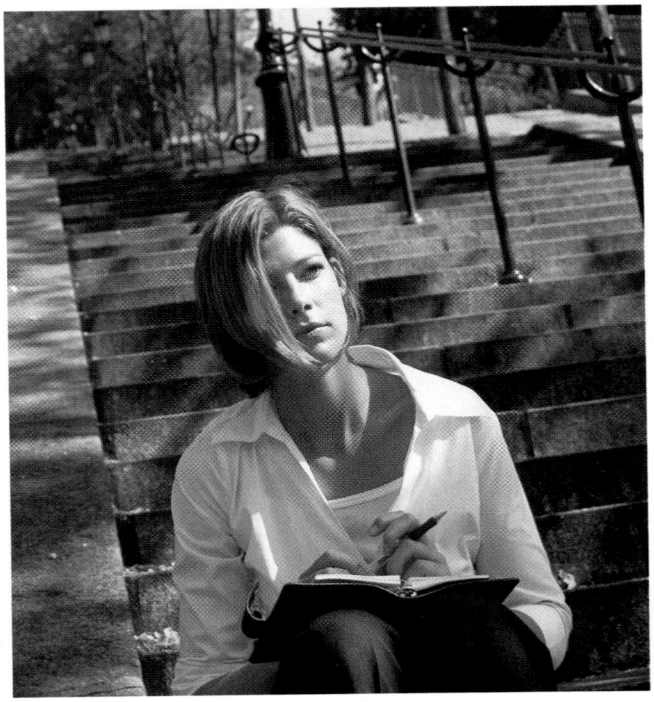

© Min Roman/Masterfile

Writing in your journal about feelings and difficulties is a simple and effective way to help control your stress. You don't need to be a journalist. Just write about *you*.

- **Exercise.** Regular physical activity can relieve stress, boost energy, lift mood, and keep stress under control. Young adults who adopt and continue regular aerobic exercise show less intense cardiovascular responses to stress, which may protect them against coronary heart disease as they age. Strength training may have similar benefits. In one study, college students who engaged in an eight-week weight training reported lower stress levels than those who participated in an aerobic dance program.
- **Journaling.** One of the simplest, yet most effective, ways to work through stress is by putting your feelings into words that only you will read. The more honest and open you are as you write, the better. College students who wrote in their journals about traumatic events felt much better afterward than those who wrote about superficial topics. Focus on intense emotional experiences and "autopsy" them to try to understand why they affected you the way they did. Rereading and thinking about your notes may reveal the underlying reasons for your response.

Defense Mechanisms

Sometimes we respond to stress or challenge with self-destructive behaviors, such as drinking or using drugs. These responses can lead to psychological problems, such as anxiety or depression, and physical problems, including psychosomatic illnesses.

Defense mechanisms, such as those described in Table 3-1, are another response to stress. These psychological devices are mental processes that help us cope with personal problems. Such responses also are not the answer to stress—and learning to recognize them in yourself will enable you to deal with your stress in a healthier way.

TABLE 3-1 Common Defense Mechanisms Used to Alleviate Anxiety and Eliminate Conflict

Defense Mechanism	Example
Denial: the refusal to accept a painful reality.	You don't accept as true the news that a loved one is seriously ill.
Displacement: the redirection of feelings from their true object to a more acceptable or safer substitute.	Instead of lashing out at a coach or a teacher, you snap at your best friend.
Projection: the attribution of unacceptable feelings or impulses to someone else.	When you want to end a relationship, you project your unhappiness onto your partner.
Rationalization: the substitution of "good," acceptable reasons for the real motivations for our behavior.	You report a classmate who has been mean to you for cheating on an exam and explain that cheating is unfair to other students.
Reaction formation: adopting attitudes and behaviors that are the opposite of what you feel.	You lavishly compliment an acquaintance whom you really despise.
Repression: the way we keep threatening impulses, fantasies, memories, feelings, or wishes from becoming conscious.	You don't "hear" the alarm after a late night, or you "forget" to take out the trash.

? FAQ What Can Help Me Relax?

Relaxation is the physical and mental state opposite that of stress. Rather than gearing up for fight or flight, our bodies and minds grow calmer and work more smoothly. We're less likely to become frazzled and more capable of staying in control. The most effective relaxation techniques include progressive relaxation, visualization, meditation, mindfulness, and biofeedback.

Progressive relaxation works by intentionally increasing and then decreasing tension in the muscles. While sitting or lying down in a quiet, comfortable setting, you tense and release various muscles, beginning with those of the hand, for instance, and then proceeding to the arms, shoulders, neck, face, scalp, chest, stomach, buttocks, genitals, and so on, down each leg to the toes. Relaxing the muscles can quiet the mind and restore internal balance.

Visualization, or **guided imagery,** involves creating mental pictures that calm you down and focus your mind. Some people use this technique to promote healing when they are ill. Visualization skills require practice and, in some cases, instruction by qualified health professionals.[11]

Meditation has been practiced in many forms over the ages, from the yogic techniques of the Far East to the Quaker silence of more modern times. Brain scans have shown that meditation activates the sections of the brain in charge of the autonomic nervous system, which governs bodily functions, such as digestion and blood pressure, that we cannot consciously control.[12] Although many studies have documented the benefits of meditation for overall health, it may be particularly helpful for people dealing with stress-related medical conditions such as high blood pressure.

Meditation helps a person reach a state of relaxation, but with the goal of achieving inner peace and harmony. There is no one right way to meditate, and many people have discovered how to meditate on their own, without even knowing what it is they are doing. Increasing numbers of college students are turning to meditation as a way of coping with stress[13] (see "You Decide"). Most forms of meditation have common elements: sitting quietly for

SAVVY CONSUMER

Can Stress-Relief Products Help?

You're stressed out, and you see an ad for a product—an oil, candle, cream, herbal tea, pill, or potion—that promises to make all your cares disappear. Should you soak in an aromatic bath, have a massage, try kava, squeeze foam balls? In most cases, you're probably not doing yourself much harm, but you aren't necessarily doing yourself much good either. Keep these considerations in mind:

- Be wary of instant cures. Regardless of the promises on the label, it's unrealistic to expect any magic ingredient or product to make all your problems disappear.
- Focus on stress-reducing behavior, rather than a product. An aromatic candle may not bring instant serenity, but if you light a candle and meditate, you may indeed feel more at peace. A scented pillow may not be a cure for stress, but if it helps you get a good night's sleep, you'll cope better the next day.
- Experiment with physical ways to work out stress. Exercise is one of the best ways to lower your stress levels. Try walking, running, swimming, cycling, kickboxing—anything physical that helps you release tension.
- Don't make matters worse by smoking (the chemicals in cigarettes increase heart rate, blood pressure, and stress hormones), consuming too much caffeine (it speeds up your system for hours), eating snacks high in sugar (it produces a quick high followed by a sudden slump), or turning to drugs or alcohol (they can only add to your stress when their effects wear off).
- Be cautious when trying "alternative" products. "Natural" products, such as herbs and enzymes, claim to have psychological effects. However, because they are not classified as drugs, these products have not undergone the rigorous scientific testing required of psychiatric medications, and little is known about their safety or efficacy. "Natural" doesn't mean risk-free. Opium and cocaine are "natural" substances that have dramatic and potentially deadly effects on the mind.

15 to 20 minutes once or twice a day, concentrating on a word or image, and breathing slowly and rhythmically. If you wish to try meditation, it often helps to have someone guide you through your first sessions. Or try tape recording your own voice (with or without favorite music in the background) and playing it back to yourself, freeing yourself to concentrate on the goal of turning the attention within.

An increasing number of colleges are offering courses on mindfulness, meditation, contemplative studies, and neurotheology (an exploration of how the brain functions during spiritual practices). Some universities offer an entire menu of mind-body programs, including yoga and mindfulness, through their counseling services. Can such courses help students handle the stresses of college life? Or do students have to develop their own unique set of coping skills?

You Decide

Mindfulness is a modern form of an ancient Asian technique that involves maintaining awareness in the present moment. You tune in to each part of your body, scanning from head to toe, noting the slightest sensation. You allow whatever you experience—an itch, an ache, a feeling of warmth—to enter your awareness. Then you open yourself to focus on all the thoughts, sensations, sounds, and feelings that enter your awareness. Mindfulness keeps you in the here and now, thinking about what is rather than about *what if* or *if only*.

Biofeedback is a method of obtaining feedback, or information, about some physiological activity occurring

defense mechanism A psychological process that alleviates anxiety and eliminates mental conflict; includes denial, displacement, projection, rationalization, reaction formation, and repression.

progressive relaxation A method of reducing muscle tension by contracting, then relaxing, certain areas of the body.

visualization, or **guided imagery** An approach to stress control, self-healing, or motivating life changes by means of seeing oneself in the state of calmness, wellness, or change.

meditation A group of approaches that use quiet sitting, breathing techniques, and/or chanting to relax, improve concentration, and become attuned to one's inner self.

mindfulness A method of stress reduction that involves experiencing the physical and mental sensations of the present moment.

biofeedback A technique of becoming aware, with the aid of external monitoring devices, of internal physiological activities in order to develop the capability of altering them.

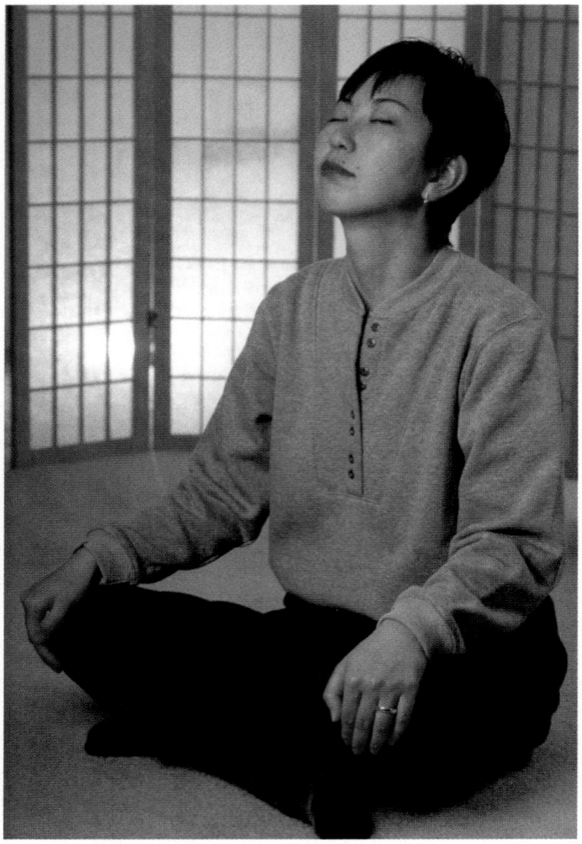

© Gary Conner/PhotoEdit

Meditation calms both mind and spirit. Sit quietly for 15 minutes and concentrate on your breath. Imagine a candle flame. Any distracting thought is a breeze that causes it to flicker.

in the body. An electronic monitoring device attached to the body detects a change in an internal function and communicates it back to the person through a tone, light, or meter. By paying attention to this feedback, most people can gain some control over functions previously thought to be beyond conscious control, such as body temperature, heart rate, muscle tension, and brain waves. Biofeedback training consists of three stages:

1. Developing increased awareness of a body state or function.
2. Gaining control over it.
3. Transferring this control to everyday living without use of the electronic instrument.

The goal of biofeedback for stress reduction is a state of tranquility, usually associated with the brain's production of alpha waves (which are slower and more regular than normal waking waves). After several training sessions, most people can produce alpha waves more or less at will.

Stress and Psychological Health

Traumatic events (such as a robbery, assault, or sudden death of a loved one) always take a toll on an individual, and it's normal to feel sad, tense, overwhelmed, angry, or incapable of coping with the ordinary demands of daily living. Usually such feelings and behaviors subside with time. The stressful event fades into the past, and those whose lives it has touched adapt to its lasting impact. But sometimes individuals remain extremely distressed and unable to function as they once did. While the majority of individuals who survive a trauma recover, at least a quarter of such individuals later develop serious psychological symptoms.

Posttraumatic Stress Disorder (PTSD)

In the past, **posttraumatic stress disorder (PTSD)** was viewed as a psychological response to out-of-the-ordinary stressors, such as captivity or combat. However, other experiences can also forever change the way people view themselves and their world. Thousands of individuals experience or witness traumatic events, such as fires or floods. PTSD is widespread, although often not recognized, in inner-city African-American communities.[14] Children, in particular, are likely to develop PTSD symptoms when they live through a traumatic event or witness a loved one or friend being assaulted.

According to research, almost half of car accident victims may develop PTSD. Individuals who were

Strategies for Change — *"Mini-Relaxation"*

Here is a quick deep-breathing exercise from Harvard psychologist Alice Domar:

- Sit upright or lie on your back.
- Place your hand just beneath your navel so you can feel the rise and fall of your belly as you breathe deeply through your nose.
- As you inhale, count slowly, saying to yourself, "one, two, three, four." Exhale slowly, counting back down from four to one.
- Do this for one minute or longer.

Strategies for Prevention — Recognize the Warning Signals of Stress Overload

- Experiencing physical symptoms, including chronic fatigue, headaches, indigestion, diarrhea, and sleep problems.
- Having frequent illness or worrying about illness.
- Self-medicating, including nonprescription drugs.
- Having problems concentrating on studies or work.
- Feeling irritable, anxious, or apathetic.
- Working or studying longer and harder than usual.
- Exaggerating, to yourself and others, the importance of what you do.
- Becoming accident-prone.
- Breaking rules, whether it's a curfew at home or a speed limit on the highway.
- Going to extremes, such as drinking too much, overspending, or gambling.

seriously injured are especially vulnerable. The main symptoms are re-experiencing the traumatic event, avoiding the site of the accident, refraining from driving in weather and road conditions similar to those on the day of the accident, and feeling a general increase in distress.[15]

In PTSD, individuals re-experience their terror and helplessness again and again in their dreams or intrusive thoughts. To avoid this psychic pain, they may try to avoid anything associated with the trauma. Some enter a state of emotional numbness and no longer can respond to people and experiences the way they once did, especially when it comes to showing tenderness or affection. Those who've been mugged or raped may be afraid to venture out by themselves.

The sooner trauma survivors receive psychological help, the better they are likely to fare. Often talking about what happened with an empathic person or someone who's shared the experience as soon as possible—preferably before going to sleep on the day of the event—can help an individual begin to deal with what has occurred. Group sessions, ideally beginning soon after the trauma, allow individuals to share views and experiences. Behavioral, cognitive, and psychodynamic therapy sometimes along with psychiatric medication, (described in Chapter 2) can help individuals suffering PTSD.[16]

Resilience

Adversity—whether in the form of a traumatic event or chronic stress—has different effects on individuals. Some people never recover and continue on a downward slide that may ultimately prove fatal. Others return, though at different rates, to their prior level of functioning. In recent years researchers have focused their attention on a particularly intriguing group: those people who not only survive stressful experiences but also thrive, that is, who actually surpass their previous level of functioning.[17]

Resilience can take many forms. A father whose child is kidnapped and killed may become a nationwide advocate for victims' rights. A student whose roommate dies in a car crash after a party may campaign for tougher laws against drunk driving. A couple whose premature baby spends weeks in a neonatal intensive care unit may find that their marriage has grown closer and stronger. Even though their experiences were painful, the individuals often look back at them as bringing positive changes into their lives.

Researchers have studied various factors that enable individuals to thrive in the face of adversity. These include:

- **An optimistic attitude.** Rather than reacting to a stressor simply as a threat, these men and women view stress as a challenge—one they believe they can and will overcome. Researchers have documented that individuals facing various stressors, including serious illness and bereavement, are more likely to report experiencing growth if they have high levels of hope and optimism.
- **Self-efficacy.** A sense of being in control of one's life can boost health, even in times of great stress.
- **Stress inoculation.** People who deal well with adversity often have had previous experiences with stress that toughened them in various ways, such as teaching them skills that enhanced their ability to cope and boosting their confidence in their ability to weather a rough patch.
- **Secure personal relationships.** Individuals who know they can count on the support of their loved ones are more likely to be resilient.
- **Spirituality or religiousness.** Religious coping may be particularly related to growth and resilience. In particular, two types seem most beneficial: spiritually based religious coping (receiving emotional reassurance and guidance from God)

posttraumatic stress disorder (PTSD) The repeated reliving of a trauma through nightmares or recollection.

and good-deeds coping (living a better, more spiritual life that includes altruistic acts).

Resilience sometimes means developing new skills simply because, in order to get through the stressful experience, people had to learn something they hadn't known how to do before—for instance, wrangling with insurance companies or other bureaucracies. By mastering such skills, they become more fit to deal with an unpredictable world and develop new flexibility in facing the unknown.

Along with new abilities comes the psychological sense of mastery. "I survived this," an individual may say. "I'll be able to deal with other hard things in the future." Such confidence keeps people actively engaged in the effort to cope and is itself a predictor of eventual success. Stress also can make individuals more aware of the fulfilling aspects of life, and they may become more interested in spiritual pursuits. Certain kinds of stressful experiences also have social consequences. If a person experiencing a traumatic event finds that the significant others in his or her life can be counted on, the result can be a strengthening of their relationship.

Organizing Your Time

We live in what some sociologists call hyperculture, a society that moves at warp speed. Information bombards us constantly. The rate of change seems to accelerate every year. Our "time-saving" devices—pagers, cell phones, modems, faxes, palm-sized organizers, laptop computers—have simply extended the boundaries of where and how we work.

As a result, more and more people are suffering from "timesickness," a nerve-racking feeling that life has become little more than an endless to-do list. The best antidote is time management, and hundreds of books, seminars, and experts offer training in making the most of the hours in the day. Yet these well-intentioned methods often fail, and sooner or later most of us find ourselves caught in a time trap.

Poor Time Management

Every day you make dozens of decisions, and the choices you make about how to use your time directly affect your stress level. If you have a big test on Monday and a term paper due Tuesday, you may plan to study all weekend. Then, when you're invited to a party Saturday night, you go. Although you set the alarm for 7:00 a.m. on Sunday, you don't pull yourself out of bed until noon. By the time you start studying, it's 4:00 p.m., and anxiety is building inside you.

How can you tell if you've lost control of your time? The following are telltale symptoms of poor time management:

- **Rushing.**
- **Chronic inability to make choices or decisions.**
- **Fatigue or listlessness.**
- **Constantly missed deadlines.**
- **Not enough time for rest** or personal relationships.
- **A sense of being overwhelmed** by demands and details and having to do what you don't want to do most of the time.

One of the hard lessons of being on your own is that your choices and your actions have consequences. Stress is just one of them. But by thinking ahead, being realistic about your workload, and sticking to your plans, you can gain better control over your time and your stress levels.

? FAQ How Can I Better Manage My Time?

Time management involves skills that anyone can learn, but they require commitment and practice to make a difference in your life. It may help to know the techniques that other students have found most useful:

- **Schedule your time.** Use a calendar or planner. Beginning the first week of class, mark down deadlines for each assignment, paper, project, and test scheduled that semester. Develop a daily schedule, listing very specifically what you will do the next day, along with the times. Block out times for working out, eating dinner, calling home, and talking with friends as well as for studying.
- **Develop a game plan.** Allow at least two nights to study for any major exam. Set aside more time for

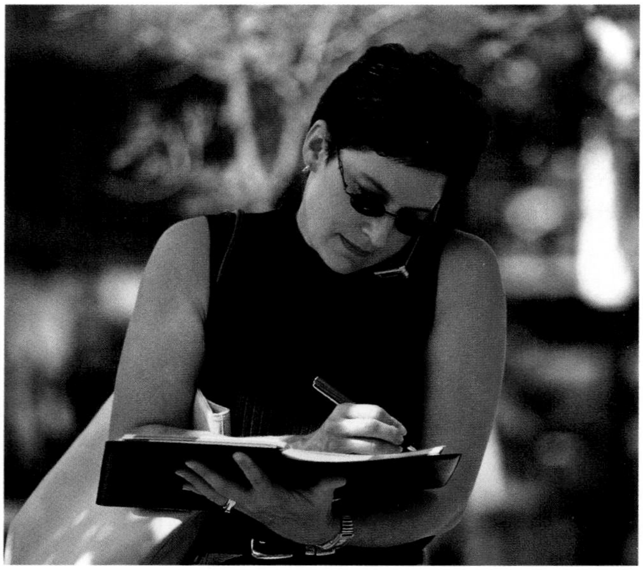

© Creatas Images/Jupiter Images

A calendar or planner is an important tool in time management. You can use it to keep track of assignment due dates, class meetings, and other "to do's."

researching and writing papers. Make sure to allow time to revise and print out a paper—and to deal with emergencies like a computer breakdown. Set daily and weekly goals for every class. When working on a big project, don't neglect your other courses. Whenever possible, try to work ahead in all your classes.

- **Identify time robbers.** For several days keep a log of what you do and how much time you spend doing it. You may discover that disorganization is eating away at your time or that you have a problem getting started. (See the following section on "Overcoming Procrastination.")
- **Make the most of classes.** Read the assignments before class rather than waiting until just before you have a test. By reading ahead of time, you'll make it easier to understand the lectures. Go to class yourself. Your own notes will be more helpful than a friend's or those from a note-taking service. Read your lecture notes at the end of each day or at least at the end of each week.
- **Develop an efficient study style.** Some experts recommend studying for 50 minutes, then breaking for 10 minutes. Small incentives, such as allowing yourself to call or visit a friend during these 10 minutes, can provide the motivation to keep you at the books longer. When you're reading, don't just highlight passages. Instead, write notes or questions to yourself in the margins, which will help you retain more information. Even if you're racing to start a paper, take a few extra minutes to prepare a workable outline. It will be easier to structure your paper when you start writing.
- **Focus on the task at hand.** Rather than worrying about how you did on yesterday's test or how you'll ever finish next week's project, focus intently on whatever you're doing at any given moment. If your mind starts to wander, use any distraction—the sound of the phone ringing or a noise from the hall—as a reminder to stay in the moment.
- **Turn elephants into hors d'oeuvres.** Cut a huge task into smaller chunks so it seems less enormous. For instance, break down your term paper into a series of steps, such as selecting a topic, identifying sources of research information, taking notes, developing an outline, and so on.
- **Keep your workspace in order.** Even if the rest of your room is a shambles, try to keep your desk clear. Piles of papers are distracting, and you can end up wasting lots of time looking for notes you misplaced or an article you have to read by morning. Try to spend the last ten minutes of the day getting your desk in order so you get a fresh start on the new day.

Overcoming Procrastination

Putting off until tomorrow what should be done today is a habit that creates a great deal of stress for many students. It also takes a surprising toll. In studies with students taking a health psychology course, researchers found that although procrastinating provided short-term benefits, including periods of low stress, the tendency to dawdle had long-term costs, including poorer health and lower grades. Early in the semester, the procrastinators reported less stress and fewer health problems than students who scored low on procrastination. However, by the end of the semester, procrastinators reported more health-related symptoms, more stress, and more visits to health-care professionals than nonprocrastinators. Students who procrastinate also get poorer grades in courses with many deadlines.

The three most common types of procrastination are putting off unpleasant things, putting off difficult tasks, and putting off tough decisions. Procrastinators are most likely to delay by wishing they didn't have to do what they must or by telling themselves they "just can't get started," which means they never do.

To get out of the procrastination trap, keep track of the tasks you're most likely to put off, and try to figure out why you don't want to tackle them. Think of alternative ways to get tasks done. If you put off library readings, for instance, is the problem getting to the library or the reading itself? If it's the trip to the library, arrange to walk over with a friend whose company you enjoy.

Do what you like least first. Once you have it out of the way, you can concentrate on the tasks you enjoy. Build time into your schedule for interruptions, unforeseen problems, and unexpected events, so you aren't constantly racing around. Establish ground rules for meeting your own needs (including getting enough sleep and making time for friends) before saying yes to any activity. Learn to live according to a three-word motto: Just do it!

LEARN IT / LIVE IT

De-Stress Your Life

College is a perfect time to learn and practice the art of stress reduction. You can start applying the techniques and concepts outlined in this chapter immediately. You may want to begin by doing some relaxation or awareness exercises. They can give you the peace of mind you need to focus more effectively on larger issues, goals, and decisions.

You needn't see stress as a problem to solve on your own. Reach out to others. As you build friendships and intimate relationships, you may find that some irritating problems are easier to put into perspective. Don't be afraid to laugh at yourself and to look for the comic or absurd aspects of a situation. In addition, you might try some simple ap-

(Continued)

proaches that can help boost your stress resistance and reslience, including the following:

- **Focusing.** Take a strain inventory of your body every day to determine where things aren't feeling quite right. Ask yourself, What's keeping me from feeling terrific today? Focusing on problem spots, such as stomach knots or neck tightness, increases your sense of control over stress.
- **Reconstructing stressful situations.** Think about a recent episode of distress; then write down three ways it could have gone better and three ways it could have gone worse. This should help you see that the situation wasn't as disastrous as it might have been and help you find ways to cope better in the future.
- **Self-improvement.** When your life feels out of control, turn to a new challenge. You might try volunteering at a nursing home, going for a long-distance bike trip, or learning a foreign language. As you work toward your new goal, you'll realize that you still can cope and achieve.

If stress continues to be a problem in your life, you may be able to find help through support groups or counseling. Your school may provide counseling services or referrals to mental health professionals; ask your health instructor or the campus health department for this information. Remember that each day of distress robs you of energy, distracts you from life's pleasures, and interferes with achieving your full potential.

3 Making This Chapter Work for You

Review Questions

1. In this text we define stress as
   a. a negative emotional state related to fatigue and similar to depression.
   b. the physiological and psychological response to any event or situation that either upsets or excites us.
   c. the end result of the general adaptation syndrome.
   d. a motivational strategy for making life changes.
2. According to the general adaptation syndrome theory, how does the body typically respond to an acute stressor?
   a. The heart rate slows, blood pressure declines, and eye movement increases.
   b. The body enters a physical state called eustress and then moves into the physical state referred to as distress.
   c. If the stressor is viewed as a positive event, there are no physical changes.
   d. The body demonstrates three stages of change: alarm, resistance, and exhaustion.
3. Over time, increased levels of stress hormones have been shown to increase a person's risk for which of the following conditions?
   a. high blood pressure, memory loss, and skin disorders
   b. stress fractures, male pattern baldness, and hypothyroidism
   c. hemophilia, AIDS, and hay fever
   d. none of the above
4. Stress levels in college students
   a. may be high due to stressors such as academic pressures, financial concerns, learning disabilities, and relationship problems.
   b. are usually low because students feel empowered living independently of their parents.
   c. are typically highest in seniors because their self-esteem diminishes during the college years.
   d. are lower in minority students because they are used to stressors such as a hostile social climate and actual or perceived discrimination.
5. Which of the following illustrates the defense mechanism of displacement?
   a. You have a beer in the evening after a tough day.
   b. You act as if nothing has happened after you have been laid off from your job.
   c. You start an argument with your sister after being laid off from your job.
   d. You argue with your boss after he lays you off from your job.
6. Which of the following situations is representative of a societal stressor?
   a. Peter has been told that his transfer application has been denied because his transcripts were not sent in by the deadline.
   b. Nia's daughter is mugged on the way home from her after-school job.
   c. Kelli's boyfriend drives her car after he had been drinking and has an accident.
   d. Joshua, who is the leading basketball player on his college varsity team, has just been diagnosed with diabetes.
7. If you are stuck in a traffic jam, which of the following actions will help reduce your stress level?
   a. deep, slow breathing
   b. honking your horn
   c. berating yourself for not taking a different route
   d. getting on your cell phone and complaining to a friend
8. A relaxed peaceful state of being can be achieved with which of the following activities?
   a. an aerobic exercise class
   b. playing a computer game

LACC Extra Credit Assignment

3. List and discuss three physical education activities that might be beneficial in reducing stress.

   c. meditating for 15 minutes
   d. attending a rap concert
9. A person suffering from posttraumatic stress disorder may experience which of the following symptoms?
   a. procrastination
   b. constant thirst
   c. drowsiness
   d. terror-filled dreams
10. To develop an efficient studying style:
   a. Schedule your study time on a calendar or planner, have a friend go to class and take notes for you, and join the chess club.
   b. Schedule your study time on a calendar or planner, write notes or questions about the material in the margins of the book, and give yourself a small break after every study hour.
   c. Read assignments before class, call a friend before studying, and plan on working for four continuous hours.
   d. Read assignments before class, skip class when studying for an exam, and have snacks on hand.

Answers to these questions can be found on page 422.

Critical Thinking

1. What reasons can you think of to account for high stress levels among college students? Consider possible social, cultural, and economic factors that may play a role.
2. Identify three stressful situations in your life and determine whether they are examples of eustress or distress. Describe both the positive and negative aspects of each situation.
3. Can you think of any ways in which your behavior or attitudes might create stress for others? What changes could you make to avoid doing so?
4. What advice might you give an incoming freshman at your school about managing stress in college? What techniques have been most helpful for you in dealing with stress? Suppose that this student is from a different ethnic group than you. What additional suggestions would you have for this student?

Media Menu

ThomsonNOW™ Go to the ThomsonNOW website at **http://www.thomsonedu.com** that will:

- Help you evaluate your knowledge of the material.
- Allow you to take an exam-prep quiz.
- Provide a Personalized Learning Plan targeting resources that address areas you should study.
- Coach you through identifying target goals for behavioral change and creating and monitoring your personal change plan throughout the semester.

INTERNET CONNECTIONS

Stress Management: A Review of Principles
www.unl.edu/stress/mgmt

This is an online series of lectures on stress management presented by Wesley E. Sime, Ph.D., M.P.H., Professor of Health and Human Performance at the University of Nebraska—Lincoln. It features information on the psychobiology of stress and relaxation, as well as the pathophysiology of stress.

How to Survive Unbearable Stress
www.teachhealth.com

This comprehensive website is written specifically for college students by Steven Burns, M.D. It features the following topics: signs of how to recognize stress, two stress surveys for adults and college students, information on the pathophysiology of stress, the genetics of stress and stress tolerance, and information on how to best manage and treat stress.

Mind Tools
www.mindtools.com/smpage.html

This site covers a variety of topics on stress management, including recognizing stress, exercise, time management, coping mechanisms, and more. The site also features a free comprehensive personal self-assessment with questions pertaining to work and home stressors, physical and behavioral signs and symptoms, as well as personal coping skills and resources.

InfoTrac College Edition Activities Log on, insert **stress management** into the Keyword search box, and limit your search to the past year. When you get the results, Mark articles to review, then Select one to read. Summarize three or four key points from the article.

You can find additional readings related to personal health with InfoTrac College Edition, an online library of more than 900 journals and publications. Follow the instructions for accessing InfoTrac College Edition that were packaged with your textbook; then search for articles using a keyword search.

For additional links, resources, and suggested readings on the InfoTrac College Edition, visit our Health and Wellness Resource Center at **http://health.wadsworth.com.**

Key Terms

The terms listed are used on the page indicated. Definitions of the terms are in the Glossary at the end of this book.

adaptive response 56
biofeedback 67
defense mechanisms 66
distress 56
eustress 56
general adaptation syndrome (GAS) 56
homeostasis 56
meditation 66
mindfulness 67
posttraumatic stress disorder (PTSD) 68
progressive relaxation 66
stress 56
stressors 56
visualization, or **guided imagery** 66

4 The Joy of Fitness

REAL HEALTH

In his first year in college, an injury sidelined Derek's basketball career. Frustrated that he had to sit out the season, he gave up his rigorous training routine. As he became immersed in other activities, Derek stopped going to the gym or working out on his own. Yet he continued to think of himself as an athlete in excellent physical condition.

On spring break, he joined his younger brothers on a neighborhood basketball court. While he wasn't surprised that his long shots were off, Derek was amazed by how quickly he got winded. In 15 minutes, he was panting for breath. "Getting old," one of his brothers joked. "Getting soft," the other teased.

Derek decided he had to get back in the game—literally. He started shooting hoops with friends and running several times a week. To build muscular strength and endurance, he worked out at the campus gym. Within a few months, Derek was feeling like his "old" self. Realizing that he also missed the challenge of competing, he joined an intramural basketball team. To his delight, his little brothers were cheering from the stands when he won the championship game with a three-pointer.

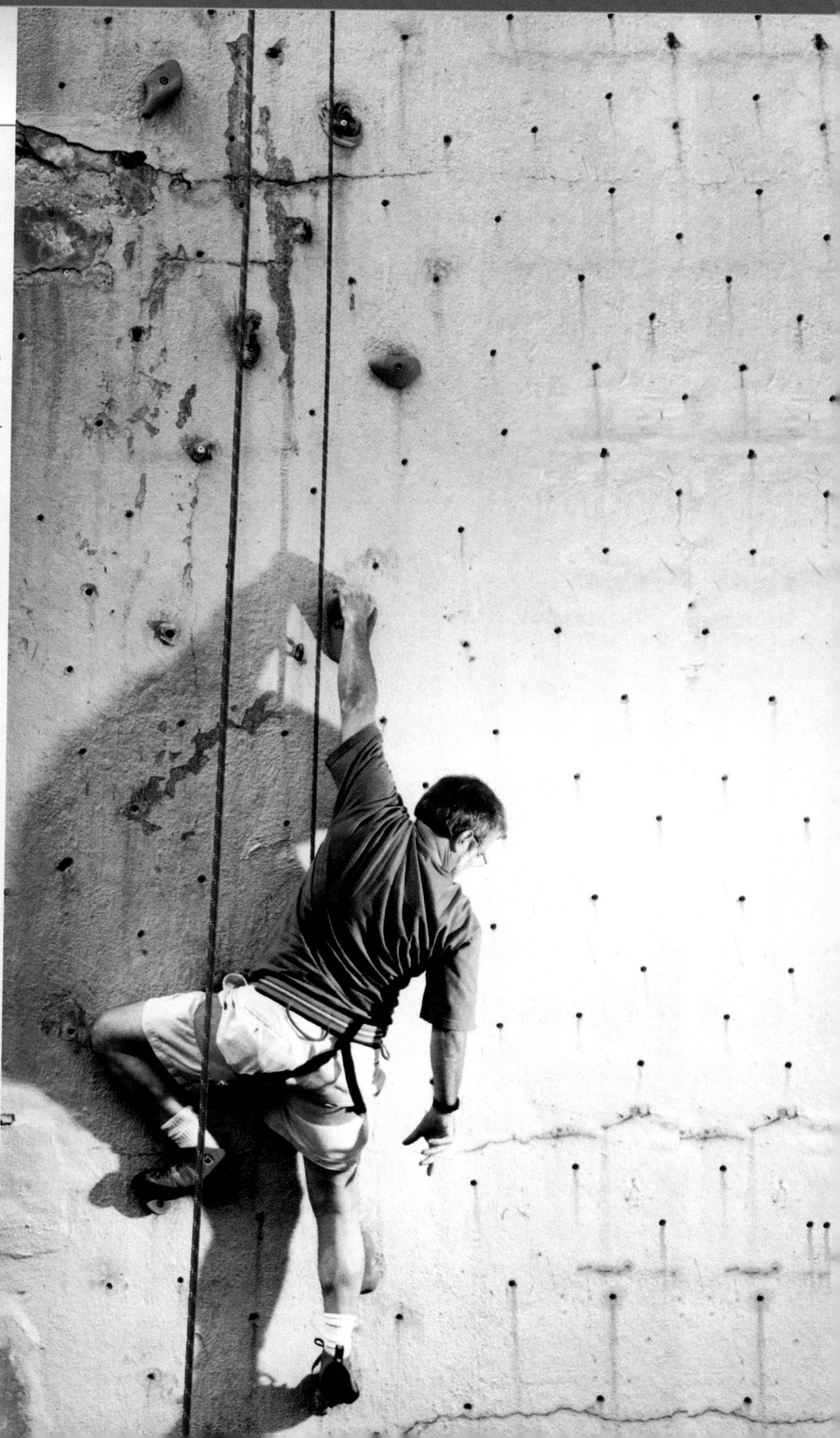

© Brian Finke/Stone/Getty Images

You are designed to move. In ways far more complex than the fastest airplane or sleekest car, your body runs, stretches, bends, swims, climbs, glides, and strides—day after day, year after year, decade after decade. While mere machines break down from constant wear and tear, your body thrives on physical activity. The more you use your body, the stronger and healthier you can become.

Often the college years represent a turning point in physical fitness. Many students, busy with classes and other commitments, devote less time to physical activity. About four in ten undergraduates do not participate in moderate or vigorous physical activity on a regular basis.[1]

The choices you make and the habits you develop now can affect how long and how well you'll live. As you'll see in this chapter, exercise yields immediate rewards: It boosts energy, improves mood, soothes stress, improves sleep, and makes you look and feel better. In the long term, physical activity slows many of the changes associated with chronological aging, such as loss of calcium and bone density, lowers the risk of certain cancers and serious chronic illnesses, and extends the lifespan.

This chapter can help you reap these benefits. It presents the latest activity recommendations, documents the benefits of exercise, describes types of exercise, and provides guidelines for getting into shape and exercising safely.

? FAQ Frequently Asked Questions

- What are the latest Exercise Guidelines for Americans? *p. 81*
- How much exercise is enough? *p. 84*
- What is the difference between stretching and warming up? *p. 97*
- How can I prevent injuries? *p. 101*

After studying the material in this chapter, you should be able to:

- **List** the five components of health-related fitness.
- **Describe** the health benefits of regular physical activity.
- **List** the different forms of cardiorespiratory activities and **describe** their potential health benefits and risks.
- **Explain** the benefits of a muscle training program and **describe** how to design a workout.
- **List** the potential health risks of strength-enhancing drugs and supplements.
- **Define** flexibility and **describe** the different types of stretching exercises.

ThomsonNOW™ Log on to ThomsonNOW at **www.thomsonedu.com/thomsonnow** to find your Behavior Change Planner and to explore self-assessments, interactive tutorials, and practice quizzes.

What is Physical Fitness?

The simplest, most practical definition of **physical fitness** is the ability to respond to routine physical demands, with enough reserve energy to cope with a sudden challenge. You can consider yourself fit if you meet your daily energy needs; can handle unexpected extra demands; and are protecting yourself against potential health problems, such as heart disease. Fitness is important both for health and for athletic performance.

Health-Related Fitness

The five health-related components of physical fitness include aerobic or cardiorespiratory endurance, muscular strength, muscular endurance, flexibility, and body composition (the ratio of fat and lean body tissue).

Cardiorespiratory fitness refers to the ability of the heart to pump blood through the body efficiently. It is achieved through aerobic exercise—any activity, such as brisk walking or swimming, in which sufficient or excess oxygen is continually supplied to the body. In other words, aerobic exercise involves working out strenuously without pushing to the point of breathlessness.

Muscular strength refers to the force within muscles; it is measured by the absolute maximum weight that you can lift, push, or press in one effort. Strong muscles help keep the skeleton in proper alignment, improve posture, prevent back and leg aches, help in everyday lifting, and enhance athletic performance. Muscle mass increases along with strength, which makes for a healthier body composition and a higher metabolic rate.

Muscular endurance is the ability to perform repeated muscular effort; it is measured by counting how many times you can lift, push, or press a given weight. Important for posture, muscular endurance helps in everyday work as well as in athletics and sports.

Flexibility is the range of motion around specific joints—for example, the stretching you do to touch your toes or twist your torso. Flexibility depends on many factors: your age, gender, and posture; how muscular you are; and how much body fat you have. As children develop, their flexibility increases until adolescence. Then a gradual loss of joint mobility begins and continues throughout adult life. Both muscles and conn[illegible] ...ch as [illegible] ...ter if not [illegible] ...ion. [illegible] ...nounts [illegible] ...r) in [illegible] ...igh [illegible] ...ions, [illegible] ...gh [illegible] ...ems, [illegible] ...r. [illegible] ...e [illegible] ...respi- [illegible] ...ular [illegible] ...tion.

Read over this
in class today

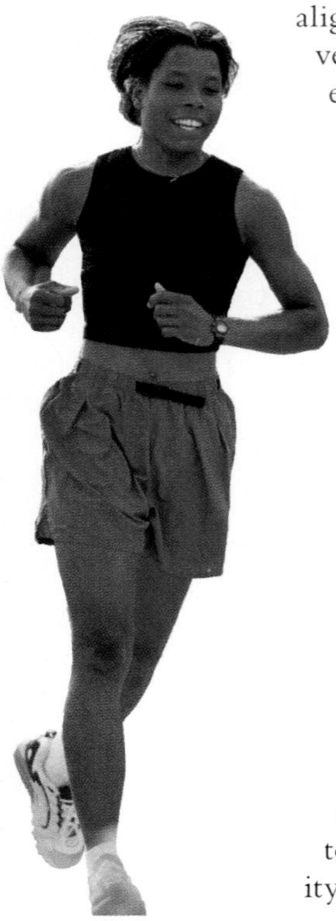

© Lori Adamski Peek/Stone/Getty Images

Fitness can enhance every dimension of your health and improve your mood and your mind as well as your body.

[illegible]

T[illegible] ...volving. Rather than focusing only on miles run or weight lifted, instructors, coaches, and consumers are pursuing a broader vision of total fitness that encompasses every dimension of health:

- **Physical.** As described later in this chapter, becoming fit reduces your risk of major diseases, increases energy and stamina, and may prolong your life.
- **Emotional.** Fitness lowers tension and anxiety, lifts depression, relieves stress, improves mood, and promotes a positive self-image.
- **Social.** Physical activities provide opportunities to meet new people and to work out with friends or family.
- **Intellectual.** Fit individuals report greater alertness, better concentration, more creativity, and improved personal health habits.
- **Occupational.** Fit employees miss fewer days of work, are more productive, and incur fewer medical costs.
- **Spiritual.** Fitness fosters appreciation for the relationship between body and mind and may lead to greater realization of your potential.
- **Environmental.** Fit individuals often become more aware of their need for healthy air and food and develop a deeper appreciation of the physical world.

Gender, Race, and Fitness

Men and women of all racial backgrounds benefit equally from fitness. However, there are some physiological differences between men and women, many of which are related to size.

♂ On average, men are 10 to 15 percent bigger than women, with roughly twice the percentage of muscle mass and half the percentage of body fat. They have more sweat glands and a greater maximum oxygen uptake. A man's bigger heart pumps more blood with each beat. His larger lungs take in 10 to 20 percent more oxygen (Figure 4-1). His longer legs cover more distance with each stride. If a man jogs along at 50 percent of his capacity, a woman has to push to 73 percent of hers to keep up.

Women have a higher percentage of body fat than men, and more is distributed around the hips and thighs; men carry more body fat around the waist and stomach.

College-age men average 15 percent body fat; college-age women, 23 percent. On average, women have 11 percent more body fat and 8 percent less muscle mass than men.

The average woman has a smaller heart and blood volume than a man. Because women have a lower concentration of red blood cells, their bodies are less effective at transporting oxygen to their working muscles during exercise.

Even though training produces the same relative increases for both genders, a woman's maximum oxygen intake remains about 25 to 30 percent lower than that of an equally well-conditioned man. In elite athletes, the gender difference is smaller: 8 to 12 percent. Because the angle of the upper leg bone (femur) to the pelvis is greater in a woman, she is less efficient at running.

In some endurance events, such as ultramarathon running and long-distance swimming, female anatomy and physiology may have some aerobic advantages. The longer a race—on land, water, or ice—the better women perform.

In absolute terms, men are 30 percent stronger, but gender differences in absolute strength do not apply to all muscle groups. Women have about 40 to 60 percent of the upper-body strength of men but 70 to 75 percent of the lower-body strength.

Racial and ethnic backgrounds also influence fitness. Among women, physical fitness levels are similar between whites and blacks, but obesity is more common among African Americans. These findings suggest that, if you are African American you may need to place even greater emphasis on improving your overall fitness to reduce your risk of heart disease.

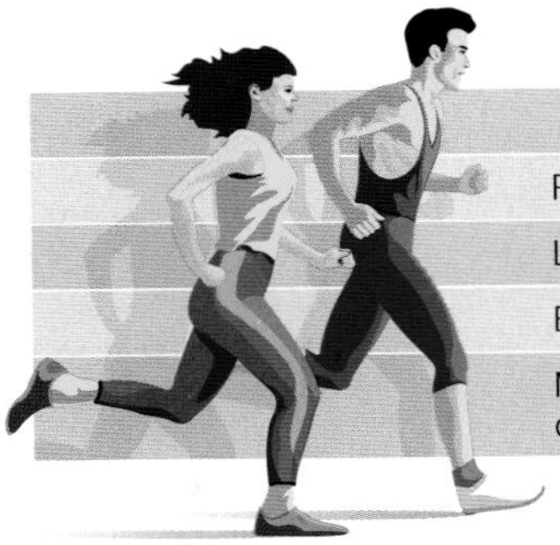

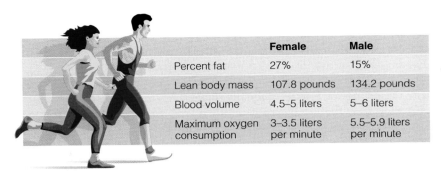

	Female	Male
Percent fat	27%	15%
Lean body mass	107.8 pounds	134.2 pounds
Blood volume	4.5–5 liters	5–6 liters
Maximum oxygen consumption	3–3.5 liters per minute	5.5–5.9 liters per minute

FIGURE 4-1 Physiological Differences Between Men and Women

The Inactivity Epidemic

One in four Americans reports no physical activity at all, according to the CDC. About half exercise occasionally, but not at the levels recommended by the National Center for Chronic Disease Prevention and Health Promotion. Only one in four adults meets the levels of physical activity recommended by federal health officials.

According to a national survey, about a third of adolescents and 14 percent of adults between ages 20 and 49 fall into the category of "low fitness" because they engage in little or no physical activity.[2] They are significantly more likely to develop diabetes, hypertension, and metabolic syndrome (discussed in Chapter 10) than those with higher fitness levels.

Many factors affect physical activity levels, including geographic location, gender, education, and income. According to the CDC, city-dwellers are more active than country folks, westerners more active than those in other regions. Men, people with higher education levels, and high-income earners work out more often.

How do Americans spend most of their leisure time? Watching television. We average more than 30 hours a week. Yet the more time spent in front of the TV, the greater the risk of obesity and related chronic diseases. Compared with other sedentary activities, such as reading, writing, or driving, watching TV lowers metabolic rate, so people burn fewer calories.

The Toll of Sedentary Living

Inactivity increases all causes of mortality, doubles the risk of cardiovascular diseases, diabetes, and obesity, and increases the risk of colon cancer, high blood pressure,

physical fitness The ability to respond to routine physical demands, with enough reserve energy to cope with a sudden challenge.

cardiorespiratory fitness The ability of the heart and blood vessels to circulate blood through the body efficiently.

muscular strength Physical power; the maximum weight one can lift, push, or press in one effort.

muscular endurance The ability to withstand the stress of continued physical exertion.

flexibility The range of motion allowed by one's joints; determined by the length of muscles, tendons, and ligaments attached to the joints.

body composition The relative amounts of fat and lean tissue (bone, muscle, organs, water) in the body.

osteoporosis, depression, and anxiety. The combination of physical inactivity and being overweight is responsible for more than 300,000 deaths a year. Epidemiologists predict that this deadly duo may soon overtake tobacco as the nation's number-one killer.

The economic impact is equally staggering: an estimated $1 trillion in health-care bills a year. As a risk factor for heart disease, physical inactivity ranks as high as elevated cholesterol, high blood pressure, or cigarette smoking.

Working Out on Campus: Student Bodies in Motion

College students aren't necessarily more active or fit than the general population. In the American College Health Assessment's National College Health Assessment survey, 40 percent of students report exercising vigorously at least three days a week.[3] (See Student Snapshot: "Working Up a Sweat on Campus.")

Men are consistently more active than women on campus. In one study at a large midwestern university, male students averaged 6.2 hours a week of moderate or vigorous exercise; female students, 5.5 hours. (By comparison, college men spend 12 hours watching TV or DVDs; women, 9.6 hours.)[4] As freshmen, both men and women report a significant drop in physical activity from high school.

Mexican-American students, both male and female, and African-American women report the lowest rates of physical activity. The most physically active men are African American; the most active women, white.

Student Snapshot

Working Up a Sweat on Campus

Students on Campus	Percentage of Students
Students who engage in moderate or vigorous activity at least 3 days a week	40%
Students who exercised to lose weight* in last 30 days	54%
Women	61%
Men	41%

*Based on surveys 47,202 students on 74 campuses.

Sources: Suminski, Richard, and Petosa, Rick. "Web-Assisted Instruction for Changing Social Cognitive Variables Related to Physical Activity." *Journal of American College Health*, Vol. 54, No. 4, January–February 2006, p. 219. American College Health Association. "American College Health Association-National College Health Assessment (ACHA-NCHA) Spring 2004 Reference Group Data Report (abridged)." *Journal of American College Health*, Vol. 54, No. 4, January–February 2006, p. 201.

Physical Activity and Health

Why Exercise?

If exercise could be packed into a pill, it would be the single most widely prescribed and beneficial medicine in the nation. Why? Because nothing can do more to help your body function at its best—a fact that not all students are aware of. In a recent survey, eight in ten undergraduates realized that physical activity can prevent heart disease and prevent and treat obesity. However, fewer than half knew that it maintains bone density and can help prevent diabetes.

As Figure 4-2 illustrates, exercise provides head-to-toe benefits. With regular activity, your heart muscles become stronger and pump blood more efficiently. Your heart rate and resting pulse slow down. Your blood pressure may drop slightly from its normal level.

Exercise thickens the bones and can slow the loss of calcium that normally occurs with age. Physical activity increases flexibility in the joints and improves digestion and elimination. It speeds up metabolism and builds lean body mass, so the body burns more calories and body fat decreases. It heightens sensitivity to insulin (a great benefit for diabetics) and may lower the risk of developing diabetes. In addition, exercise enhances clot-dissolving substances in the blood, helping to prevent strokes, heart attacks, and pulmonary embolisms (clots in the lungs), and it helps lower the risk of certain cancers. Regular exercise can actually extend your lifespan and sharpen your memory and mind.

Healthier Heart and Lungs

Regular physical activity makes blood less likely to clot and cause a stroke or heart attack. Sedentary people are about twice as likely to die of a heart attack as people who are physically active. Although rigorous exercise somewhat increases the risk of sudden cardiac death for men, regular physical activity lowers the overall danger, especially in women.[5] (See Chapter 10 for a discussion of heart disease.)

Exercise also lowers levels of the indicators of increased risk of heart disease, such as high cholesterol and C-reactive protein, which is discussed in Chapter 10.[6] Exercise itself, even without weight loss, may reduce the risk of developing the prediabetic condition called metabolic syndrome, which if untreated can lead to type 2 diabetes and increase the risk of heart disease.[7]

In addition to its effects on the heart, exercise makes the lungs more efficient. The lungs take in more oxygen, and their vital capacity (the maximum amount

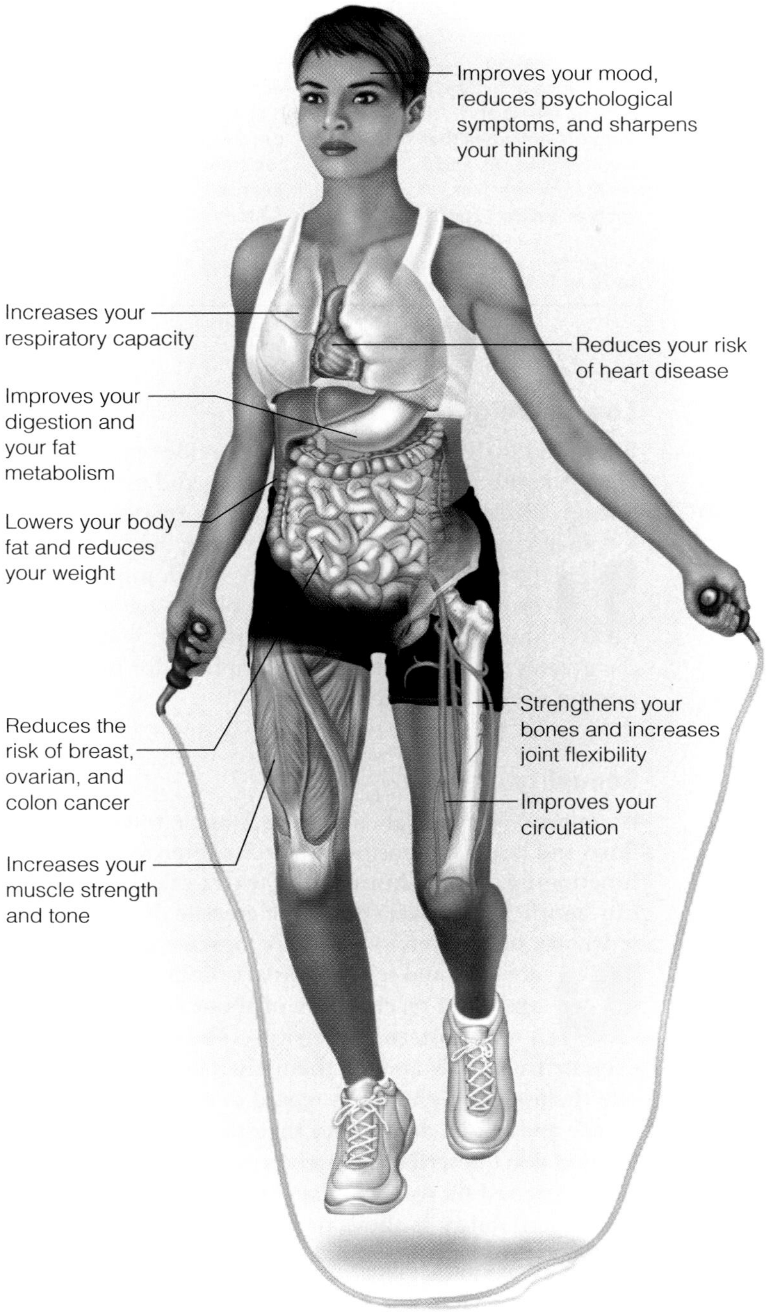
Improves your mood, reduces psychological symptoms, and sharpens your thinking
Increases your respiratory capacity
Reduces your risk of heart disease
Improves your digestion and your fat metabolism
Lowers your body fat and reduces your weight
Strengthens your bones and increases joint flexibility
Reduces the risk of breast, ovarian, and colon cancer
Improves your circulation
Increases your muscle strength and tone

FIGURE 4-2 The Benefits of Exercise
Regular physical activity enhances your overall physical and mental health and helps prevent disease.

of air volume the lungs can take in and expel) increases, providing more energy for you to use.

Even in young men, physical fitness is associated with improvements in blood pressure and the makeup of blood fats, including cholesterol and triglycerides. Exercise, along with a healthy weight, keeps blood fats at healthy levels over time. Prolonged, sustained endurance training prevents the stiffening of the heart muscle once thought to be an inevitable consequence of aging.

Protection Against Cancer

As discussed in Chapter 6, fatness increases the risk of several cancers; fitness decreases it. The evidence for exercise's protective effects is strongest for colon and rectal cancer, possibly because it enhances digestion and elimination. Physical activity also lowers the risk of breast and ovarian cancer in women. Breast cancer patients who perform the equivalent of three to five hours of walking a week live longer and reduce their *risk* of dying.[8]

In a study that followed more than 5000 men and women for more than 20 years, fitness was a strong predictor of cancer death rates for men, but not for women. The fittest men had the lowest cancer death rates. But for women, body weight, as measured by body mass index (BMI, discussed later in the chapter), proved more significant.

Less Risk of Disease

Moderate exercise correlates with a reduced number of sick days. Researchers speculate that exercise may enhance immune function by reducing stress hormones like cortisol that can dampen resistance to disease.

Women who walk briskly for 35 to 45 minutes five days a week experience half the number of sick days with cold symptoms as inactive women. While moderate exercise seems to bolster a person's immune system, heavy training may increase the risk of upper respiratory tract infections for endurance athletes.

Moderate exercise, combined with a balanced diet and weight loss, can cut in half the risk of developing diabetes among those at high risk. For individuals with type 2 (non-insulin-dependent) diabetes, intense aerobic exercise and strength training help control blood sugar levels.

Brighter Mood

Exercise makes people feel good from the inside out. Exercise boosts mood, elevates self-esteem, increases energy, reduces anxiety, improves concentration and alertness, enables people to handle stress better, and may help ward off dementia.[9] During long workouts, some people experience what is called "runner's high," which may be the result of increased levels of mood-elevating brain chemicals called **endorphins.**

Better Mental Health and Functioning

Exercise is an effective—but underused—treatment for mild to moderate depression and may help in treating other mental disorders. Regular, moderate exercise, such as walking, running, or lifting weights, three times a week, has proved helpful for depression and anxiety disorders, including panic attacks.[10] Exercise is as effective as medication in improving mood and also helps prevent relapse.

According to numerous long-term studies, physically fit adults perform better on cognitive tests than their less fit peers. Improving cardiorespiratory fitness reduces the harmful effects of aging on brain structures as well as on memory and other functions.

Better Bones

By 2020, one in two Americans over age 50 may suffer **osteoporosis**—a condition in which bones lose their mineral density and become susceptible to injury. Most are unaware that their bone health is in jeopardy. Four times as many men and almost three times as many women actually have osteoporosis than realize they do.[11]

You may think that weak, brittle bones are a problem only for the elderly. However, 2 percent of college-age women have osteoporosis; another 15 percent have already sustained significant losses in bone density and are at high risk of osteoporosis. Women who did not participate in high school sports are seven times more likely to have low bone density than those who did. The college women at greatest risk often are extremely skinny and maintain their low weights and slim looks by dieting and by avoiding exercise so as not to increase their muscle mass. Some eliminate dairy products, an important source of calcium, from their diets. Depo-Provera, a method of birth control that consists of hormone injections every three months, also is associated with low bone density, especially with long-term use. (See Chapter 8 on contraception.)

What are the best exercises to boost bone density? According to a study of college women, high-impact aerobics, such as step exercising, "may offer the quickest route to building bone in young women." Resistance exercises such as squats, leg presses, and calf presses strengthened leg muscles but had no effect on bone density.[12] The American College of Sports Medicine recommends moderate- to high-intensity weight-bearing activities to maintain bone mass in adults (Table 4-1).[13]

TABLE 4-1 RX: Healthy Bones

Mode	Intensity	Frequency	Duration
Weight-bearing endurance activities, such as tennis and jogging; activities that involve jumping; and resistance exercise, such as weight lifting	Moderate to high	Weight-bearing activities, 3 to 5 times per week; resistance exercise, 2 or 3 times per week	30 to 60 minutes

Source: "Physical Activity and Bone Health." Position Stand, American College of Sports Medicine, www.acsm-/msse.org.

Lower Weight

For individuals on a diet, exercise provides extra benefits: A combination of dietary change and moderate- to high-level intensity exercise leads to greater weight loss than either alone. Dieters who work out lose more fat than lean muscle tissue, which improves their body composition. College-age men who start exercising lose abdominal fat, which poses the greatest risk to health. (See Chapter 6 for information on exercise and weight control.)

Sexuality

By improving physical endurance, muscle tone, blood flow, and body composition, exercise improves sexual functioning. Simply burning 200 extra calories a day can significantly lower the risk of erectile dysfunction in sedentary men. Exercise also may increase sexual drive, activity, and sexual satisfaction in people of all ages. In a recent study of about 400 students at a southeastern university, college students who exercise frequently and see themselves as physically fit rate themselves higher with regard to sexual performance and sexual desirability than those who exercise less and don't describe themselves as fit. All the men who exercised six to seven days per week rated their sexual desirability as above or much above average.[14]

Benefits for Students

Unlike middle-aged and older individuals, traditional-age college students cite improved fitness as the number-one advantage that exercise offers, followed by improved appearance and muscle tone. Undergraduates who recognize the benefits of exercise are more likely to be physically active than those who focus on barriers to working out.

Will exercise improve your grades? Not necessarily. A study at two Texas universities found that the fittest students didn't necessarily have higher GPAs. However, increasing their level of physical fitness did have a positive impact on the GPAs of the female students.

A More Active Old Age

Exercise slows the changes that are associated with advancing age: loss of lean muscle tissue, increase in body fat, and decrease in work capacity. In addition to lowering the risk of heart disease and stroke, exercise also helps older men and women retain the strength and mobility needed to live independently. Even in old age, exercise boosts strength and stamina, lessens time in wheelchairs, and improves outlook and sense of control.

Longer Life

Capacity for exercise has proved a better predictor of whether a man would die in the next few years than other risk factors, such as high blood pressure, high total cholesterol, or smoking. Formerly sedentary people, even the elderly, who begin to exercise live longer, on average, than those who remain inactive. However, for active people, light to moderate exercise won't do it—only vigorous exercise reduces the risk of dying of heart disease and of premature death from other causes.

? FAQ What Are the Latest Exercise Guidelines for Americans?

Because inactivity is so hazardous to our well-being, public health officials have tried many approaches to get Americans moving. Rather than emphasizing vigorous cardiorespiratory or aerobic activity, a landmark report by the Surgeon General in 1996 recommended 30 minutes of moderate intensity exercise—such as brisk walking, bicycling, and gardening—on all or most days of the week.

The most recent federal Dietary Guidelines call for more physical activity for added health benefits:

- Engage in regular physical activity and reduce sedentary activities to promote health, psychological well-being, and a healthy body weight.
  - To reduce the risk of chronic disease in adulthood: Engage in at least 30 minutes of moderate-intensity physical activity, above usual activity, at work or home on most days of the week.
  - For most people, greater health benefits can be obtained by engaging in physical activity of more vigorous intensity or longer duration.
  - To help manage body weight and prevent gradual, unhealthy body weight gain in adulthood: Engage in approximately 60 minutes of moderate- to vigorous-intensity activity on most days of the week while not exceeding caloric intake requirements.
  - To sustain weight loss in adulthood: Participate in at least 60 to 90 minutes of daily moderate-intensity physical activity while not exceeding caloric intake requirements. Some people may need to consult with a health-care provider before participating in this level of activity.
- Achieve physical fitness by including cardiovascular conditioning, stretching exercises for flexibility, and resistance exercises or calisthenics for muscle strength and endurance."[15]

YOUR LIFE COACH

Motivating Yourself to Move

Before you move a muscle, you need to be motivated. You may never even have thought about becoming more active. You may be thinking about getting into shape—someday. You may exercise, but not on a regular basis. Or you may have started working out in the last six months.

Each of these statements applies to a different stage of motivational readiness for change, discussed in Chapter 1. In studies on increasing activity in adults, researchers have found that strategies tailored to an individual's stage of readiness for change are effective in boosting motivation and getting people moving.[16]

One thing is clear: College students don't become more active simply because teachers or coaches ask or urge them to get moving.[17] Colleges and universities can encourage exercise by environmental means, for instance, by creating recreational trails for walking, jogging, and biking.[18] Web-based instruction materials that help students develop skills for planning, organizing, and maintaining physical activities also have proved useful.[19]

However, the most effective motivators are intrinsic (that, is they come from within the individual) rather than extrinsic (stemming from external goals or pressures). College students, according to a recent study, are more likely to pursue a sport—either individually or as part of a team—for intrinsic motives, such as enjoyment and feeling competent, but to exercise for extrinsic motives, such as improving their appearance. Male and female students differ in their reasons for playing a sport or being physically active. Men rank challenge, competition, social recognition, strength, and endurance as their primary motivators. Women consistently rank one incentive—weight management—higher than men.[20]

Both cognitive and behavioral strategies are effective in motivating change. Cognitive strategies, such as learning about the risks of remaining sedentary, typically work best in the contemplation and preparation stages.

endorphins Mood-elevating, pain-killing chemicals produced by the brain.

osteoporosis A condition common in older people in which the bones become increasingly soft and porous, making them susceptible to injury.

Strategies for Change — Get Yourself Going

What would most motivate you to get moving? Make a list, and identify which motivators are intrinsic or extrinsic. Then try the following strategies to follow through:

- **Sign up for a fitness class,** such as spinning or step aerobics, so that exercise is built into your weekly schedule.
- **Go to gym with friends.** "Even if it's rainy and cold, I know they're waiting for me so I go," one women explained.
- **Find a fun workout.** "I love working out when it's something different—like water aerobics, ice skating, or swing dance," said one student.
- **Join a team—or root for one.** College sports, whether competitive or informal, can help maintain fitness levels. So can cheerleading, which has become so physically demanding that college cheerleaders recently scored as high a fitness levels as college athletes.

Behavioral strategies, such as keeping athletic shoes in the car or in a locker at the gym, are most effective at the action stage. Take the Self-Survey: "Physical Activity Stages of Change Questionnaire" in the Self-Assessment Booklet to find out your readiness for change to a more active life.

The Principles of Exercise

Your body is literally what you make of it. Superbly designed for multiple uses, it adjusts to meet physical demands. If you need to sprint for a bus, your heart will speed up and pump more blood. Beyond such immediate, short-term adaptations, physical training can produce long-term changes in heart rate, oxygen consumption, and muscle strength and endurance. Although there are limits on the maximum levels of physical fitness and performance that any individual can achieve, regular exercise can produce improvements in everyone's baseline wellness and fitness.

As you begin the process of working toward total fitness, it's important to keep in mind the principles of exercise, discussed next.

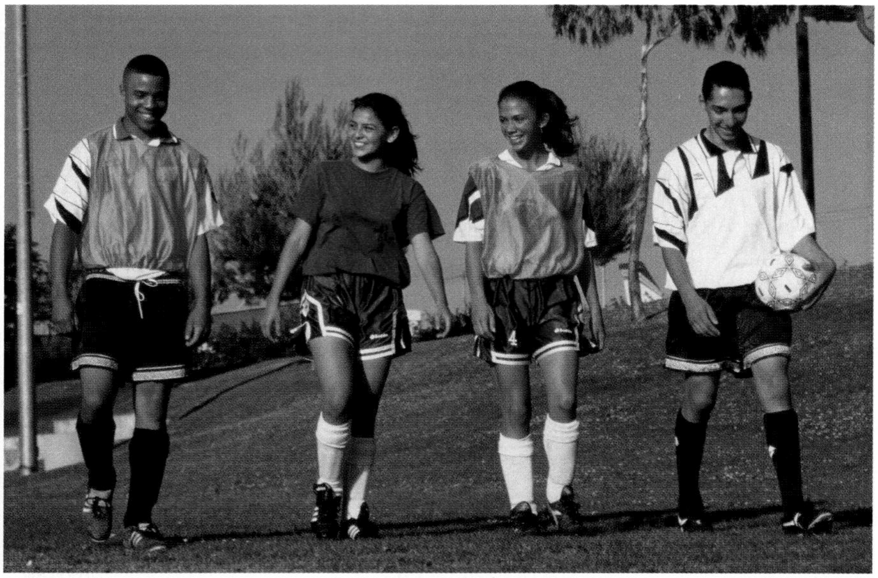

College men and women have different motives for participating in a sport or engaging in regular exercise. What would motivate you to join a team?

Overload Principle

The overload principle requires a person exercising to provide a greater stress or demand on the body than it's usually accustomed to handling. For any muscle, including the heart, to get stronger, it must work against a greater-than-normal resistance or challenge. To continue to improve, you need further increases in the demands—but not too much too quickly. **Progressive overloading**—gradually increasing physical challenges—provides the benefits of exercise without the risk of injuries (Figure 4-3).

Overloading is specific to each body part and to each component of fitness. Leg exercises develop only the lower limbs; arm exercises, only the upper limbs. This is why you need a comprehensive fitness plan that includes a variety of exercises to develop different parts of the body. If you play a particular sport, you also need training to develop sports-specific skills, such as a strong, efficient stroke in swimming.

FITT

Although low-intensity activity can enhance basic health, you need to work harder—that is, at a greater intensity—to improve fitness. Whatever exercise you do, there is a level, or threshold, at which fitness begins to improve; a target zone, where you can achieve maximum benefits; and an upper limit, at which potential risks outweigh any further benefits. The acronym **FITT** sums up the four dimensions of progressive overload: *frequency* (how often you exercise), *intensity* (how hard), *time* (how long), and *type* (specific activity) (Table 4-2).

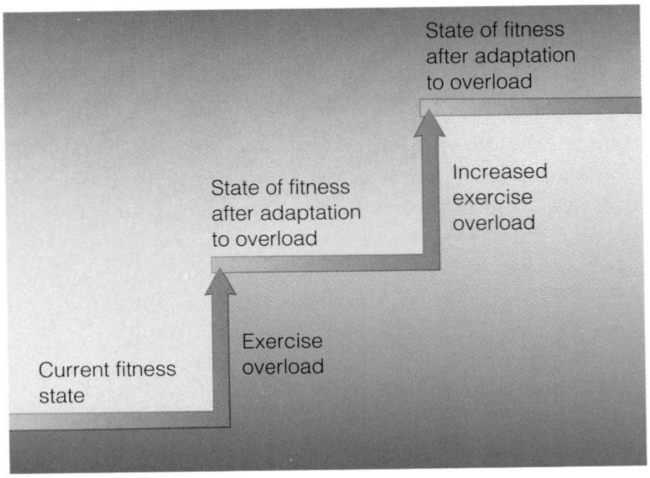

FIGURE 4-3 The Overload Principle

By increasing frequency, intensity, or duration, you will improve your level of fitness. Once your body adapts (becomes comfortable) to the demands, you can again apply the overload principle to achieve a higher level of fitness.

Frequency

To attain and maintain physical fitness, you need to exercise regularly, but the recommended frequency varies with different types of exercise and with an individual's fitness goals. Health officials urge Americans to engage in moderate-intensity aerobic activity most days and in resistance and flexibility training two or three days a week.

Intensity

Exercise intensity varies with the type of exercise and with personal goals. To improve cardiorespiratory fitness, you need at a minimum to increase your heart rate to a target zone (the level that produces benefits). To develop muscular strength and endurance, you need to increase the amount of weight you lift or the resistance you work against and/or the number of repetitions. For enhanced flexibility, you need to stretch muscles beyond their normal length.

overload principle Providing a greater stress or demand on the body than it is normally accustomed to handling.

progressive overloading Gradually increasing physical challenges once the body adapts to the stress placed upon it to produce maximum benefits.

FITT A formula that describes the frequency, intensity, type, and length of time for physical activity.

TABLE 4-2 Guidelines for Physical Fitness: The FITT Principle

	Cardiorespiratory	Strength	Flexibility
	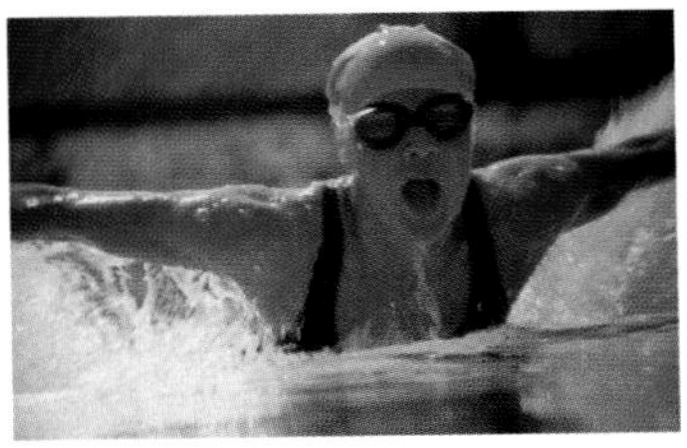 © 2000 PhotoDisc, Inc.	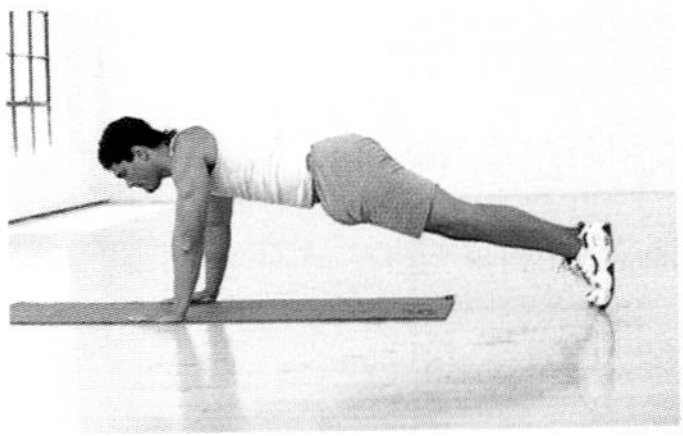 David Hanover	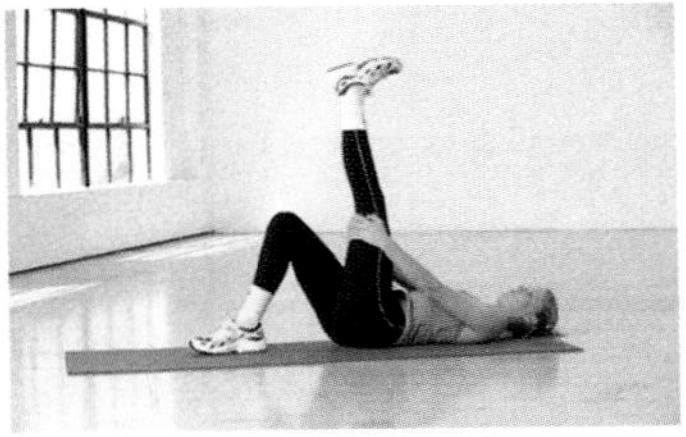 David Hanover
Frequency: Most days of the week. Start with three days and gradually increase frequency.	Almost every day	2 to 3 days per week	A minimum of 2 to 3 days per week
Intensity: Start at low to moderate intensity and gradually increase to more vigorous efforts over several weeks.	60 to 85 percent of maximum heart rate	Enough to enhance muscle strength and improve body composition	Enough to develop and maintain a full range of motion
Time: 30 to 60 minutes, using a gradual progression.	20 to 60 minutes	8 to 12 repetitions of 8 to 10 different exercises (minimum)	4 repetitions of 10 to 30 seconds per muscle group (minimum)
Type of activity: Start with low-impact activities (walking, cycling, low-impact aerobics, water exercise); resistance or weight training; flexibility exercises.	Aerobic activity that uses large-muscle groups and can be maintained continuously	Resistance activity that is performed at a controlled speed and through a full range of motion	Stretching activity that uses the major muscle groups

Source: Adapted from American College of Sports Medicine, "Position Stand: The Recommended Quantity and Quality of Exercise for Developing and Maintaining Cardiorespiratory and Muscular Fitness, and Flexibility in Healthy Adults." *Medicine and Science in Sports and Exercise*, Vol. 30, 1998, pp. 975-991; and from Kyle McInnis et al., "Counseling for Physical Activity in Overweight and Obese Patients." *American Family Physician*, Vol. 67, No. 6, March 15, 2003, p. 1254.

Time (Duration)

The amount of time, or duration, of your workouts is also important, particularly for cardiorespiratory exercise. As noted in Table 4-2, the American College of Sports Medicine recommends 30 to 45 minutes of aerobic exercise, preceded by 5 to 10 minutes of warm-up and followed by 5 to 10 minutes of stretching. However, experts have found similar health benefits from a single 30-minute session of moderate exercise as from several shorter sessions throughout the day. Duration and intensity are interlinked. If you're exercising at high intensity (biking or running at a brisk pace, for instance), you don't need to exercise as long as when you're working at lower intensity (walking or swimming at a moderate pace). For muscular strength and endurance and for flexibility, duration is defined by the number of sets or repetitions rather than total time.

Type (Specificity)

The **specificity principle** refers to the body's adaptation to a particular type of activity or amount of stress placed upon it. Jogging, for instance, trains the heart and lungs to work more efficiently and strengthens certain leg muscles. However, it does not build upper body strength or enhance flexibility.

Reversibility Principle

The **reversibility principle** is the opposite of the overload principle. Just as the body adapts to greater physical demands, it also adjusts to lower levels. If you stop exercising, you can lose as much as 50 percent of your fitness improvements within two months. If you have to curtail your usual exercise routine because of a busy schedule, you can best maintain your fitness by keeping the intensity constant and reducing frequency or duration. The principle of reversibility is aptly summed up by the phrase, "Use it or lose it."

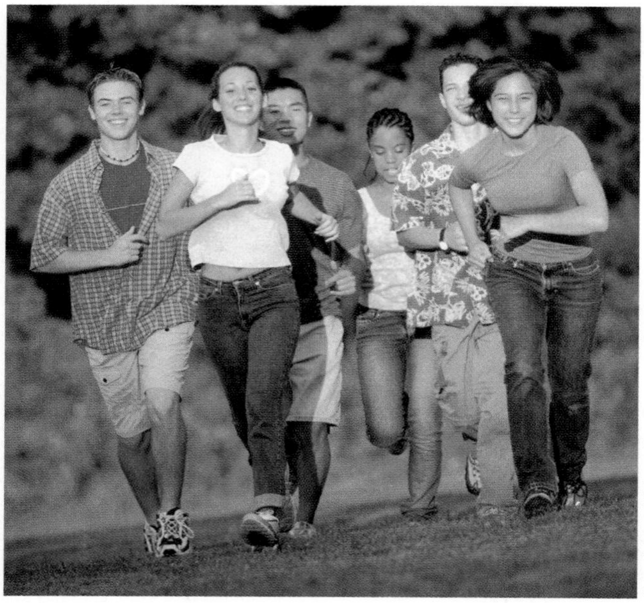

© Jon Feingersh/Masterfile

The goal of exercise isn't to become a competitive athlete but to improve your well-being and achieve your maximum fitness potential.

? FAQ How Much Exercise Is Enough?

The answer depends on your reasons for working out. If you want to feel better, boost your energy, tone your muscles, condition your heart, strengthen your bones, protect your heart, and lower your risk of major diseases, leading medical authorities, including the American College of Sports Medicine, the U.S. Surgeon General, and Health Canada's Physical Activity Guide to Healthy Active Living, recommend a minimum of 30 to 60 minutes of moderate activity (such as walking at a speed of three to four miles per hour) most days of the week. According to the most recent research, a minimum of 150 minutes a week of moderate-intensity exercise lifts men and women out of the "low-fitness" category and lowers their risk of cardiovascular disease and diabetes, regardless of weight or body composition.

While half an hour of exercise five days a week is good, according to a recent review of current research, working out more often and more intensely can yield more health dividends, including improved muscular strength and endurance. You may also need to exercise longer and harder to maintain a healthy weight and lose excess pounds. As discussed on page 81, the latest Exercise Guidelines for Americans concludes that individuals who've lost weight may need to exercise 60 to 90 minutes a day to keep off the pounds.[21] Vigorous physical activity (such as jogging or spinning) burns calories more rapidly per unit of time than moderate activities like walking. It doesn't matter if your goal is to improve fitness or avoid fatness. The same strategy—regular physical activity—is the key to both.

Improving Cardiorespiratory Fitness

Cardiorespiratory endurance refers to the ability of the heart, lungs, and circulatory system to deliver oxygen to muscles working rhythmically over an extended period of time. Unlike muscular endurance (discussed later in this chapter), which is specific to individual muscles, cardiorespiratory endurance involves the entire body. **Aerobic exercise,** which improves cardiorespiratory endurance, can take many forms, but all involve working strenuously without pushing to the point of breathlessness. A person who builds up good aerobic capacity can maintain long periods of physical activity without great fatigue.

In **anaerobic exercise,** the amount of oxygen taken in by the body cannot meet the demands of the activity. This quickly creates an oxygen deficit that must be made up later. Anaerobic activities are high in intensity but short in duration, usually lasting only about ten seconds to two minutes. An example is sprinting the quarter-mile, which leaves even the best-trained athletes gasping for air. In *nonaerobic exercise,* such as bowling, softball, or doubles tennis, there is frequent rest between activities. Because the body can take in all the oxygen it needs, the heart and lungs don't get much of a workout.

Target Heart Rate

To use your pulse, or heart rate, as a guide, feel your pulse in the carotid artery in your neck. Slightly tilt your head back and to one side. Use your middle finger or forefinger, or both, to feel for your pulse. (Do not use your thumb; it has a beat of its own.) To determine your heart rate, count the number of pulses you feel for 10 seconds and multiply that number by six, or count for 30 seconds and multiply that number by two. Learn to recognize the pulsing of your heart when you're sitting or lying down. This is your **resting heart rate.**

Start taking your pulse during, or immediately after, exercise, when it's much more pronounced than when you're at rest. Three minutes after heavy exercise, take your pulse again. The closer that reading is to your resting heart rate, the better your condition. If it takes a long time for your pulse to recover and return to its resting level, your body's ability to handle physical stress is poor. As you continue working out, however, your pulse will return to normal much more quickly.

You don't want to push yourself to your maximum heart rate, yet you must exercise at about 60 to 85 percent of that maximum to get cardiorespiratory benefits from your training. This range is called your **target heart rate.** If you don't exercise intensely enough to raise your heart rate at least this high, your heart and lungs won't reap the most benefit from the workout. If you push too hard, and exercise at or near your absolute maximum heart rate, you run the risk of placing too great a burden on your heart. Figure 4-4 shows the target heart rate for various ages and activities. Find your age at the bottom of the figure and move up the grid to find your target heart rate for "aerobic workout."

You can also use the following steps to determine your maximum heart rate and target heart rate (in beats per minute):

1. Maximum heart rate: Subtract your age from 220. So if you are 20, your maximum heart rate is $220 - 20 = 200$ beats per minute.

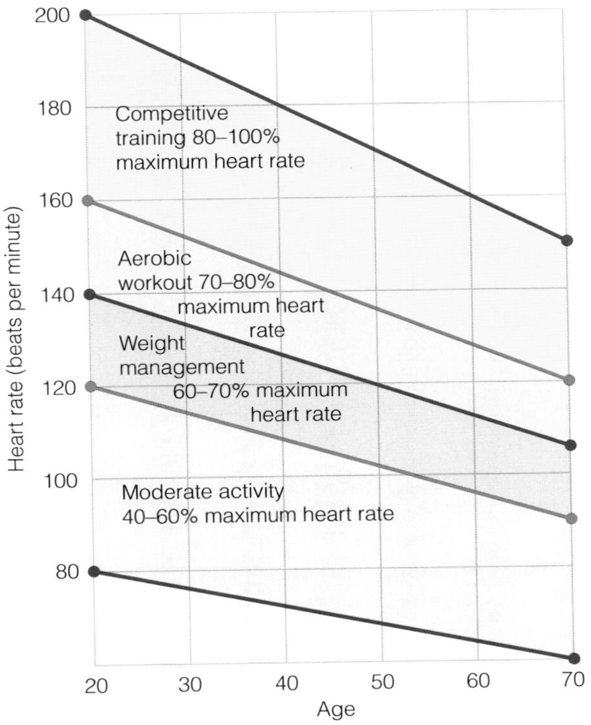

FIGURE 4-4 Target Heart Rates for Different Ages and Various Levels of Activity
Your maximum heart rate is 220 minus your age.

2. Lower-limit target heart rate: Multiply your maximum heart rate by 0.6. So if you are 20, your lower-limit target heart rate is $200 \times 0.6 = 120$ beats per minute.
3. Upper-limit target heart rate. Multiply your maximum heart rate by 0.85. If you are 20, your upper-limit target heart rate is $200 \times 0.85 = 170$.

Your target heart rate range is between your lower and upper limits.

According to the American College of Sports Medicine, for most people, exercising at the lower end of the target heart rate range for a long time is more beneficial

specificity principle Each part of the body adapts to a particular type and amount of stress placed upon it.

reversibility principle The physical benefits of exercise are lost through disuse or inactivity.

aerobic exercise Physical activity in which sufficient or excess oxygen is continually supplied to the body.

anaerobic exercise Physical activity in which the body develops an oxygen deficit.

resting heart rate The number of heartbeats per minute during inactivity.

target heart rate Sixty to eighty-five percent of the maximum heart rate; the heart rate at which one derives maximum cardiovascular benefit from aerobic exercise.

than exercising at the higher end of the range for a short time. If your goal is losing weight, exercise at 60 to 70 percent of your maximum heart rate in order to burn fat calories. To improve aerobic endurance and strengthen your heart, work at 70 to 80 percent of your maximum heart rate. Competitive athletes may train at 80 to 100 percent of their maximum heart rate (see Figure 4-4).

Designing an Aerobic Workout

Whatever activity you choose, your aerobic workout should consist of several stages: a warm-up, an aerobic activity, and a cool-down.

Warm-Up

Just as you don't get in your car and immediately gun your engine to 60 miles per hour, you shouldn't do the same with your body. You need to prepare your cardiorespiratory system for a workout, speed up the blood flow to your lungs, and increase the temperature and elasticity of your muscles and connective tissue to avoid injury.

After reviewing more than 350 scientific studies, the American College of Sports Medicine (ACSM) concluded that preparing for sports or exercise should involve a variety of activities and not be limited to stretching alone. They found little to no relationship between stretching and injuries or postexercise pain. A better option, according to the ACSM, is a combination of warm-up, strength training, and balance exercises.

Aerobic Activity

The two key components of this part of your workout are intensity and duration. As described in the previous section, you can use your target heart rate range to make sure you are working at the proper intensity. The current recommendation is to keep moving for 30 to 60 minutes, either in one session or several briefer sessions, each lasting at least 10 minutes.

Cool-Down

After you've pushed your heart rate up to its target level and kept it there for a while, the worst thing you can do is slam on the brakes. If you come to a sudden stop, you put your heart at risk. When you stand or sit immediately after vigorous exercise, blood can pool in your legs. You need to keep moving at a slower pace to ensure an adequate supply of blood to your heart. Ideally, you should walk for 5 to 10 minutes at a comfortable pace before you end your workout session.

Your Long-Term Fitness Plan

One of the most common mistakes people make is to push too hard too fast. Often they end up injured or discouraged and quit entirely. If you are just starting an aerobic program, think of it as a series of phases: beginning, progression, and maintenance:

- **Beginning (4-6 weeks).** Start slow and low (in intensity). If you're walking, monitor your heart rate and aim for 55 percent of your maximum heart rate. Another good rule of thumb to make sure you're moving at the right pace: If you can sing as you walk, you're going too slow; if you can't talk, you're going too fast.
- **Progression (16-20 weeks).** Gradually increase the duration and/or intensity of your workouts. For instance, you might add 5 minutes every two weeks to your walking time. You also can gradually pick up your pace, using your target heart rate as your guide. Keep a log of your workouts so you can chart your progress until you reach your goal.
- **Maintenance (lifelong).** Once you've reached the stage of exercising for an hour every day, you may want to develop a repertoire of aerobic activities you enjoy. Combine or alternate activities to avoid monotony and keep up your enthusiasm (cross-training).

Aerobic Options

You have lots of choices for aerobic exercise, so experiment. Focus on one for a few weeks; alternate different activities on different days; try something new every month.

Walk the Walk

More men and women are taking to their feet. Some are casualties of high-intensity sports and can no longer withstand the wear and tear of rigorous workouts. Others want to shape up, slim down, or ward off heart disease and other health problems. (Figure 4-5 shows good walking technique.) The good news for all is that walking is good exercise. Research has demonstrated that walking reduces the risk of cardiorespiratory disease—in some studies, as much as vigorous activity does.

Walking has also proved to be one of the safest and most effective ways of preventing bone and joint disorders in obese individuals.

Why Walk? One major study of women, the Nurses Health Study, found that women who walk briskly three hours a week are as well protected from heart disease as women who spend an hour and a half a week in more vigorous activities, such as aerobics or running. Women engaged in either form of exercise had a rate of heart attacks 30 to 40 percent lower than that of sedentary women.

Walking also protects men's hearts, whether they're healthy or have had heart problems. Men who regularly engage in light exercise, including walking, have a significantly lower risk of death than their sedentary counterparts.

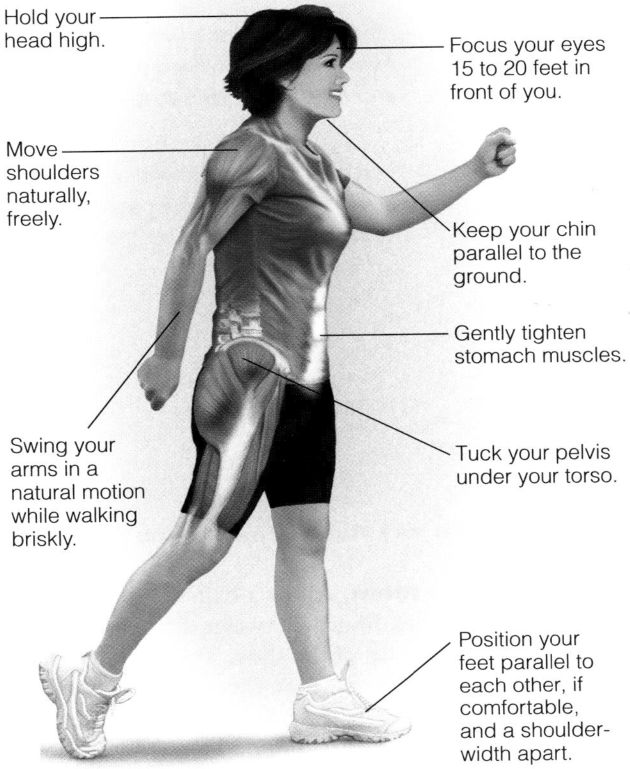

Hold your head high.
Focus your eyes 15 to 20 feet in front of you.
Move shoulders naturally, freely.
Keep your chin parallel to the ground.
Gently tighten stomach muscles.
Swing your arms in a natural motion while walking briskly.
Tuck your pelvis under your torso.
Position your feet parallel to each other, if comfortable, and a shoulder-width apart.

FIGURE 4-5 Good Walking Technique

Source: Mayo Clinic, www. mayoclinic. com. © Mayo Foundation for Medical Education and Research. All rights reserved.

America on the Move How many steps do you walk every day? The typical adult averages about 5310 steps; a child from 11,000 to 13,000. According to the American College of Sports Medicine, college students who used a pedometer to count their daily steps took an average of 7700 steps per day. This falls short of the 10,000 steps recommended as part of the national "America on the Move" program.

How far is 10,000 steps? The average person's stride length is approximately 2.5 feet long. That means it takes just over 2000 steps to walk 1 mile, and 10,000 steps is close to 5 miles. Wearing a pedometer is an easy way to track your steps each day. Start by wearing the pedometer every day for one week. Put it on when you get up in the morning and wear it until bedtime. Record your daily steps in a log or diary. By the end of the week, you can calculate your average daily steps. To increase your steps, add 500 daily steps every week until you reach 10,000.

Why 10,000 steps? According to researchers' estimates, you take about 5000 steps just to accomplish your daily tasks. Adding about 2000 steps brings you to a level that can improve your health and wellness. Another 3000 steps can help you lose excess pounds and prevent weight gain. People who walk at least 10,000 steps a day are more likely to have healthy weights. In addition, 10,000 steps generally translates into 30 minutes of activity, the minimum recommended by the U.S. Surgeon General.

Treadmills are a good alternative to outdoor walks—and not just in bad weather. They keep you moving at a certain pace, they're easier on the knees, and they allow you to exercise in a climate-controlled, pollution-free environment—a definite plus for many city dwellers. Holding onto the handrails while walking on a treadmill reduces both heart rate and oxygen consumption, so you burn fewer calories. Experts advise slowing the pace if necessary so you can let go of the handrails while working out.

Jogging and Running

The difference between jogging and running is speed. You should be able to carry on a conversation with someone on a long jog or run; if you're too breathless to talk, you're pushing too hard.

If your goal is to enhance aerobic fitness, long, slow, distance running is best. If you want to improve your speed, try *interval training*—repeated hard runs over a certain distance, with intervals of relaxed jogging in between. Depending on what suits you and what your training goals are, you can vary the distance, duration, and number of fast runs, as well as the time and activity between them.

If you have been sedentary, it's best to launch a walking program before attempting to jog or run. Start by walking for 15 to 20 minutes three times a week at a comfortable pace. Continue at this same level until you no longer feel sore or unduly fatigued the day after exercising. Then increase your walking time to 20 to 25 minutes, speeding up your pace as well.

When you can handle a brisk 25-minute walk, alternate fast walking with slow jogging. Begin each session walking, and gradually increase the amount of time you spend jogging. If you feel breathless while jogging, slow down and walk. Continue to alternate in this manner until you can jog for 10 minutes without stopping. If you gradually increase your jogging time by 1 or 2 minutes with each workout, you'll slowly build up to 20 or 25 minutes per session. For optimal fitness, you should jog at least three times a week.

How to Buy the Right Athletic Shoe Footwear has come a long way from the days of canvas sneakers. With so many new materials and high-tech options, choosing the right shoe for working out can be confusing. The best shoes aren't necessarily the most expensive but the ones that fit you best. Here are some basic guidelines:

- **Choose the right shoe for your sport.** If you're a walker or runner, you want maximum overall shock absorption for the foot, with extra cushioning in the heel and under the ball of the foot (the metatarsal

Strategies for Change — The Right Way to Walk and Run

Here are some guidelines for putting your best foot forward, whether you are walking or running:

- Maintain good posture. Keep your back straight, your head up, and your eyes looking straight ahead. Hold your arms slightly away from your body—your elbows should be bent slightly so that your forearms are almost parallel to the ground.
- Use the heel-to-toe method. The heel of your leading foot should touch the ground before the ball or toes of that foot do. Push off the ball of your foot, and bend your knee as you raise your heel. You should be able to feel the action in your calf muscles.
- Pump your arms back and forth. This burns more calories and gives you an upper-body workout as well.
- Do not walk or run on the balls of your feet. This produces soreness in the calves because the muscles must contract for a longer time. Avoid running on hard surfaces and making sudden stops and turns.
- End your walk or run with a cool-down period. Let your pace become more leisurely for the last 5 minutes.

area) to prevent pain, burning, and tenderness. If you also participate in other types of exercise, consider "cross-trainers," shoes that are flexible enough in the front for running but provide the side-to-side, or lateral, control you need for aerobics or tennis.

- **Check out the shoe.** A "slip-lasted" shoe, made by sewing together the upper like a moccasin and gluing it to the sole, is lightweight and flexible. A "board-lasted" shoe has a leather, nylon mesh, or canvas upper sewn to a cardboardlike material, which provides more support and control. A "combination-last" shoe offers the advantages of both and works well for a variety of foot types (Figure 4-6).
- **Shop late.** Try on shoes at the end of the day or after a workout, when your foot size is at its maximum (sometimes half a shoe size larger than in the morning). Wear socks similar to those you'll wear for workouts.
- **Give your toes room.** Allow a half-inch, or the width of your index finger, between the end of your longest toe and the tip of the shoe. Try on both shoes. If one foot is larger than the other, buy the larger size.
- **Check the width.** A shoe should be as wide as possible across the forefoot without allowing the heel to slip. Lace up the shoe completely and walk or jog a few steps to make sure the shoes are comfortable.
- **Replace shoes when they lose their cushioning.** After about 300 to 500 miles of running or 300 hours of aerobic activity, your shoes are no longer absorbing the pounding and jarring of your sport. Don't put yourself at increased risk of knee and ankle injuries.

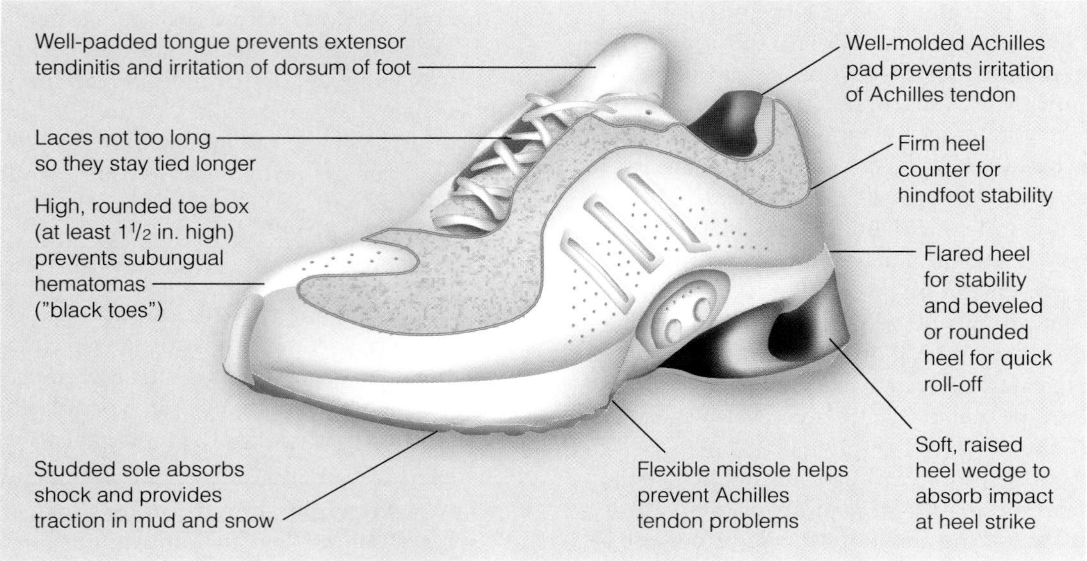
Well-padded tongue prevents extensor tendinitis and irritation of dorsum of foot
Laces not too long so they stay tied longer
High, rounded toe box (at least 1 1/2 in. high) prevents subungual hematomas ("black toes")
Studded sole absorbs shock and provides traction in mud and snow
Flexible midsole helps prevent Achilles tendon problems
Well-molded Achilles pad prevents irritation of Achilles tendon
Firm heel counter for hindfoot stability
Flared heel for stability and beveled or rounded heel for quick roll-off
Soft, raised heel wedge to absorb impact at heel strike

FIGURE 4-6 What to Look for When You Buy Running Shoes

Other Aerobic Activities

Because variety is the spice of an active life, many people prefer different forms of aerobic exercise. All can provide many health benefits. Among the popular options:

- **Swimming.** For aerobic conditioning, you have to swim laps using the freestyle, butterfly, breaststroke, or backstroke. (The sidestroke is too easy.) You must also be a good enough swimmer to keep churning through the water for at least 20 minutes. Your heart will beat more slowly in water than on land, so your heart rate while swimming is not an accurate guide to exercise intensity. Try to keep up a steady pace that's fast enough to make you feel pleasantly tired, but not completely exhausted, by the time you get out of the pool.
- **Cycling.** Bicycling, indoors and out, can be an excellent cardiovascular conditioner, as well as an effective way to control weight—provided you aren't just along for the ride. If you coast down too many hills, you'll have to ride longer up hills or on level ground to get a good workout. An 18-speed bike can make pedaling too easy unless you choose gears carefully. To gain aerobic benefits, mountain bikers have to work hard enough to raise their heart rates to their target zone and keep up that intensity for at least 20 minutes.
- **Spinning.™** Spinning is a cardiovascular workout for the whole body that utilizes a special stationary bicycle. Led by an instructor, a group of bikers listens to music, and modifies their individual bike's resistance and their own pace according to the rhythm. An average spinning class lasts 45 minutes.
- **Cardio kick-boxing.** Also referred to as kick-boxing or boxing aerobics, this hybrid of boxing, martial arts, and aerobics offers an intense total-body workout. An hour of kick-boxing burns an average of 500 to 800 calories, compared to 300 to 400 calories in a typical step aerobics class.
- **Rowing.** Whether on water or a rowing machine, rowing provides excellent aerobic exercise as well as working the upper and lower body and toning the shoulders, back, arms, and legs. Correct rowing techniques are important to avoid back injury.
- **Skipping rope.** Essentially a form of stationary jogging with some extra arm action thrown in, skipping rope is excellent as both a heart conditioner and a way of losing weight. Always warm up before starting and cool down afterward.
- **Aerobic dancing.** This activity combines music with kicking, bending, and jumping. A typical class (you can also dance at home to a video or TV program) consists of stretching exercises and sit-ups, followed by aerobic dances and cool-down exercises. "Soft," or low-impact, aerobic dancing doesn't put as much strain on the joints as "hard," or high-impact, routines.
- **Step training, or bench aerobics.** "Stepping" combines step, or bench, climbing with music and choreographed movements. Basic equipment consists of a bench 4 to 12 inches high. The fitter you are, the higher the bench—but the higher the bench, the greater the risk of knee injury.
- **Stair-climbing.** You could run up the stairs in an office building or dormitory, but most people use stair-climbing machines available in home models and at gyms and health clubs.
- **Inline skating.** Inline skating can increase aerobic endurance and muscular strength and is less stressful on joints and bones than running or high-impact aerobics. Skaters can adjust the intensity of their workout by varying the terrain.
- **Tennis.** As with other sports, tennis can be an aerobic activity—depending on the number of players and their skill level. In general, a singles match requires more continuous exertion than playing doubles.

Building Muscular Fitness

Although aerobic workouts condition your insides (heart, blood vessels, and lungs), they don't exercise many of the muscles that shape your outsides and provide power when you need it. Strength workouts are important because they enable muscles to work more efficiently and reliably. Conditioned muscles function more smoothly and contract somewhat more vigorously and with less effort. With exercise, muscle tissue becomes firmer and can withstand much more strain—the result of toughening the sheath protecting the muscle and developing more connective tissue within it (Figure 4-7).

The two dimensions of muscular fitness are strength and endurance. Muscular strength is the maximal force that a muscle or group of muscles can generate for one movement. Muscular endurance is the capacity to sustain repeated muscle actions. Both are important. You need strength to hoist a shovelful of snow—and endurance so you can keep shoveling the entire driveway.

The latest research on fat-burning shows that the best way to reduce your body fat is to add muscle-strengthening exercise to your workouts. Muscle tissue is your very best calorie-burning tissue, and the more you have, the more calories you burn, even when you are resting. You don't have to become a serious bodybuilder. Using handheld weights (also called *free weights*) two or three times a week is enough. Just be sure you learn how to use them properly, because you can tear or strain muscles if you don't practice the proper weight-lifting techniques. As more people have begun to lift weights, injuries have soared.

A balanced workout regimen of muscle building and aerobic exercise does more for you than just burn

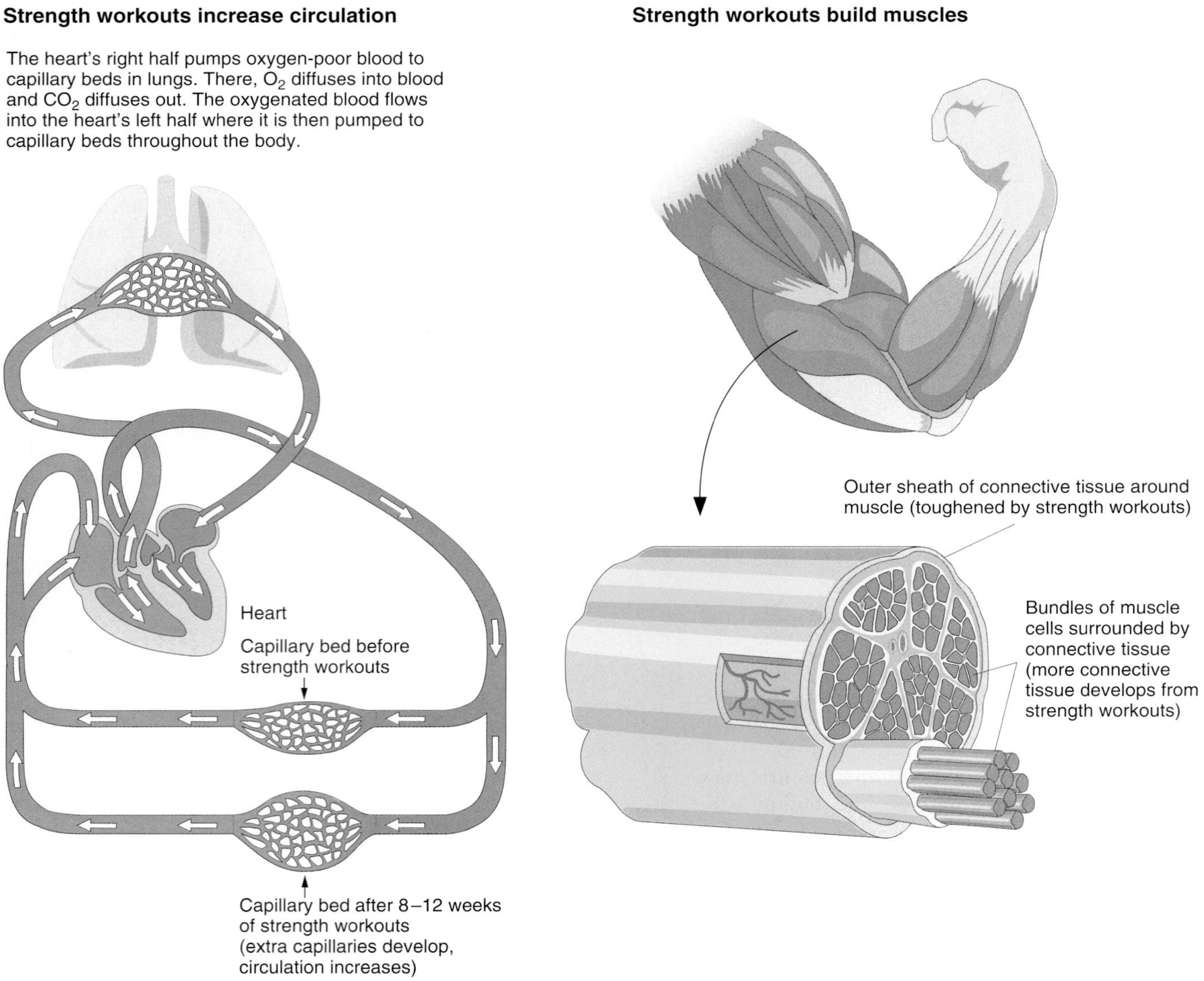
Strength workouts increase circulation
The heart's right half pumps oxygen-poor blood to capillary beds in lungs. There, O_2 diffuses into blood and CO_2 diffuses out. The oxygenated blood flows into the heart's left half where it is then pumped to capillary beds throughout the body.
Heart
Capillary bed before strength workouts
Capillary bed after 8–12 weeks of strength workouts (extra capillaries develop, circulation increases)
Strength workouts build muscles
Outer sheath of connective tissue around muscle (toughened by strength workouts)
Bundles of muscle cells surrounded by connective tissue (more connective tissue develops from strength workouts)

FIGURE 4-7 Benefits of Strength Training on the Body
Strength training increases blood circulation and oxygen supply to body tissues and develops muscles.

fat. It gives you more endurance by promoting better distribution of oxygen to your tissues and increasing the blood flow to your heart.

Strength training has particular benefits for women: As numerous studies have documented, it makes their muscles stronger, their bodies leaner, and their bones more resistant to falls. In young women, it boosts self-esteem, body image, and emotional well-being. In middle-aged and older women, it enhances self-concept, boosts psychological health, and prevents weight gain.

Muscles at Work

Your muscles never stay the same. If you don't use them, they atrophy, weaken, or break down. If you use them rigorously and regularly, they grow stronger. The only way to develop muscles is by demanding more of them than you usually do. This is called **overloading.** (Remember the overload principle?) As you train, you have to gradually increase the number of repetitions or the amount of resistance and work the muscle to temporary fatigue. That's why it's important not to quit when your muscles start to tire. Progressive overload—steadily increasing the stress placed on the body—builds stronger muscles.

Yous need to exercise differently for strength than for endurance. *To develop strength,* do a few repetitions with heavy loads. As you increase the weight your muscles must move, you increase your strength. *To increase endurance,* you do many more repetitions with lighter loads. If your muscles are weak and you need to gain strength in your upper body, you may have to work for weeks to do a half-dozen regular push-ups. Then you

© Blend Images/Alamy

You can use everyday objects as well as weights to strengthen your muscles.

can start building endurance by doing as many push-ups as you can before collapsing in exhaustion.

Muscles can do only two things: contract or relax. As they do so, skeletal muscles either pull on bones or stop pulling on bones. All exercise involves muscles pulling on bones across a joint. The movement that takes place depends on the structure of the joint and the position of the muscle attachments involved.

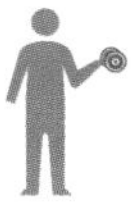

In an **isometric** contraction, the muscle applies force while maintaining an equal length. The muscle contracts and tries to shorten but cannot overcome the resistance. An example is pushing against an immovable object, like a wall, or tightening an abdominal muscle while sitting. The muscle contracts, but there is no movement. Push or pull against the immovable object, with each muscle contraction held for 5 to 8 seconds; repeat five to ten times daily.

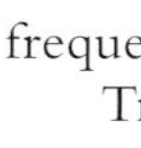

An **isotonic** contraction involves movement, but the muscle tension remains the same. In an isotonic exercise, the muscle moves a moderate load several times, as in weight lifting or calisthenics. The best isotonic exercise for producing muscular strength involves high resistance and a low number of repetitions. On the other hand, you can develop the greatest flexibility, coordination, and endurance with isotonic exercises that incorporate lower resistance and frequent repetitions.

True **isokinetic** contraction is a constant speed contraction. Isokinetic exercises require special machines that provide resistance to overload muscles throughout the entire range of motion.

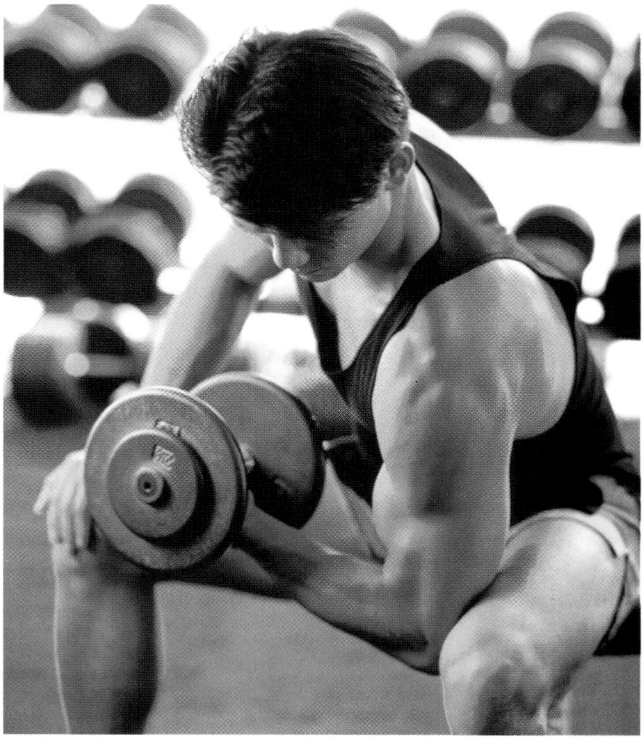

© Jurgen Reisch/Stone/Getty Images

Various types of weight training, including free weights build muscular strength and endurance.

Designing a Muscle Workout

A workout with weights should exercise your body's primary muscle groups: the *deltoids* (shoulders), *pectorals* (chest), *triceps* and *biceps* (back and front of upper arms), *quadriceps* and *hamstrings* (front and back of thighs), *gluteus maximus* (buttocks), *trapezius* and *rhomboids* (back), and *abdomen* (Figure 4-8). Various machines and free-weight routines focus on each muscle group, but the principle is always the same: Muscles contract as you raise and lower a weight, and you repeat the lift-and-lower routine until the muscle group is tired.

A weight training program is made up of **reps** (the single performance, or **repetition,** of an exercise, such

overloading Method of physical training involving increasing the number of repetitions or the amount of resistance gradually to work the muscle to temporary fatigue.

isometric Of the same length; exercise in which muscles increase their tension without shortening in length, such as when pushing an immovable object.

isotonic Having the same tension or tone; exercise requiring the repetition of an action that creates tension, such as weight lifting or calisthenics.

isokinetic Having the same force; exercise with specialized equipment that provides resistance equal to the force applied by the user throughout the entire range of motion.

rep (or **repetition**) In weight training, a single performance of a movement or exercise.

as lifting 50 pounds one time) and **sets** (a *set* number of repetitions of the same movement, such as a set of 20 push-ups). You should allow your breath to return to normal before moving on to each new set. Pushing yourself to the limit builds strength. Although the ideal number of sets in a resistance training program remains controversial, recent evidence suggests that multiple sets lead to additional benefits in short- and long-term training in young and middle-aged adults.

Maintaining proper breathing during weight training is crucial. To breathe correctly, inhale when muscles are relaxed and exhale when you push or lift. Don't ever hold your breath, because oxygen flow helps prevent muscle fatigue and injury.

No one type of equipment—free weight or machine—has a clear advantage in terms of building fat-free body mass, enhancing strength and endurance, or improving a sport-specific skill. Each type offers benefits but also has drawbacks.

Free weights offer great versatility for strength training. With dumbbells, for example, you can perform a variety of exercises to work specific muscle groups, such as the chest and shoulders. Machines, in contrast, are much more limited; most allow only one exercise.

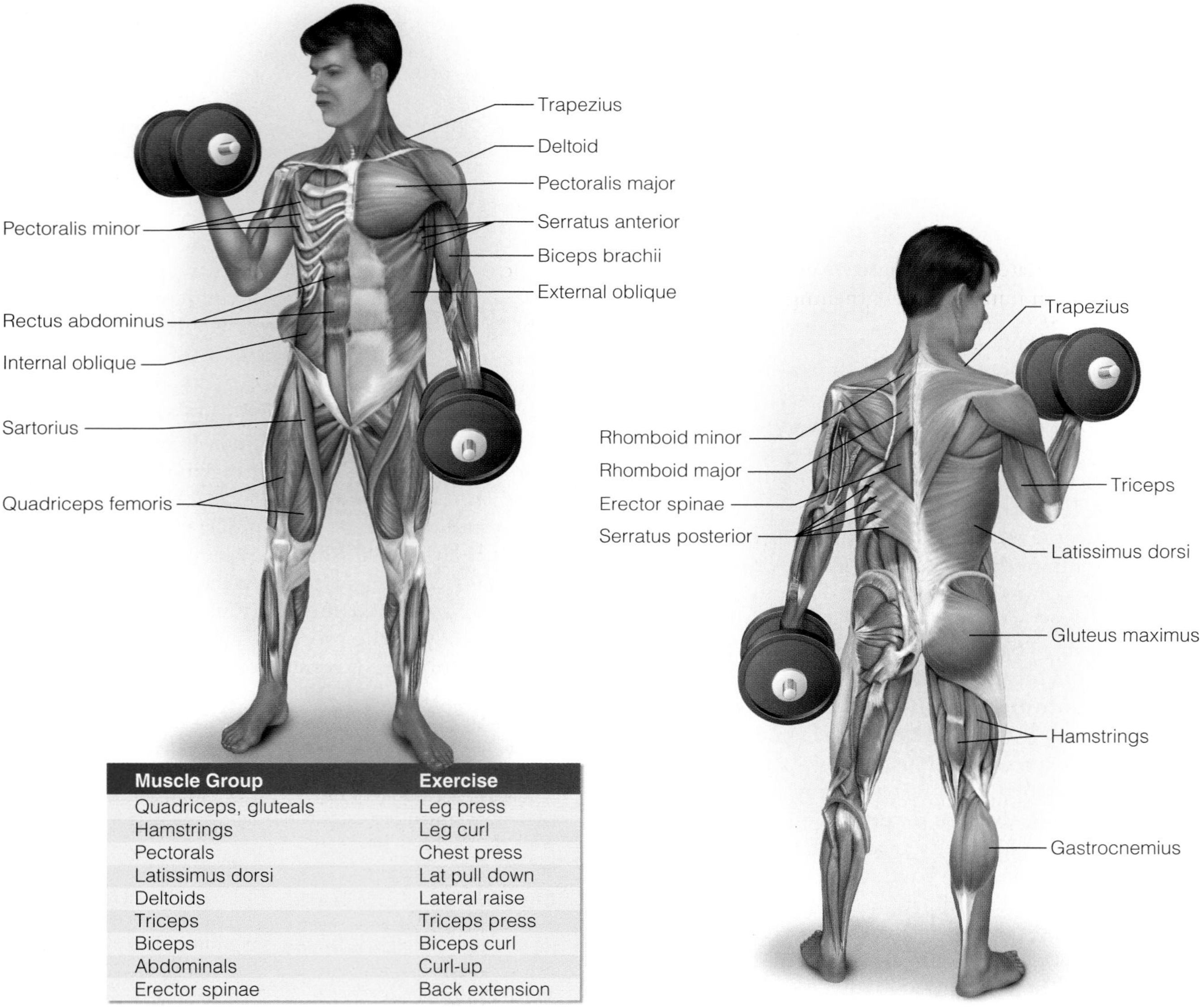

Muscle Group	Exercise
Quadriceps, gluteals	Leg press
Hamstrings	Leg curl
Pectorals	Chest press
Latissimus dorsi	Lat pull down
Deltoids	Lateral raise
Triceps	Triceps press
Biceps	Biceps curl
Abdominals	Curl-up
Erector spinae	Back extension

FIGURE 4-8 Primary Muscle Groups
Different exercises can strengthen and stretch different muscle groups.

Strategies for Prevention: Working with Weights

If you plan to work with free weights, here are some guidelines for using them safely and effectively:

- Don't train alone—for safety's sake. Work with a partner so you can serve as spotters for each other and help motivate each other as well.
- Always warm up before weight training; also be sure to stretch after training.
- Breathe! Holding your breath during exertion can produce a dangerous rise in blood pressure.
- Begin with relatively light weights (50 percent of the maximum you can lift), and increase the load slowly until you find the weight that will cause muscle failure at anywhere from eight to twelve repetitions. (Muscle failure is the point during a workout at which you can no longer perform or complete a repetition through the entire range of motion.)
- In the beginning, don't work at maximum intensity. Increase your level of exertion gradually over two to six weeks to allow your body to adapt to new stress without soreness.
- Always train your entire body, starting with the larger muscle groups. Don't focus only on specific areas, although you may want to concentrate on your weakest muscles.
- Always use proper form. Unnecessary twisting, lurching, lunging, or arching can cause serious injury. Remember, quality matters more than quantity. One properly performed set of lifts can produce a greater increase in strength and muscle mass than many sets of improperly performed lifts.
- Work through the full range of motion. Be careful not to hyperextend or overextend.

Strength-training machines have several advantages. They ensure correct movement for a lift, which helps protect against injury and prevent cheating when fatigue sets in. They isolate specific muscles, which is good for rehabilitating an injury or strengthening a specific body part. Because they offer high-tech options like varying resistance during the lifting motion, they can tax muscles in ways that a traditional barbell cannot.

Recovery

The American College of Sports Medicine recommends a minimum of eight to ten exercises involving the major muscle groups two to three days a week. Remember that your muscles need sufficient time to recover from a weight-training session. Never work a sore muscle, because soreness may indicate that too-heavy weights have caused tiny tears in the fibers. Allow no less than 48 hours, but no more than 96 hours, between training sessions, so your body can recover from the workout and you avoid overtraining. Workouts on consecutive days do more harm than good because the body can't recover that quickly. Strength training twice a week at greater intensity and for a longer duration can be as effective as working out three times a week. However, your muscles will begin to atrophy if you let more than three or four days pass without exercising them.

Core Strength Conditioning

"Core strength," a popular trend in exercise and fitness, refers to the ability of the muscles to support your spine and keep your body stable and balanced. When you have good core stability, the muscles in your pelvis, lower back, hips, and abdomen work in harmony. This improves your posture, breathing, appearance, and performance in sports, while reducing your risk of muscle strain. When your core is weak, you become more susceptible to lower back pain and injury.

The major muscles of your core include the transverse abdominis, the deepest of the abdominal muscles; the external and internal obliques on the side and front of the abdomen around your waist; and the rectus abdominis, a long muscle that extends along the front of the abdomen. Strengthening all of your core muscles provides stability, improves balance, and protects you from injury.

Performance-Enhancing Drugs

Performance-enhancing substances include any compounds taken to increase strength, power, speed, or endurance (ergogenic) or to change body weight or composition for the sake of boosting athletic performance. Approximately 1 to 3 million people in the United States have used these substances, including an estimated 4.7 percent of boys and 1.6 percent of girls.[22]

The discovery that many Major League Baseball players have used drugs to improve their power and performance set off a national scandal. But professional and amateur athletes

sets In weight training, the number of repetitions of the same movement or exercise.

Strategies for Prevention — Watch out for "Pump Fiction"

Shape up in seven days! Burn calories without breaking a sweat! A brand-new body in minutes a day!

Too good to be true? Absolutely. Advertisers promise no-sweat, no-effort ways to fitness with pills, potions, flab-melting belts, and thigh-slimming paddles. These claims amount to nothing more than what the American Council on Exercise calls "pump fiction." The benefits of fitness are real and well documented, but the only way to reap them is through regular exercise.

Here are some specific guidelines:

- **Be wary** of any program or product that promises "easy" or "effortless" results. Athletes in peak condition might use them without breaking a sweat. Chances are that you, like most people, won't.
- **Watch out for "spot" reducers.** You can't lose a "spare tire" or firm flabby thighs by targeting only that area of your body. You need to lose weight and tone your entire body.
- **Read the fine print.** Often it states that the results are based not just on the device but on dieting and exercise as well.
- **Don't believe testimonials** or celebrity endorsements. Slim, trim, smiling celebrities are paid well for their enthusiasm.
- **Be skeptical** of dramatic "before and after" photos. With today's technology, you never know if photos were doctored or if the results lasted.
- **Check the details** on warranties, guarantees, and return policies. The ads may promise a "30-day money-back guarantee" but fail to mention hefty shipping costs.

aren't the only ones turning to drugs to reshape their bodies. Young men use them to look more buff and muscular. Older men try them to fight the effects of aging. All face serious risks to their hearts, liver, reproductive systems, and psychological well-being. (See Savvy Consumer: "What You Should Know About Performance-Boosting Drugs.")

College athletes are among the groups most likely to use performance-enhancing drugs. To stop sports doping, some suggest more rigorous drug testing of athletes and immediate suspension if they test positive. Others urge stiff fines and dismissal of coaches who turn a blind eye on athletes' drug use. Should colleges and athletic associations focus on identifying and punishing students who take performance-boosting drugs? Or should they focus on the coaches and trainers who tolerate or endorse this practice?

You Decide

Becoming More Flexible

Flexibility is the characteristic of body tissues that determines the **range of motion** achievable without injury at a joint or group of joints. There are two types of flexibility: static and dynamic. **Static flexibility**—the type most people think of as flexibility—refers to the ability to assume and maintain an extended position at one end point in a joint's range of motion. **Dynamic flexibility,** by comparison, involves movement. It is the ability to move a joint quickly and fluidly through its entire range of motion with little resistance. The static flexibility in the hip joint determines whether you can do a split; dynamic flexibility is what would enable you to perform a split leap.

Static flexibility depends on many factors, including the structure of a joint and the tightness of the muscles, tendons, and ligaments attached to it. Dynamic flexibility is influenced by static flexibility but also depends on additional factors, such as strength, coordination, and resistance to movement.

Genetics, age, gender, and body composition all influence how flexible you are. Girls and women tend to be more flexible than boys and men to a certain extent because of hormonal and anatomical differences. The way females and males use their muscles and the activities they engage in can also have an effect. Over time, the natural elasticity of muscles, tendons, and joints decreases in both genders, resulting in stiffness.

The Benefits of Flexibility

Just as cardiorespiratory fitness benefits the heart and lungs and muscular fitness builds endurance and strength, a stretching program produces unique benefits, including enhancement of the ability of the respiratory, circulatory, and neuromuscular systems to cope with the stress and demands of our high-pressure world (Figure 4-9). Among the other benefits of flexibility are:

- **Prevention of injuries.** Flexibility training stretches muscles and increases the elasticity of joints. Strong, flexible muscles resist stress better than weak or inflexible ones. Adding flexibility to a training program for sports such as soccer, football, or tennis can reduce the

SAVVY CONSUMER

What You Should Know about Performance-Boosting Drugs

Here's what we know—and don't know—about the most widely used performance boosters.

Anabolic steroids are synthetic derivatives of the male hormone testosterone that promote the growth of skeletal muscle and increase lean body mass. Taken orally, applied in creams, or injected, anabolic steroids are typically used in cycles of weeks or months, rather than continuously.

Anabolic steroids have been reported to increase lean muscle mass, strength, and ability to train longer and harder, but they pose serious health hazards, including liver tumors, jaundice (yellowish pigmentation of skin, tissues, and body fluids), fluid retention, high blood pressure, decreased immune function, and severe acne. Men may experience shrinking of the testicles, reduced sperm count, infertility, baldness, and development of breasts. Women may experience growth of facial hair, acne, changes in or cessation of the menstrual cycle, enlargement of the clitoris, and deepened voice. In women, these changes are irreversible. In men, side effects may be reversible once abuse stops. In adolescents, steroids may bring about a premature halt in skeletal maturation.

Anabolic steroid abuse may lead to aggression and other psychiatric side effects. Many users report feeling good about themselves while on anabolic steroids, but researchers report that anabolic steroid abuse can cause wild mood swings including maniclike symptoms leading to "'roid rage," or violent, even homicidal, episodes. Researchers have reported that users may suffer from paranoid jealousy, extreme irritability, delusions, and impaired judgment stemming from feelings of invincibility. Stopping the drugs abruptly can lead to depression.

- **Androstenedione ("andro").** This testosterone precursor is normally produced by the adrenal glands and gonads. Manufacturers claim that androstenedione improves testosterone concentration, increases muscular strength and mass, helps reduce body fat, enhances mood, and improves sexual performance. Studies have shown that supplemental androstenedione doesn't increase testosterone and muscles don't get stronger with andro use. Andro has been classified as a controlled substance, making its use illegal.
- **Creatine.** This amino acid is made by the body and stored predominantly in skeletal muscle. Creatine serves as a reservoir to replenish adenosine triphosphate (ATP), a substance involved in energy production. Some studies show creatine may increase strength and endurance. Other effects on the body remain unknown.

  The Food and Drug Administration has warned consumers to consult a physician before taking creatine supplements. Creatine may cause dehydration and heat-related illnesses, reduced blood volume, and electrolyte imbalances. Some athletes drink quantities of water hoping to avoid such effects. However, many coaches forbid or discourage creatine use because its long-term effects remain unknown.
- **GBL (gamma butyrolactone).** This unapproved drug is being studied as a treatment for narcolepsy, a disabling sleep disorder. Nevertheless, it is marketed on the Internet and in some professional gyms as a muscle-builder and performance-enhancer. The Food and Drug Administration has warned consumers to avoid any products containing GBL, noting that they have been associated with at least one death and several incidents in which users became comatose or unconscious.

rate of injuries by as much as 75 percent. In one study of competitive runners, weekly stretching sessions significantly reduced the incidence of low-back pain.

- **Relief of muscle strain.** Muscles tighten as a result of stress or prolonged sitting. If you study or work in one position for several hours, you'll often feel stiffness in your back or neck. Stretching helps relieve this tension and enables you to work more effectively.
- **Relaxation.** Flexibility exercises are great stress-busters that reduce mental strain, slow the rate of breathing, and reduce blood pressure.

range of motion The fullest extent of possible movement in a particular joint.

static flexibility The ability to assume and maintain an extended position at one end point in a joint's range of motion.

dynamic flexibility The ability to move a joint quickly and fluidly through its entire range of motion with little resistance.

anabolic steroids Drugs derived from testosterone and approved for medical use, but often used by athletes to increase their musculature and weight.

- **Relief of soreness after exercise.** Many people develop delayed-onset muscle soreness (DOMS) one or two days after they work out. This may be the result of damage to the muscle fibers and supporting connective tissue.
- **Improved posture.** Bad posture can create tight, stressed muscles. If you slump in your chair, for instance, the muscles in the front of your chest may tighten, causing those in the upper spine to overstretch and become loose.

Stretching

When you stretch a muscle, you are primarily stretching the connective tissue. The stretch must be intense enough to increase the length of the connective tissue without tearing it.

Static stretching involves a gradual stretch held for a short time (10 to 30 seconds). A shorter stretch provides little benefit; a longer stretch does not provide additional benefits. Since a slow stretch provokes less of a reaction from the stretch receptors, the muscles can safely stretch farther than usual. Fitness experts most often recommend static stretching because it is both safe and effective. An example of such a stretch is letting your hands slowly slide down the front of your legs (keeping your knees in a soft, unlocked position) until you reach your toes and holding this final position for several seconds before slowly straightening up. You should feel a pull, but not pain, during this stretch.

In **passive stretching,** your own body, a partner, gravity, or a weight serves as an external force or resistance to help your joints move through their range of motion. You can achieve a more intense stretch and a greater range of motion with passive stretching. There is a greater risk of injury, however, because the muscles themselves are not controlling the stretch.

Active stretching involves stretching a muscle by contracting the opposing muscle (the muscle on the opposite side of the limb). This method allows the muscle to be stretched farther with a low risk of injury.

Ballistic stretching is characterized by rapid bouncing movements, such as a series of up-and-down bobs as you try again and again to touch your toes with your hands. These bounces can stretch the muscle fibers too far, causing the muscle to contract rather than

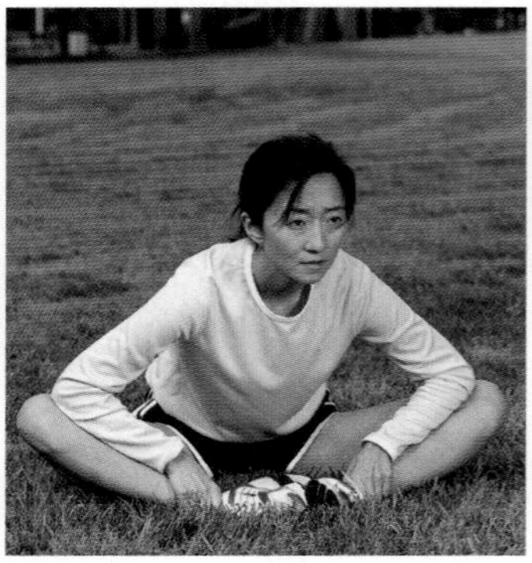

(a) Foot pull for the groin and thigh muscles

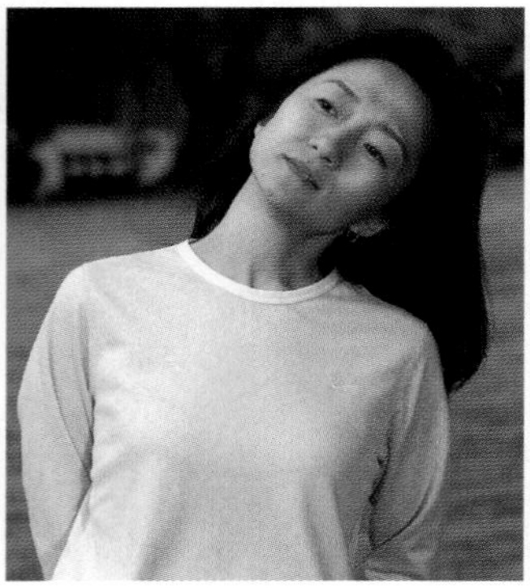

(b) Lateral head tilt

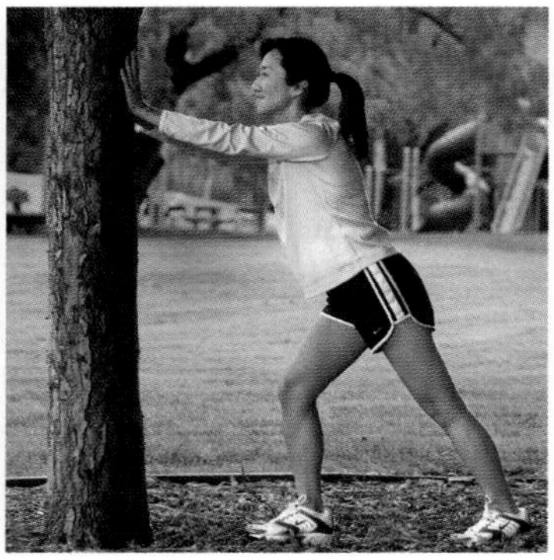

(c) Wall stretch for the Achilles tendon

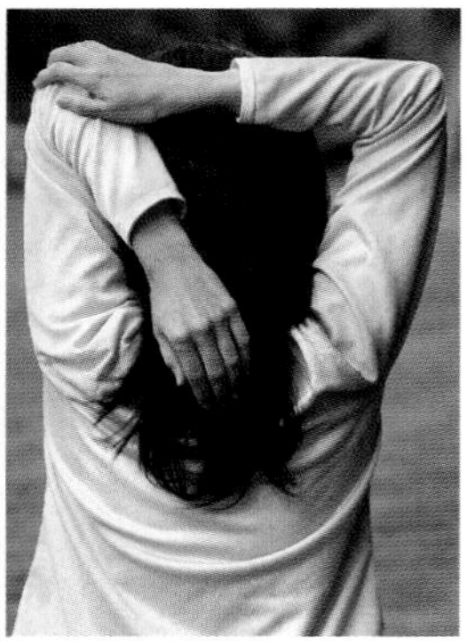

(d) Triceps stretch for the upper arm and shoulder

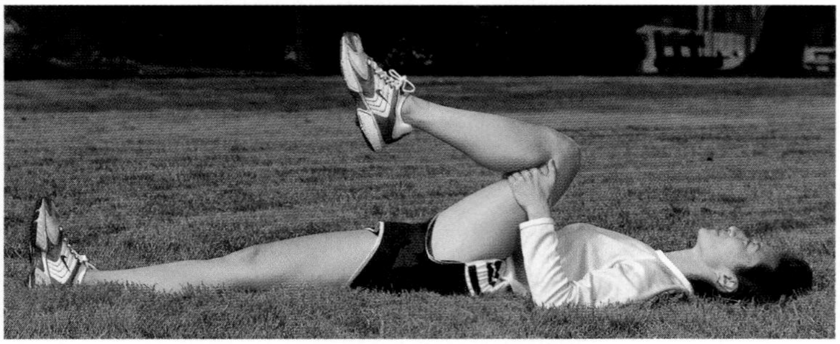

(e) Knee-chest pull for lower back muscles

Matthew Farruggio (all)

FIGURE 4-9 Some Simple Stretching Exercises

(a) Sit on the ground and bend your legs so that the soles of your feet touch. Pull your feet closer as you press on your knees with your elbows. Hold for 10 seconds; repeat. **(b)** Gently tilt your head to each side. Repeat several times. **(c)** Stand 3 feet from a wall or post with your feet slightly apart. Keeping your heels on the ground, lean into the wall. Hold for 10 seconds; repeat. **(d)** Place your right hand behind your neck and grasp above the elbow with your left hand. Gently pull the elbow back. Repeat with the left elbow. **(e)** Lying on your back, clasp one knee and pull it toward your chest. Hold for 15–30 seconds; repeat with the other knee.

Strategies for Prevention — How to Avoid Stretching Injuries

Before you begin, increase your body temperature by slowly marching or running in place. Sweat signals that you're ready to start stretching.

- Don't force body parts beyond their normal range of motion. Stretch to the point of tension, back off, and hold for ten seconds to a minute.
- Do a minimum of four repetitions of each stretch, with equal repetitions on each side.
- Don't hold your breath. Continue breathing slowly and rhythmically throughout your stretching routine.
- Don't attempt to stretch a weak or injured muscle.
- Start small. Work the muscles of the smaller joints in the arms and legs first and then work the larger joints like the shoulders and hips.
- Stretch individual muscles before you stretch a group of muscles, for instance, the ankle, knee, and hip before a stretch that works all three.
- Don't make any quick, jerky movements while stretching. Stretches should be gentle and smooth.
- Certain positions can be harmful to the knees and lower back. In particular, avoid stretches that require deep knee bends or full squats, because they can harm your knees and lower back.

stretch. Because of its potential dangers, fitness experts generally recommend against ballistic stretching.

? FAQ What Is the Difference Between Stretching and Warming Up?

Warming up means getting the heart beating, breaking a sweat, and readying the body for more vigorous activity. Stretching is a specific activity intended to elongate the muscles and keep joints limber, not simply a prelude to a game of tennis or a three-mile run. According to a review of recent studies, the value of stretching varies with different activities. While it does not prevent injuries from jogging, cycling, or swimming, stretching may be beneficial in sports, like soccer and football, that involve bouncing and jumping.

For aerobic activities, one of the best times to stretch is after an aerobic workout. Your muscles will be warm, more flexible, and less prone to injury. In addition, stretching after aerobic activity can help a fatigued muscle return to its normal resting length and possibly helps reduce delayed muscle soreness.

Mind-Body Approaches

Yoga, Pilates, and t'ai chi, increasingly popular on campuses and throughout the country, can help reduce stress, enhance health and wellness, and improve physical fitness.

Yoga

One of the most ancient of mind-body practices, *yoga* comes from the Sanskrit word meaning "union." Traditionally associated with religion, yoga consists of various breathing and stretching exercises that unite all aspects of a person.

Once considered an exotic pursuit, yoga has gained acceptance as part of a comprehensive stress management and fitness program. Scientific studies have demonstrated its benefits, which include:

- **Improved flexibility,** which may offer protection from back pain and injuries.
- **Protection of joints** because yoga postures take joints through their full range of motion, providing a fresh supply of nutrients to joint cartilage.
- **Stronger, denser bones** from yoga's weight-bearing postures.
- **Enhanced circulation,** which also boosts the supply of oxygen throughout the body.
- **Lower blood pressure.**
- **Lower levels of the stress hormone cortisol,** which (as discussed in Chapter 3) can affect the immune system, interfere with memory, and increase the risk of depression and osteoporosis.
- **Lower blood sugar in people with diabetes,** which reduces the risk of complications.
- **Reduced pain** in people with back problems, arthritis, carpal tunnel syndrome, fibromyalgia, and other chronic problems.

static stretching A gradual stretch held for a short time of 10 to 30 seconds.

passive stretching A stretching technique in which an external force or resistance (your body, a partner, gravity, or a weight) helps the joints move through their range of motion.

active stretching A technique that involves stretching a muscle by contracting the opposing muscle.

ballistic stretching Rapid bouncing movements.

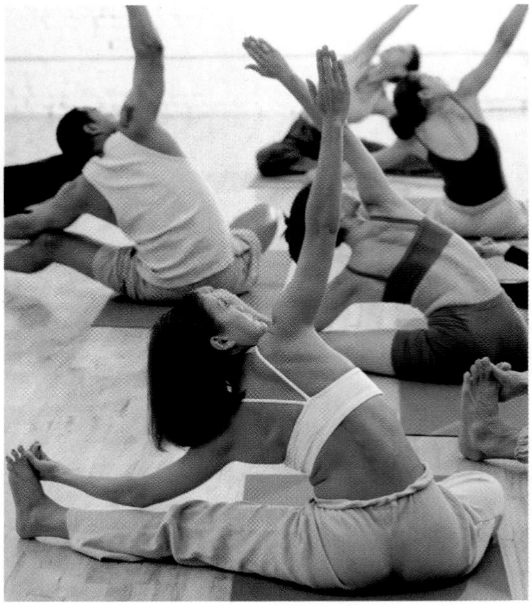

Yoga, one of the most ancient mind-body practices, has many health benefits.

Pilates

Increasingly used to complement aerobics and weight training, Pilates exercises improve flexibility and joint mobility and strengthen the core by developing pelvic stability and abdominal control. Pilates-trained instructors offer "mat" or "floor" classes that stress the stabilization and strengthening of the back and abdominal muscles. Fitness centers also may offer training on Pilates equipment, primarily a device called the Reformer, a wooden contraption with various cables, pulleys, springs, and sliding boards attached that is used for a series of progressive, range-of-motion exercises. Unlike exercise techniques that emphasize numerous repetitions in a single direction, Pilates exercises involve very few, but extremely precise, repetitions in several planes of motion.

T'ai Chi

This ancient Chinese practice, designed to exercise body, mind, and spirit, gently works muscles, focuses concentration, and improves the flow of "qi" (often spelled "chi"), the vital life energy that sustains health. Popular with all ages, from children to seniors, t'ai chi is easy to learn and perform. Because of its focus on breathing and flowing gestures, t'ai chi is sometimes described as "meditation in motion."

Physicians may recommend t'ai chi for those with musculoskeletal disorders like arthritis to improve flexibility and build muscle strength gently and gradually.

Body Composition

Body composition, the fifth component of fitness, can tell you a lot about risk for cardiovascular disease and diabetes.

A combination of regular exercise and good nutrition is the best way to maintain a healthy body composition. Aerobic exercise helps by burning calories and increasing metabolic rate (the rate at which the body uses calories) for several hours after a workout. Strength training increases the proportion of lean body tissue by

Strategies for Prevention — Back Talk

Back pain is the second-most common health problem among college students (allergies rank first), according to the National College Health Assessment. Your risk of lower back pain is higher if you smoke or if you're overstressed, overweight, or out of shape. Here are some ways to prevent back problems now and in the future:

- When standing, shift your weight from one foot to the other. If possible, place one foot on a stool, step, or railing 4 to 6 inches off the ground. Hold in your stomach, tilt your pelvis toward your back, and tuck in your buttocks to provide crucial support for the lower back.
- Because sitting places more stress on the lower back than standing, try to get up from your seat at least once an hour to stretch or walk around. Whenever possible, sit in a straight chair with a firm back. Avoid slouching in overstuffed chairs or dangling your legs in midair. When driving, keep the seat forward so that your knees are raised to hip level; your right leg should not be fully extended. A small pillow or towel can help support your lower back.
- Sleep on a flat, firm mattress. The best sleep position is on your side, with one or both knees bent at right angles to your torso. The pillow should keep your head in line with your body so that your neck isn't bent forward or to the side.
- When lifting, bend at the knees, not from the waist. Get close to the load. Tighten your stomach muscles, but don't hold your breath. Let your leg muscles do the work.

building muscle mass, which also increases the metabolic rate.

Experts debate which measure of body composition—body mass index (BMI), waist circumference, or waist-to-hip ratio—is the best indicator of central or visceral obesity, which increases the risk of heart disease, metabolic syndrome, diabetes, and other illnesses.

Body Mass Index (BMI)

Body mass index (BMI), a ratio between weight and height, is a mathematical formula that correlates with body fat. You can determine your BMI from Figure 4-10. A healthy BMI ranges from 18.5 to 24.9.

A BMI of 25 or greater defines **overweight** and marks the point at which excess weight increases the risk of disease. If your BMI is between 25 and 29.9 (23.4 for Asians), your weight is undermining the quality of your life. You suffer more aches and pains. You find it harder to perform everyday tasks. You run a greater risk of serious health problems.

A BMI of 30 or greater defines **obesity** and marks the point at which excess weight increases the risk of death. If your BMI is between 30 and 34.9 (class 1 obesity), you face all the preceding dangers plus one more: dying. The risk of premature death increases even more if your BMI is between 35 and 39.9 (class 2 obesity). A BMI of 40 or higher indicates class 3 or severe obesity (Table 4-3).

Doctors use BMI to determine whether a person is at risk for weight-related diseases like diabetes. However, using BMI as an assessment tool has limitations. Muscular individuals, including athletes and body builders, may be miscategorized as overweight or obese because they have greater lean muscle mass. BMI also does not

body mass index (BMI) A mathematical formula that correlates with body fat; the ratio of weight to height squared.

overweight A condition of having a BMI between 25.0 and 29.9.

obesity The excessive accumulation of fat in the body; class 1 obesity is defined by a BMI between 30 and 34.9; class 2 obesity is defined by a BMI between 35 and 39.9; class 3, or severe obesity, is a BMI of 40 or higher.

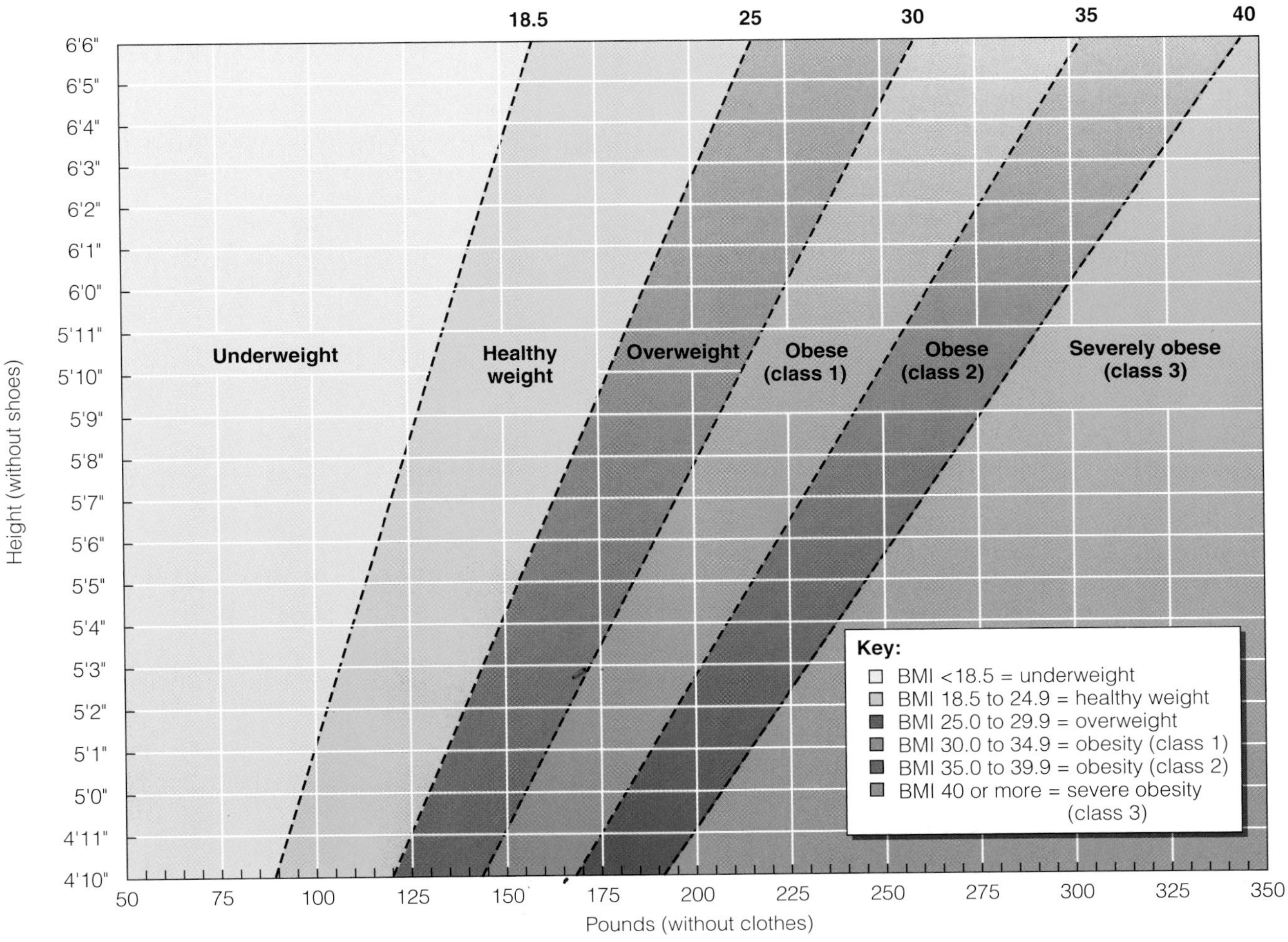

FIGURE 4-10 BMI Values Used to Assess Weight for Adults

TABLE 4-3 Undergraduate BMIs

Students	BMIs			
	Healthy	Over-weight	Obese	Under-weight
White	62%	23%	12%	4%
Black	60%	27%	18%	4%
Hispanic/Latino	55%	28%	14%	4%
Asian/ Pacific Islander	65%	20%	5%	11%

*Based on a survey of 16,832 students.
Source: American College Health Association. American College Health Association-National College Health Assessment (ACHA-NCHA) Web Summary. Updated April 2006. Available at www.acha.org/projects_programs/ncha_sampledata.cfm.

reliably reflect body fat, an independent predictor of health risk, and is not useful for growing children, women who are pregnant or nursing, or the elderly. In addition, BMI, which was developed in Western nations, may not accurately indicate the risk of obesity-related diseases in Asian men and women.

Waist Circumference

Even if your scale shows that you haven't gained a lot of weight, your waist may widen—particularly if you've been under stress. Because of the physiological impact of stress hormones, fat accumulates around your midsection in times of tension and turmoil.

A widening waist or "apple" shape is a warning signal. In women, a wider waist correlates with high levels of harmful blood fats, such as LDL cholesterol and triglycerides.[23] In both sexes, abdominal fat, unlike fat in the thighs or hips, increases the risk of high blood pressure, type 2 diabetes, high cholesterol, and metabolic syndrome (a perilous combination of overweight, high blood pressure, and high levels of cholesterol and blood sugar, discussed in Chapter 15).

To measure your waist circumference, place a tape measure around your bare abdomen just above your hip bone. Be sure that the tape is snug but does not compress your skin. Relax, exhale, and measure.

When is a waist too wide? Various studies have produced different results, but the general guideline is that a waist measuring more than 35 inches in a woman or more than 40 inches in a man signals greater health risks. These waist circumferences indicate "central" obesity, which is characterized by fat deposited deep within the central abdominal area of the body. Such "visceral" fat is more dangerous than "subcutaneous" fat just below the skin because it moves more readily into the bloodstream and directly raises levels of harmful cholesterol.

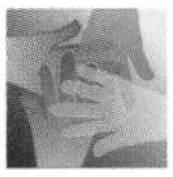

Body composition varies with race and ethnicity. Asians, for instance, may be more likely and African Americans less likely to accumulate visceral fat than Caucasians.

Waist-to-Hip Ratio

Another way of determining your health risk is your **waist-to-hip ratio (WHR)**. In addition to measuring your waist, measure your hips at the widest part. Divide your waist measurement by your hip measurement. For women, a ratio of 0.80 or less is considered safe; for men, the recommended ratio is 0.90 or less. For both men and women, a 1.0 or higher is considered "at risk" or in the danger zone for undesirable health consequences, such as heart disease and other ailments associated with being overweight.

Men of all ages are more prone to develop the "apple" shape characteristic of central obesity; women in their reproductive years are more likely to accumulate fat around the hips and thighs and acquire a pear shape (Figure 4-11).

When men and women diet, men lose more visceral fat located around the abdominal area. This weight loss produces more cardiovascular benefits for men, including a decrease in triglycerides (fats circulating in the blood) and an increase in the "good" form of cholesterol, high-density lipoprotein (HDL).

Safe and Healthy Workouts

Whenever you work out, you don't want to risk becoming sore or injured. Starting slowly when you begin any new fitness activity is the smartest strategy. Keep a simple diary to record the time and duration of each workout. Get accustomed to an activity first and then begin to work harder or longer. In this way, you strengthen your musculoskeletal system so you're less likely to be injured, you lower the cardiovascular risk, and you build the exercise habit into your schedule.

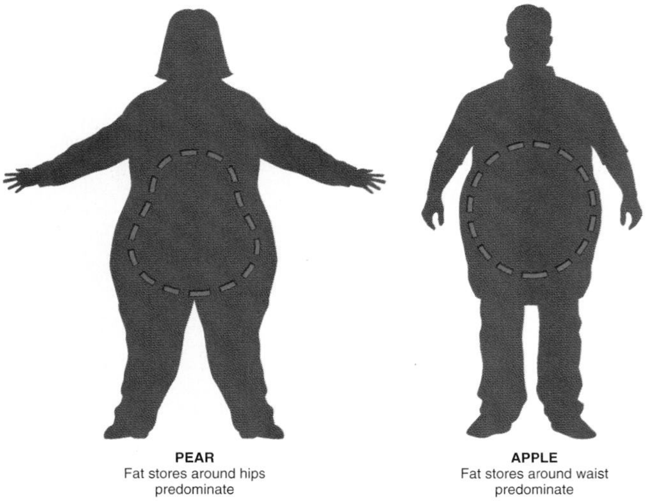

FIGURE 4-11 Pear-Shaped Versus Apple-Shaped Bodies

Strategies for Prevention — Heeding Heat

- Increase your fluid intake during hot temperatures by two to four glasses of cool fluids each hour. Cold beverages can cause stomach cramps; alcoholic beverages can cause you to lose more fluid.
- Cool off with a cool shower or sponge bath.
- Move into an air-conditioned environment.
- Wear lightweight clothing.
- Check weather conditions. The National Weather Service has produced a Heat Index chart that can be accessed online at www.crh .noaa.gov/pub/ heat.php.

Thinking of Temperature

Prevention is the wisest approach to heat and cold problems. And knowing what can go wrong is part of that preventive approach.

Handling Heat

Heat cramps are caused by profuse sweating and the consequent loss of electrolytes (salts). They occur most often during exercise in hot weather. Salty snacks and sports beverages like Gatorade can help, but be aware that sports drinks can be very high in calories.

Heat exhaustion and *heat stroke* are most likely to occur when both temperature and humidity are high, because sweat does not evaporate as quickly, preventing the body from releasing heat quickly. Other conditions that limit the body's ability to regulate temperature are old age, fever, obesity, dehydration, heart disease, poor circulation, sunburn, and drug and alcohol use. Heat exhaustion is a mild from of heat-related illness.The signs of heat exhaustion are heavy sweating, paleness, muscle cramps, tiredness, weakness, dizziness, headache, nausea or vomiting, and/or fainting.Your pulse rate or heart rate may be fast and weak, and your breathing fast and shallow.

A heat stroke can occur when the body temperature rises to 106 degrees Fahrenheit or higher within 10 to 15 minutes. A heat stroke is a medical emergency that can be fatal. The warning signs are extremely high temperature; red, hot, and dry skin; rapid, strong pulse; throbbing headache; dizziness; nausea; confusion or unconsciousness.

If you think someone might have heat stroke, you should take him or her to a cool, shady place quickly, and call a doctor. Remove unnecessary clothing and bathe or spray the victim with cool water. People with heat stroke may seem confused. They may have seizures or go into a coma.

Coping with Cold

The tips of the toes, fingers, ears, nose, and chin and the cheeks are most vulnerable to exposure to high wind speeds and low temperatures, which can result in *frostnip*. The best early treatment is warming the area by firm, steady pressure with a warm hand; blowing on it with hot breath; holding it against your body; or immersing it in warm (not hot) water.

More severe is *frostbite*. There are two types of frostbite: *superficial* and *deep*. Superficial frostbite, the freezing of the skin and tissues just below the skin, is characterized by a waxy look and firmness of the skin, although the tissue below is soft. Initial treatment should be to slowly rewarm the area.

Deep frostbite, the freezing of skin, muscle, and even bone, requires medical treatment. It usually involves the tissues of the hands and feet, which appear pale and feel frozen. Keep the victim dry and as warm as possible on the way to a medical facility. Cover the frostbitten area with a dry, sterile dressing.

When body temperature falls below 95 degrees Fahrenheit, the body is incapable of rewarming itself. This state is known as **hypothermia.** The first sign of hypothermia is severe shivering. Then the victim becomes uncoordinated, drowsy, listless, and confused and is unable to speak properly. Symptoms become more severe as body temperature continues to drop, and coma or death can result. Hypothermia requires emergency medical treatment.

? FAQ How Can I Prevent Injuries?

According to the American Physical Therapy Association, the most common exercise-related injury sites are the knees, feet, back, and shoulders, followed by the ankles and hips. **Acute injuries**—sprains, bruises, and pulled muscles—are the result of sudden trauma, such as a fall or collision. **Overuse injuries,** on the other hand,

waist-to-hip ratio (WHR) The proportion of one's waist circumference to one's hip circumference.

hypothermia An abnormally low body temperature; if not treated appropriately, coma or death could result.

acute injuries Physical injuries, such as sprains, bruises, and pulled muscles, which result from sudden traumas, such as falls or collisions.

overuse injuries Physical injuries to joints or muscles, such as strains, fractures, and tendinitis, which result from overdoing a repetitive activity.

Strategies for Prevention — Protecting Yourself from the Cold

- Dress appropriately. Choose several layers of loose clothing made of wool, cotton, down, or synthetic down. Make sure your head, feet, and hands are well protected. A pair of cotton socks inside a pair of wool socks will keep your feet warm.
- Don't go out in the cold after drinking. Alcohol can make you more susceptible to cold and can impair your judgment and sense of time.
- When snowshoeing or cross-country skiing, always let a responsible person know where you're heading and when you expect to be back. Stick to marked trails.
- Carry a small emergency kit that includes waterproof matches, a compass, a map, high-energy food, and water.
- Don't eat snow; it could lower your body temperature.

are the result of overdoing a repetitive activity, such as running. When one particular joint is overstressed—such as a tennis player's elbow or a swimmer's shoulder—tendinitis, an inflammation at the point where the tendon meets the bone, can develop.

Men and women may be vulnerable to different types of injuries. Studies of male and female college basketball and soccer players have shown that gender differences in the neuromuscular control of the knee places female athletes at higher risk for knee injuries. Balance training may reduce the risk.

To prevent exercise-related problems before they happen, use common sense and take appropriate precautions, including the following:

- **Get proper instruction** and, if necessary, advanced training from knowledgeable instructors.
- **Make sure you have good equipment** and keep it in good condition. Know how to check and do at least basic maintenance on the equipment yourself. Always check your equipment prior to each use (especially if you're renting it).
- **Always make sure that stretching** and exercises are preventing, not causing, injuries.
- **Use reasonable protective measures,** including wearing a helmet when cycling or skating.
- For some sports, such as boating, **always go with a buddy.**
- **Take each outing seriously**—even if you've dived into this river a hundred times before, even if you know this mountain like you know your own backyard. Avoid the unknown under adverse conditions (for example, hiking unfamiliar terrain during poor weather or kayaking a new river when water levels are unusually high or low) or when accompanied by a beginner whose skills may not be as strong as yours.
- **Never combine alcohol or drugs with any sport.**

Taking Care of Injuries

Sooner or later most active people suffer an injury. Although most are minor, they all require attention. Ignoring a problem or trying to push through the pain can lead to more serious complications.

PRICE

If you develop aches and pains beyond what you might expect from an activity, stop. Never push to the point of fatigue. If you do, you could end up with sprained or torn muscles. Follow the PRICE prescription for coping with an exercise injury (Figure 4-12):

- **P**rotect the area with an elastic wrap, a sling, splint, cane, crutches, or an air cast.
- **R**est to promote tissue healing. Avoid activities that cause pain, swelling, or discomfort.
- **I**ce the area immediately, even if you're seeking medical help (don't put the ice pack directly on the skin). Repeat every two or three hours while you're awake for the first 48 to 72 hours. Cold reduces pain, swelling, and inflammation in injured muscles, joints, and connecting tissues and may slow bleeding if a tear has occurred.
- **C**ompress the area with an elastic bandage until the swelling stops. Begin wrapping at the end farthest from your heart. Loosen the wrap if the pain increases, the area becomes numb, or swelling is occurring below the wrapped area.
- **E**levate the area above your heart, especially at night. Gravity helps reduce swelling by draining excess fluid.

After 48 hours, if the swelling is gone, you may apply warmth or gentle heat, which improves the blood flow and speeds healing.

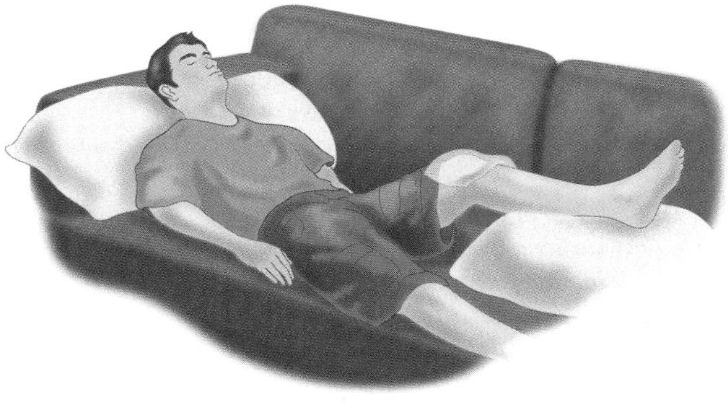

FIGURE 4-12 PRICE: How to Cope with an Exercise Injury

Overtraining

About half of all people who start an exercise program drop out within six months. One common reason is that they **overtrain,** pushing themselves to work too intensely too frequently. Signs of overdoing it include persistent muscle soreness, frequent injuries, unintended weight loss, nervousness, and an inability to relax. Overtraining for endurance sports like marathon running can damage the lungs and intensify asthma symptoms. You may find yourself unable to complete a normal workout or to recover after a normal workout.

If you develop any of the symptoms of overtraining, reduce or stop your workout sessions temporarily. Make gradual increases in the intensity of your workouts. Allow 24 to 48 hours for recovery between workouts. Make sure you get adequate rest. Check with a physical education instructor, coach, or trainer to make sure your exercise program fits your individual needs.

overtrain Working muscles too intensely or too frequently, resulting in persistent muscle soreness, injuries, unintended weight loss, nervousness, and an inability to relax.

LEARN IT / LIVE IT

Shaping Up

This chapter has given you the basic information you need to launch a fitness program. However, you're more likely to succeed if you create a plan and follow it. These basic steps can help you determine where you are now and how to get to where you want to be.

- **Evaluate your readiness for change.** Use the Self-Survey "Physical Activity Stages of Change Questionnaire" in the Self-Assessment Booklet to determine your stage of behavioral change. Don't expect to progress directly from one stage to another just once. Most people "recycle" several times before a change becomes permanent.
- **Consider your fitness goals.** Do you have an overall conditioning goal, such as losing weight? Or do you have a training goal, such as preparing for a 5K race or the tryouts for the volleyball team? Break down your goal into smaller "step" goals that lead you toward it.
- **Think through your personal preferences.** What are your physical strengths and weaknesses? Do you have good upper body strength but easily get winded? Do you have a stiff back? Do your allergies flare up when you exercise outdoors? By paying attention to your needs, likes, and dislikes, you can choose activities you enjoy—and are more likely to continue.
- **Schedule exercise into your daily routine.** If you can, block out a half-hour for working out at the beginning of the day, between classes, or in the evening. Write it into your schedule as if it were a class or doctor's appointment. If you can't find 30 minutes, look for two 15-minute or three 10-minute slots that you can use for "mini-workouts." Once you've worked out a schedule, write it down. A written plan encourages you to stay on track.
- **Assemble your gear.** Make sure you put your athletic shoes in your car or in the locker at the gym. Lay out the clothes you'll need to shoot hoops or play racquetball.
- **Start slowly.** If you are just beginning regular activity or exercise, begin at a low level. If you have an injury, disability, or chronic health problem, be sure you get medical clearance from a physician.
- **Progress gradually.** If you have not been physically active, begin by incorporating a few minutes of physical activity into each day, building up to 30 minutes or more of moderate-intensity activities. If you have been active but not as often or as intensely as recommended, become more consistent. Continue to increase the frequency, intensity, and duration of your workouts.
- **Take stock.** After a few months of leading a more active life, take stock. Think of how much more energy you have at the end of the day. Ask yourself if you're feeling any less stressed, despite the push and pull of daily pressures. Focus on the unanticipated rewards of exercise. Savor the

(Continued)

exhilaration of an autumn morning's walk; the thrill of feeling newly toughened muscles bend to your will; or the satisfaction of a long, smooth stretch after a stressful day. Enjoy the pure pleasure of living in the body you deserve.

4 Making This Chapter Work for You

Review Questions

1. Mary Ann takes a step aerobics class three times a week. Which component of physical fitness does her exercise routine emphasize?
   a. muscular strength and endurance
   b. flexibility
   c. cardiorespiratory fitness
   d. body composition
2. Which of the following statements is true?
   a. Inactivity does not affect health until middle age.
   b. Total fitness includes emotional and social dimensions of health in addition to the physical.
   c. Men and women have the same physiological capacities.
   d. Total fitness is one dimension of physical fitness.
3. The benefits of regular physical activity include
   a. decreased bone mass.
   b. lowered risk of shin splints.
   c. enhanced immune response.
   d. altered sleep patterns.
4. To motivate yourself to stick to an exercise program:
   a. Watch professional athletic competitions.
   b. Set a long-term goal, then break it down into short-term goals that can be achieved in a few months.
   c. Keep a detailed record of all the times that you avoided working out.
   d. Join an expensive health club so that you feel pressured to get your money's worth.
5. Michael started a walking program two weeks ago. Which of these workouts would you recommend to him for aerobic exercise?
   a. 5 minutes of brisk walking, 30 minutes of flexibility exercises, 5 minutes of brisk walking
   b. 5 minutes of stretching, 15 minutes of slow walking, 5 minutes of brisk walking, 15 minutes of slow walking
   c. 10 minutes of slow walking, 35 minutes of brisk walking, 5 minutes of slow walking
   d. 10 minutes of stretching, 45 minutes of slow walking
6. The new Exercise Guidelines for Americans recommend all of these *except*
   a. Engage in at least 30 minutes of moderate-intensity physical activity on most days of the week.
   b. Engage in physical activity of more vigorous intensity or longer duration for greater health benefits.
   c. Engage in 60 minutes of moderate- to vigorous-intensity activity on most days of the week to prevent gradual weight gain.
   d. Engage in 120 minutes of vigorous-intensity activity to get really fit.
7. For any muscle to get stronger, it must work against a greater-than-normal resistance. This is called the
   a. reversibility principle.
   b. overload principle.
   c. FITT principle.
   d. principle of compound interest.
8. A regular flexibility program provides which of the following benefits?
   a. stronger heart and lungs
   b. relief of muscle strain and soreness
   c. increased strength and endurance
   d. increased bone mass and leaner muscles
9. If you are a healthy weight,
   a. you are always hungry.
   b. your BMI is between 18.5 and 24.9.
   c. your waist measurement is 25 to 28 inches.
   d. your waist-to-hip ratio is greater than 1.0.
10. Which of the following precautions could help to prevent a serious sports injury from occurring?
    a. Wear swimming goggles when doing laps to decrease the irritating effects of chlorine.
    b. Wear knee pads when cycling to prevent knee gashes if you fall off your bicycle.
    c. To eliminate persistent muscle soreness, increase the frequency and/or time period of your workout.
    d. Wear a helmet, wrist guards, and knee pads when inline skating to help prevent fractures and head injuries.

Answers to these questions can be found on page 422.

Critical Thinking

1. Allison knows that exercise is good for her health, but she figures she can keep her weight down by dieting and worry about her heart and health when she gets older. "I look good. I feel okay. Why should I bother exercising?" she asks. What would you reply?
2. College athletes have died unexpectedly from heart-related problems. The American Heart Association has identified guidelines to screen competitive athletes. Does your school follow these guidelines? If not, what precautions are taken to protect young athletes?
3. Your younger brother Andre is hoping to get a starting position on his high school football team. Practices began in July. You are aware that a couple of other players

LACC Extra Credit Assignment

4. List what physical education activities you participated in during high school and what if any you participate in today. Is it enough and if not, why?

have suffered heat-related incidences, but according to Andre, these players just weren't tough enough. What can you do to help your brother protect his health?

4. Research is mixed on whether stretching can decrease delayed-onset muscle soreness. Do you think a placebo effect can occur in studies on exercise and training as it does in research on medications? Why?

Media Menu

ThomsonNOW™ Go to the ThomsonNOW website at **http://www.thomsonedu.com** that will:

- Help you evaluate your knowledge of the material.
- Allow you to take an exam-prep quiz.
- Provide a Personalized Learning Plan targeting resources that address areas you should study.
- Coach you through identifying target goals for behavioral change and creating and monitoring your personal change plan throughout the semester.

INTERNET CONNECTIONS

American Council on Exercise
www.acefitness.org

This website features information for the general public as well as for certified fitness trainers. The comprehensive site includes health and fitness news headlines, Fit Facts information sheets, a question and answer site, whole body exercise workouts, daily fitness tips, discussion boards, newsletters, and information on ACE certification.

American Alliance for Health, Physical Education, Recreation and Dance
www.aahperd.org

This organization provides legislative advocacy for healthy lifestyles through high-quality programs in health and physical education. The website features consumer news, career links, a listing of graduate programs, research, and a link for the International Electronic Journal of Health Education.

Shape Up America
www.shapeup.org/fitness.html

At this site, you can perform a battery of physical fitness assessments, including activity level, strength, flexibility, and an aerobic fitness test. You get started by entering your weight, height, age, and gender and then take a quick screening test to assess your physical readiness for physical activity. Your final results in each area will be based on your personal data.

Just Move
www.justmove.org

At this website sponsored by the American Heart Association, after a free registration, you can access an interactive exercise diary where you can keep track of your own exercise progress. In addition, an information resource called My Fitness provides recommendations for optimizing your exercise program to match your lifestyle as well as a list of health and fitness resources.

InfoTrac College Edition Activities Log on, insert **cardiorespiratory fitness** into the Keyword search box, and limit your search to the past year. When you get the results, mark articles to review, then select one to read. Summarize three or four key points from the article.

You can find additional readings related to personal health with InfoTrac College Edition, an online library of more than 900 journals and publications. Follow the instructions for accessing InfoTrac College Edition that were packaged with your textbook; then search for articles using a keyword search.

For additional links, resources, and suggested readings on the InfoTrac College Edition, visit our Health and Wellness Resource Center at **http://health.wadsworth.com.**

Key Terms

The terms listed are used on the page indicated. Definitions of the terms are in the Glossary at the end of this book.

active stretching 96
acute injuries 101
aerobic exercise 84
anabolic steroids 95
anaerobic exercise 85
ballistic stretching 96
body composition 76
body mass index (BMI) 99
cardiorespiratory fitness 76
dynamic flexibility 94
endorphins 80
FITT 83
flexibility 76
hypothermia 101
isokinetic 91
isometric 91
isotonic 91
muscular endurance 76
muscular strength 76
obesity 99
osteoporosis 80
overload principle 82
overloading 90
overtrain 103
overuse injuries 101
overweight 99
passive stretching 96
physical fitness 76
progressive overloading 82
range of motion 94
reps (or repetition) 91
resting heart rate 85
reversibility principle 84
sets 92
specificity principle 84
static flexibility 94
static stretching 96
target heart rate 85
waist-to-hip ratio (WHR) 100

5 Personal Nutrition

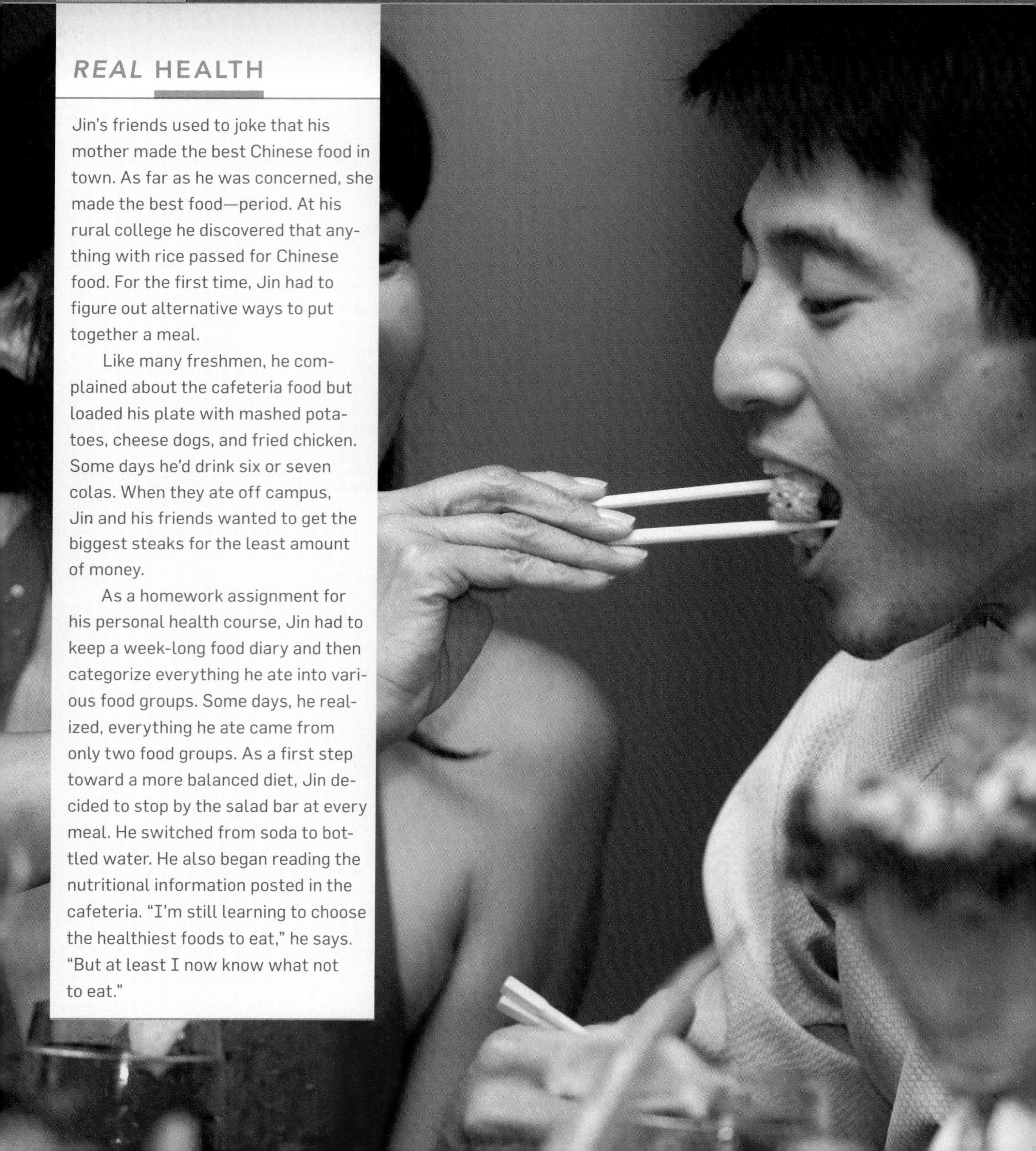

REAL HEALTH

Jin's friends used to joke that his mother made the best Chinese food in town. As far as he was concerned, she made the best food—period. At his rural college he discovered that anything with rice passed for Chinese food. For the first time, Jin had to figure out alternative ways to put together a meal.

Like many freshmen, he complained about the cafeteria food but loaded his plate with mashed potatoes, cheese dogs, and fried chicken. Some days he'd drink six or seven colas. When they ate off campus, Jin and his friends wanted to get the biggest steaks for the least amount of money.

As a homework assignment for his personal health course, Jin had to keep a week-long food diary and then categorize everything he ate into various food groups. Some days, he realized, everything he ate came from only two food groups. As a first step toward a more balanced diet, Jin decided to stop by the salad bar at every meal. He switched from soda to bottled water. He also began reading the nutritional information posted in the cafeteria. "I'm still learning to choose the healthiest foods to eat," he says. "But at least I now know what not to eat."

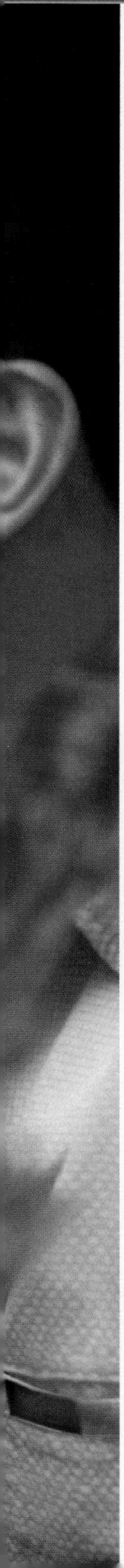

We are indeed what we eat—and it shows in everything from our stamina and strength to the sheen in our hair and the glow in our cheeks. Eating well helps us live and feel well.

As demonstrated by the science of **nutrition,** the field that explores the connections between our bodies and the foods we eat, our daily diet affects how long and how well we live. Poor diet and a sedentary lifestyle are culprits in about 400,000 of the two million annual deaths in the United States. Unhealthy eating contributes to many health problems, including heart disease, high blood pressure, high cholesterol, type 2 diabetes, obesity, osteoporosis, iron deficiency, anemia, and digestive disorders.

Adopting healthy eating behaviors could eliminate an estimated 16 percent of deaths in men and 9 percent of deaths in women. A high-quality diet also enhances day-to-day health, vitality, energy, and sense of well-being. But making healthy food choices isn't easy. In 1900, people in the United States could choose from about 500 different foods; today, we can choose from more than 50,000.

This chapter can help you make good choices. It presents the most recent dietary guidelines for Americans and translates the latest scientific research into specific advice designed both to promote health and to prevent chronic disease. By learning more about nutrients, food groups, eating patterns, nutrition labels, and sefety practices, you can nourish your body with foods that not only taste good but also are good for you.

? FAQ Frequently Asked Questions

- How many calories do I need? *p. 108*
- Should I switch to low-carb foods? *p. 110*
- Are low-fat diets good for you or not? *p. 113*
- Should I take supplements? *p. 118*
- Do men and women have different nutritional needs? *p. 123*
- What should I know about vegetarian diets? *p. 125*
- What should I look for on nutrition labels? *p. 127*
- How can I find snacks that are good for me? *p. 130*
- What causes food poisoning? *p. 130*

After studying the material in this chapter, you should be able to:

- **List** the basic nutrients necessary for a healthy body and **describe** their functions.
- **Describe** the key themes of the USDA MyPyramid System.
- **List** five specific nutrition guidelines of the MyPyramid system.
- **Explain** how to interpret the nutritional information provided on food labels.
- **List** the food safety hazards and **describe** prevention measures.

nutrition The science devoted to the study of dietary needs for food and the effects of food on organisms.

ThomsonNOW™ Log on to ThomsonNOW at **www.thomsonedu.com/thomsonnow** to find your Behavior Change Planner and to explore self-assessments, interactive tutorials, and practice quizzes.

What You Need to Know About Nutrients

Every day your body needs certain **essential nutrients** that it cannot manufacture for itself. They provide energy, build and repair body tissues, and regulate body functions. The six classes of essential nutrients, which are discussed in this section, are water, protein, carbohydrates, fats, vitamins, and minerals (Table 5-1).

Water makes up about 60 percent of the body and is essential for health and survival. Besides water, we also need energy to live, and we receive our energy from the carbohydrates, proteins, and fats in the foods we eat. The digestive system (Figure 5-1) breaks down food into these **macronutrients.** They are the nutrients required by the human body in the greatest amounts. The amount of energy that can be derived from the macronutrients is measured in **calories.** There are 9 calories in every gram of fat and 4 calories in every gram of protein or carbohydrate. The other two essential nutrients—the vitamins and minerals—are called **micronutrients** because our bodies need them in only very small amounts.

Your need for macronutrients depends on how much energy you expend. Because fats, carbohydrates, and protein can all serve as sources of energy, they can, to some extent, substitute for one another in providing calories. Adults, according to federal standards, should get 45 to 65 percent of calories from carbohydrates, 20 to 35 percent from fat, and 10 to 35 percent from protein. Children's fat intake should be slightly higher: 25 to 40 percent of their caloric intake.

To eat well without overeating, choose foods that are "nutrient-dense," that is, foods that provide the most nutritional value. For example, both a cup of nonfat milk and an ounce and a half of cheddar cheese provide about 300 mg of calcium, but the milk offers the same amount of calcium for half the calories. Foods that are extremely low in nutrient density—such as potato chips, candy, and soft drinks—are "empty," delivering only calories with few, if any, nutrients.

? FAQ How Many Calories Do I Need?

Calories are the measure of the amount of energy that can be derived from food. How many calories you need depends on your gender, age, body-frame size, weight, percentage of body fat, and your **basal metabolic rate (BMR)**—the number of calories needed to sustain your

TABLE 5-1 The Essential Nutrients

	Sources	Functions
Water	Liquids, fruits, and vegetables	Carries nutrients and removes waste; dissolves amino acids, glucose, and minerals; cleans body by removing toxins; regulates body temperature
Proteins	Meat, poultry, fish, eggs, beans, nuts, cheese, tofu, vegetables, some fruits, pastas, breads, cereal, and rice	Help build new tissue to keep hair, skin, and eyesight healthy; build antibodies, enzymes, hormones, and other compounds; provide fuel for body
Carbohydrates	Grains, cereal, pasta, fruits and vegetables, nuts, milk, and sugars	Provide energy
Fats		
Saturated Fats	Red meat, dairy products, egg yolks, coconut and palm oils, shortening, stick margarine, baked goods	Provide energy; trigger production of cholesterol (see Chapter 10)
Unsaturated Fats	Some fish; avocados; olive, canola, and peanut oils	Also provide energy, but trigger more "good" cholesterol production and less "bad" cholesterol production (see Chapter 10)
Vitamins	Fruits, vegetables, grains, some meat and dairy products	Facilitate use of other nutrients; involved in regulating growth, maintaining tissue, and manufacturing blood cells, hormones, and other body components
Minerals	Many foods	Help build bones and teeth; aid in muscle function and nervous system activity; assist in various body functions including growth and energy production

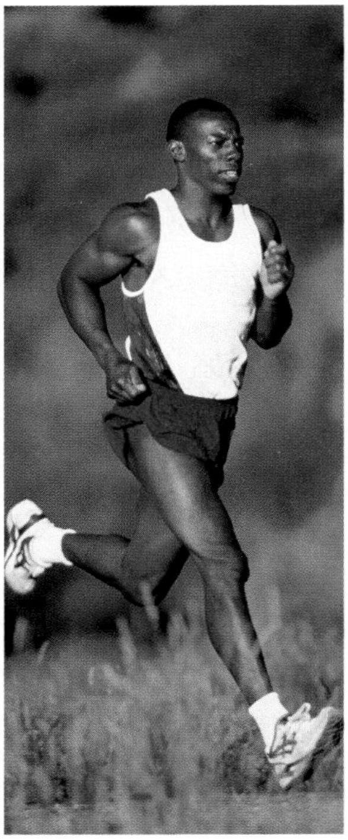

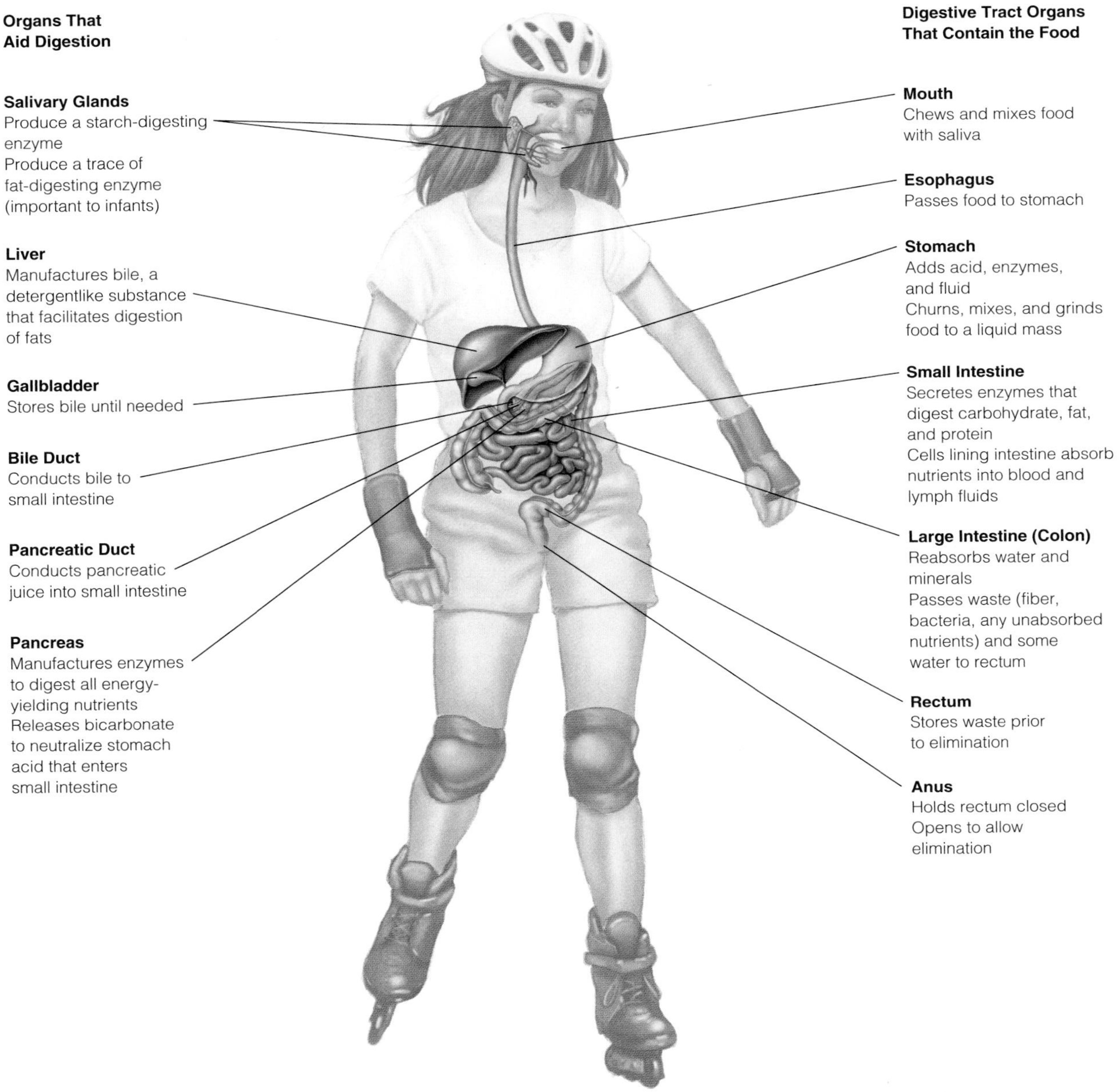
Organs That Aid Digestion
Salivary Glands
Produce a starch-digesting enzyme
Produce a trace of fat-digesting enzyme (important to infants)
Liver
Manufactures bile, a detergentlike substance that facilitates digestion of fats
Gallbladder
Stores bile until needed
Bile Duct
Conducts bile to small intestine
Pancreatic Duct
Conducts pancreatic juice into small intestine
Pancreas
Manufactures enzymes to digest all energy-yielding nutrients
Releases bicarbonate to neutralize stomach acid that enters small intestine
Digestive Tract Organs That Contain the Food
Mouth
Chews and mixes food with saliva
Esophagus
Passes food to stomach
Stomach
Adds acid, enzymes, and fluid
Churns, mixes, and grinds food to a liquid mass
Small Intestine
Secretes enzymes that digest carbohydrate, fat, and protein
Cells lining intestine absorb nutrients into blood and lymph fluids
Large Intestine (Colon)
Reabsorbs water and minerals
Passes waste (fiber, bacteria, any unabsorbed nutrients) and some water to rectum
Rectum
Stores waste prior to elimination
Anus
Holds rectum closed
Opens to allow elimination

FIGURE 5-1 The Digestive System
The organs of the digestive system break down food into nutrients that the body can use.

body at rest. Your activity level also affects your calorie requirements. Regardless of whether you consume fat, protein, or carbohydrates, if you take in more calories than required to maintain your size and don't work them off in some sort of physical activity, your body will convert the excess to fat (see Chapter 6). On average, daily calorie needs are:

- Most women, some older adults, children ages two to six: 1,600
- Average adult: 2,000
- Most men, active women, teenage girls, older children: 2,200
- Active men, teenage boys: 2,800

essential nutrients Nutrients that the body cannot manufacture for itself and must obtain from food.

macronutrients Nutrients required by the human body in the greatest amounts, including water, carbohydrates, proteins, and fats.

calorie The amount of energy required to raise the temperature of 1 gram of water by 1 degree Celsius. In everyday usage related to the energy content of foods and the energy expended in activities, a calorie is actually the equivalent of a thousand such calories, or a kilocalorie.

micronutrients Vitamins and minerals needed by the body in very small amounts.

basal metabolic rate (BMR) The number of calories required to sustain the body at rest.

Water

Water, which makes up 85 percent of blood, 70 percent of muscles, and about 75 percent of the brain, performs many essential functions: It carries nutrients, maintains temperature, lubricates joints, helps with digestion, rids the body of waste through urine, and contributes to the production of sweat, which evaporates from the skin to cool the body. Research has correlated high fluid intake with a lower risk of kidney stones, colon cancer, and bladder cancer.

You lose about 64 to 80 ounces of water a day—the equivalent of eight to ten 8-ounce glasses—through perspiration, urination, bowel movements, and normal exhalation. You lose water more rapidly if you exercise, live in a dry climate or at a high altitude, drink a lot of caffeine or alcohol (which increase urination), skip a meal, or become ill. To assure adequate water intake, nutritionists advise drinking a minimum of 64 ounces, enough so that your urine is not dark in color. Healthy individuals can get adequate hydration from beverages other than plain water, including juice and soft drinks.

Protein

Critical for growth and repair, **proteins** form the basic framework for our muscles, bones, blood, hair, and fingernails. Supplying 4 calories per gram, they are made of combinations of 20 **amino acids,** 9 of which we must get from our diet because the human body cannot produce them. These are called *essential amino acids.*

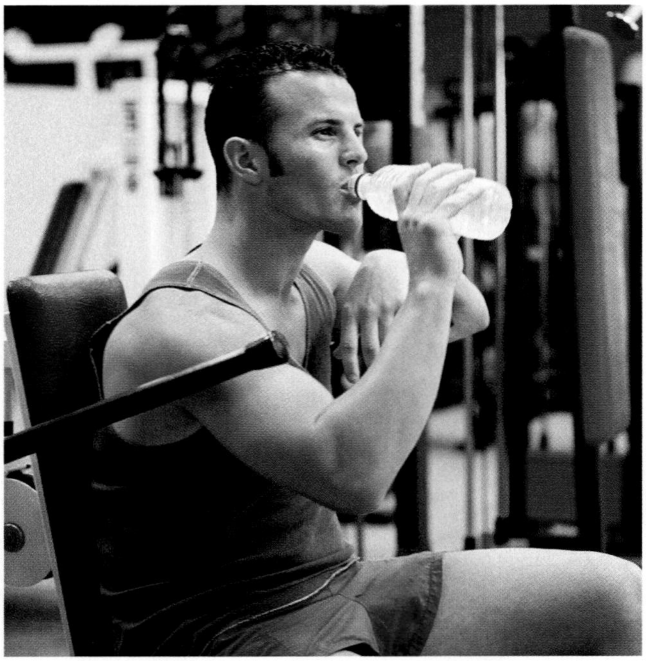

© Banana Stock/Jupiter Images

Water is an essential nutrient. Remember: Each day you must replace the amount you use.

Animal proteins—meat, fish, poultry, and dairy products—are **complete proteins** that provide the nine essential amino acids. Grains, dry beans, and nuts are **incomplete proteins** that may have relatively low levels of one or two essential amino acids but fairly high levels of others. Combining incomplete proteins, such as beans and rice, ensures that the body gets sufficient protein. The recommended level of protein intake is 0.8 gram per kilogram of body weight for adults.

Carbohydrates

Carbohydrates are organic compounds that provide our brains and bodies with *glucose,* their basic fuel. The major sources of carbohydrates are plants—including grains, vegetables, fruits, and beans—and milk. There are two types: *simple carbohydrates* (sugars) and *complex carbohydrates* (starches and fiber). All provide 4 calories per gram. Both adults and children should consume at least 130 grams of carbohydrates each day, the minimum needed to produce enough glucose for the brain to function.

Forms of Carbohydrates

Simple carbohydrates include *natural sugars*, such as the lactose in milk and the fructose in fruit, and *added sugars* that are found in candy, soft drinks, fruit drinks, pastries, and other sweets. Those whose diets are higher in added sugars typically have lower intakes of other essential nutrients.

Complex carbohydrates include grains, cereals, vegetables, beans, and nuts. Americans, however, get most of their complex carbohydrates from refined grains, which have been stripped of fiber and many nutrients.

Far more nutritious are whole grains, which are made up of all components of the grain: the *bran* (or fiber-rich outer layer), the *endosperm* (middle layer), and the *germ* (the nutrient-packed inner layer). Increasing whole-grain consumption has become a public health priority, and the 2005 Dietary Guidelines recommend that Americans increase their consumption of whole-grain foods.[1] Individuals who eat whole-grain products each day have about a 15 to 25 percent reduction in death from all causes, including heart disease and cancer.

? FAQ Should I Switch to Low-Carb Foods?

The popularity of diets that restrict carbohydrate intake, such as the Atkins diet discussed in Chapter 6, prompted an explosion in products touted as "low-carb." You can get low-carb versions of everything from beer to bread. However, the Food and Drug Administration (FDA), which regulates health claims on food labels in the

United States, hasn't defined what "low-carb" means. Words like "low-carb," "carb-wise," or "carb-free" are marketing terms created by manufacturers to sell their products.

Although many people may buy low-carbohydrate foods because they believe that they're healthier, that isn't necessarily the case. A low-carb nutrition bar, for instance, may be high in saturated fat and calories. Since low-carb food products are relatively new on grocery shelves, no one knows their long-term hazards. Some cause digestive symptoms because food companies often replace the carbohydrates in a cookie or cracker with substances such as the sweetener sorbitol, which can cause diarrhea or stomach cramps.

Dieters often buy low-carb products in order to lose weight. According to proponents of low-carbohydrate diets, if carbohydrates raise blood sugar and insulin levels and cause weight gain, a decrease in carbs should result in lower blood sugar and insulin levels—and weight loss. With limited carbohydrates in the diet, the body would break down fat to provide needed energy.

Some people do lose weight when they switch to low-carb foods, but the reasons are probably that they consume fewer calories, lose water weight, and have decreased appetite because of a buildup of ketones (a by-product of fat metabolism) in the blood.[2] As discussed in Chapter 6, a low-carb diet can lead to fairly rapid weight loss but is no easier to maintain over the long run than any other diet.

Glycemic Index and Glycemic Load

The glycemic index is a ranking of carbohydrates, gram for gram, based on their immediate effect on blood glucose (sugar) levels. Carbohydrates that break down quickly during digestion and trigger a fast, high glucose response have the highest glycemic index rating. Those that break down slowly, releasing glucose gradually into the bloodstream, have low glycemic index ratings. Potatoes, which raise blood sugar higher and faster than apples, for instance, earn a higher glycemic-index rating than apples. Glycemic index does not account for the amount of food you typically eat in a serving.

Glycemic load is a measure of how much a typical serving size of a particular food raises blood glucose. For example, the glycemic index of table sugar is high, but you use so little to sweeten your coffee or tea that its glycemic load is low.[3]

Some diets are based on the theory that high-glycemic-index foods raise blood sugar and insulin levels and cause weight gain, while low-glycemic-index foods lower your blood sugar and insulin levels so you'll lose weight. Although some people do lose weight on low-glycemic diets, this theory has not been scientifically proved. Experts are dubious because many factors play a role in how much blood glucose rises, including age and weight. And people typically don't eat single foods at a meal, but a combination of foods that affect blood sugar differently.

Fiber

Dietary fiber is the nondigestible form of complex carbohydrates occurring naturally in plant foods, such as leaves, stems, skins, seeds, and hulls. **Functional fiber** consists of isolated, nondigestible carbohydrates that may be added to foods and that provide beneficial effects in humans. Total fiber is the sum of both.

The various forms of fiber enhance health in different ways: They slow the emptying of the stomach, which creates a feeling of fullness and aids weight control. They interfere with absorption of dietary fat and cholesterol, which lowers the risk of heart disease and stroke in both middle-aged and elderly individuals. In addition, fiber helps prevent constipation, diverticulosis (a painful inflammation of the bowel), and diabetes. The link between fiber and colon cancer is complex. Some studies have indicated that increased fiber intake reduces risk; others found no such correlation.

The Institute of Medicine has set the first-ever recommendations for daily intake levels of total fiber (dietary plus functional fiber): 38 grams of total fiber for men and 25 grams for women. For men and women over 50 years of age, who consume less food, the recommendations are, respectively, 30 and 21 grams. The American Dietetic Association recommends 25 to 35 grams of dietary fiber a day, much more than the amount Americans typically consume.

Good fiber sources include wheat and corn bran (the outer layer); leafy greens; the skins of fruits and root vegetables; oats, beans, and barley; and the pulp, skin, and seeds of many fruits and vegetables, such as apples and strawberries (Table 5-2). Because sudden increases in fiber can cause symptoms like bloating and gas, ex-

proteins Organic compounds composed of amino acids; one of the essential nutrients.

amino acids Organic compounds containing nitrogen, carbon, hydrogen, and oxygen; the essential building blocks of proteins.

complete proteins Proteins that contain all the amino acids needed by the body for growth and maintenance.

incomplete proteins Proteins that lack one or more of the amino acids essential for protein synthesis.

carbohydrates Organic compounds, such as starches, sugars, and glycogen, that are composed of carbon, hydrogen, and oxygen, and are sources of bodily energy.

simple carbohydrates Sugars; like all carbohydrates, they provide the body with glucose.

complex carbohydrates Starches, including cereals, fruits, and vegetables.

dietary fiber The nondigestible form of carbohydrates found in plant foods, such as leaves, stems, skins, seeds, and hulls.

functional fiber Isolated, nondigestible carbohydrates with beneficial effects in humans.

TABLE 5-2 Putting Fiber into Meals and Snacks

High-Fiber Options for Breakfast		
Whole-grain toast		2 g per slice
Bran cereal:		
Bran flakes	1 cup	7 g
All Bran	1/3 cup	10 g
Raisin bran	3/4 cup	5 g
Oat bran	1/3 cup	5 g
Bran muffin, with fruit	1 small	3 g
Strawberries	10	2 g
Raspberries	1/2 cup	3 g
Banana	1 medium	2 g
Lunches that Include Fiber		
Whole-grain bread		2 g per slice
Baked beans	1/2 cup	10 g
Carrot	1 medium	2 g
Raisins	1/4 cup	2 g
Peas	1/2 cup	6 g
Peanut butter	2 tablespoons	2 g
Fiber on the Menu for Supper		
Brown rice	1/2 cup	2 g
Potato	1 medium	3 g
Dried cooked beans	1/2 cup	8 g
Broccoli	1/2 cup	3 g
Corn	1/2 cup	5 g
Tomato	1 medium	2 g
Green beans	1/2 cup	3 g
Fiber-Filled Snacks		
Peanuts	1/4 cup	3 g
Apple	1 medium	2 g
Pear	1 medium	4 g
Orange	1 medium	3 g
Prunes*	3	2 g
Sunflower seeds	1/4 cup	2 g
Popcorn	2 cups	2 g

*Prunes contain fiber, but their laxative effect is primarily due to a naturally occurring chemical substance that causes an uptake of fluid into the intestines and the contraction of muscles that line the intestines.

Source: Brown, Judith E. *Nutrition Now*, 4th ed. Belmont, CA: Wadsworth, 2005.

perts recommend gradually adding more fiber to your diet with an additional serving or two of vegetables, fruit, or whole wheat bread.

Fats

Fats carry the fat-soluble vitamins A, D, E, and K; aid in their absorption in the intestine; protect organs from injury; regulate body temperature; and play an important role in growth and development. They provide 9 calories per gram—more than twice the amount in carbohydrates or proteins.

Both high- and low-fat diets can be unhealthy. When people eat very low levels of fat and very high levels of carbohydrates, their levels of high-density lipoprotein, the so-called *good cholesterol,* decline. On the other hand, high-fat diets can lead to obesity and its related health dangers, discussed in Chapter 6.

Forms of Fat

Saturated fats and **unsaturated fats** are distinguished by the type of fatty acids in their chemical structures. Unsaturated fats can be divided into monounsaturated or polyunsaturated, again depending on their chemical structure. All dietary fats are a mix of saturated and unsaturated fats but are predominantly one or the other. Unsaturated fats, like oils, are likely to be liquid at room temperature and saturated fats, like butter, are likely to be solid. In general, vegetable and fish oils are unsaturated, and animal fats are saturated.

Olive, soybean, canola, cottonseed, corn, and other vegetable oils are unsaturated fats. Olive oil is considered a good fat and one of the best vegetable oils for salads and cooking. Used for thousands of years, this staple of the Mediterranean diet, discussed later in this chapter, has been correlated with a lower incidence of heart disease, including strokes and heart attacks.

Fish oils are rich in omega-3 fatty acids, which make molecules such as prostaglandins that may enhance cardiovascular health. Long touted as "good" fats with numerous health benefits, omega-3 fatty acids may not live up to expectations. An extensive analysis of 89 studies on omega-3 fatty acids and their impact on cardiovascular disease, cancer, and stroke concluded that they do not improve health outcomes for the general population, although they do not cause harm or increase health risks.[4] Yet another large study yielded different findings, concluding that people who had higher intake of these fatty acids had lower death rates, primarily because of decreased heart attacks and strokes.[5]

Saturated fats can increase the risk of heart disease and should be avoided as much as possible. In response to consumer and health professionals' demand for less saturated fat in the food supply, many manufacturers switched to partially hydrogenated oils.

The process of hydrogenation creates unsaturated fatty acids called **trans fat.** They are found in some margarine products and most foods made with partially hydrogenated oils, such as baked goods and fried foods. Even though trans fats are unsaturated, they appear similar to saturated fats in terms of raising cholesterol levels. Epidemiological studies have suggested a possible link between cardiovascular disease risk and high intakes of trans fats, and researchers have concluded that they are, gram for gram, twice as damaging as saturated fat. There is no safe level for trans fats, which occur naturally in meats as well as in foods prepared with partially hydrogenated vegetable oils.

To cut down on both saturated and trans fats, choose soybean, canola, corn, olive, safflower, and sunflower oils, which are naturally free of trans fats and lower in saturated fats. Look for reduced-fat, low-fat, fat-free, and trans fat-free versions of baked goods, snacks, and other processed foods. Table 5-3 compares saturated fat content and calories for some typical foods.

TABLE 5-3 Comparing Saturated Fat and Calorie Content

Food	Saturated Fat Content (grams)	Calories
Cheese (1 oz.)		
Regular cheddar cheese	6.0	114
Low-fat cheddar cheese	1.2	49
Ground beef (3 oz. cooked)		
Regular ground beef (25% fat)	6.1	236
Extra lean ground beef (5% fat)	2.6	148
Milk (1 cup)		
Whole milk (3.24%)	4.6	146
Low-fat (1%) milk	1.5	102
Breads (1 medium)		
Croissant	6.6	231
Bagel, oat bran (4″)	0.2	227
Frozen desserts (1/2 cup)		
Regular ice cream	4.9	145
Frozen yogurt	2.0	110
Table spreads (1 tsp.)		
Butter	2.4	34
Trans fat-free soft margarine	0.7	25
Chicken (3 oz. cooked)		
Fried chicken (leg)	3.3	212
Chicken breast	0.9	140
Fish (3 oz.)		
Fried fish	2.8	195
Baked fish	1.5	129

Source: ARS Nutrient Database for Standard Reference, *Dietary Guidelines for Americans 2005*, USDHHS, USDA, www.healthierus.gov/dietary guidelines.

? FAQ Are Low-Fat Diets Good for You or Not?

Some people began questioning the value of low-fat diets after a major study challenged the conventional belief that cutting dietary fat could reduce the risk of disease. The Women's Health Initiative (WHI), a landmark clinical trial that followed more than 48,000 postmenopausal women for eight years, showed women who reduced their fat intake from 38 percent of daily calories to 29 percent had similar rates of breast cancer,[6] colon cancer,[7] and cardiovascular disease[8] as those who did not change their fat intake.

Yet this study's surprising findings are far from conclusive. Some researchers argue that the women did not cut their fat intake enough—that is, to the recommended 20 percent. A greater reduction might have led to greater benefits.[9] Furthermore, the average age of the study participants was 62 so the reduction in fat was not only too little, but too late. Cutting back on fat at a younger age or for a longer time might provide more benefits.

The WHI also did not distinguish between good and bad fats. If the women substituted "healthy" monounsaturated and polyunsaturated fats (from vegetable oils, nuts, and fish) for unhealthy saturated and trans fats (found in meat, processed foods, and some dairy products), the results might have been quite different.

The women on the low-fat diets did experience minor reductions in breast cancer rates and cholesterol levels, as well as slightly fewer cases of pre-cancerous growths in the colon.[10] These findings could have been due to chance, but more significant improvement may emerge over time. Most of the women were overweight or obese; none were told to lose weight or exercise. Excess pounds and a sedentary lifestyle may cancel out the benefits of a low-fat diet.

Unless you are a postmenopausal woman, the results of the WHI may not apply to you. A low-fat diet may not protect anyone entirely from heart disease, breast cancer, or colon cancer. But as part of a healthy lifestyle, it may well lower your risk of these illnesses.[11]

Vitamins and Minerals

Vitamins, which help put proteins, fats, and carbohydrates to use, are essential to regulating growth, maintaining tissue, and releasing energy from foods. Together with the enzymes in the body, they help produce the right chemical reactions at the right times. They're also involved in the manufacture of blood cells, hormones, and other compounds.

The body produces some vitamins, such as vitamin D, which is manufactured in the skin after exposure to sunlight. Other vitamins must be ingested.

Vitamins A, D, E, and K are fat-soluble; they are absorbed through the intestinal membranes and stored in the body.

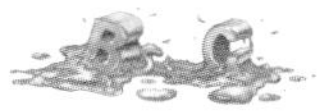

The B vitamins and vitamin C are water-soluble; they are absorbed directly into the blood and then used up or washed out of the body in urine and sweat. They must be replaced daily. Table 5-4 summarizes key information about the vitamins.

Antioxidants are substances that prevent the harmful effects caused by oxidation within the body. They include vitamins C, E, and beta-carotene (a form of vitamin A), as well as compounds like carotenoids and flavonoids. All share a common enemy: renegade oxygen

saturated fat A chemical term indicating that a fat molecule contains as many hydrogen atoms as its carbon skeleton can hold. These fats are normally solid at room temperature.

unsaturated fat A chemical term indicating that a fat molecule contains fewer hydrogen atoms than its carbon skeleton can hold. These fats are normally liquid at room temperature.

trans fat Fat formed when liquid vegetable oils are processed to make table spreads or cooking fats; also found in dairy and beef products; considered to be especially dangerous dietary fats.

vitamins Organic substances that are needed in very small amounts by the body and carry out a variety of functions in metabolism and nutrition.

antioxidants Substances that prevent the damaging effects of oxidation in cells.

TABLE 5-4 Key Information About Vitamins

Vitamin/Recommended Intake per Day	Significant Sources	Chief Functions	Signs of Severe, Prolonged Deficiency	Signs of Extreme Excess
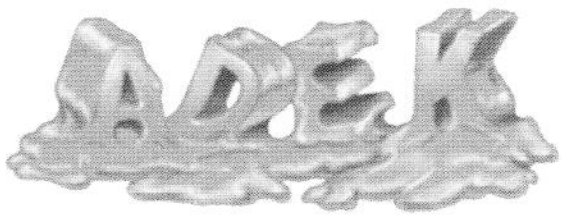				
Fat-Soluble Vitamins				
Vitamin A Males 19–50: 900 μg Females 19–50: 700 μg	Fortified milk, cheese, cream, butter, fortified margarine, eggs, liver; spinach and other dark, leafy greens, broccoli, deep orange fruits (apricots, cantaloupes) and vegetables (carrots, sweet potatoes, pumpkins)	Antioxidant; needed for vision, health of cornea, epithelial cells, mucous membranes, skin health, bone and tooth growth, reproduction, immunity	Anemia, painful joints, cracks in teeth, tendency toward tooth decay, diarrhea, depression, frequent infections, night blindness, keratinization, corneal degeneration, rashes, kidney stones	Nosebleeds, bone pain, growth retardation, headaches, abdominal cramps and pain, vomiting, diarrhea, weight loss, overreactive immune system, blurred vision, fatigue, irritability, hair loss, dry skin
Vitamin D Males 19–50: 5 μg Females 19–50: 5 μg	Fortified milk or margarine, eggs, liver, sardines; exposure to sunlight	Mineralization of bones (promotes calcium and phosphorus absorption)	Abnormal growth, misshapen bones (bowing of legs), soft bones, joint pain, malformed teeth	Raised blood calcium, excessive thirst, headaches, irritability, loss of appetite, weakness, nausea, kidney stones, deposits in arteries
Vitamin E Males 19–50: 15 mg Females 19–50: 15 mg	Polyunsaturated plant oils (margarine, salad dressings, shortenings), green and leafy vegetables, wheat germ, whole-grain products, nuts, seeds	Antioxidant; needed for stabilization of cell membranes, regulation of oxidation reactions	Red blood cell breakage, anemia, muscle degeneration, difficulty walking, leg cramps	Augments the effects of anticlotting medication; general discomfort; blurred vision
Vitamin K Males 19–50: 120 μg Females 19–50: 90 μg	Green leafy vegetables, cabbage-type vegetables, soybeans, vegetable oils	Synthesis of blood-clotting proteins and proteins important in bone mineralization	Hemorrhage	Interference with anticlotting medication; jaundice
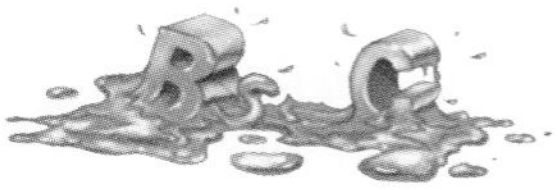				
Water-Soluble Vitamins				
Vitamin B^{6} Males 19–50: 1.3 mg Females 19–50: 1.3 mg	Meats, fish, poultry, liver, legumes, fruits, whole grains, potatoes, soy products	Part of a coenzyme used in amino acid and fatty acid metabolism, helps make red blood cells	Anemia, depression, abnormal brain wave pattern, convulsions, skin rashes	Impaired memory, irritability, headaches, numbness, damage to nerves, difficulty walking, loss of reflexes
Vitamin B^{12} Males 19–50: 2.4 μg Females 19–50: 2.4 μg	Animal products (meat, fish, poultry, milk, cheese, eggs)	Part of a coenzyme used in new cell synthesis, helps maintain nerve cells	Anemia, nervous system degeneration progressing to paralysis, hypersensitivity	None known
Vitamin C Males 19–50: 90 mg Females 19–50: 75 mg	Citrus fruits, cabbage-type vegetables, dark green vegetables, cantaloupe, strawberries, peppers, lettuce, tomatoes, potatoes, papayas, mangoes	Antioxidant, collagen synthesis (strengthens blood vessel walls, forms scar tissue, matrix for bone growth), amino acid metabolism, strengthens resistance to infection, aids iron absorption	Anemia, pinpoint hemorrhages, frequent infections, bleeding gums, loosened teeth, muscle degeneration and pain, joint pain, blotchy bruises, failure of wounds to heal	Nausea, abdominal cramps, diarrhea, excessive urination, headache, fatigue, insomnia, rashes; deficiency symptoms may appear at first on withdrawal of high doses

TABLE 5-4 (continued)

Vitamin/Recommended Intake per Day	Significant Sources	Chief Functions	Signs of Severe, Prolonged Deficiency	Signs of Extreme Excess
Thiamin Males 19–50: 1.2 mg Females 19–50: 1.1 mg	Pork, ham, bacon, liver, whole grains, legumes, nuts; occurs in all nutritious foods in moderate amounts	Part of a coenzyme used in energy metabolism, supports normal appetite and nervous system function	Edema, enlarged heart, nervous/muscular system degeneration, difficulty walking, loss of reflexes, mental confusion	None reported
Riboflavin Males 19–50: 1.3 mg Females 19–50: 1.1 mg	Milk, yogurt, cottage cheese, meat, leafy green vegetables, whole-grain or enriched breads and cereals	Part of a coenzyme used in energy metabolism, supports normal vision and skin health	Cracks at corner of mouth, magenta tongue, hypersensitivity to light, reddening of comea, skin rash	None reported
Niacin Males 19–50: 16 mg Females 19–50: 14 mg	Milk, eggs, meat, poultry, fish, whole-grain and enriched breads and cereals, nuts, and all protein-containing foods	Part of a coenzyme used in energy metabolism	Diarrhea, black smooth tongue, irritability, loss of appetite, weakness, dizziness, mental confusion, flaky skin rash on areas exposed to sun	Nausea, vomiting, painful flush and rash, sweating, liver damage
Folate Males 19–50: 400 µg Females 19–50: 400 µg	Leafy green vegetables, legumes, seeds, liver, enriched breads, cereal, pasta, and grains	Part of coenzyme needed for new cell synthesis	Anemia, heartburn, frequent infections, smooth red tongue, depression, mental confusion	Masks Vitamin B_{12} deficiency
Panothenic acid Males 19–50: 5 mg Females 19–50: 5 mg	Widespread in foods	Part of coenzyme used in energy metabolism	Vomiting, intestinal distress, insomnia, fatigue	Water retention (rate)
Biotin Males 19–50: 30 µg Females 19–50: 30 µg	Widespread in foods	Used in energy metabolism, fat synthesis, amino acid metabolism, and glycogen synthesis	Abnormal heart action, loss of appetite, nausea, depression, muscle pain, drying of facial skin	None reported

Source: Adapted from Sizer, Frances, and Ellie Whitney. *Nutrition: Concepts and Controversies,* 10th ed. Belmont, CA: Wadsworth, 2006.

cells called free radicals released by normal metabolism as well as by pollution, smoking, radiation, and stress.

Diets high in antioxidant-rich fruits and vegetables have been linked with lower rates of esophageal, lung, colon, and stomach cancer. Nevertheless, scientific studies have not proved conclusively that any specific antioxidant, particularly in supplement form, can prevent cancer.

Carbon, oxygen, hydrogen, and nitrogen make up 96 percent of our body weight. The other 4 percent consists of **minerals** that help build bones and teeth, aid in muscle function, and help our nervous systems transmit messages. Every day we need about a tenth of a gram (100 milligrams) or more of the major minerals: sodium, potassium chloride, calcium, phosphorus, magnesium, and sulfur. We also need about a hundredth of a gram (10 milligrams) or less of each of the trace minerals: iron (although premenopausal women need more), zinc, selenium, molybdenum, iodine, copper, manganese, fluoride, and chromium. (See Table 5-5 on page 116 for key information on minerals.)

Americans get adequate amounts of most nutrients. However, the 2005 Advisory Committee for Dietary Guidelines reported that intakes of several nutrients are low enough to be of concern. Are you getting enough of these nutrients?

- **For adults:** vitamins A, C, and E, calcium, magnesium, potassium, and fiber.
- **For children:** vitamin E, calcium, magnesium, potassium, and fiber.

Among the groups at highest risk of nutritional deficiencies are:

- **Teenage girls.**
- **Women of child-bearing age** (iron and folic acid).
- **Persons over age 50** (vitamin B_{12}).
- **The elderly, persons with dark skin,** and those who do not get adequate exposure to sunshine (vitamin D).[12]

Calcium

Calcium, the most abundant mineral in the body, builds strong bone tissue throughout life and plays a vital role in blood clotting

minerals Naturally occurring inorganic substances, small amounts of some being essential in metabolism and nutrition.

TABLE 5-4 Key Information About Vitamins

Mineral	Significant Sources	Chief Functions	Signs of Severe, Prolonged Deficiency	Signs of Extreme Excess
Major Minerals				
Sodium	Salt, soy sauce, processed foods	Needed to maintain fluid balance and acid-base balance in body cells; critical to nerve impulse transmission	Mental apathy, poor appetite, muscle cramps	High blood pressure
Potassium	All whole foods: meats, milk, fruits, vegetables, grains, legumes	Needed to maintain fluid balance and acid-base balance in body cells; needed for muscle and nerve activity	Muscle weakness, mental confusion, paralysis	Irregular heartbeat, heart attack; muscular weakness
Chloride	Salt, soy sauce, processed foods	Aids in digestion; needed to maintain fluid balance and acid-base balance in body cells	Muscle cramps, apathy, poor appetite, growth failure in children	Vomiting
Calcium	Milk and milk products, oysters, small fish (with bones), tofu, greens, legumes	Component of bones and teeth, needed for muscle and nerve activity, blood clotting	Stunted growth in children, adult bone loss (osteoporosis)	Constipation; calcium deposits in kidneys, liver; decreased absorption of other minerals
Phosphorus	All animal tissues	Component of bones and teeth, energy formation, needed to maintain cell membranes	Loss of appetite, muscle weakness, impaired growth	Loss of calcium from bones
Magnesium	Nuts, legumes, whole grains, dark green vegetables, seafoods, chocolate, cocoa	Component of bones and teeth, nerve activity, energy and protein formation	Stunted growth in children, weakness, muscle spasms, personality changes	Diarrhea, dehydration, impaired nerve activity
Sulfur	All protein-containing foods	Component of certain amino acids; stabilizes protein shape	None known; protein deficiency would occur first	Depresses growth in animals
Trace Minerals				
Iron	Red meats, fish, poultry, shellfish, eggs, legumes, dried fruits	Aids in transport of oxygen, component of myoglobin, energy formation	Anemia, weakness, fatigue, pale appearance, reduced attention span, developmental delays in children	Vomiting, abdominal pain, blue coloration of skin, shock, heart failure, diabetes
Zinc	Protein-containing foods: fish, shellfish, poultry, grains, vegetables	Protein reproduction, component of insulin	Growth failure, delayed sexual maturation, slow wound healing	Nausea, vomiting, weakness, fatigue, metallic taste in mouth
Selenium	Meats and seafood, eggs, grains	Acts as an antioxidant in conjunction with vitamin E	Anemia, muscle pain and tenderness, heart failure	Hair and fingernail loss, weakness, liver damage, garlic or metallic breath
Molybdenum	Dried beans, grains, dark green vegetables, liver, milk and milk products	Aids in oxygen transfer from one molecule to another	Rapid heartbeat and breathing, nausea, vomiting, coma	Loss of copper from the body, joint pain, growth failure, anemia, gout
Iodine	Iodized salt, milk and milk products, seaweed, seafood, bread	Component of thyroid hormones that helps regulate energy production and growth	Goiter, cretinism in newborns (mental retardation, hearing loss, growth failure)	Pimples, goiter, decreased thyroid function
Copper	Organ meats, whole grains, nuts and seeds, seafood, drinking water	Component of enzymes involved in the body's utilization of iron and oxygen	Anemia, nerve and bone abnormalities in children, growth retardation	Vomiting, diarrhea, liver disease
Manganese	Whole grains, coffee, tea, dried beans, nuts	Formation of body fat and bone	Weight loss, rash, nausea and vomiting	Infertility in men, disruptions in the nervous system, muscle spasms
Fluoride	Fluoridated water, foods, and beverages; tea; shrimp; crab	Component of bones and teeth (enamel)	Tooth decay and other dental diseases	Fluorosis, brittle bones, mottled teeth, nerve abnormalities
Chromium	Whole grains, liver, meat, beer, wine	Glucose utilization	Poor blood glucose control, weight loss	Kidney and skin damage

Source: Adapted from Brown, Judith E. *Nutrition Now*, 4th ed. Belmont, CA: Wadsworth, 2005; Sizer, Frances, and Ellie Whitney. *Nutrition: Concepts and Controversies*, 10th ed. Belmont, CA: Wadsworth, 2006.

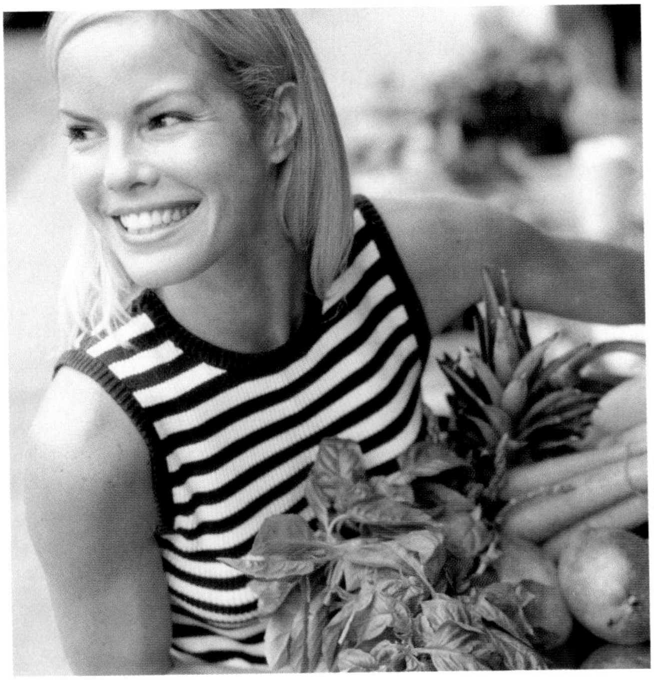

© LWA-Stephen Welstead/CORBIS

Antioxidants are found in vegetables and fruit. By eating an orange at breakfast and half a carrot for lunch, you will have all the antioxidants you need for the day.

and muscle and nerve functioning. Pregnant or nursing women need more calcium to meet the additional needs of their babies' bodies. Calcium may also help control high blood pressure, prevent colon cancer in adults, and promote weight loss. Adequate calcium and vitamin D intake during childhood, adolescence, and young adulthood is crucial to prevent *osteoporosis,* the bone-weakening disease that strikes one of every four women over the age of 60.

National health organizations are promoting greater calcium consumption among college students, particularly women, to increase bone density and safeguard against osteoporosis.

In both men and women, bone mass peaks between the ages of 25 and 35. Over the next 10 to 15 years, bone mass remains fairly stable. At about age 40, bone loss equivalent to 0.3 to 0.5 percent per year begins in both men and women. Women may experience greater bone loss, at a rate of 3 to 5 percent, at the time of menopause. This decline continues for approximately five to seven years and is the primary factor leading to postmenopausal osteoporosis.

The higher an individual's peak bone mass, the longer it takes for age- and menopause-related bone loss to increase the risk of fractures. Osteoporosis is less common in groups with higher peak bone mass—men versus women, blacks versus whites.

Calcium is a special concern for African Americans who, as a group, have a higher risk for high blood pressure and obesity than the rest of the population but, on average, consume less than one serving of dairy foods a day. In fact, more than 80 percent of African Americans fail to get their daily recommended amount of calcium.

Calcium and vitamin D supplements in healthy postmenopausal women provide a modest benefit in preserving bone mass and preventing hip fractures, but do not prevent other types of fractures or colorectal cancer, according to the results of a major clinical trial, part of the Women's Health Initiative, which studied more than 36,000 women over age 50.[13] Others have questioned the value of calcium supplementation in younger adults and children as well. A combination of regular exercise, dietary calcium, and vitamin D may be the best prescription for building and preserving strong bones.

The question of whether increased calcium intake can help in weight loss remains controversial. In a large study of middle-aged men, those who increased their total calcium intake gained more weight, but consumption of low-fat dairy products was not significantly associated with weight change.[14]

Sodium

Sodium helps maintain proper fluid balance, regulates blood pressure, transmits muscle impulses, and relaxes muscles. Excess sodium isn't a problem for most healthy people, but for those who are sodium-sensitive—as many as 30 percent of the population—too much sodium contributes to high blood pressure.

The National Heart, Lung, and Blood Institute recommends less than 2.4 grams (2,400 milligrams) of sodium a day, the equivalent of about one teaspoon of table salt a day. For someone with high blood pressure, a daily intake of less than 1,500 mg of sodium is better for lowering blood pressure.

Blacks, who have higher rates of high blood pressure and diseases related to hypertension, such as stroke and kidney failure, tend to be more sensitive to salt than nonblacks. African Americans also have lower intakes of calcium and potassium—both of which can protect against heart disease.[15]

Phytochemicals

Phytochemicals, compounds that exist naturally in plants, serve many functions, including helping a plant protect itself from bacteria and disease. Some phytochemicals such as solanine, an insect-repelling chemical found in the leaves and stalks of potato plants, are natural toxins, but many are beneficial to humans. Flavonoids, found in apples, strawberries, grapes, onions, green and black tea, and red wine, may

phytochemicals Chemicals suc as indoles, coumarins, and capsaicin, which exist naturally i plants and have disease-fighting properties.

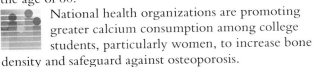

decrease atherosclerotic plaque and DNA damage related to cancer development. Phytochemicals are associated with a reduced risk of heart disease, certain cancers, age-related macular degeneration, adult-onset diabetes, stroke, and other diseases. However, in Western societies, research has shown neither an increase nor decrease in breast cancer with consumption of phytochemicals.

? FAQ Should I Take Supplements?

Since vitamins and minerals in food are good for you, you might figure that taking more in the form of dietary supplements would be even better. That's exactly why many people—half of all Americans, by some estimates—have taken vitamin pills, often in high doses, especially after studies confirmed the benefits of antioxidants in food, particularly vitamins C and E. But recent research indicates that larger-than-recommended doses of vitamins do not reduce the risk of heart disease, cancer, and dementia—and may do more harm than good.

In major trials with nearly 140,000 randomized participants, antioxidant vitamins were essentially of no benefit in preventing cardiovascular disease or cancer. In a 12-year study of nearly 40,000 women, vitamin E failed to show any protective effects against cardiovascular problems or breast, lung, and colon cancer.[16] It is not yet known if it might be beneficial for men. In other studies, antioxidant supplements did not reduce heart disorders or death rates, nor did they help people who already had diabetes or blood vessel disease.[17] Super-high doses of vitamin E also have not helped people with mild cognitive impairment, an early stage of Alzheimer's disease.[18]

High doses of vitamins carry potential risks. Certain antioxidants can interfere with the efficacy of cholesterol-lowering medications. High doses of vitamin E may increase the chances of earlier death. In cancer patients, those taking large doses had an increased risk of a new cancer.[19]

In particular, the fat-soluble vitamins, primarily A and D, can build up in our bodies and cause serious complications, such as damage to the kidneys, liver, or bones. Large doses of water-soluble vitamins, including the B vitamins, may also be harmful. Excessive intake of vitamin B_6 (pyridoxine), often used to relieve premenstrual bloating, can cause neurological damage, such as numbness in the mouth and tingling in the hands. (An excessive amount in this case is 250 to 300 times the recommended dose.) High doses of vitamin C can produce stomachaches and diarrhea. Niacin, often taken in high doses to lower cholesterol, can cause jaundice, liver damage, and irregular heartbeats as well as severe, uncomfortable flushing of the skin.

If you do feel a need for vitamins, choose a multivitamin supplement that does not exceed the recommended doses listed in Tables 5-4 and 5-5.

Using the MyPyramid System

Making healthy choices about what and how to eat isn't easy. However, the federal government is trying to help. In its most recent edition of *Nutrition and Your Health: Dietary Guidelines for Americans,* the U.S. Departments of Health and Human Services and of Agriculture provide science-based advice both to promote wellness and to reduce the risk of major chronic diseases. The MyPyramid Food Guidance System (Figure 5-2) translates the guidelines into a personalized, balanced, total diet.

The key themes of MyPyramid are:

- **Variety.** Eating foods from all food groups and subgroups.
- **Proportionality.** Eating more of some foods (fruits, vegetables, whole grains, fat-free or low-fat milk products) and less of others (foods high in saturated or trans fats, added sugars, cholesterol, salt, and alcohol). Critics of the new pyramid point out that the guidelines still do not take a hard enough line on the amount of refined starches or red meat in the American diet.
- **Moderation.** Choosing forms of foods that limit intake of saturated or trans fats, added sugars, cholesterol, salt, and alcohol.
- **Activity.** Being physically active every day.
- **Personalization.** To make the most of the new MyPyramid system, you need to go online to www.mypyramid.gov. By filling in your age, gender, and typical level of activity, you will be linked to one of twelve versions of the pyramid, ranging from 1,000 to 3,200 daily calories. You can print out your customized pyramid and use it as a dietary guide. Track what you eat for a week to see how it compares with the recommendations, and go back to the website for specific suggestions.

Critics of the new MyPyramid charge that it does not go far enough in urging Americans to cut back on harmful fats and simple carbohydrates and also lumps together various protein sources (red meat, poultry, fish, and beans) as equally healthy.[20] However, national surveys show that a large majority of Americans have heard of the revised guidelines and had a generally positive reaction. About a third said they would change their habits, another third said they might change, and a third said they wouldn't alter their lifestyles.[21]

The following guidelines are based on the MyPyramid system.

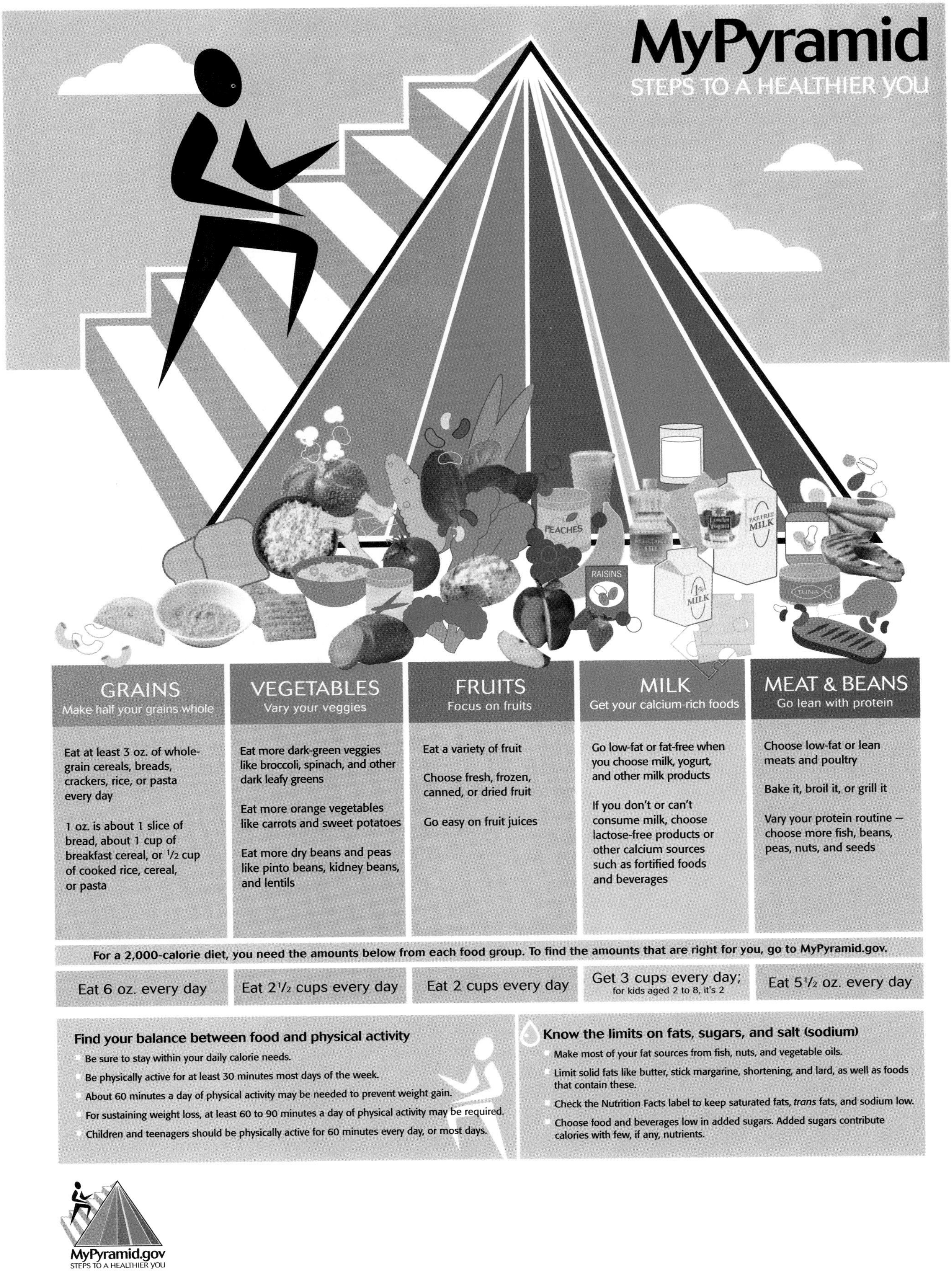
MyPyramid
STEPS TO A HEALTHIER YOU
PEACHES
RAISINS
TUNA
FAT-FREE MILK
1% MILK
GRAINS
Make half your grains whole
Eat at least 3 oz. of whole-grain cereals, breads, crackers, rice, or pasta every day
1 oz. is about 1 slice of bread, about 1 cup of breakfast cereal, or 1/2 cup of cooked rice, cereal, or pasta
VEGETABLES
Vary your veggies
Eat more dark-green veggies like broccoli, spinach, and other dark leafy greens
Eat more orange vegetables like carrots and sweet potatoes
Eat more dry beans and peas like pinto beans, kidney beans, and lentils
FRUITS
Focus on fruits
Eat a variety of fruit
Choose fresh, frozen, canned, or dried fruit
Go easy on fruit juices
MILK
Get your calcium-rich foods
Go low-fat or fat-free when you choose milk, yogurt, and other milk products
If you don't or can't consume milk, choose lactose-free products or other calcium sources such as fortified foods and beverages
MEAT & BEANS
Go lean with protein
Choose low-fat or lean meats and poultry
Bake it, broil it, or grill it
Vary your protein routine — choose more fish, beans, peas, nuts, and seeds
For a 2,000-calorie diet, you need the amounts below from each food group. To find the amounts that are right for you, go to MyPyramid.gov.
Eat 6 oz. every day
Eat 2 1/2 cups every day
Eat 2 cups every day
Get 3 cups every day; for kids aged 2 to 8, it's 2
Eat 5 1/2 oz. every day
Find your balance between food and physical activity
Be sure to stay within your daily calorie needs.
Be physically active for at least 30 minutes most days of the week.
About 60 minutes a day of physical activity may be needed to prevent weight gain.
For sustaining weight loss, at least 60 to 90 minutes a day of physical activity may be required.
Children and teenagers should be physically active for 60 minutes every day, or most days.
Know the limits on fats, sugars, and salt (sodium)
Make most of your fat sources from fish, nuts, and vegetable oils.
Limit solid fats like butter, stick margarine, shortening, and lard, as well as foods that contain these.
Check the Nutrition Facts label to keep saturated fats, trans fats, and sodium low.
Choose food and beverages low in added sugars. Added sugars contribute calories with few, if any, nutrients.
MyPyramid.gov
STEPS TO A HEALTHIER YOU

FIGURE 5-2 The MyPyramid Food Guidance System

Consume a Variety of Foods

The six colors on the MyPyramid graphic represent the five food groups—grains, vegetables, fruits, milk, and meat and beans—and oils. The greater the variety of colors and of foods you choose, the more likely you are to obtain the nutrients you need—see Table 5-6. In general, the USDA recommends a diet that is high in fruits and vegetables, whole grains, and nonfat or low-fat milk products that provides amounts of nutrients (including potassium and fiber) that can help reduce the risk of chronic disease and is low in saturated fat, cholesterol, added sugars, trans fat, and sodium.

Manage Your Weight

As discussed in Chapter 6, you must expend as much energy (calories) as you take in to stay at the same weight. Among the best ways to balance this energy equation are limiting portion sizes (discussed later in this chapter), substituting nutrient-dense foods (such as raw vegetables or low-fat soups) for nutrient-poor foods (such as candy and cake), and limiting added sugars, solid fats, and alcoholic beverages.

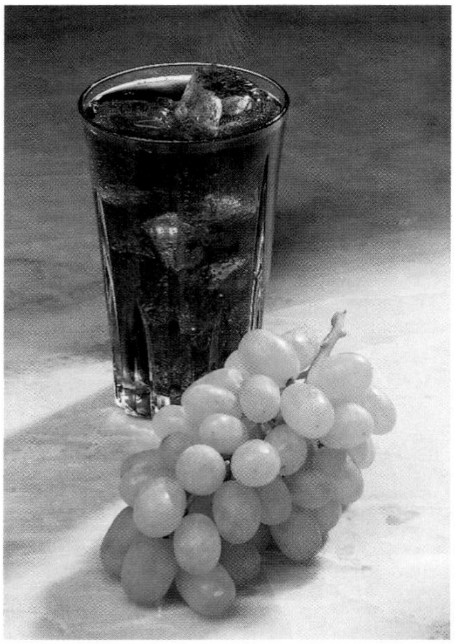

© Polara Studios Inc.

This cola and bunch of grapes each provide about 150 calories, but the nutrient-dense grapes offer a trace of protein, some vitamins, minerals, and fiber. The cola beverage offers only "empty" calories from sugar without any other nutrients.

Get Physical Every Day

As discussed in Chapter 4, regular physical activity helps maintain a healthy weight and reduces risk for several chronic diseases. While 30 minutes of moderate physical activity (such as walking at a pace of three or four miles an hour) on most days provides important benefits, exercising more often and more intensely yields additional health dividends. Many adults need up to 60 minutes of moderate to vigorous physical activity—the equivalent of 150 to 200 calories, depending on body size, daily to prevent unhealthy weight gain. Men and women who have lost weight may need 60 to 90 minutes to keep off excess pounds. Children and teenagers require at least 60 minutes of moderate physical activity every day.

Increase Foods from Certain Food Groups

Greater consumption of fruits and vegetables (5 to 13 servings or 2½ to 6½ cups per day, depending on how many calories you burn) may reduce the risk of stroke, certain cancers, and type 2 diabetes (vegetables more so than fruit) as well as helping reach and maintain a healthy weight (Figure 5-3). The more fruits and vegetables men and women consume, the lower their levels of harmful low-density lipoprotein (LDL) cholesterol. Plant-based foods also reduce the risk of rectal cancer in both men and women (Table 5-7).

Among the ways to increase your fruit and vegetable intake:

- **Toss fruit into a green salad** for extra flavor, variety, color, and crunch.
- **Start the day with a daily double:** a glass of juice and a banana or other fruit on cereal.
- **Buy pre-cut vegetables** for snacking or dipping (instead of chips).
- **Make or order sandwiches** with extra tomatoes or other vegetable toppings.

Consuming at least three servings (the equivalent of 3 ounces) of whole grains per day can reduce the risk of diabetes and coronary heart disease and maintain a healthy weight. To increase your intake of grains:

- **Check labels of rolls and bread,** and choose those with at least 2 to 3 grams of fiber per slice.
- **Add brown rice or barley** to soups.
- **Choose whole-grain,** ready-to-eat cereals.

To get more dairy products with less fat, try the following:

- **Substitute fat-free sour cream** or nonfat, plain yogurt for sour cream.
- **Add low-fat milk** instead of water to oatmeal and hot cereals.
- **Eat cereals with added calcium** and with milk.
- **Top salads or soups with low-fat shredded cheese.**

TABLE 5-6 Nutrient Contributions of Each Food Group

Food Group	Major Contribution(s)[1]	Substantial Contribution(s) (>10% of total)[2]		
Fruit Group	Vitamin C	Thiamin Vitamin B_6 Folate	Copper Potassium Carbohydrate	Magnesium Fiber
Vegetable Group	Vitamin A Potassium	Vitamin E Vitamin C Thiamin Niacin Vitamin B_6	Magnesium Iron Zinc Copper Carbohydrate	Folate Calcium Phosphorus Fiber Alpha-linolenic acid
Vegetable Subgroups:				
Dark green vegetables		Vitamin A Vitamin C		
Orange vegetables	Vitamin A			
Legumes		Folate Copper	Fiber	
Starchy vegetables		Vitamin B_6 Copper		
Other vegetables			Vitamin C	
Grain Group	Thiamin Folate Magnesium Iron Copper Carbohydrate Fiber	Vitamin A Riboflavin Niacin Vitamin B_6 Vitamin B_{12} Calcium	Phosphorus Zinc Potassium Protein Linoleic acid Alpha-linolenic acid	
Grain Subgroups:				
Whole grains	Folate (tie) Magnesium Iron Copper Carbohydrate (tie) Fiber	Thiamin Riboflavin Niacin Vitamin B_6	Vitamin B_{12} Phosphorus Zinc Protein	
Enriched grain	Folate (tie) Thiamin Carbohydrate (tie)	Riboflavin Niacin	Iron Copper	
Meat, Poultry, Fish, Eggs, and Nuts Group	Niacin Vitamin B_6 Zinc Protein	Vitamin E Thiamin Riboflavin Vitamin B_{12} Phosphorus	Magnesium Iron Copper Potassium Linoleic acid	
Milk Group	Riboflavin Vitamin B_{12} Calcium Phosphorus	Vitamin A Thiamin Vitamin B_6 Magnesium	Zinc Potassium Carbohydrate Protein	
Oils and Soft Margarines	Vitamin E Linoleic acid Alpha-linolenic acid			

1. *Major contribution* means that the food group or subgroup provides more of the nutrient than any other single food group, averaged over all calorie levels. When two food groups or subgroups provide equal amounts, it is noted as a tie.
2. A *substantial contribution* means that the food group or subgroup provides 10% or more of the total amount of the nutrient in the food patterns, averaged over all calorie levels.
Source: Dietary Guidelines for Americans 2005. USDHHS, USDA, www.healthierus.gov/dietaryguidelines.

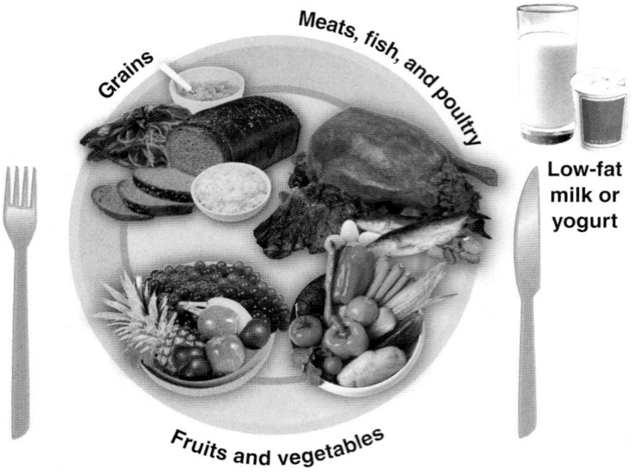

FIGURE 5-3 Fill Half Your Plate with Fruits and Vegetables

TABLE 5-7 Which Fruits and Vegetables[1] Provide the Most Nutrients?

Sources of Vitamin A (carotenoids)
Bright orange vegetables like carrots, sweet potatoes, and pumpkin
Dark green leafy vegetables such as spinach, collards, and turnip greens
Bright orange fruits like mango, cantaloupe, and apricots
Sources of Vitamin C
Citrus fruits and juices, kiwi fruit, strawberries, and cantaloupe
Broccoli, peppers, tomatoes, cabbage, and potatoes
Leafy greens such as romaine, turnip greens, and spinach
Sources of Folate
Cooked dried beans and peas
Oranges and orange juice
Deep green leaves like spinach and mustard greens
Sources of Potassium
Baked white or sweet potato, cooked greens (such as spinach), winter (orange) squash
Bananas, plantains, many dried fruits, and orange juice

1. Often, the fruits and vegetables with brighter colors have the higher content of vitamins and minerals.
Source: Dietary Guidelines for Americans 2005. USDHHS, USDA, www.healthierus.gov/dietaryguidelines.

Be Finicky About Fats

Reducing saturated fat, trans fat, and cholesterol can lower harmful LDL cholesterol and your risk of heart disease. You should keep saturated fat below 10 percent of total calories, trans fat as low as possible, and cholesterol intake below 300 mg per day. Your total fat intake should make up no more than 20 to 35 percent of calories. For children ages 2 and 3, recommended minimum fat intake is 30 percent of calories; for those between ages 4 and 18, it is 25 percent.

To keep within these limits:

- **Restrict animal fats** (such as those in cheese, milk, butter, ice cream, and other full-fat dairy products, fatty meat, bacon, sausage, poultry skin and fat).
- **Cut back** on foods made with partially hydrogenated vegetable oils.
- **Limit your intake** of eggs and organ meats.

As noted earlier, recent research has challenged the health benefits of omega-3 fats. However, foods containing these fats are generally healthful ones: oily fish (such as salmon or sardines), flaxseed, walnuts, and canola oils. You should continue to include them in your diet about two times a week. Choose safer fish varieties with lower mercury content, such as salmon, canned light tuna (rather than albacore), shrimp, and catfish. Do not eat swordfish, shark, large mackerel, and tilefish.

Omega-3 fatty acids are especially important for the proper development of the nervous system in the fetus. Omega-3s also play a role in nervous system development in young children. This poses a dilemma because while oily fish are a great source of omega-3s, they are also the ones highest in mercury and potentially other toxic substances such as dioxins. Pregnant and nursing women and children should limit their consumption of oily fish and always choose the safer varieties.

Choose Carbohydrates Wisely

Eating more fruits, vegetables, whole grains, and nonfat or low-fat milk and dairy products is a healthful way to get the carbohydrates you need. Fiber-rich choices—an apple rather than apple juice, for example—have the added benefit of promoting digestive health and reduce the risk of type 2 diabetes and heart disease.

The new guidelines do not include a specific message about sugar but caution against "added" sugars, those added to foods during processing or preparation or at the table. Recent research has implicated sugar-sweetened beverages as a culprit in weight gain. Carbohydrates (including sucrose, glucose, fructose, lactose, and starch) also can increase the risk of dental cavities. Drinking fluoridated water and/or using fluoride-containing dental hygiene products can protect your teeth.

To make sure your grains are whole, choose foods that name one of the following whole-grain ingredients first on the label's ingredient list: brown rice, bulgur, graham flour, oatmeal, whole-grain corn, whole oats, whole rye, whole wheat, wild rice. Foods labeled multi-grain, stone-ground, 100% wheat, cracked wheat, seven-grain, or bran are usually not whole-grain products.

Limit Salt

Reducing salt in your diet is one way to lower your blood pressure and reduce your risk of stroke, heart disease, and kidney disease. Another effective strategy is to eat more foods rich in potassium, which blunts the effects of salt on blood pressure, may decrease bone loss, and reduces the risk of kidney stones.

The USDA guidelines recommend less than 2,300 mg of sodium per day. Many people, including those with hypertension, blacks, and older adults, should reduce their salt intake even more and increase potassium to at least 4,700 mg.

To reduce sodium intake:

- **Look for labels that say "low sodium."** They contain 140 mg or less of sodium per serving.
- **Learn to use spices and herbs rather than salt** to enhance the flavor of food.
- **Go easy on condiments** such as soy sauce, pickles, olives, ketchup, and mustard, which can add a lot of salt to your food.
- **Always check the amount of sodium** in processed foods, such as frozen dinners, packaged mixes, cereals, salad dressings, and sauces. The amount in different types and brands can vary widely.

If You Drink Alcoholic Beverages, Do So in Moderation

As discussed in Chapter 12, alcohol has different effects on health for different age groups. In middle-aged and older adults, one to two drinks a day seem to lower the risk of dying, primarily because moderate alcohol consumption protects against heart disease. Compared with nondrinkers, however, women who consume one alcoholic beverage per day appear to have a slightly higher risk of breast cancer. For younger people, alcohol provides little, if any, health benefits and increases the risk of traumatic injury and death. At any age, heavy drinking contributes to automotive accidents and deaths, assaults, liver disease, and other health problems.

MyPyramid includes a category for "discretionary calories," which can be used on fats, added sugar, alcohol, or more food from any food group. However, most people, especially those who are not physically active, "earn" very small discretionary calorie allowances, usually no more than 100 to 300 calories a day.[22]

Keep Food Safe to Eat

See page 130 for an in-depth discussion of food safety. The key steps you can take to ensure food safety and prevent a problem with foodborne illnesses are:

- **Thoroughly wash hands,** contact surfaces, and fruits and vegetables (but not meat and poultry).
- **Separate raw, cooked, and ready-to-eat foods** while shopping, preparing, or storing.
- **Cook foods to a safe temperature.**
- **Chill (refrigerate) perishable foods promptly.**

The Way We Eat

Just as there is no one perfect food, there is no one eating pattern that suits all people of all ages and backgrounds at all times. Your ethnic background and family makeup influenced the way you ate as a child. In college, you probably will find yourself eating in different—and not necessarily better—ways. Because the United States is so diverse, you also will have the opportunity to sample the cuisines of many cultures.

? FAQ Do Men and Women Have Different Nutritional Needs?

Men and women do not need to eat different foods, but their nutritional needs are different. Because most men are bigger and taller than most women, they consume more calories. Eating more means it's easier for them to get the nutrients they need, even though many don't make the wisest food choices.

Women, particularly those who restrict their caloric intake or are chronically dieting, are more likely to develop specific deficiencies. Calcium is one example. Many teenage girls and young women under age 30 do not consume the recommended 800 to 1,200 milligrams of calcium daily and may be at increased risk of bone-weakening osteoporosis.[23]

Many women also get too little iron. Even in adolescence, girls are more prone to iron deficiency than boys; some suffer memory and learning impairments as a result. In adult women, menstrual blood loss and poor eating habits can lead to low iron stores, which puts them at risk for anemia. According to U.S. Department of Agriculture research, most women consume only 60 percent of the recommended 15 milligrams of iron per day. (The recommendation for men is 10 milligrams.) Regular blood tests can monitor a woman's iron status.

Both genders should increase their fruit and vegetable intake to ensure that they are getting adequate amounts of vitamins and fiber in their daily diet.

Here are some gender-specific strategies for better nutrition:

- **Men should cut back on fat** and meat in their diets, two things they eat too much.
- **Women should increase their iron intake** by eating meat (iron from animal sources is absorbed better than that from

vegetable sources) or a combination of meat and vegetable iron sources together (for example, a meat and bean burrito). Those with iron deficiencies should consult a physician. Because large doses of iron can be toxic, iron supplements should be taken only with medical supervision.

- **Women should consume more calcium-rich** foods, including low-fat and nonfat dairy products, leafy greens, and tofu. Women who cannot get adequate amounts of calcium from their daily diet should take calcium supplements. This is not advised for all men because of a possible connection between calcium and prostate cancer.
- **Women who could become pregnant should take a multivitamin** with 400 micrograms of **folic acid,** which helps prevent neural tube defects such as spina bifida. Folic acid is also useful to men because it may cut the risk of heart disease, stroke, and colon cancer.

Nutrition 101: The Eating Habits of College Students

Often on their own for the first time, college students typically change their usual eating patterns. In one recent survey, 59 percent of freshmen said their diet had changed since they began college. When they are making meal choices, the top two influences on students are price and convenience, with nutrition coming in third (see Student Snapshot: "Why Students Choose the Foods They Do").

According to various national samples, many students do not consume adequate amounts of fruits and vegetables and consume too many fried and fast foods. In one study that followed students through their freshman and sophomore years, more than half remained in the precontemplation stage for adopting healthier eating behaviors throughout this time. Only 30 percent of the students consumed at least five fruits and vegetables daily; more than half reported eating high-fat fried or fast foods at least three times during the previous week.[24]

Perhaps because they don't get five daily servings of fruit and vegetables, students also fall short in fiber intake. When 144 undergraduates at a four-year university completed three-day food intake reports, only 19 met the recommended 20 to 35 grams per day of dietary fiber: 13 percent of the women and 16 percent of the men.[25]

The same holds true for consumption of healthful omega-3 polyunsaturated fats, such as fish oils. In a recent study of 51 college-aged women, 84 percent failed to meet the recommended levels for adequate intake. Only the small percentage consuming higher-than-recommended levels for total fat intake met or exceeded the recommended amounts of beneficial fats.[26]

Some colleges are doing their part to improve student nutrition. Many post nutritional information in dining halls; some have expanded their offerings to include more salads, fewer fried foods, and more ethnic dishes.

Student Snapshot

Why Students Choose The Foods They Do

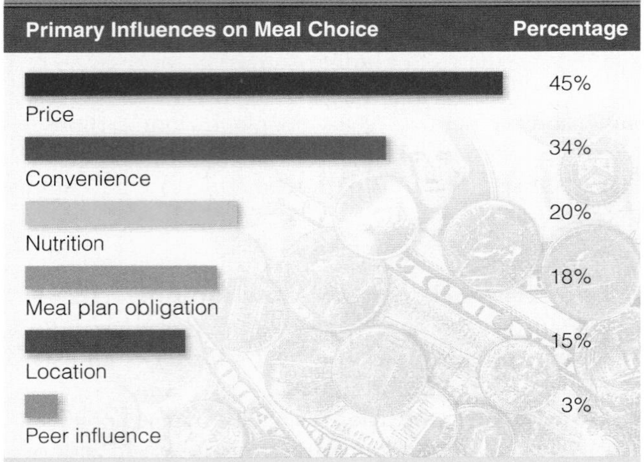

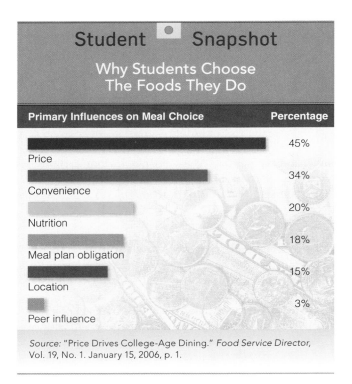

Source: "Price Drives College-Age Dining." *Food Service Director,* Vol. 19, No. 1. January 15, 2006, p. 1.

Dietary Diversity

Whatever your cultural heritage, you have probably sampled Chinese, Mexican, Indian, Italian, and Japanese foods. If you belong to any of these ethnic groups, you may eat these cuisines regularly. Each type of ethnic cooking has its own nutritional benefits and potential drawbacks.

Mediterranean Diet

Several years ago epidemiologists noticed something unexpected in the residents of regions along the Mediterranean Sea: a lower incidence of deaths from heart disease. Scientists have identified antioxidants in red wine and olive oil that may account for the beneficial effects on the heart of the Mediterranean diet, which features lots of fruits and vegetables, legumes, nuts, and grains. Meat is used mainly as a condiment rather than as a main course, and fish, yogurt, and low-fat feta cheese are the predominant animal foods. The diet is relatively high in fat, but the main source is olive oil, an unsaturated fat.

Ethnic Cuisines

The cuisine served in Mexico features rice, corn, and beans, which are low in fat and high in nutrients. However, the dishes Americans think of as Mexican are far less healthful. Burritos, especially when topped with cheese and sour cream, are very high in fat. Although guacamole has a high fat content, it contains mostly monounsaturated fatty acids, a better form of fat.

African-American cuisine traces some of its roots to food preferences from west Africa (for example, peanuts, okra, and black-eyed peas), as well as to traditional American foods, such as fish, game, greens, and sweet potatoes. It uses many nutritious vegetables, such as collard greens and sweet potatoes, as well as legumes. However, some dishes include high-fat food products such as peanuts and pecans or involve frying, sometimes in saturated fat.

The mainland Chinese diet, which is plant-based, high in carbohydrates, and low in fats and animal protein, is considered one of the healthiest in the world. However, Chinese restaurants here serve more meat and sauces than are generally eaten in China. According to laboratory tests of typical take-out dishes from Chinese restaurants, many have more fats and cholesterol than hamburger or egg dishes from fast-food outlets.

Traditional French cuisine, which includes rich, high-fat sauces and dishes, has never been considered healthful. Yet, nutritionists have been stumped to explain the so-called French paradox. Despite a diet high in saturated fats, the French have had one of the lowest rates of coronary artery disease in the world. The French diet increasingly resembles the American diet, but French portions tend to be one-third to one-half the size of American portions.

Many Indian dishes highlight healthful ingredients such as vegetables and legumes (beans and peas). However, many also use *ghee* (a form of butter) or coconut oil; both are rich in harmful saturated fats. The best advice in an Indian restaurant is to ask how each dish is prepared. Good choices include *daal* or *dal* (lentils), *karbi* or *karni* (chickpea soup), and *chapati* (tortilla-like bread).

The traditional Japanese diet is very low in fat, which may account for the low incidence of heart disease in Japan. Dietary staples include soybean products, fish, vegetables, noodles, and rice. A variety of fruits and vegetables are also included in many dishes. However, Japanese cuisine is high in salted, smoked, and pickled foods. Watch out for deep-fried dishes such as tempura and salty soups and sauces.

? FAQ What Should I Know About Vegetarian Diets?

Not all vegetarians avoid all meats. Some, who call themselves *lacto-ovo-pesco-vegetarians,* eat dairy products, eggs, chicken, and fish but not red meat. **Lacto-vegetarians** eat dairy products as well as grains,

folic acid A form of folate used in vitamin supplements and fortified foods.

lacto-vegetarians People who eat dairy products as well as fruits and vegetables (but not meat, poultry, or fish).

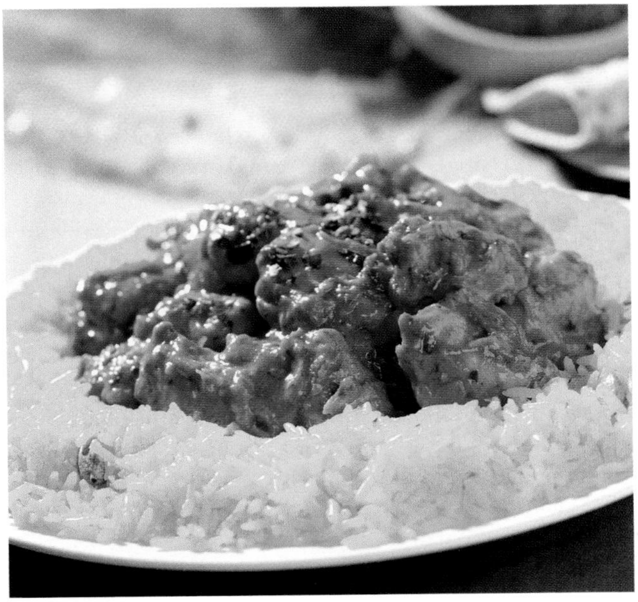

© Corbis

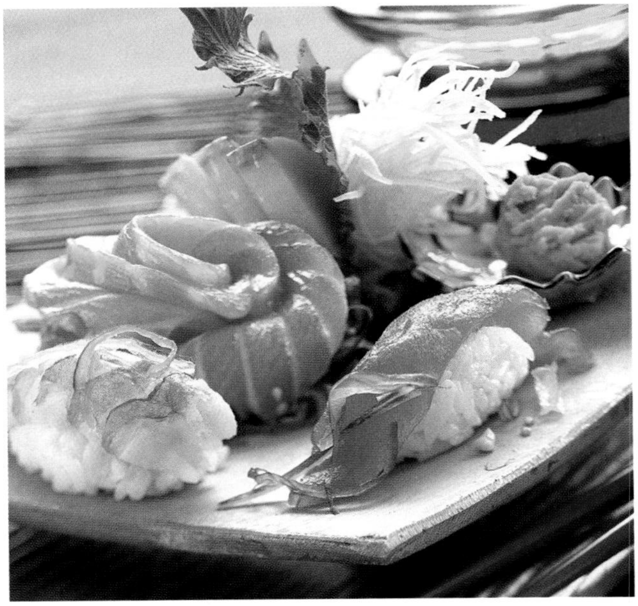

© David Chasey/Photodisc Red/Getty Images

In today's ethnically diverse United States, all-American food ranges from Indian to Japanese. The vegetables and legumes in the Indian diet are healthy and high in protein, but too much saturated fat can cancel some of the benefits. The Japanese diet is high in seafood and rice and low in fats, cheese, and meat.

fruits, and vegetables; **ovo-lacto-vegetarians** also eat eggs. Pure vegetarians, called **vegans,** eat only plant foods; often they take vitamin B_{12} supplements because that vitamin is normally found only in animal products. If they select their food with care, vegetarians can get sufficient amounts of protein, vitamin B_{12}, iron, and calcium without supplements.

The key to getting sufficient protein from a vegetarian diet is understanding the concept of **complementary proteins.** Meat, poultry, fish, eggs, and dairy products are *complete proteins* that provide the nine essential amino acids—substances that the human body cannot produce itself. *Incomplete proteins,* such as legumes or nuts, may have relatively low levels of one or two essential amino acids but fairly high levels of others. By combining complementary protein sources, you can make sure that your body makes the most of the nonanimal proteins you eat. Many cultures rely heavily on complementary foods for protein. In Middle Eastern cooking, sesame seeds and chickpeas are a popular combination; in Latin American dishes, beans and rice, or beans and tortillas; in Chinese cuisine, soy and rice.

According to the 2005 Dietary Guidelines, vegetarians can best meet their nutrient needs by paying special attention to protein, iron, vitamin B_{12}, calcium, and vitamin D. Instead of a 6-ounce serving of meat, they can substitute one egg, 1.5 ounces of nuts, or two-thirds cup of legumes. Those who avoid milk because of its lactose content may obtain all the nutrients of milk by using lactose-reduced milk or eating other calcium-rich foods, such as broccoli, calcium-fortified orange juice, and fortified soy milk.[27]

Vegetarian diets have proven health benefits. Studies show that vegetarians' cholesterol levels are low, and vegetarians are seldom overweight. As a result, they're less apt to be candidates for heart disease than those who consume large quantities of meat. Vegetarians also have lower incidences of breast, colon, and prostate cancer; high blood pressure; and osteoporosis.

Fast Food: Nutrition on the Run

On any given day, about 25 percent of adults in the United States go to a fast-food restaurant. The typical American consumes three hamburgers and four orders of french fries every week. Not all fast foods are junk foods—that is, high in calories, sugar, salt, and fat and low in beneficial nutrients (Table 5-8). But while it's not all bad, fast food has definite disadvantages. A meal in a fast-food restaurant may cost twice as much as the same meal prepared at home and may provide half your daily calorie needs. The fat content of many items is extremely high. A Burger King Whopper with cheese contains 723 calories and 48 grams of fat, 18 grams from saturated fat. A McDonald's Sausage McMuffin with egg has 517 calories and 33 grams of fat, 13 grams from saturated fat. Many fast-food chains have switched from beef tallow or lard to unsaturated vegetable oils for frying, but the total fat content of the foods remains the same.

YOUR LIFE COACH

Taking Charge of What You Eat

You can't control what you don't know. Because of the Nutrition Labeling and Education Act, food manufacturers must provide information about fat, calories, and ingredients in large type on packaged food labels, and they must show how a food item fits into a daily diet of 2,000 calories. The law also restricts nutritional claims for terms such as *healthy, low-fat,* and *high-fiber.*

At one university, almost two-thirds of the freshmen reported that they were aware of the nutrition labels posted in the dining commons. One-third used them to help make food choices. Female students were significantly more likely to base their food choices on the labels than the men. Students primarily checked overall good/balanced nutrition content of foods, calories, fat, saturated fat, and protein. Their top reason for checking labels: to be healthy now.[28]

In evaluating food labels and product claims, keep in mind that while individual foods vary in their nutritional value, what matters is your total diet. If you eat too much of any one food—regardless of what its label states—you may not be getting the variety and balance of nutrients that you need.

Portions and Servings

Consumers often are confused by what a *serving* actually is, especially since many American restaurants have super-sized the amount of food they put on their customers' plates. The average bagel has doubled in size in the last ten to fifteen years. A standard fast-food serving of french fries is larger in the United States than in the United Kingdom.

A food-label *serving* is a specific amount of food that contains the quantity of nutrients described on the Nutrition Facts label. A *portion* is the amount of a specific food that an individual eats at one time. Portions can be bigger or smaller than the servings on food labels. According to nutritionists, "marketplace portions"—the actual amounts served to customers—are two to eight times larger than the standard serving sizes defined by the USDA. In fast-food chains, today's portions are two to five times larger than the original sizes. As studies have shown, people presented with larger

TABLE 5-8 Healthier Fast Food Choices

Arby's®	Calories	Fat (g)	Percent Fat	Protein (g)	Carb (g)
Roast Chicken Salad	160	2.5	13	20	15
Grilled Chicken Salad	210	4.5	19	30	14
Light Grilled Chicken	280	5	17	23	33
Light Roast Chicken Deluxe	260	5	17	23	33
Light Roast Turkey Deluxe	260	5	17	23	33
Burger King®					
BK Broiler Chicken Sandwich	267	8	27	22	25
Frozen Yogurt, Vanilla	120	3	22.5	2	20
Frozen Yogurt, Chocolate	130	3	20.8	3	21
Salad, Chunky Chicken	142	4	25.4	20	8
Side Salad	25	0	0	1	5
Jack In The Box®					
Hamburger	250	9	32	12	31
Chicken Fajita Pita	330	11	30	24	35
KFC®					
Original Recipe, Whole Wing	140	10	15	9	5
Orignimal Recipe, Drumstick	140	9	13	13	4
Extra Crispy, Whole Wing	220	15	23	10	10
Extra Crispy, Drumstick	195	12	19	15	7
Hot & Spicy, Whole Wing	210	25	23	10	9
Hot & Spicy, Drumstick	175	10	17	13	9
McDonald's®					
English Muffin	140	2	10	4	25
Chicken McGrill w/o mayo	340	7	19	26	45
Hamburger	280	10	32	12	35
Taco Bell®					
Bean Burrito	380	12	28.9	13	55
Grilled Chicken Burrito	410	15	32.9	50	17
Wendy's®					
Jr. Hamburger	270	9	30	14	34
Grilled Chicken Sandwich	300	7	20	24	36
Chili, small	210	7	28	15	21

portions eat 30 to 50 percent more than they otherwise would.

If you are trying to balance your diet or control your weight, it's important to keep track of the size of your portions so that you do not exceed recommended servings. For instance, a 3-ounce serving of meat is about the size of a pack of playing cards—see Figure 5-4. If you eat a larger amount, count it as more than one serving.

? FAQ What Should I Look For on Nutrition Labels?

As Figure 5-5 shows, the Nutrition Facts on food labels present a wealth of information—if you know what to look for. The label focuses on those nutrients most clearly associated with disease risk and health: total fat, saturated fat, cholesterol, sodium, total carbohydrate, dietary fiber, sugar, and protein.

- **Calories.** Calories are the measure of the amount of energy that can be derived from food. Science defines a *calorie* as the amount of energy required to raise the temperature of 1 gram of water by 1 degree Celsius. In the laboratory, the caloric content of food is measured in 1,000-calorie units called *kilocalories.* The calorie referred to in everyday usage is actually the equivalent of the laboratory kilocalorie.

  The Nutrition Facts label lists two numbers for calories: calories per serving and calories from fat per serving. This allows consumers to calculate how many calories they'll consume and to determine the percentage of fat in an item.
- **Serving size.** Rather than the tiny portions manufacturers sometimes used in the past to keep down the number of calories per serving, the new labels reflect more realistic portions. Serving sizes, which have been defined for approximately 150 food categories, must be the same for similar products (for example, different brands of potato chips) and for similar products within a category (for example, snack foods such as pretzels, potato chips, and popcorn). This makes it easier to compare the nutritional content of foods.
- **Daily Values (DVs).** DVs refer to the total amount of a nutrient that the average adult should aim to get or not exceed on a daily basis. The DVs for cholesterol, sodium, vitamins, and minerals are the same for all adults. The DVs for total fat, saturated fat, carbohydrate, fiber, and protein are based on a 2,000-calorie daily diet—the amount of food ingested by many American men and active women.
- **Percent Daily Values (%DVs).** The goal for a full day's diet is to select foods that together add up to 100 percent of the DVs. The %DVs show

ovo-lacto-vegetarians People who eat eggs, dairy products, and fruits and vegetables (but not meat, poultry, or fish).

vegans People who eat only plant foods.

complementary proteins Incomplete proteins that, when combined, provide all the amino acids essential for protein synthesis.

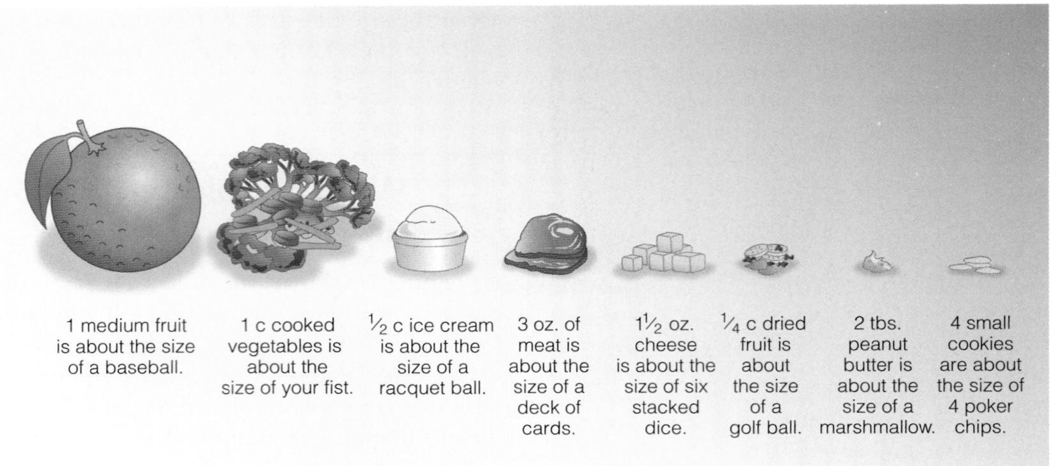

FIGURE 5-4 Quick and Easy Estimates of Portion Sizes

how a particular food's nutrient content fits into a 2,000-calorie diet. Individuals who consume (or should consume) fewer than 2,000 total calories a day have to lower their DVs for total fat, saturated fat, and carbohydrates. For example, if their caloric intake is 10 percent less than 2,000 calories, they would lower the DV by 10 percent. Similarly, those who consume more than 2,000 calories should adjust the DVs upward.

- **Calories per gram.** The bottom of the food label lists the number of calories per gram for fat, carbohydrates, and protein.

People zero in on different figures on the food label—for example, calories if they're watching their weight, specific ingredients if they have food allergies. Among the useful items to check are the following:

- **Calories from fat.** Get into the habit of calculating the percentage of fat calories in a food before buying or eating it.
- **Total fat.** Since the average person munches on 15 to 20 food items a day, it's easy to overload on fat. Saturated fat and trans fat numbers deserve special attention because of their reported link to several diseases.
- **Cholesterol.** Cholesterol is made by and contained in products of animal origin only. Many high-fat products, such as potato chips, contain 0 percent cholesterol because they're made from plants and are cooked in vegetable fats. However, if the vegetable fats are hydrogenated, the resulting trans fat is more harmful to the heart than cholesterol.
- **Sugars.** There is no Daily Value for sugars because health experts have yet to agree on a daily limit. The figure on the label includes naturally present sugars, such as lactose in milk and fructose in fruit, as well as those added to the food, such as table sugar, corn syrup, or dextrose.
- **Fiber.** A "high-fiber" food has 5 or more grams of fiber per serving. A "good" source of fiber provides at least 2.5 grams. "More" or "added" fiber means at least 2.5 grams more per serving than similar foods—10 percent more of the DV for fiber.
- **Calcium.** "High" equals 200 milligrams (mg) or more per serving. "Good" means at least 100 mg, while "more" indicates that the food contains at least 100 mg more calcium—10 percent more of the DV—than the item usually would have.
- **Sodium.** Most of us routinely get more sodium than we need. Read labels carefully to avoid excess sodium, which can be a health threat.
- **Vitamins.** A Daily Value of 10 percent of any vitamin makes a food a "good" source; 20 percent qualifies it as "high" in a certain vitamin.

Nutrition labeling for fresh produce, fish, meat, and poultry remains voluntary. Packages too small for a full-sized label must provide an address or phone number so that cosumers can obtain information from the manufacturer.

Functional Foods

As the American Dietetic Association has noted, all foods are functional at some physiological level. However, the term *functional* generally applies to a food specifically created to have health-promoting benefits. The International Food Information Council defines functional foods as those "that provide health benefits beyond basic nutrition."

Some manufacturers are adding biologically active components such as beta-carotene to food products and promoting them as functional foods. However, the amounts added are often too low to have any effect, and many such foods are high-sugared drinks and snack foods. More research is needed to evaluate their claims of health benefits.

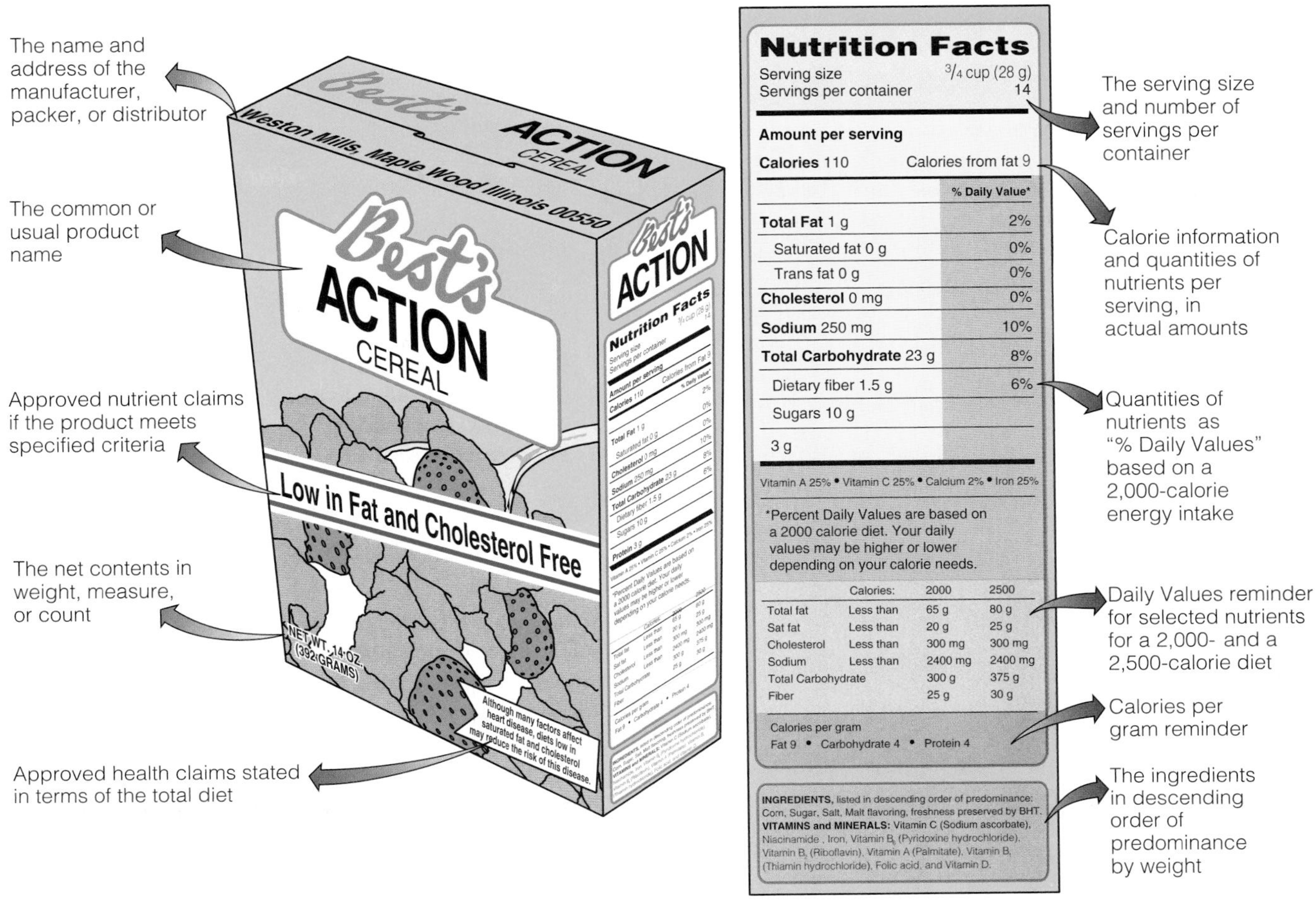

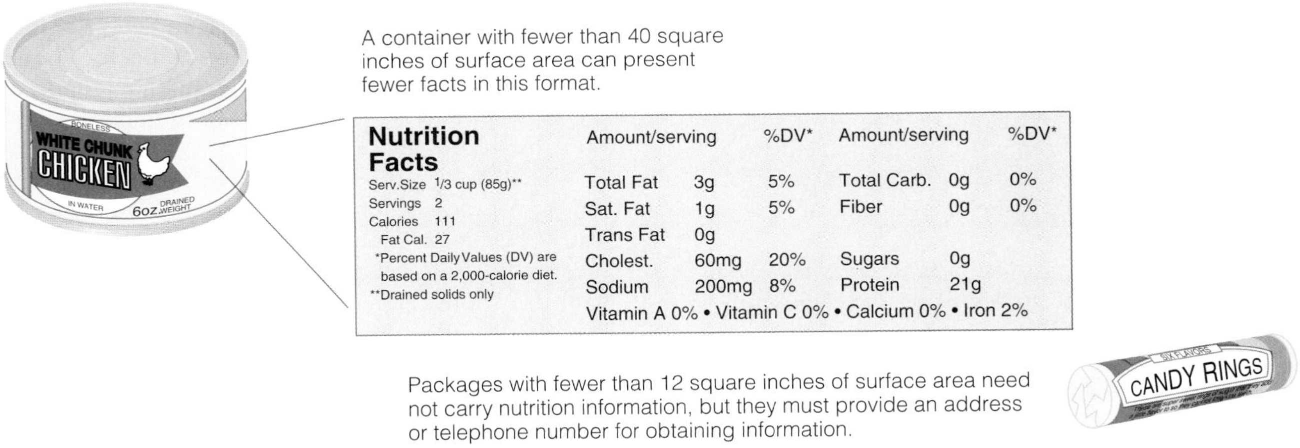

BONELESS
WHITE CHUNK CHICKEN
IN WATER
6OZ. DRAINED WEIGHT
A container with fewer than 40 square inches of surface area can present fewer facts in this format.
Nutrition Facts
Serv.Size 1/3 cup (85g)**
Servings 2
Calories 111
Fat Cal. 27
*Percent Daily Values (DV) are based on a 2,000-calorie diet.
**Drained solids only
Amount/serving %DV* Amount/serving %DV*
Total Fat 3g 5% Total Carb. 0g 0%
Sat. Fat 1g 5% Fiber 0g 0%
Trans Fat 0g
Cholest. 60mg 20% Sugars 0g
Sodium 200mg 8% Protein 21g
Vitamin A 0% • Vitamin C 0% • Calcium 0% • Iron 2%
Packages with fewer than 12 square inches of surface area need not carry nutrition information, but they must provide an address or telephone number for obtaining information.
CANDY RINGS

FIGURE 5-5 Understanding Nutrition Labels
The Nutrition Facts label lists the essential nutrient content of packaged food as well as the amount of potentially harmful substances such as fat and sodium.

? FAQ How Can I Find Snacks That Are Good for Me?

Snacking has become more widespread on campuses, as in other places. College students snack primarily "to satisfy hunger"; the second-most common reason is "no time for meals." Other reasons for munching between meals: "for energy," "to be sociable," and "to relieve stress." One-third snack at 9:00 p.m. or later.

In response to consumer demands for smart snack choices, food manufacturers are offering "better-for-you" options that are lower in salt and sugar or free of trans fatty acids and artificial colors. Some new snack items touted as healthy options, such as sugar-free chocolate or organic potato chips, offer little nutritional value. Meat-based snacks, increasingly popular among young men, also can be high in fat and sodium. Read labels carefully, and be sure to check total calories and fat.

A best-for-you option is fruit, such as bananas, apples, or berries, rich in vitamins, low in calories, and packed with fiber. Other nutritious snacks include nuts, trail mix, granola bars, yogurt, sunflower seeds, soy nuts, and dried fruit (such as cranberries). If you enjoy fruit juice, buy 100 percent fruit juice without added sugar. Limit yourself to one serving of these calorie-rich beverages a day.[29]

If you rely on snacks to keep you energized throughout the day, take time to plan in advance so you have choices other than the nearest vending machine. Try to prepare snacks from different food groups: low- or no-fat milk and a few graham crackers, for instance, or celery sticks with peanut butter and raisins. Save part of one meal—half of your breakfast bagel or lunch sandwich—to eat a few hours later. If you're trying to add fiber to your diet, eat high-fiber snacks, such as prunes, popcorn, or sunflower seeds.

Some advocates of healthier eating recommend banning junk food, such as candy bars and chips, from campus vending machines and cafeterias. Others argue that universities should not try to dictate what students can or cannot eat. Should schools take such steps to encourage healthier eating, or should students have the right to make their own food choices?

You Decide

Food Safety

Foodborne illnesses cause an estimated 76 million illnesses, 325,000 hospitalizations, and 5,000 deaths in the United States every year. Three organisms—*Salmonella, Listeria,* and *Toxoplasma*—are responsible for more than 75 percent of these deaths. Although most foodborne infections cause mild illness, severe infections and serious complications—including death—do occur.

Fight BAC!

To improve food safety awareness and practices, government and private agencies have developed the Fight Bac! campaign, which identifies four key culprits in foodborne illness:

- **Improper cooling**
- **Improper hand washing**
- **Inadequate cooking**
- **Failure to avoid cross-contamination.**[30]

? FAQ What Causes Food Poisoning?

Salmonella is a bacterium that contaminates many foods, particularly undercooked chicken, eggs, and sometimes processed meat. Eating contaminated food can result in salmonella poisoning, which causes diarrhea and vomiting. The Centers for Disease Control and Prevention (CDC) estimates 40,000 reported cases of salmonella poisoning a year; the actual number of cases could be anywhere from 400,000 to 4 million. The FDA has warned consumers about the dangers of unpasteurized orange juice because of the risk of salmonella contamination.

Another bacterium, *Campylobacter jejuni,* may cause even more stomach infections than salmonella. Found in water, milk, and some foods, campylobacter poisoning causes severe diarrhea and has been implicated in the growth of stomach ulcers.

Bacteria can also cause illness by producing toxins in food. *Staphylococcus aureus* is the most common culprit. When cooked foods are cross-contaminated with the bacteria from raw foods and not stored properly, staph infections can result, causing nausea and abdominal pain anywhere from thirty minutes to eight hours after ingestion.

Even many healthy foods can pose dangers. The FDA has urged consumers to avoid eating raw sprouts because of the risk of getting sick. Sprouts, particularly alfalfa and clover, can be contaminated by salmonella or *E. coli* bacteria, which can cause nausea, diarrhea, and cramping in healthy adults. Children and senior citizens can experience serious symptoms that lead to kidney failure and compromised immune systems. The FDA advises people to either cook sprouts before eating them or request that they be left off sandwiches and other food ordered in restaurants. Homegrown sprouts can also present a risk if they come from contaminated seeds.

Strategies for Prevention — Protecting Yourself from Food Poisoning

- Always wash your hands with liquid or clean bar soap before handling food. Rub your hands vigorously together for 10 to 15 seconds; the soap combined with the scrubbing action dislodges and removes germs.
- When preparing fresh fruits and vegetables, discard outer leaves, wash under running water, and when possible, scrub with a clean brush or hands. Do not wash meat or poultry.
- To avoid the spread of bacteria to other foods, utensils, or surfaces, do not allow liquids to touch or drip onto other items. Wipe up all spills immediately.
- Clean out your refrigerator regularly. Throw out any leftovers stored for three or four days.

An uncommon but sometimes fatal form of food poisoning is **botulism,** caused by the *Clostridium botulinum* organism. Improper home-canning procedures are the most common cause of this potentially fatal problem.

There have been several outbreaks of listeriosis, caused by the bacteria **listeria,** commonly found in deli meats, hot dogs, soft cheeses, raw meat, and unpasteurized milk. Although rare, listeriosis can be life-threatening. At greatest risk are pregnant women, infants, and those with weakened immune systems. You can reduce your risk by cooking meats and leftovers thoroughly and by washing everything that may come into contact with raw meat.

"Hamburger Disease"/ Barbecue Syndrome

Barbecue syndrome is the common name for a type of food poisoning caused by the bacteria *verotoxigenic E. coli,* or VTEC. People who develop this syndrome frequently report that they ate ground beef hamburgers prior to getting sick. Other kinds of undercooked meat and poultry and drinking unpasteurized milk or unchlorinated water also are culprits.

Symptoms, which can range from mild to life-threatening, usually develop within two to ten days and include severe stomach cramps, vomiting, and a mild fever. Most people recover within seven to ten days. Proper handling and cooking of food can practically eliminate hamburger disease.

Pesticides

Plants and animals naturally produce compounds that act as pesticides to aid in their survival. The vast majority of the pesticides we consume are therefore natural, not added by farmers or food processors. *Commercial pesticides* save billions of dollars of valuable crops from pests, but they also may endanger human health and life.

Fearful of potential risks in pesticides, many consumers are purchasing **organic** foods. The term *organic* refers to foods produced without the use of commercial chemicals at any stage. Independent groups now certify foods before they can be labeled organic. Foods that are truly organic are cleaner and have much lower levels of residues than standard commercial produce. There's no guarantee that the organic produce you buy at a grocery or health-food store is more nutritious than other produce. However, buying organic foods is one way in which you can work toward a healthier environment.

Food Allergies

As many as one in four Americans experience some adverse reaction to a particular food.[31] Food allergies are more common in children than adults.

Physicians disagree as to which foods are the most common triggers of food allergies. Cow's milk, eggs, seafood, wheat, soybeans, nuts, seeds, and chocolate have all been identified as culprits. The symptoms they provoke vary. One person might sneeze if exposed to an irritating food; another might vomit or develop diarrhea; others might suffer headaches, dizziness, hives, or a rapid heart-beat. Symptoms may not develop for up to

botulism Possibly fatal food poisoning caused by a type of bacterium that grows and produces its toxin in the absence of air and is found in improperly canned food.

listeria A bacterium commonly found in deli meats, hot dogs, and soft cheeses that can cause an infection called listeriosis.

organic Term designating food produced with, or production based on the use of, fertilizers originating from plants or animals, without the use of pesticides or chemically formulated fertilizers.

72 hours, making it hard to pinpoint which food was responsible.

If you suspect that you have a food allergy, see a physician with specialized training in allergy diagnosis. Medical opinion about the merits of many treatments for food allergies is divided. Once you've identified the culprit, the wisest and sometimes simplest course is to avoid it.

Nutritional Quackery

The American Dietetic Association describes nutritional quackery as a growing problem for unsuspecting consumers. Because so much nutritional nonsense is garbed in scientific-sounding terms, it can be hard to recognize bad advice when you get it. One basic rule: If the promises of a nutritional claim sound too good to be true—

SAVVY CONSUMER

Spotting Nutrition Misinformation

- Don't believe everything you read. A quick way to spot a bad nutrition self-help book is to look in the index for a diet to prevent or treat rheumatoid arthritis (none exists). If you find one, don't buy the book.
- Before you try any new nutritional approach, check with your doctor or a registered dietitian or call the American Dietetic Association's consumer hot line, (800)366-1655.
- Don't believe ads or advisers basing their nutritional recommendations on hair analysis, which is not accurate in detecting nutritional deficiencies.
- Be wary of anyone who recommends megadoses of vitamins or nutritional supplements, which can be dangerous. High doses of vitamin A, which some people take to clear up acne, can be toxic.
- Question personal testimonies about the powers of some magical-seeming pill or powder, and be wary of "scientific articles" in journals that aren't reviewed by health professionals.
- Be wary of any nutritional supplements sold in health stores or through health and body-building magazines. These products may contain ingredients that have not been tested and proved safe.

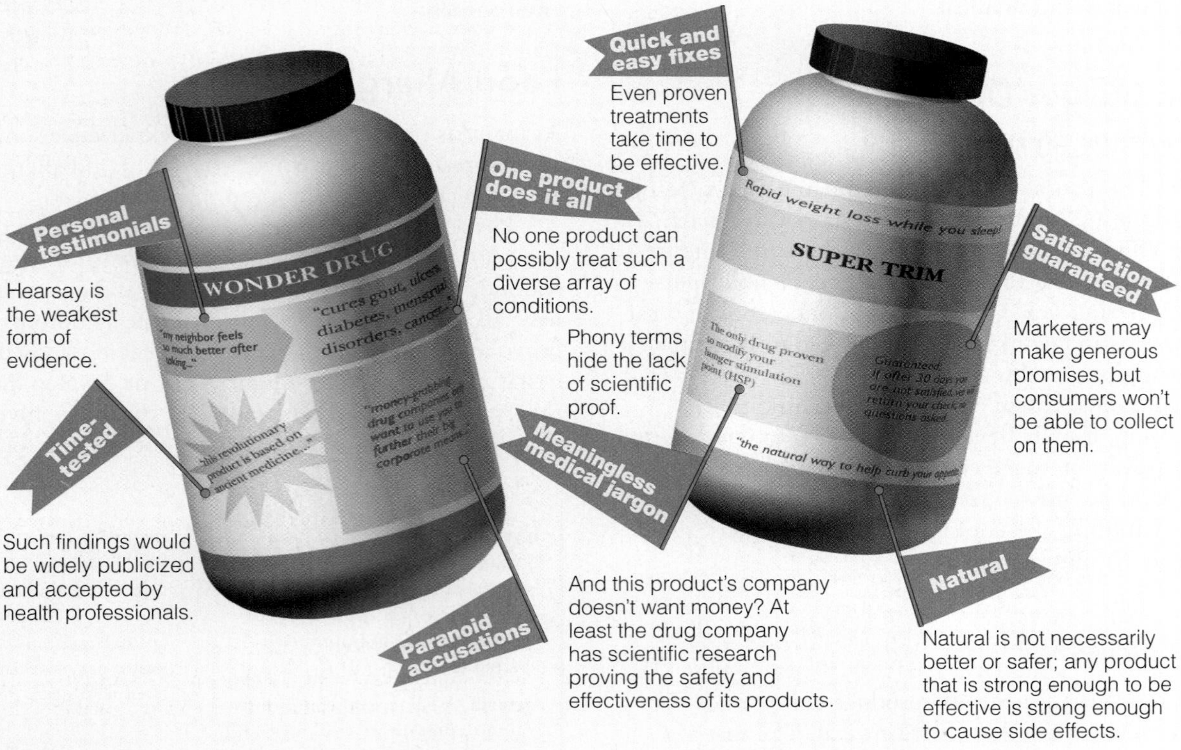

Personal testimonials
Hearsay is the weakest form of evidence.
Time-tested
Such findings would be widely publicized and accepted by health professionals.
WONDER DRUG
"cures gout, ulcers, diabetes, menstrual disorders, cancer..."
"my neighbor feels so much better after taking..."
"this revolutionary product is based on ancient medicine..."
One product does it all
No one product can possibly treat such a diverse array of conditions.
Paranoid accusations
And this product's company doesn't want money? At least the drug company has scientific research proving the safety and effectiveness of its products.
Quick and easy fixes
Even proven treatments take time to be effective.
Rapid weight loss while you sleep!
SUPER TRIM
The only drug proven to modify your hunger stimulation point (HSP)
"the natural way to help curb your appetite"
Meaningless medical jargon
Phony terms hide the lack of scientific proof.
Satisfaction guaranteed
Marketers may make generous promises, but consumers won't be able to collect on them.
Natural
Natural is not necessarily better or safer; any product that is strong enough to be effective is strong enough to cause side effects.

they probably are (see Savvy Consumer: "Spotting Nutrition Misinformation").

If you seek the advice of a nutrition consultant, carefully check his or her credentials and professional associations. Because licensing isn't required in all states, almost anyone can use the label "nutritionist," regardless of qualifications. Be wary of diplomas from obscure schools and organizations that allow anyone who pays dues to join. (One physician obtained a membership for his dog!) A registered dietitian (R.D.), who has a bachelor's degree and specialized training (including an internship) and who passed a certification examination, is usually a member of the American Dietetic Association (ADA), which sets the standard for quality in diets. A nutrition expert with an M.D. or Ph.D. generally belongs to the ADA, the American Institute of Nutrition, or the American Society of Clinical Nutrition; all have stringent membership requirements.

LEARN IT / LIVE IT

Making Healthy Food Choices

As nutritional knowledge expands and evolves, it's easy to be confused by changing advice on which foods to avoid and which to eat. But even though research may challenge or change thinking on a specific food, some basic principles always apply.

- **Eat breakfast.** Easy to prepare breakfasts include cold cereal with fruit and low-fat milk, whole-wheat toast with peanut butter, yogurt with fruit, or whole-grain waffles.
- **Don't eat too much of one thing.** Your body needs protein, carbohydrates, fat, and many different vitamins and minerals, such as vitamins C and A, iron, and calcium, from a variety of foods.
- **Eat more grains, fruits, and vegetables.** These foods give you carbohydrates for energy, plus vitamins, minerals, and fiber. Try breads such as whole-wheat, bagels, and pita. Spaghetti and oatmeal are also in the grain group.
- **Don't ban any food.** Fit in a higher-fat food, like pepperoni pizza, at dinner by choosing lower-fat foods at other meals. And don't forget about moderation. If two pieces of pizza fill you up, don't eat a third.
- **Make every calorie count.** Load up on nutrients, not on big portions. Choosing foods that are nutrient dense will help protect against disease and keep you healthy.

5 Making This Chapter Work for You

Review Questions

1. The classes of essential nutrients include which of the following?
   a. amino acids, antioxidants, fiber, and cholesterol
   b. proteins, calcium, calories, and folic acid
   c. carbohydrates, minerals, fat, and water
   d. iron, whole grains, fruits, and vegetables
2. Which type of fat is *not* considered a threat to heart health?
   a. omega-3 fatty acids
   b. trans fat
   c. triglycerides
   d. saturated fats
3. Antioxidants
   a. are nutrients important in the production of hemoglobin.
   b. are substances added to foods to make them more flavorful or physically appealing.
   c. are suspected triggers of food allergies.
   d. are substances that prevent the harmful effects of free radicals.
4. The MyPyramid system can be personalized to your age, gender, and activity level at www.MyPyramid.gov. Besides personalization, the MyPyramid system has these themes:
   a. variety, proportionality, moderation, and activity
   b. variety, bulimia, activity
   c. variety, moderation, activity, and food safety
   d. variety, moderation, activity, and correct food labeling
5. The MyPyramid system includes this recommendation:
   a. Make half your grains whole.
   b. Go lean with protein.
   c. Focus on fruits.
   d. All of the above.
6. The 2005 Dietary Guidelines for Americans include:
   a. Decrease intake of added sugars.
   b. Increase consumption of olive oil.
   c. Control calorie intake to manage body weight.
   d. Eat dessert no more than three days a week.
7. Food labels on packaged foods include all of the following *except*
   a. total weight of the package.
   b. total amount of nutrients contained in the food.
   c. the percent of nutrient Daily Values provided in the food.
   d. serving size.

8. Since Sam plays poker, it's been easy for him to remember that a recommended serving of 3 ounces of meat means a piece of meat about the size of
   a. one deck of cards.
   b. eight poker chips.
   c. two decks of cards.
   d. a roll of quarters.
9. Some vegetarians may
   a. include chicken and fish in their diets.
   b. avoid vitamin B_{12} supplements if they eat only plant foods.
   c. eat only legumes or nuts because these provide complete proteins.
   d. have high cholesterol levels because of the saturated fats in fruits and vegetables.
10. Common causes of foodborne infections include which of the following?
    a. the influenza virus
    b. *Salmonella* and *E. coli* bacteria
    c. avian flu virus
    d. pesticides

Answers to these questions can be found on page 422.

Critical Thinking

1. Which alternative or ethnic diet do you think has the best tasting food? Which is the most healthy? Why?
2. Is it possible to meet nutritional requirements on a limited budget? Have you ever been in this situation? What would you recommend to someone who wanted to eat healthfully on $30 a week?
3. Consider the number of times a week you eat fast food. How much money would you have saved if you had eaten home-prepared meals? Which fast foods could you have selected that would have provided more nutritional value?

Media Menu

ThomsonNOW™ Go to the ThomsonNOW website at **http://www.thomsonedu.com** that will:

- Help you evaluate your knowledge of the material.
- Allow you to take an exam-prep quiz.
- Provide a Personalized Learning Plan targeting resources that address areas you should study.
- Coach you through identifying target goals for behavioral change and creating and monitoring your personal change plan throughout the semester.

INTERNET CONNECTIONS

U.S. Food and Nutrition Information Center
www.nal.usda.gov/fnic/

This comprehensive governmental website features reports and scientific studies on a variety of nutrition information, including the 2005 USDA Dietary Guidelines, an updated Food Guide Pyramid, dietary supplements, dietary assessment, food composition searchable databases, educational brochures, historical food guides, and a topics "A-Z" section.

USDA Center for Nutrition Policy and Promotion
www.usda.gov/cnpp/

This interactive site sponsored by the United States Center for Nutrition Policy and Promotion features the Interactive Health Eating Index, an online dietary assessment that enables you to receive a personalized score on the overall quality of your diet, on a daily basis, based on the recommendations of the Food Guide Pyramid. This tool provides you with information on total fat, cholesterol, sodium, and other nutrients. You can also download a series of brochures featuring dietary guidelines as well as healthy recipes.

Nutrient Analysis Tool
http://nat.crgq.com

This site, provided as a public service by the Food Science and Human Nutrition Department at the University of Illinois, features a free nutrient analysis interactive program that calculates the amount of calories, carbohydrates, protein, fat, vitamins, minerals, and fiber in the foods that make up your daily diet.

Cyberkitchen
www.nhlbi.nih.gov/chd/Tipsheets/cyberkit.htm

This interactive site helps you discover how much you are really eating with an activity on comparing standard serving sizes versus real serving sizes. You also can provide personal information regarding your age, gender, height, weight, and activity level, and the Cyberkitchen will provide you with a healthy diet plan to meet your weight management goals. It's fun and educational.

InfoTrac College Edition Activities Log on, insert **nutrition** into the Keyword search box, and limit your search to the past year. When you get the results, Mark articles to review, then Select one to read. Summarize three or four key points from the article.

You can find additional readings related to personal health with InfoTrac College Edition, an online library of more than 900 journals and publications. Follow the instructions for accessing InfoTrac College Edition that were packaged with your textbook; then search for articles using a keyword search.

For additional links, resources, and suggested readings on the InfoTrac College Edition, visit our Health and Wellness Resource Center at **http://health .wadsworth.com.**

Key Terms

The terms listed are used on the page indicated. Definitions of the terms are in the Glossary at the end of this book.

amino acids 110
antioxidants 113
basal metabolic rate (BMR) 108

Healthy and Delicious Recipes

Chili

INGREDIENTS:

- 2 tsp canola oil
- 1 medium yellow onion
- 1 large red pepper, deseeded and chopped
- 1 jalapeno chile pepper, deseeded and chopped
- 1 large carrot, chopped
- 2 tbsp chili powder
- 1 tbsp cumin
- 3/4 pound extra-lean ground beef
- 1 15-ounce can crushed tomatoes
- 1 15-ounce can low sodium black beans, drained
- 2 cups frozen sweet corn

PREPARATION:

Heat oil in a large Dutch oven on medium heat. Add onion, red pepper, jalapeno pepper and carrot. Sauté for 5 minutes, until onion has softened. Sprinkle chili powder and cumin over the vegetables and stir for 1 minute.

Crumble in ground beef; cook on medium-high until no longer pink. Add canned tomatoes and black beans. Turn down heat and simmer for 15 minutes. Add sweet corn and cook for a further 5 minutes.
Serve with a dollop of fat free sour cream or a light sprinkling (1-2 tbsp) of reduced fat Jack cheese.
Serves 6-8
Per Serving: Calories 279, Calories from Fat 53, Total Fat 5.7g (sat 1.8g), Cholesterol 35mg, Sodium 304mg, Carbohydrate 37mg, Fiber 9.3g, Protein 19.4g

---

Yogurt-Chicken Kebabs

This is a simple and delicious way to prepare chicken. If you use wooden skewers, soak them for 30 minutes before using, to prevent them burning. I also cover the skewer ends with foil wrap, too. I like to serve these with some quick-cooking rice or couscous.

INGREDIENTS:

- 4 6-ounce skinless, boneless chicken breasts
- 3/4 cup low fat plain yogurt
- 2 tbsp fresh lemon juice

- 1 tbsp ground cumin

PREPARATION:

Cut chicken breasts into chunks. Thread on to presoaked wooden skewers and place in a large glass dish. Combine yogurt, lemon juice and cumin. Spoon over skewered chicken. Cover and marinate for 4-6 hours.
Preheat broiler and spray broiler pan with nonstick cooking spray.

Place skewers on broiler pan and broil for 10 minutes, turning once halfway through.
Serve on a rice pilaf, fruited couscous or quinoa
Serves 4.
Per Serving: Calories 214, Calories from Fat 28, Total Fat 3.1g (sat 1.1g), Cholesterol 101mg, Sodium 146mg, Carbohydrate 4.6g, Fiber 0.2g, Protein 4.2g

---

Orange Glazed Turkey Tenders

2 teaspoons olive oil
1 pound turkey tenders
1/2 teaspoon salt
1/4 teaspoon ground black pepper
1/3 cup orange marmalade
2 tablespoons red wine vinegar
1 tablespoon peeled & grated fresh ginger
1 small navel orange cut into wedges
1 teaspoon parsley

1. In a non-stick skillet, heat oil on medium temperature until hot.
2. Place turkey tenders in skillet and sprinkle with salt and pepper.
3. Cook tenders until they are slightly browned on the outside and have lost the pink color on the inside. This will take about 4 minutes on each side.
4. While tenders are cooking, mix marmalade, vinegar and ginger in a small bowl.
5. Add this mixture to the skillet containing the turkey heat to a boil. Upon reaching the boiling point your delicious turkey entrée is ready for garnish.
6. Garnish with the orange wedges & parsley to serve.

Serves: 4
Each serving about 220 calories, 27g protein, 20g carbohydrate, 4g total fat (1g saturated) 68mg cholesterol, 340mg sodium.

Optional: Serve with boiled small red potatoes.
Tip: Many grocers refer to turkey tenders as turkey cutlets or vice versa.

Veggie Enchiladas

2 packages (10 oz. each) frozen chopped spinach, thawed
1 ½ cups sliced mushrooms
1 can (15 oz.) pinto beans, rinsed and drained
3 tsp. chili power, divided
¼ tsp. red pepper flakes
1 can (8oz.) low sodium tomato sauce
2 Tbsp. water
½ tsp. hot pepper sauce
8 (8-inch) corn tortillas
1 cup (4oz.) shredded Monterey Jack cheese
dash of salt

1.In a large skillet combine spinach, mushrooms, beans, 2 tsp. chili powder and red pepper flakes over medium heat.
2. Cook 5 minutes, stirring often. Remove from heat.
3. Combine tomato sauce, water, remaining 1 tsp. Chili powder and pepper sauce in a pie pan. Stir.
4. Dip tortillas into tomato sauce mixture and stack on wax paper.
5. Divide spinach filling into 8 portions. Spoon onto centers of tortillas.
6. Roll up and place tortillas in microwavable dish.
7. Spread tomato mixture over enchiladas.
8. Cover dish with vented plastic wrap. Microwave at medium for about 10 minutes.
9. Sprinkle with cheese. Microwave at Medium for about 1 minute or until cheese is melted.

Makes 4 servings. Per Serving: Calories 385, Total Fat 11g, Cholesterol 25mg, Sodium 741mg, Carbohydrates 55g, Dietary Fiber 2g, Protein 22g.

Fiesta Skillet Spaghetti

1/2 tsp olive oil
1 lb ground chicken breast, skinless
1/2 c onions, chopped
1/2 c bell peppers, chopped
15 ozs tomato sauce
4 c water
1 env taco seasoning mix
8 ozs thin spaghetti, uncooked
1/2 c fat-free cheddar cheese, shredded

Heat oil in a 12" skillet over medium heat. Add chicken, onions, and bell peppers. Cook until chicken is no longer pink and vegetables are tender. Stir in water, tomato sauce and taco seasoning mix. Bring to a boil. Add the uncooked spaghetti. Reduced heat covered and simmer until spaghetti is tender, about 25 minutes. Sprinkle with cheese.

6 servings; 290 Calories; 2g Fat; 23g Protein; 38g Carbohydrate; 44mg Cholesterol; 899mg Sodium

---

Rotini and Tuna Salad

Salad:
12 ozs tuna in water, drained and flaked
2 1/2 c rotini pasta, uncooked
1 c frozen green peas, thawed and cooked
1 c celery, sliced
1/2 c bell peppers, chopped
1/2 c onions, chopped

Dressing:
1 c fat-free mayonnaise
3 tbsps lemon juice, bottled
1/2 tsp thyme
1/8 tsp salt
1/8 tsp black pepper

Cook pasta according to directions on package. Rinse pasta with cold water and drain. For the salad combine pasta, tuna, peas, celery, bell peppers, and onions in a mixing bowl. Mix well. For the dressing combine mayonnaise, lemon juice, thyme, salt, and black pepper. Mix well. Gently stir dressing into the salad. Cover and refrigerate 1 hour.

8 servings; 197 Calories; 1g Fat; 16g Protein; 31g Carbohydrate; 13mg Cholesterol; 599mg Sodium

---

GOURMET SPINACH SALAD

2 teaspoons lemon juice, fresh
1 teaspoon olive oil
2 tablespoons white wine vinegar
4 cups of spinach leaves
2 large tomatoes, chopped
1/4 cup goat cheese, crumbled
1 tablespoon pine nuts, toasted
Salt & pepper to taste

1. Whisk lemon juice, oil and vinegar together. Add salt & pepper to taste.
2. In a large bowl toss spinach leaves with dressing.
3. Add the tomatoes and goat cheese, mix gently to flavor entire salad.
4. Sprinkle pine nuts over entire surface of salad.

Approximate Nutritional Breakdown:

Servings (4)
Fat 3.9g, Calories 79, Protein 8g, Carb 7g, Cholesterol 15mg, Sodium 87mg

*Note: A non-fat salad dressing can be used in place of the oil and vinegar to lower the fat and calories in this recipe.

CREAMY COLESLAW

1/2 cup plain low-fat yogurt
2 tablespoons Dijon mustard
1 tablespoon water
2 teaspoons low-fat mayonnaise
2 teaspoons fresh lemon juice
6 cups thinly sliced cabbage (about 1 large)
4 medium carrots, shredded
1 cup thinly sliced red onion (about 1 large)
1/2 teaspoon dill seeds

Whisk together yogurt, mustard, water, mayonnaise, and lemon juice in a large bowl. Add remaining ingredients and toss to combine well. Season coleslaw with salt and pepper. Coleslaw may be made 1 day ahead and chilled if covered.

Serves 6. Each serving about 68.1 calories and 1.1 gram fat (15% of calories from fat)

Creamy Potato & Green Onion Soup

1 1/2 cups water
6 Medium potatoes, peeled & cubed
2 Stalks celery, sliced (1 cup)
1/4 cup water
1 cup skim milk
3/4 tsp. salt
1/4 tsp. white pepper
2 green onions with tops (sliced finely)

1. Bring 1 1/2 cups water to boiling, add potatoes & celery, cover and bring to boil again. Reduce heat and simmer until potatoes are tender. 20 minutes or so.
2. Drain liquid into blender and 3 cups of cooked vegetables, add 1/4 cup of water. Cover and blend until smooth (1 minute)
3. Place pureed vegetables back into sauce pan with remaining potatoes & celery. Stir in remaining ingredients, heat, stirring occasionally, until hot.
4. Garnish with garlic toast!

1 serving: l05 calories (10 calories from fat) 1 g fat (1 g saturated, 5 mg cholesterol, 330 mg

sodium, 23 g carbohydrate (2 g dietary fiber)

TORTILLA SOUP

1/2 c onions - chopped
4 ozs green chilies - chopped
4 c chicken broth
2 c long-grain white rice - cooked
10 ozs tomatoes and green chilies - undrained
5 ozs chicken breast strips - cooked and cubed
1 tbsp lime juice
low-fat tortilla chips

In a large saucepan, cook onions and chilies until tender. Add broth, rice, tomatoes, and chicken cubes. Mix well. Bring to a boil. Reduce heat. Cover and simmer for 20 minutes. Stir in lime juice. Top each serving with tortilla chips.

10 servings; 169 Cal; 1g Fat; 7g Pro; 32g Carb; 9mg Chol; 796mg Sodium

---

MEATBALL SOUP

1/2 cup regular long-grain rice
2 cans (13 3/4 to 14 1/2 ounces each) chicken broth
3 medium carrots, sliced
3 medium celery stalks, sliced
5 ounces washed spinach (half 10-ounce bag)
8 frozen lean meatballs, thawed and sliced
shredded or grated Parmesan cheese (optional)

In 1-quart saucepan, heat 1 cup water to boiling over high heat. Add rice, heat to boiling. Reduce heat to low, cover and simmer 15 to 20 minutes until water is absorbed and rice is tender. Meanwhile, in 4-quart saucepan, heat chicken broth and 2 cups water to boiling over high heat. Add carrots and celery, heat to boiling. Reduce heat to low, cover and simmer 5 to 7 minutes, until vegetables are tender. Stir in spinach, rice, and sliced meatballs, heat through. Serve soup with Parmesan cheese if you like.

Without Parmesan cheese per serving: About 300 calories, 25 g protein, 30 g carbohydrate, 7 g total fat (3 g saturated), 51 mg cholesterol, 1010 mg sodium.

DEVIL'S DELIGHT COOKIES

1/4 c margarine softened
1/2 c Fat-Free Buttermilk
1 tsp pure vanilla extract

2 egg whites whipped
1 1/2 c unbleached flour
1/2 c cocoa powder sifted
2/3 c granulated sugar
1 tsp baking soda
1/4 tsp salt
2 tsps powdered sugar sifted

Preheat oven to 350. Prepare baking sheets with cooking spray; set aside. In a mixing bowl, combine margarine, buttermilk, vanilla extract, and egg whites. In another mixing bowl, combine flour, cocoa powder, sugar, baking soda, and salt. Mix wet ingredients with dry ingredients just until moistened. Drop dough by tablespoonfuls, 2" apart onto prepared baking sheets. Bake for 7 minutes. Sprinkle with powdered sugar.

30 servings; 58 Calories; 2g Fat (26% calories from fat); 1g Protein; 10g Carbohydrate; 0mg Cholesterol; 77mg Sodium

---

Baked Apples

1 Granny Smith Apple
2 Tablespoons Grape Nuts Cereal
2 Tablespoons Sugar

1. Wash apple(s) and core.
2. Place apple(s) right side up in a medium sized baking dish.
3. Layer the sugar and Grape Nuts in the apple until the core is full to slightly overflowing.
4. Sprinkle 2 teaspoons of water on each apple.
5. Add a little water to the bottom of the baking dish.
6. Bake at 350 degrees for about 45 minutes or until apples are soft.

Serving Size: 1 Apple
Calories 223, Protein 1.8g, Carbohydrates 57.1, Fat 0g, Cholesterol 0mg.

Chocolate Banana Muffin

3/4 cup whole wheat flour
1 cup all purpose flour
3/4 cup cocoa powder
1 teaspoon baking powder
2 teaspoons baking soda
1 teaspoon salt
1 1/2 cups sugar
1 1/2 bananas
2 eggs
1 cup coffee (regular or decaffeinated)

1 cup nonfat milk
1 teaspoon vanilla extract

1. Spray non-stick muffin pan with vegetable oil and set aside. Preheat oven to 300 degrees.
2. Sift cocoa powder, baking powder and baking soda together.
3. Puree the sugar, bananas and eggs.
4. Mix the sifted ingredients with the remaining dry ingredients.
5. Combine coffee, milk and vanilla extract with the banana mixture.
6. Add the wet and dry mixtures together.
7. Bake at 300 degrees for about 15-20 minutes.
8. Muffins are done when you push on the top of muffin and it springs back. Cool for twenty minutes.

Optional: Sprinkle with confectioners' sugar.

Yield: Makes 22, 1/2 ounce muffins.
Per Serving: Calories 240; Fat 2.5 gm; Saturated Fat 0.9 gm; Cholesterol 36 mg; Sodium 452 mg; Carbohydrate 54 gm; Dietary fiber 4 gm; Sugars 35 gm; Protein 5 gm.

PUMPKIN SPICE BREAD

1 c unbleached flour

1 c whole wheat flour
1 c brown sugar, packed
1 tbsp baking powder
2 tsps cinnamon
1/2 tsp nutmeg
1/4 tsp baking soda
1/4 tsp ginger
1/4 tsp cloves
1 15 oz canned pumpkin
1/2 c skim milk
2 egg whites, whipped
1/3 c fat-free sour cream

1. Preheat oven to 350°.
2. Prepare a bundt pan with cooking spray, set aside.
3. Combine flour, brown sugar, baking powder, baking soda, cinnamon, nutmeg, ginger and cloves in a large mixing bowl.
4. In a medium mixing bowl, combine pumpkin, skim milk, egg whites and sour cream.
5. Spoon the pumpkin mixture into the flour mixture and mix just until moistened.
6. Pour batter into prepared pan. Bake 60 minutes.

18 servings; 112 Cal, less than one gram Fat, 3g Pro, 28g Carb, 1mg Chol, 116mg Sod

Note: The following pans may be used in place of the bundt: 4 mini loaf pans, 12 muffin pans, 1-9 x 5" loaf pan, 1-9 x 13" baking pan, or 2-8 x 8" baking pans.

SUGAR & SPICE ZUCCHINI BREAD

1 c unbleached flour

½ c wheat flour
1 c granulated sugar
2 tsps cinnamon
1/2 tsp baking soda
1/2 tsp nutmeg
1/4 tsp baking powder
1 c zucchini -- unpeeled and grated
1/4 c fat-free sour cream
1 egg white -- whipped
1/2 tsp lemon peel -- grated

Preheat oven at 350. Prepare pan a 8 x 4x 2" loaf pan with cooking spray and flour; set aside. In a bowl, combine flour, sugar, cinnamon, baking soda, nutmeg, and baking powder. In another bowl, combine zucchini, sour cream, egg white, and lemon peel. Combine dry ingredients with wet ingredients just until moistened. Pour batter into prepared pan. Bake 60 minutes.

16 servings; 92 Calories; less than one gram Fat (1% calories from fat); 2g Protein; 22g Carbohydrate; 0mg Cholesterol; 53mg Sodium

---

CREAMED CORN BREAD

1 cup cornmeal
1/2 cup whole wheat flour
1 tablespoon baking powder
1-3 tablespoons sugar
1/2 teaspoon salt
1/3 cup applesauce
3/4 cup skim milk
2 egg whites
1 15-ounce can creamed corn, optional

Preheat oven to 425 degrees. Lightly spray an 8" by 8" cake pan (or equivalent iron skillet or other oven-proof pan) with vegetable oil and put into the oven to preheat. Mix all ingredients together in a large bowl, pour batter into heated pan and bake for 20 minutes.

9 servings: Per Serving Cal 127; Fat 1 gm; Sat Fat 0.1 gms; Chol 0.4 mgs; Sod 444 mgs; Carb 27.7 gms; Dietary Fib 2.4 gms; Sug 5 gms; Pro 4.3 gms. This recipe is 7% fat.

LACC Extra Credit Assignment

5. List what you eat in a 24 hour day. To the side list what percentages are fat, protein, and carbohydrate, and to the side of that the total calories consumed. Include breakfast, lunch, dinner, and snacks. At the bottom add the total number of calories for all.

botulism 131
calories 108
carbohydrates 110
complementary proteins 126
complete proteins 110
complex carbohydrates 110
dietary fiber 111
essential nutrients 108
folic acid 124
functional fiber 111
incomplete proteins 110
lacto-vegetarians 125
listeria 131
macronutrients 108
micronutrients 108
minerals 115
nutrition 107
organic 131
ovo-lacto-vegetarians 126
phytochemicals 117
proteins 110
saturated fats 112
simple carbohydrates 110
trans fat 112
unsaturated fats 112
vegans 126
vitamins 113

6 Taking Control of Your Weight

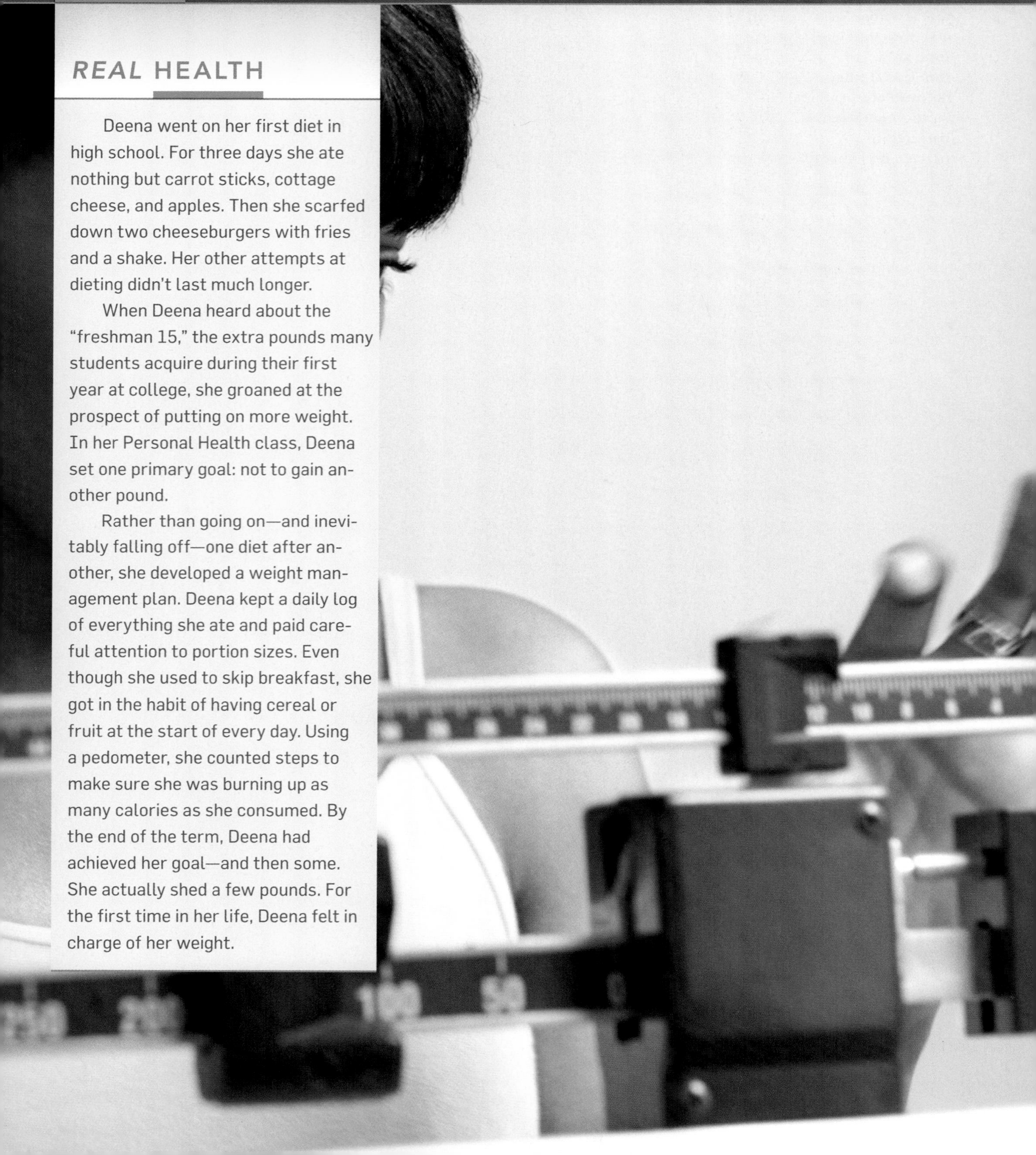

REAL HEALTH

Deena went on her first diet in high school. For three days she ate nothing but carrot sticks, cottage cheese, and apples. Then she scarfed down two cheeseburgers with fries and a shake. Her other attempts at dieting didn't last much longer.

When Deena heard about the "freshman 15," the extra pounds many students acquire during their first year at college, she groaned at the prospect of putting on more weight. In her Personal Health class, Deena set one primary goal: not to gain another pound.

Rather than going on—and inevitably falling off—one diet after another, she developed a weight management plan. Deena kept a daily log of everything she ate and paid careful attention to portion sizes. Even though she used to skip breakfast, she got in the habit of having cereal or fruit at the start of every day. Using a pedometer, she counted steps to make sure she was burning up as many calories as she consumed. By the end of the term, Deena had achieved her goal—and then some. She actually shed a few pounds. For the first time in her life, Deena felt in charge of her weight.

For the first time in history, more than half of the people on the planet are overweight. Obesity, as headlines blare and health experts warn, is emerging as the number-one public health problem of the twenty-first century. Approximately 127 million adults in the United States are overweight; 60 million are obese; and 9 million are severely obese.[1]

Excess weight has become an epidemic. Two-thirds of American adults, up from fewer than half 20 years ago, are overweight. About one in every three American adults is obese. Among children under 5 years old, one in four is overweight.[2]

Once viewed as a cosmetic problem, fat now is recognized as a crippler and killer. Excess weight weakens hearts; raises blood pressure; clogs arteries; strains backs and joints; increases the risk of diabetes, stroke, and certain cancers; and steals years of productive life. The earlier the weight gain, the greater the danger it poses. Obesity at age 20 can cut 20 years off a person's life. Even moderate overweight at age 40 can subtract 3 to 7 years from life expectancy.

This chapter explains how we grew so big, tells what obesity is and why excess pounds are dangerous, describes current approaches to weight loss, discusses diets that work (and some that don't), offers practical guidelines for exercise and behavioral approaches to losing weight, and examines unhealthy eating patterns and eating disorders. Regardless of your current weight, you will find insights and skills you will need for healthy weight management throughtout your life.

? FAQ Frequently Asked Questions

- How did we get so fat? *p. 138*
- Is my weight healthy? *p. 143*
- I'm too thin: How can I gain weight? *p. 145*
- Why do I overeat? *p. 146*
- Can a person be fit and fat? *p. 152*
- Who develops eating disorders? *p. 157*

After studying the material in this chapter, you should be able to:

- **List** the factors besides genetics that have contributed to the global increase in overweight and obesity.
- **Identify** the main health risks of excess weight.
- **Assess** various approaches to weight loss.
- **Design** a personal plan for sensible weight management.
- **Identify** and **describe** the symptoms and dangers associated with eating disorders.

ThomsonNOW™ Log on to ThomsonNOW at **www.thomsonedu.com/thomsonnow** to find your Behavior Change Planner and to explore self-assessments, interactive tutorials, and practice quizzes.

The Global Epidemic

An estimated 1.1 billion people around the world—seven in ten of the Dutch and Spanish, two in three Americans and Canadians, and one in two Britons, Germans, and Italians—are overweight or obese. In Europe, excess weight ranks as the most common childhood disorder. Since 1980, obesity rates have tripled in parts of Eastern Europe, the Middle East, China, and the Pacific Islands. In many poor countries, obesity is common among city dwellers, while people in rural areas remain underweight and malnourished.

The World Health Organization, in its first global diet, exercise, and health program to combat obesity, recommends that governments promote public knowledge about diet, exercise, and health; offer information that makes healthy choices easier for consumers to make; and require accurate, comprehensible food labels.[3] Although ultimately each individual decides what and how much to eat, policy makers agree that governments also must act to reverse the obesity epidemic.

Exposure to a Western lifestyle seems to bring out susceptibility to excess weight. Obesity is much more common among the Pima Indians of Arizona compared to Pimas living in Mexico, who have maintained a more traditional lifestyle, with more physical activity and a diet lower in fat and richer in complex carbohydrates. Native Hawaiians who follow a more traditional diet and lifestyle also have lower rates of obesity and cardiovascular disease.

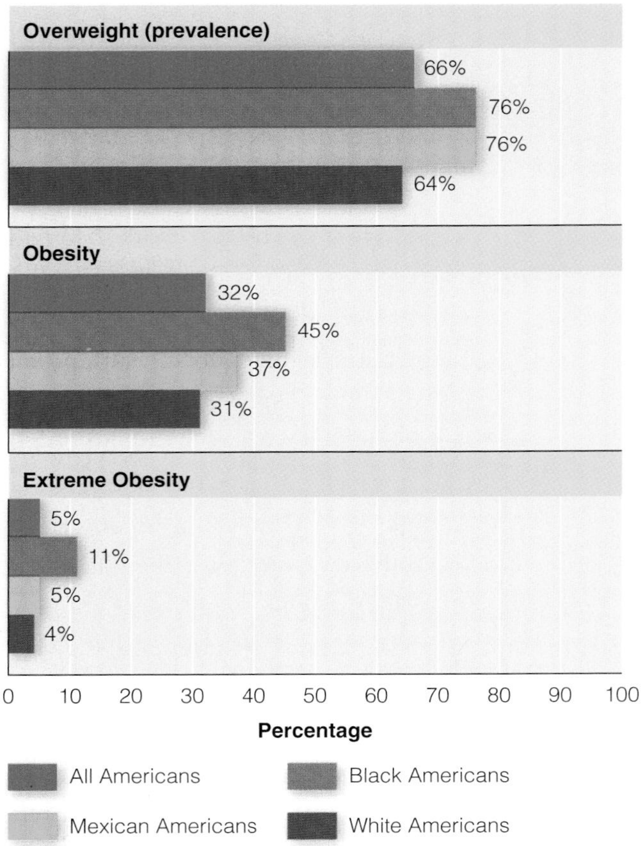

FIGURE 6-1 Weight Problems by Race/Ethnic Group

Source: Ogden, Cynthia, et al. "Prevalence of Overweight and Obesity in the United States, 1999–2004." *Journal of the American Medical Association*, Vol. 295, No. 13, April 5, 2006, pp. 1549.

Supersized Nation

Since 1980, the obesity rate has tripled for children and adolescents. The prevalence of obesity among men has increased significantly since 1999, rising to 31 percent. The rate of obesity among women has remained the same: 33 percent. About 3 percent of men and 7 percent of women are extremely obese. Men and women between ages 20 and 39 have the lowest rate of obesity: 29 percent. Among 40- to 59-year-olds, 37 percent are obese, as are 31 percent of those over age 60.[4]

Obesity rates vary by ethnic groups as well as by gender and age. About 30 percent of white Americans are obese, compared with 45 percent of African Americans and 37 percent of Mexican Americans (Figure 6-1). In some Native American communities, up to 70 percent of all adults are dangerously overweight. Differences in metabolic rates may be one factor.

Weight problems are starting earlier than ever. About one in four children between ages two and five is overweight or at risk of becoming overweight. Among those between ages six to eleven, the percentage rises to 37 percent. About one in three teenagers falls into this category.[5]

Not all Americans are equally likely to be overweight or obese. As Figure 6-2 shows, the southern states have the highest concentration of obese residents. Mississippi is home to the county with the highest percentage of people with a body mass index (BMI) between 30 and 40. (BMI, as discussed in Chapter 4, is defined as the ratio between weight and height that correlates with percentage of body fat.)

? FAQ How Did We Get So Fat?

A variety of factors, ranging from behavior to environment to genetics, played a role in the increase in overweight and obesity. They include:

1. **More calories.** Bombarded by nonstop commercials for taste treats, tempted by foods in every form to munch and crunch, Americans are eating more—some 200 to 400 calories more a day than they did several decades ago. Many of these extra calories come from refined carbohydrates, which can raise levels of heart-damaging blood fats called

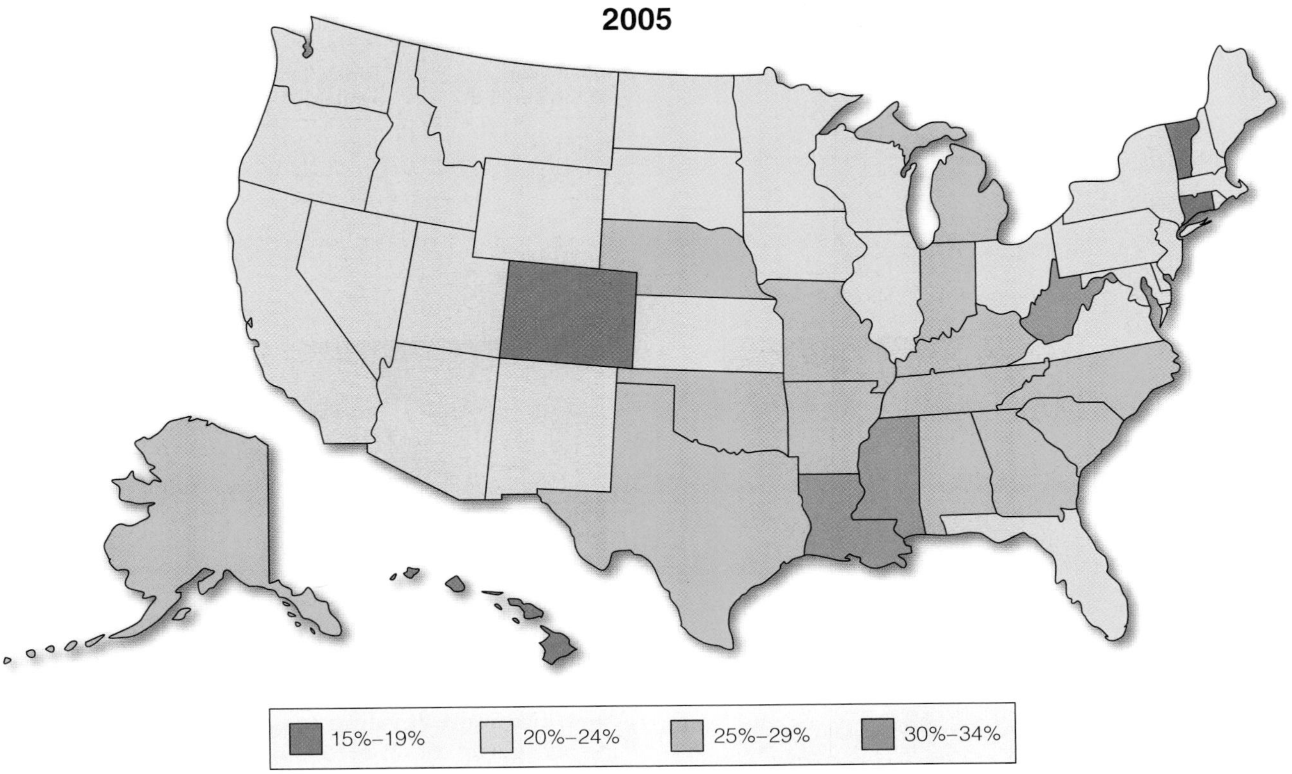

FIGURE 6-2 Obesity in the United States
This map shows the percentage of people in each state who are obese—they have a body mass index between 30 and 40.
Source: Data from National Center for Chronic Disease Prevention and Health Promotion, 2006.

triglycerides and increase the risk of diabetes as well as obesity.

2. **Bigger portions.** As Table 6-1 shows, the size of many popular restaurant and packaged foods has increased two to five times during the past 20 years. Some foods, like chocolate bars, have grown more than ten times since they were first introduced. Popular 64-ounce sodas can pack a whopping 800 calories. According to studies of appetite and satiety, people presented with larger portions eat up to 30 percent more than they otherwise would.
3. **Fast food.** Young adults who eat frequently at fast-food restaurants gain more weight and develop metabolic abnormalities that increase their risk of diabetes in early middle age. In a recent study, those who ate fast food at least twice a week gained an extra 10 pounds and had a twofold greater increase in insulin resistance, a risk factor for diabetes. The men in the study visited fast-food restaurants more often than the women; blacks did so more frequently than whites.[6]
4. **Physical inactivity.** As Americans eat more, they exercise less. Experts estimate that most adults expend 200 to 300 fewer calories than people did 25 years ago. The most dramatic drop in physical activity often occurs during the college years.
5. **Passive entertainment.** Television is a culprit in an estimated 30 percent of new cases of obesity. TV viewing may increase weight in several ways: It takes up time that otherwise might be spent in physical activities. It increases food intake since people tend to eat more while watching TV. And compared with sewing, reading, driving, or other relatively sedentary pursuits, watching television lowers metabolic rate so viewers burn fewer calories. The combination of watching television (at least two and one-half hours a day) and eating fast food more than twice a week triples the risk of obesity, according to a 15-year study of more than 3,700 white and black young adults.
6. **Modernization.** The growth of industry and technology has led to an abundance of food, less need for physical activity, urbanization, labor-saving devices, and a more sedentary lifestyle. Suburban sprawl directly contributes to obesity, according to a recent study. People who live in neighborhoods where they must drive to get anywhere are significantly more likely to be obese than those who can easily walk to their destinations.

TABLE 6-1 Supersized Portions

Food/Beverage	Original Size (year introduced)	Today (largest available)
Budweiser (bottle)	7 oz. (1976)	40 oz.
Nestle's Crunch	1.6 oz. (1938)	5 oz.
Soda (Coca Cola)	6.5 oz. (1916)	34 oz.
French fries (Burger King)	2.6 oz. (1954)	6.9 oz.
Hamburger (McDonald's); (beef only)	1.6 oz. (1955)	8 oz.

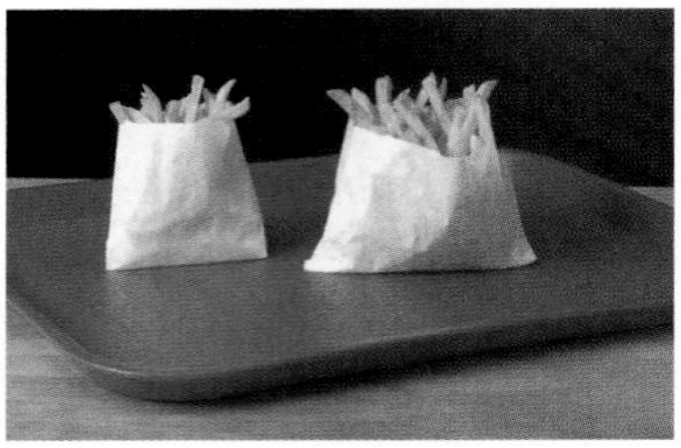

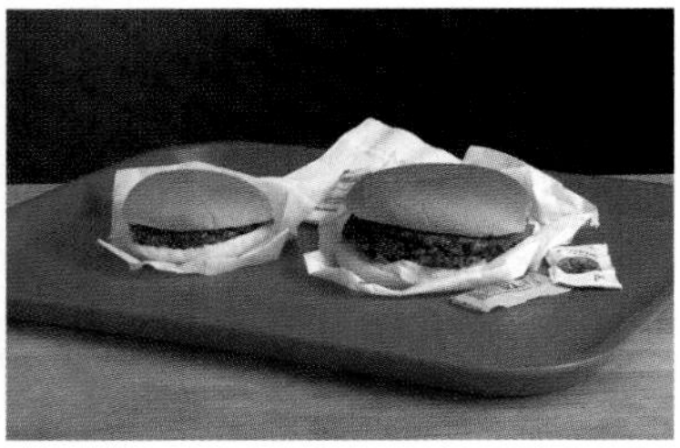

Source: "Are Growing Portion Sizes Leading to Expanding Waistlines?" American Dietetic Association, www.eatright.org.

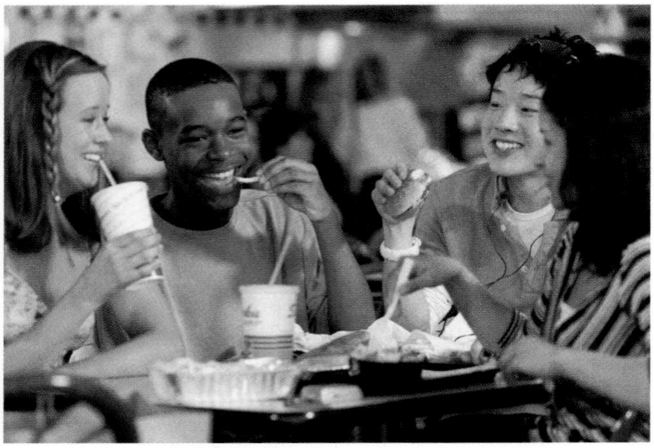

Round-the-clock snacking, fast-food restaurants around every corner, and hours in front of the TV have all contributed to the increase in overweight and obesity.

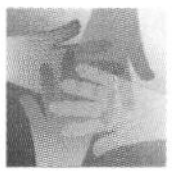

7. **Socioeconomics.** The less money you make, the more likely you are to be overweight. One in four adults below the poverty level is obese, compared with one in six in households earning $67,000 or more. Minorities are at even greater risk. One in three poor African Americans is obese.
8. **Prenatal factors.** A woman's weight before conception and weight gain during pregnancy influence her child's weight. A substantial number of children are prone to gaining weight because their mothers developed gestational diabetes during their pregnancies. Children born to obese women are more than twice as likely to be overweight by age four.
9. **Childhood development.** Today's children don't necessarily eat more food than in the past, but they eat more high-fat, high-calorie foods and they exercise much, much less. On days when they eat fast food, youngsters consume an average of 187 more calories per day. Fewer than half of grade schoolers participate in daily physical education classes. Many spend five hours or more a day in front of a computer or television screen.
10. **Genetics.** Although scientists have identified genes involved in appetite and metabolism, they have not found a genetic cause for obesity. It may be that various genes contribute a small increase in risk or that rare abnormalities in many genes create a predisposition to weight gain and obesity.
11. **Emotional influences.** Obese people are neither more nor less psychologically troubled than others. Psychological problems, such as irritability, depression, and anxiety, are more likely to be the result of obesity than the cause. As discussed later in this chapter, emotions do play a role in weight problems. Just as some people reach for a drink or a drug when they're upset, others cope by overeating, bingeing, or purging.

Body Image

Throughout most of history, bigger was better. The great beauties of centuries past, as painted by such artistic masters as Rubens and Renoir, were soft and fleshy, with rounded bellies and dimpled thighs. Culture often shapes views of beauty and health.

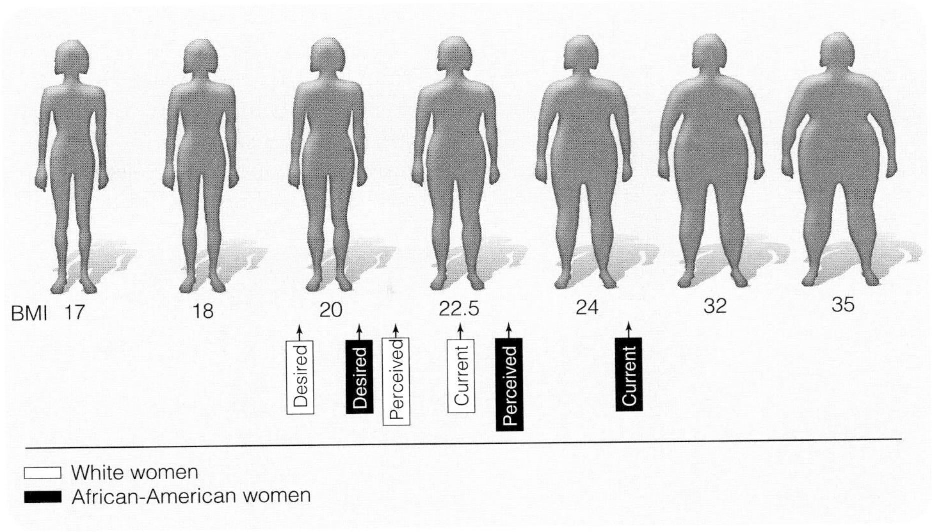

FIGURE 6-3 Body Dissatisfaction in African-American and White Students
In a study of 630 undergraduates, both African-American and white women perceived themselves to be smaller than they actually were—and wished to be even smaller. However, the white students saw themselves as and desired to be considerably smaller than did the African-American women. Both African-American and white men rated the silhouette depicting a BMI of 20 as the most desirable.
Source: "Body Dissatisfaction Among College Students." *Nutrition Research Newsletter,* Vol. 21, No. 3, March 2002, p. 9.

Many developing countries still regard a full figure, rather than a thin one, as the ideal. Fattening huts, in which brides-to-be eat extra food to plump up before marriage, still exist in some African cultures. Among certain Native American tribes of the Southwest, if a girl is thin at puberty, a fat woman places her foot on the girl's back so she will magically gain weight and become more attractive.

Influenced by the media, many Americans are paying more attention to their body images than ever before—and at a younger age. In a study of high school girls, those who regularly read women's health and fitness magazines, which may present unrealistic physical ideals, were more likely to go on low-calorie diets, take pills to suppress their appetites, use laxatives, or force themselves to vomit after eating. In other research, girls who watched a lot of television and expressed concern about slimness and popularity were more dissatisfied with their bodies than girls involved in sports.

Boys' body images also are influenced by media images depicting superstrong, highly muscular males.

Being overweight for a long period of time has a cumulative negative impact on body image. In a study of 266 college women, those who described themselves as "always overweight" ranked much lower in current body self-esteem than those with more recent weight problems.

College students of different ethnic and racial backgrounds, including Asians, express as much—and sometimes more—concern about their body shape and weight as whites. In a study of university students, African-American and Caucasian men were similar in their ideals for body size and in their perceptions of their own shapes. As shown in Figure 6-3, both African-American and white women perceived themselves as smaller than they actually were and desired an even smaller body size. However, the African-American women were more accepting of larger size. (BMI, or body mass index, is discussed in Chapter 4.)

Male and Female Body Image

Although women generally report a more negative body image, many men are dissatisfied with their bodies but for different reasons. Often they want either to lose or gain weight or to gain muscle and bulk. Women compare their appearance to others more frequently than men and worry more that others will think negatively about their looks. Yet appearance matters just as much to men, who are just as likely as women to engage in efforts to improve their bodies.[7]

Women have long been bombarded by the media with idealized images of female bodies that bear little resemblance to the way most women look. Increasingly, more advertisements and men's magazines are featuring idealized male bodies. Sleek, strong, and sculpted, they too do not resemble the bodies most men inhabit. The gap between reality and ideal is getting bigger for both genders.

When college men and women step on a scale or look in a mirror, they react in different ways. In a study of 525 undergraduates, the women failed to see themselves as underweight, even

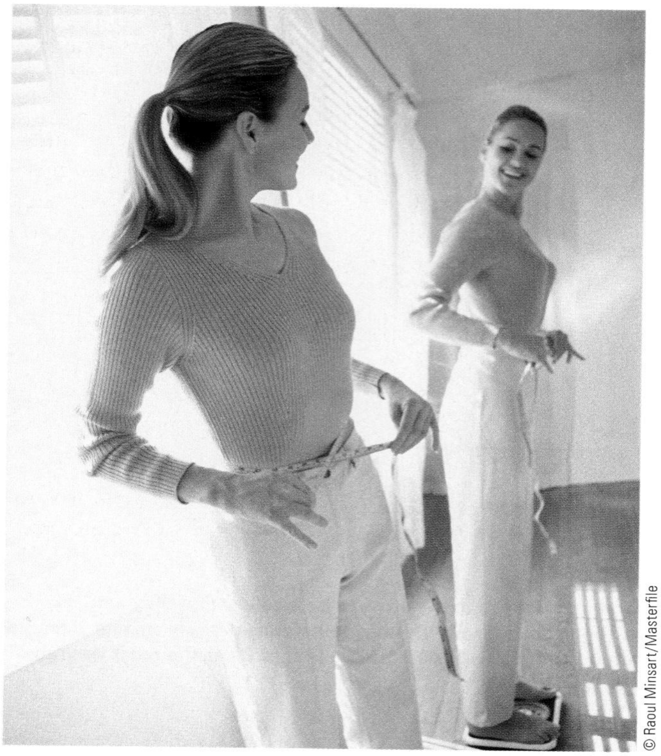

© Raoul Minsart/Masterfile

How do you decide what your ideal body size is?

when they were, and perceived themselves as overweight, even when they were not. Many of the women who considered themselves normal weight nonetheless desired to be thinner. Men in the study generally saw themselves as underweight, even when they were not. Most desired to be heavier, though not obese.

The greater the discrepancy between a woman's current view of her body shape and the ideal she considers most attractive to men, the more likely she is to worry about how others will view her and to doubt her ability to make a desirable impression. Such "social physique anxiety" occurs often in women who feel they do not measure up to what they or others consider most desirable in terms of weight or appearance. Women with high BMIs and greater body-related anxiety may exercise to become thinner or more attractive. Those reporting the greatest distress because of body image are at highest risk of disordered eating or actual eating disorders (discussed on page 157).

Understanding Weight Problems

Weight problems don't develop overnight. Fat accumulates meal by meal, day by day, pound by pound. Ultimately, all weight problems are the result of a prolonged energy imbalance—of consuming too many calories and burning too few in daily activities.

How many calories you need depends on your gender, age, body-frame size, weight, percentage of body fat, and your *basal metabolic rate (BMR)*—the number of calories needed to sustain your body at rest. Your activity level also affects your calorie requirements. Regardless of whether you consume fat, protein, or carbohydrates, if you take in more calories than required to maintain your size and don't work them off in some sort of physical activity, your body will convert the excess to fat.

The average American consumes about one million calories a year. Given that number, what difference does an extra 100-calorie soda or 300-calorie brownie make? A lot, because the extra calories that you don't burn every day accumulate, adding an average of 2 to 4 pounds to your weight every year.

Weight and the College Student

Obesity rates have increased most rapidly among 18- to 29-year-olds. About one in three college students may be overweight or obese (see Student Snapshot: "The

Strategies for Change — *How to Boost Your Body Esteem*

Whatever your weight or shape, here are some ways to improve your body image:

- Start walking with more bounce in your step.
- Focus on the parts of your body you like. Take pride in your powerful shoulders or large eyes.
- Treat yourself with the respect you'd like to receive from others.
- Don't put yourself down or joke about your weight.
- Work with hand weights. As you build your muscles, your sense of strength and self-confidence also will grow.
- Don't put off special plans, such as learning to kayak or signing up for an exchange program, until you reach a certain magical weight: Do what you want to do *now*.
- Pull your shoulders back, suck in your stomach, and stand up straight. You'll look and feel better.

Student Snapshot
The Weight of Student Bodies

Body Mass Index

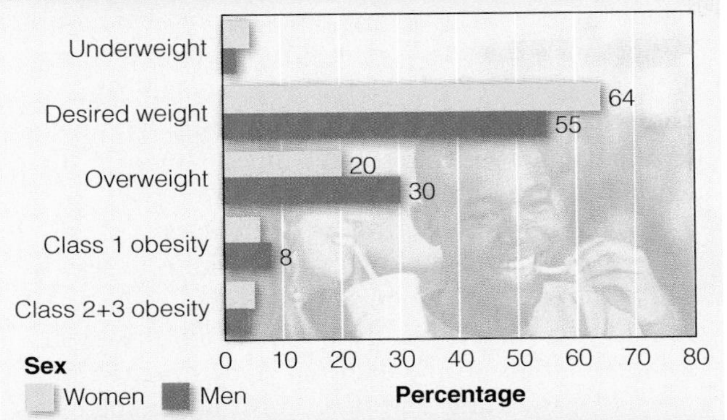

© SuperStock/Alamy

Self Description of Weight

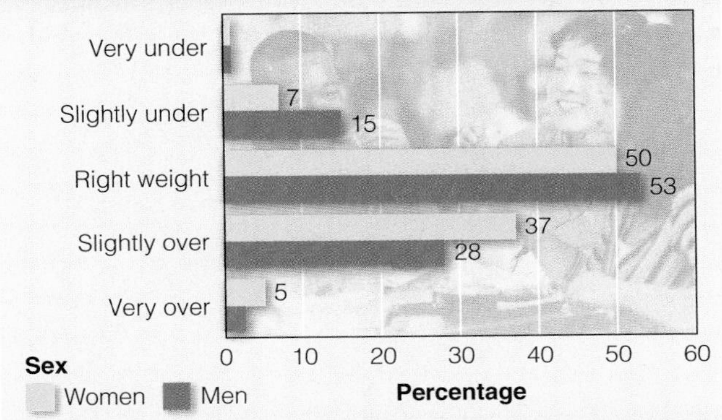

© White Packert/Photonica/Getty Images

*Based on a survey of 16,832 students.
Source: American College Health Association. American College Health Association – National College Health Assessment (ACHA-NCHA) Web Summary. Updated April 2006. Available at www. acha .org/projects_programs/ncha_sampledata.cfm.

Weight of Student Bodies")[8]. One in five college students has an unhealthy weight as well as at least one risk factor for metabolic disorder, an important cause of cardiovascular disease (discussed in Chapter 10).

As many students discover, it's easy to gain weight on campuses, which are typically crammed with vending machines, fast-food counters, and cafeterias serving up hearty meals. But the infamous *freshman 15,* the extra pounds acquired in the first year at college, seems to be a myth. Several studies have documented much lower weight gains, ranging from 2.45 to 7 pounds.

? FAQ Is My Weight Healthy?

Rather than relying on a range of ideal weights for various heights, as they did in the past, medical experts use various methods to assess body composition and weight. The best indicators of weight-related health risks are Body Mass Index (BMI); waist circumference (WC); and waist-to-hip ratio (WHR). (All are discussed in depth in Chapter 4.)

If you have a BMI higher than 25, you are **overweight** and at greater risk of health problems. If your BMI is between 30 and 34.9, you have class 1 **obesity**. If it is between 35 and 39.9, you have class 2 obesity. Both indicate increased risk of dying of weight-related problems. A BMI over 40 signifies class 3 or severe obesity and poses the greatest threat to health and longevity.[9]

If you're a young adult, even mild to moderate over-weight poses a threat to your health because it puts you at risk for gaining even more weight—and for

overweight A condition of having a BMI between 25.0 and 29.9.

obesity The excessive accumulation of fat in the body; class 1 obesity is defined by a BMI between 30.0 and 34.9; class 2 obesity by a BMI between 35.0 and 39.9; class 3 or severe obesity by a BMI of 40 or higher.

Strategies for Prevention — *Holding the Line on College Weight Gain*

- **Plan meals.** Most campus cafeterias post the week's menus in advance. Plan which items you will eat before you see or smell high-fat dishes.
- **Don't linger.** If you use the cafeteria as a social gathering place, you may end up eating with two or three different groups of people. Set a time limit to eat—then leave.
- **Plan alternative behaviors.** People who eat when they are stressed or bored need substitute activities ready when they need them. Make a list of things you can do—shower, phone a friend, take a hike—when stress strikes.
- **Eat at "home."** If the dormitory has a small kitchen, cook some healthful dishes and invite friends to join you.
- **Take advantage of physical activity programs.** Many college students become less active during their years in college. Aim to maintain or increase the amount of exercise you did in high school. Join a biking club, take a salsa class, learn yoga.

facing greater health risks. Obesity has been implicated as a culprit in rising rates of disability among younger Americans as well as a factor in chronic health problems. If you are older than a traditional-aged student, the risks to your health are more immediate.

Health Dangers of Excess Weight

The federal government has recognized obesity as a serious, potentially fatal disease. This designation cleared the way for insurance coverage for obesity treatments, rather than just for the medical problems it can cause. The effects of obesity on health are the equivalent of 20 years of aging. They include increased risk of cardiovascular disease, diabetes, and cancer, as well as disability, rheumatoid arthritis, sleep apnea, gout, and liver disease (Figure 6-4). Total medical costs, both direct and indirect, amount to more than $117 billion a year.[10]

The Impact on the Body

The incidence of diabetes, gallstones, hypertension, heart disease, and colon cancer increases with the degree of overweight in both sexes. Those with BMIs of 35 or more are approximately 20 times more likely to develop diabetes. Individuals who are overweight but not obese, with BMIs between 25 and 29.9, are significantly more likely than leaner women to develop gallstones, high blood pressure, high cholesterol, and heart disease. Overweight men and women are at least three times more likely to suffer knee injuries that require surgery to repair.

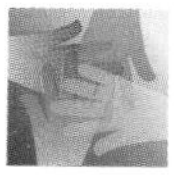

Health risks may vary in different races, ethnic groups, and at-risk populations. Even relatively small amounts of excess fat—as little as 5 pounds—can add to the dangers in those already at risk for hypertension and diabetes. According to the National Heart, Lung, and Blood Institute, being overweight, even if not obese, increases the risk of heart failure. Obesity also causes alterations in various measures of immune function and increases the risk of kidney stones and disease.

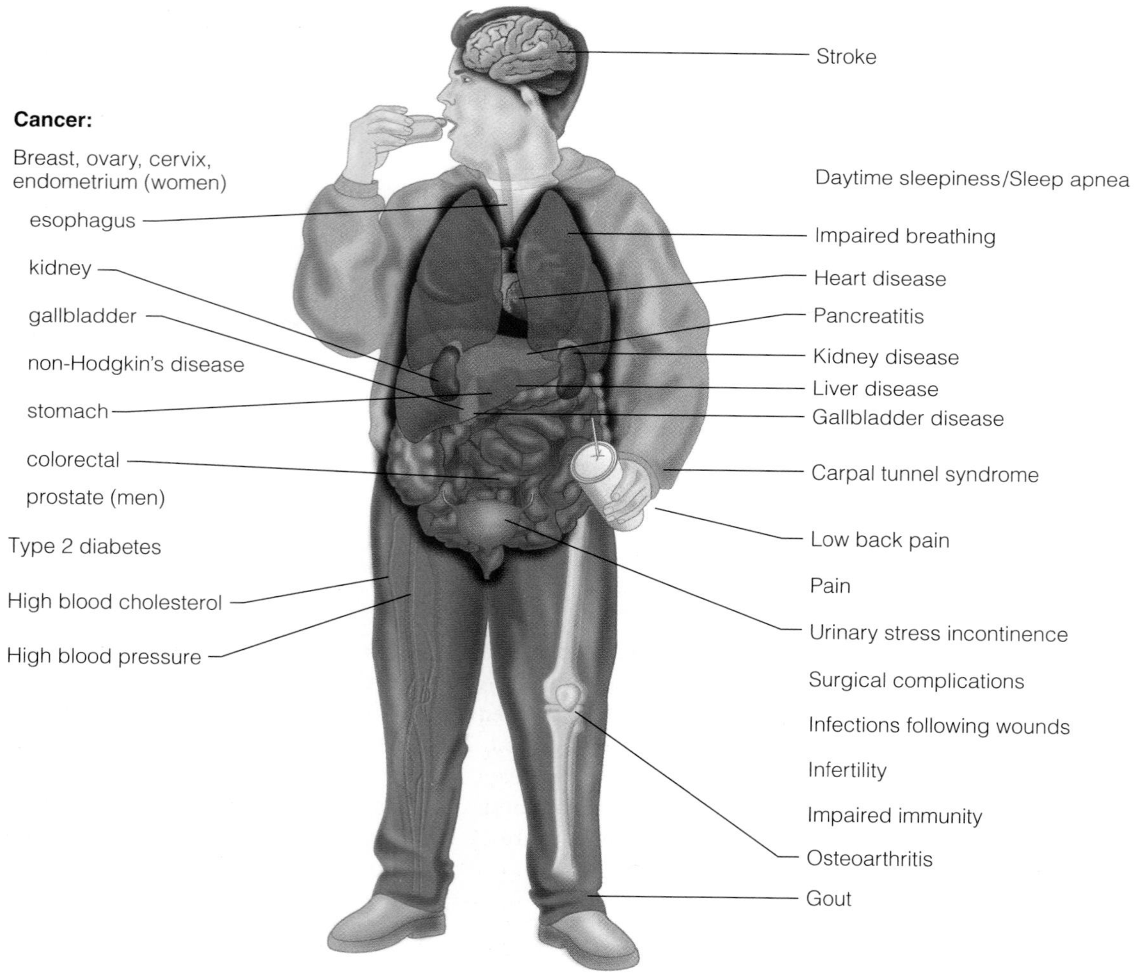

FIGURE 6-4 Health Dangers of Excess Weight

Overweight young adults have a 70 percent chance of becoming overweight or obese adults. They are two to three times more likely to have high total cholesterol levels and more than 43 times more likely to have cardiovascular disease risk factors such as elevated blood pressure. They also have a higher prevalence of type 2 diabetes.

Major diseases linked to obesity include:

- **Type 2 diabetes.** More than 80 percent of people with type 2 diabetes are overweight. Although the reasons are not known, being overweight may make cells less efficient at using sugar from the blood. This then puts stress on the cells that produce insulin (a hormone that carries sugar from the blood to cells) and makes them gradually fail. You can lower your risk for developing type 2 diabetes by losing weight and increasing the amount of physical activity you do. If you have type 2 diabetes, losing weight and becoming more physically active can help you control your blood sugar levels and may allow you to reduce the amount of diabetes medication you take.
- **Heart disease and stroke.** People who are overweight are more likely to suffer from high blood pressure, high levels of triglycerides (blood fats) and harmful LDL cholesterol, and low levels of beneficial HDL cholesterol. In addition, people with more body fat have higher blood levels of substances that cause inflammation, which may raise heart disease risk. Losing 5 to 15 percent of your weight can lower your chances for developing heart disease or having a stroke.

  People who both smoke and are obese are at especially high risk of cardiovascular disease. Although some smokers have felt that they couldn't lose weight until they stopped smoking, researchers have found that weight loss among smokers is possible and beneficial, leading to a reduction in other risk factors, such as lower blood pressure and lower cholesterol.
- **Cancer.** Excess weight may account for 14 percent of all cancer deaths in men and 20 percent of those in women. Losing weight, researchers estimate, could prevent as many as one of every six cancer deaths. Excess weight has been linked to cancers of the colon and rectum, kidney, esophagus, and gallbladder; non-Hodgkin's lymphoma; multiple myeloma; and cancers of the pancreas and liver, the breast, uterus, cervix, and ovary (in women), and the stomach and prostate (in men).

Body size and higher BMI are linked with increased risk of breast cancer in premenopausal women and in postmenopausal women not using hormone replacement therapy.

Too much body fat can influence cancer in several ways: It increases the amount of estrogen in the blood, raising the risk of cancers of the female reproductive system. It raises the levels of insulin, which prompts the body to create a hormone that causes cells to multiply. Acid reflux, which can cause cancer of the esophagus, occurs more frequently in heavy men and women. Obesity also makes cancer harder to diagnose and treat.

Excess pounds affect people around the clock. Overweight and obese individuals sleep less than those with normal weights. (See Chapter 2 for a discussion of sleep.) The lost sleep could add to the risk of medical problems.

Life Expectancy

Obesity kills. Researchers attribute 112,000 to 280,000 deaths every year to excess weight.[11] Your weight in early adulthood and middle age can have an impact on how long and how well you live. Overweight and obesity after age 30 increase the risk of hospitalization and of dying from cardiovascular disease and diabetes later in life, even in individuals with no risk factors for heart disease (discussed in Chapter 10) and in those with just one risk factor.[12]

The Emotional Toll

In our calorie-conscious and thinness-obsessed society, obesity also affects quality of life, including sense of vitality and physical pain. Many see it as a psychological burden, a sign of failure, laziness, or inadequate willpower. Overweight men and women often blame themselves for becoming heavy and feel guilty and depressed as a result. In fact, the psychological problems once considered the cause of obesity may be its consequence.

Weight may affect risky sexual behaviors among college students. In a study of almost 1,000 undergraduates, sexually active women with the highest BMIs were more likely to have sex with a casual partner, to have multiple same-sex partners, and to recall being intoxicated at the time of their most recent sexual intercourse. There was no correlation between men's weight and their sexual behavior.[13]

? FAQ I'm Too Thin: How Can I Gain Weight?

Being underweight is not an uncommon problem, particularly among adolescent and young adult men as well as among those who diet excessively or suffer from an eating disorder (discussed on page 157). If you lose weight suddenly and don't know the reason, talk to a doctor. Rapid weight loss can be an early symptom of a health problem.

If you're trying to put on pounds, you need to do the opposite of dieters: Consume more calories than you burn. But as with losing weight, you should try to gain weight in healthy ways. Here are some suggestions:

- **Eat more of a variety of foods** rather than more high-fat, high-calorie foods. Get no more than 30 percent of your daily calories from fat. A higher percentage poses a threat to your heart and your health.

- **If your appetite is small, eat more frequently.** Try for five or six smaller meals rather than a big lunch and dinner.
- **Choose some calorie-rich foods,** such as dried fruits rather than fresh ones. Add nuts and cheese to salads and main dishes.
- **Drink juice** rather than regular or diet soda.
- **Try adding a commercial liquid meal** replacement as a snack.
- **Exercise regularly** to build up both appetite and muscle.

People who are overweight or obese often earn less money, miss out on job opportunities, and get passed over for promotions. In addition, they may be the targets of jokes and disparaging remarks. Is weight discrimination a real problem in our society? Or is it understandable that some may think less of individuals who are extremely overweight?

You Decide

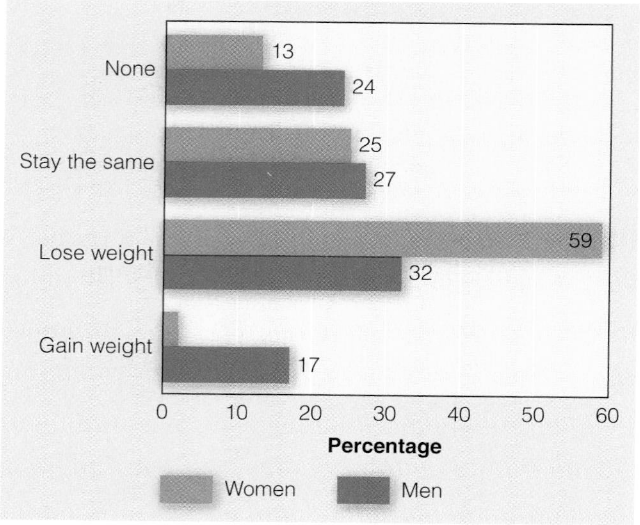

FIGURE 6-5 Student Intentions About Their Weight

*Based on a survey of 16,832 students.
Source: American College Health Association. American College Health Association-National College Health Assessment (ACHA-NCHA) Web Summary. Updated April 2006. Available at www.acha.org/projects_programs/ncha_sampledata.cfm.

A Practical Guide to Weight Loss

As Figure 6-5 shows, more than half of college women and about a third of college men intend to lose weight.[14] Readiness to change is the key to successful weight loss. However, individuals vary in their readiness to change their diets, increase their physical activity, and seek professional counseling. Take the Self Survey in the Self-Assessment Booklet to determine your readiness to lose weight.

? FAQ Why Do I Overeat?

The answer lies not just in the belly but in the brain. Both **hunger,** the physiological drive to consume food, and **appetite,** the psychological desire to eat, influence and control our desire for food. Scientists have discovered appetite receptors within the brain that specifically respond to hunger messengers carried by hormones produced in the digestive tract (Figure 6-6).

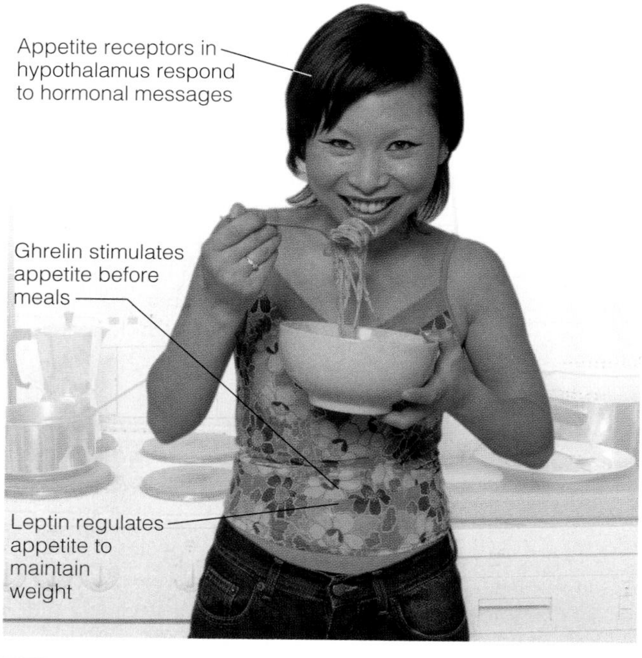

© Betsie Van der Meer/Stone/Getty Images

FIGURE 6-6 Hormones Help Regulate Our Appetites

Appetite usually begins with the fear of the unpleasant sensation of hunger. We learn to avoid hunger by eating a certain amount of food at certain times of the day, just as dogs in the laboratory learn to avoid electric shocks by jumping at the sound of a warning bell. But appetite is easily led into temptation. In one famous experiment, psychologists bought bags of high-calorie goodies—peanut butter, marshmallows, chocolate-chip cookies, and salami—for their test rats. The animals ate so much on this "supermarket diet" that they gained more weight than any laboratory rats ever had before. The snack-food diet that fattened up these rats was particularly high in fats. Biologists speculate that creamy, buttery, or greasy foods may cause internal changes that increase appetite and, consequently, weight.

A hormone called leptin, produced by fat cells, sends signals to the brain that affect appetite. When leptin levels are normal, people eat just enough to maintain weight. When leptin is low, the brain responds as if fat stores had been depleted and slows down metabolism. This may be one reason why it is so difficult to lose weight by dieting alone.

Other hormones made in the stomach also influence how hungry we feel. One is ghrelin, a natural appetite stimulant. When given shots of ghrelin, people become very hungry and eat 30 percent more than they normally would. Ghrelin typically rises before meals and falls afterward. Dieters tend to have high levels of ghrelin, as if their bodies were trying to stimulate appetite so they regain lost fat.

We stop eating when we feel satisfied; this is called **satiety,** a feeling of fullness and relief from hunger. The neurotransmitter serotonin has been shown to produce feelings of satiety. In addition, several peptides, released from the digestive tract as we ingest food, may signal the brain to stop or restrict eating. However, it takes 20 minutes for the brain to register fullness.

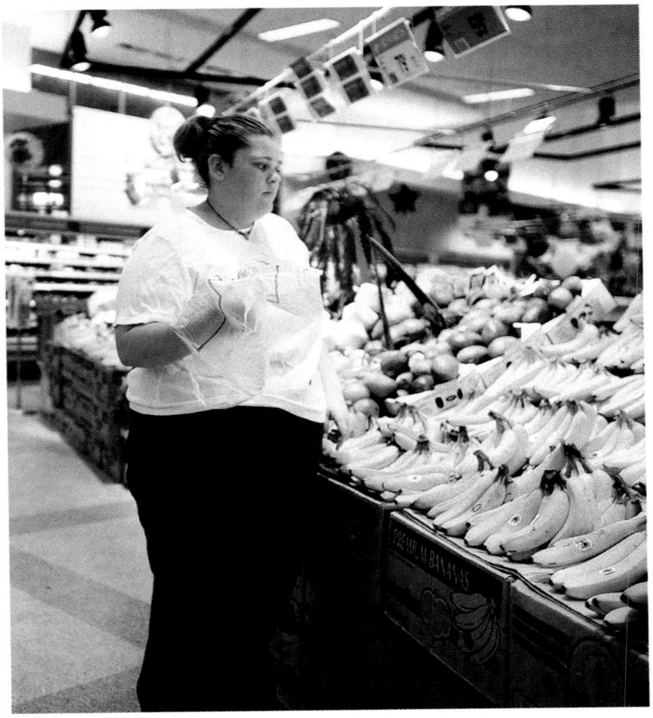

Today's Goal: Have fruit instead of dessert at lunch.

Weight Loss Diets

Never before have so many had so much to lose. More than two-thirds of Americans—77 percent of women and 63 percent of men—are either dieting or struggling to maintain their weight. You've probably heard that 95 percent of people who lose weight gain it all back. That widely quoted statistic, based on a small study from 1959, is no longer true, if it ever was. Diets can and do work. Tens of thousands of dieters have lost excess pounds and maintained lower, healthier weights. Although many regain some weight, most manage to keep off about two-thirds of the weight lost by dieting for at least a year.

Which Weight Loss Diet Works Best?

You've seen the commercials and read the claims that a popular new diet can pare away pounds. Don't believe the hype. According to a review of commercial weight loss programs, there is little scientific evidence to back up any claims that popular diets help overweight individuals slim down.[15] In almost any program, people lose weight because they are paying more attention to their food choices and limiting their calories (Table 6-2).

Diets do work—for a while. Low-calorie (1,000 to 1,200 calories daily) and very low-calorie diets produce similar results a year later. Physical activity alone leads to a weight loss of about 2 to 3 percent of initial weight and reduces abdominal fat. A combination of diet and physical activity, particularly along with behavioral therapy, produces greater reductions in weight and abdominal fat than either approach alone. "High-intensity" programs, which provide person-to-person contact more than once a month, are more effective than those with less frequent contact.

In a year-long "battle of the bulge," researchers compared four popular diets: Atkins, Weight Watchers, The Zone, and Ornish. All produced similar results, including a weight loss of about 7 pounds and a lowering of heart disease risk factors—but only in those who stuck with the program. Nearly half of the dieters dropped out before the year was up because the diets were too hard to follow or weren't working. The Atkins and Ornish plans had the highest dropout rates.[16] In another study, Weight Watchers dieters who regularly attended the program lost approximately 5 percent of their body weight in three to six months. Those on very low-calorie diets who finished the program lost up to 25 percent of their initial weight but were at high risk of regaining at least half of it back.[17]

Because of the high relapse rate, researchers are searching for ways to motivate dieters and sustain weight loss for five to ten years. In the meantime, the best treatment of obesity is

hunger The physiological drive to consume food.

appetite A desire for food, stimulated by anticipated hunger, physiological changes within the brain and body, the availability of food, and other environmental and psychological factors.

satiety A feeling of fullness after eating.

TABLE 6-2 How Consumer Reports Rates the Diets

Better ◉ ◓ ○ ◒ ● Worse

Diet	Price[1]	Overall Score	Nutrition	Analytical Results: 6 mo. Weight loss	6 mo. Dropout rate	1 year Weight loss	1 year Dropout rate	Average Daily Calories	Nutritional Content (Percentage of Calories): Fat	Saturated fat	Carbohydrates	Protein	Grams of fiber/1,000cal	Fruits & veggies (daily servings)
In performance order:														
1 Weight Watchers	$10–13 per week	◓	◉	○	◓	○	◓	1,450	24	7	56	20	20	11
2 Slim-Fast	$2–3 per day (bars or drinks)	◓	◉	◓	◓	◓	●	1,540	22	6	57	21	21	12
3 Zone (men's menu) (*The Zone*, by Barry Sears Ph.D., with Bill Lawren)[2]	$25.00	◓	◉	○	○	○	◒	1,660	27	7	42	30	21	17
4 Ornish (*Eat More, Weigh Less*, by Dean Ornish M.D.)	$15.00	○	○	○	●	◓	●	1,520	6	1	77	16	31	17
5 Atkins Ongoing Weight Loss (OWL) (*Dr. Atkins' New Diet Revolution*, by Robert C. Atkins M.D.)[3]	$13.95	◒	●	◓	○	○	◒	1,520	60	20	11	29	12	6
6 Atkins Induction (*Dr. Atkins' New Diet Revolution*, by Robert C. Atkins M.D.)	$13.95	◒	●	◓	○	○	◒	1,640	61	19	8	31	8	6
Not Rated: Insufficient Study Data (diets listed in alphabetical order)														
7 eDiets	$12–32 per month	—	◉	—	—	—	—	1,450	23	5	53	24	19	12
8 Jenny Craig	$6–7.65 per week, $11–15 per day (food)	—	◉	—	—	—	—	1,520	18	7	62	20	16	6
9 South Beach Phase One (*The South Beach Diet*, by Arthur Agatston M.D.)	$24.95	—	◒	—	—	—	—	1,530	51	14	15	34	9	12
10 South Beach Phase Two (*The South Beach Diet*, by Arthur Agatston M.D.)	$24.95	—	◓	—	—	—	—	1,340	39	9	38	22	19	13
11 Volumetrics (*The Volumetrics Eating Plan*, by Barbara Rolls Ph.D.)	$25.95	—	◉	—	—	—	—	1,500	23	7	55	22	20	14

[1] Except where noted, price is for the book.
[2] Women's menu similar but about 1,300 calories.
[3] Studies of Atkins used first the induction and then the ongoing diet plans, so our 6-month and 1-year results include both phases.
Source: "Rating the Diets from Atkins to Zone" © 2005 by Consumers Union of U.S., Inc. Yonkers, NY 10703–1057, a nonprofit organization. Reprinted with permission from the June 2005 issue of Consumer Reports® for educational purposes only. No commercial use or reproduction permitted. www.ConsumerReports.org®.

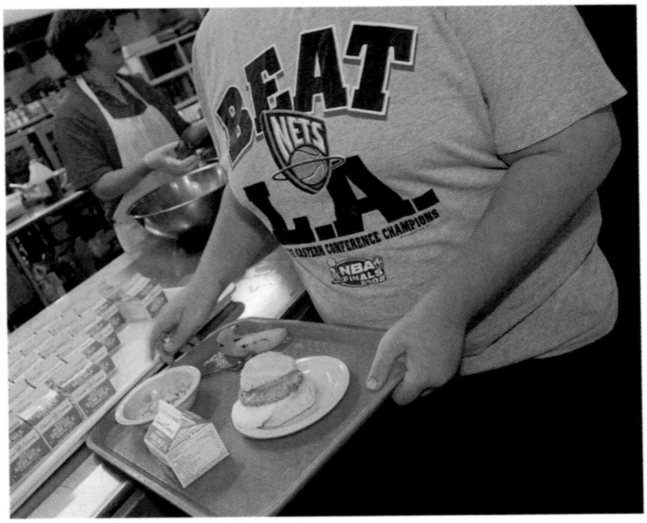

© Radhika Chalasani/Corbis

The foods you choose at every meal of every day can affect both your weight and your health.

a "low-fad" approach, with an emphasis on healthy food choices and regular physical activity.

Low-Carbohydrate Diets

An estimated 17 million Americans have tried a low-carb diet in the last year. The diet popularized by the late Dr. Robert Atkins is high in protein and extremely low in carbohydrates. Followers of the Atkins diet eat unlimited amounts of meat, eggs, and cheese and cut back on bread, pasta, crackers, cakes, cookies, and other carbohydrates. Because they avoid many high-calorie foods and fill up on proteins, which take longer to digest, these dieters typically lose weight without feeling hungry.

Particularly in the initial stages, followers of the Atkins diet may consume 40 percent of their calories in fat, much of it saturated. For years professional groups such as the American Dietetic Association and the American Heart Association warned that low-carb, high-fat weight loss plans like the Atkins diet pose serious health dangers, primarily because the high fat content may increase the risk of heart disease, diabetes, stroke, and kidney and liver disease.

In a year-long study, those on a low-carb diet lost more weight in the first six months, but at the end of the year their weight loss was comparable to the participants on a low-fat diet, whose weight declined slowly but steadily.

Diets such as Sugar Busters! and the Glucose Revolution distinguish between "correct" carbs (fruits, vegetables, and whole grains) and "harmful" ones (refined sugars and processed grains). Other popular diets call for specific proportions of nutrients. For instance, the Zone diet advocates meals and snacks that consist of 40 percent carbohydrate, 30 percent fat, and 30 percent protein. Dieters may lose weight because they're paying more attention to what they eat and making better food choices. However, approaches like this generally make smart eating more complicated than it has to be.

Low-Fat Diets

Various diets reduce daily fat intake—some to 25 to 30 percent of calories; others, such as the Dean Ornish program, to less than 10 percent. The Ornish diet has proved effective in reversing atherosclerotic buildup. Low-fat diets also may enhance the immune response.

As discussed in Chapter 5, the final reports of the Women's Health Initiative, the landmark clinical trial that followed more than 48,000 postmenopausal women for eight years, showed women who reduced their fat intake to 29 percent had similar rates of breast cancer,[18] colon cancer,[19] and cardiovascular disease[20] as those who did not change their fat intake. The long-term impact on younger individuals who reduce dietary fat, particularly saturated fat, even more is not known.[21]

Low-Calorie Diets

Any diet that restricts calories will lead to weight loss. "There is no substitute for the simple formula that 'calories in must equal calories out' in order to control weight," said the FDA Deputy Commissioner when the agency's Obesity Working Group issued its report in 2004 and called for more focus on calories. The Department of Health and Human Services has launched a public education campaign, similar to earlier stop-smoking initiatives, that emphasizes the simple message, Calories count.

Cutting back 500 to 1,000 calories a day typically leads to a loss of 1 to 2 pounds a week and an average weight loss of about 8 percent of body weight in six months. Expert groups, such as the American Society for Clinical Nutrition, the North American Association for the Study of Obesity, and the National Heart, Lung, and Blood Institute Obesity Education Initiative, recommend going no lower than 1,000 to 1,200 calories a day for women and 1,200 to 1,600 calories for men.

Very Low-Calorie Diets Very low-calorie diets, which provide fewer than 800 calories a day, lead to rapid weight loss but pose serious, potentially deadly health risks. Whenever people cut back drastically on calories, they immediately lose several pounds because of a loss of fluid. As soon as they return to a more normal way of eating, they regain this weight.

On a very low-calorie diet, as much as 50 percent of the weight you lose may be muscle (so you'll actually look flabbier). Because your heart is a muscle, it may become so weak that it no longer can pump blood through your body. In addition, your blood pressure may plummet, causing dizziness, light-headedness, and

Strategies for Change — Designing a Diet

There is no one perfect diet that will work for everyone who needs to lose weight. "Experiment with various methods for weight control," suggests Dr. Walter Willett of the Harvard School of Public Health. "Patients should focus on finding ways to eat that they can maintain indefinitely rather than seeking diets that promote rapid weight loss." In other words, design an eating plan that you can stick with for the rest of your life.

Whether you decide to focus on carbohydrates, fat, or calories, the following strategies can help you get to and maintain a healthy weight:

- Avoid "bad" fats, including trans fats and partially hydrogenated fats.
- Consume "good" fats, such as omega-3 fatty acids, every day.
- Eat fewer "bad" carbohydrates, such as sugar and white flour.
- Eat more "good" carbs, including fruits, vegetables, legumes, and unrefined grains like whole-wheat flour and brown rice.
- Opt for quality over quantity. Eating a smaller amount of something delicious and nutritious can be far more satisfying than larger portions of junk foods.
- Exercise more. The key to balancing the equation between calories consumed and calories used is physical activity.

fatigue. You may develop nausea and abdominal pain. You may lose hair. If you're a woman, your menstrual cycle may become irregular, or you may stop menstruating altogether. As you lose more water, you also lose essential vitamins, and your metabolism slows down. Even reaction time slows, and crash dieters may not be able to respond as quickly as usual.

Once you go off an extreme diet—as you inevitably must—your metabolism remains slow, even though you're no longer restricting your food intake. The human body appears to alter its energy use to compensate for weight loss. These metabolic changes may make it harder for people to maintain a reduced body weight after dieting.

Avoiding Diet Traps

Whatever your eating style, there are only two effective strategies for losing weight: eating less and exercising more. Unfortunately, most people search for easier alternatives that almost invariably turn into dietary dead ends or unexpected dangers (see Savvy Consumer: "How to Spot a Dubious Diet"). Three common traps to avoid are diet pills, diet foods, and the yo-yo syndrome.

Diet Pills

In their search for a quick fix to weight problems, millions of people have tried often risky remedies. In the 1920s, some women swallowed patented weight loss capsules that turned out to be tapeworm eggs. In the 1960s and 1970s, addictive amphetamines were common diet aids. In the 1990s, appetite suppressants known as fen-phen became popular. They were taken off the market after being linked to heart valve problems.

In the last decade dieters tried ephedra products for weight loss, but a major study reported more than 16,000 adverse events associated with the use of ephedra-containing dietary supplements, including heart palpitations, tremors, and insomnia. The study also found little evidence that ephedra is effective in boosting physical activities and weight loss. The Food and Drug Administration has prohibited the sale of dietary supplements containing ephedra, because they present an unreasonable risk of illness or injury.

Diet Foods

According to the Calorie Control Council, 90 percent of Americans choose some foods labeled "light." But even though these foods keep growing in popularity, Americans' weight keeps rising. There are several reasons: Many people think choosing a food that's lower in calories, fat-free, or light gives them a license to eat as much as they want. What they don't realize is that many foods that are low in fat are still high in sugar and calories. Refined carbohydrates, rapidly absorbed into the bloodstream, raise blood glucose levels. As they fall, appetite increases.

Diet products, including diet sodas and low-fat foods, are a very big business. Many people rely on meal replacements, usually shakes or snack bars, to lose or keep off weight. If used appropriately—as actual replacements rather than supplements to regular meals and snacks—they can be a useful strategy for weight loss. Yet people who use these products often gain weight because they think that they can afford to add high-calorie treats to their diets.

What about the artificial sweeteners and fake fats that appear in many diet products? Nutritionists caution to use them in moderation and not to substitute them for basic foods, such as grains, fruits, and vegetables.

Foods made with fat substitutes may have fewer grams of fat, but they don't necessarily have significantly fewer calories. Many people who consume reduced-fat, fat-free, or sugar-free sodas, cookies, chips, and other snacks often cut back on more nutritious foods, such as fruits and vegetables. They also tend to eat more of the low- or no-fat foods so that their daily calorie intake either stays the same or actually increases.

The Yo-Yo Syndrome

On-and-off-again dieting, especially by means of very low-calorie diets (under 800 calories a day), can be self-defeating and dangerous. Some studies have shown that weight cycling may make it more difficult to lose weight or keep it off (Figure 6-7). Repeated cycles of rapid weight loss followed by weight gain may even change food preferences. Chronic crash dieters often come to prefer foods that combine sugar and fat, such as cake frosting.

To avoid the yo-yo syndrome and overcome its negative effects: Exercise. Researchers at the University of Pennsylvania found that when overweight women who also exercised went off a very low-calorie diet, their metabolism did not stay slow but bounced back to the appropriate level for their new, lower body weight. The reason may be exercise's ability to preserve muscle tissue. The more muscle tissue you have, the higher your metabolic rate.

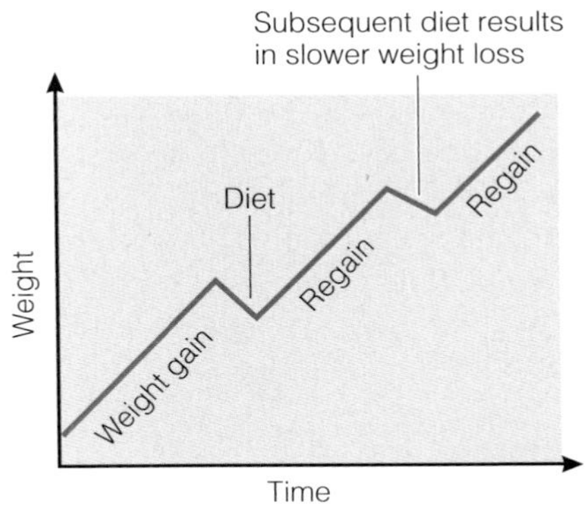

FIGURE 6-7 Weight-Cycling Effect of Repeated Dieting
Each round of dieting is typically followed by a rebound leading to a greater weight gain.

If you've been losing (and regaining) the same 5 or 10 pounds for years, try the following suggestions for long-term success:

- **Set a danger zone.** Once you've reached your desired weight, don't let your weight climb more than 3 or 4 pounds higher. Take into account normal fluctuations, but watch out for an upward trend. Once you hit your upper weight limit, take action immediately rather than waiting until you gain 10 pounds.

SAVVY CONSUMER

How to Spot a Dubious Diet

The National Council Against Health Fraud cautions dieters to watch for these warnings of dangerous or fraudulent programs.

- Promises of very rapid weight loss.
- Claims that the diet can eliminate "cellulite" (a term used to describe dimply fatty tissue on the arms and legs).
- "Counselors" who are really salespersons pushing a product or program.
- No mention of any risks associated with the diet.
- Unproven gimmicks, such as body wraps, starch blockers, hormones, diuretics, or "unique" pills or potions.
- No maintenance program.

If you hear about a new diet that promises to melt away fat, don't try it until you get answers to the following questions:

- Does it include a wide variety of nutritious foods?
- Does it provide at least 1,200 calories a day?
- Is it designed to reduce your weight by one-half to two pounds per week?
- Does it emphasize moderate portions?
- Does it use foods that are easy to find and prepare?
- Can you follow it wherever you eat—at home, work, restaurants, or parties?
- Is its cost reasonable?

If the answer to any of these questions is no, don't try the diet; then ask yourself one more question: Is losing weight worth losing your well-being?

- **Be patient.** Think of weight loss as a road trip. If you're going across town, you expect to get there in 20 minutes. If your destination is 400 miles away, you know it'll take longer. Give yourself the time you need to lose weight safely and steadily.
- **Try, try again.** Dieters don't usually keep weight off on their first attempt. The people who eventually succeed don't give up. Through trial and error, they find a plan that works for them.

Physical Activity

Unplanned daily activity, such as fidgeting or pacing, can make a difference in preventing weight gain. Scientists use the acronym **NEAT**—for **nonexercise activity thermogenesis**—to describe such "nonvolitional" movement and have verified that it can be an effective way of burning calories. In a study of ten lean and ten mildly obese people—all self-confessed couch potatoes—the thinner ones sat an average of two hours less and moved and stood more often than the heavier individuals.[22] Small steps such as taking the stairs for a flight or two or parking farther away can make a difference.[23]

Although physical activity and exercise can prevent weight gain and improve health, usually it does not lead to significant weight loss. However, when combined with diet, exercise ensures that you lose fat rather than muscle and helps keep off excess pounds. Moderate exercise, such as 30 to 60 minutes of daily physical activity, has proved effective in reducing the risk of heart disease and other health threats. Although there are no definitive data, experts generally agree that more exercise—an estimated 60 to 90 minutes daily of moderately intense activity—is necessary to prevent weight gain. Recommending such higher levels of activity to overweight men and women does indeed lead to more exercise—and more lasting weight loss.

Exercise has other benefits: It increases energy expenditure, builds up muscle tissue, burns off fat stores, and stimulates the immune system. Exercise also may reprogram metabolism so that more calories are burned during and after a workout.

An exercise program designed for both health benefits and weight loss should include both aerobic activity and resistance training. People who start and stick with an exercise program during or after a weight loss program are consistently more successful in keeping off most of the pounds they've shed.

? FAQ Can a Person be Fat and Fit?

Most people assume that fitness comes in only one size: small. That's not necessarily so. There is considerable controversy over how to define a healthy weight. But individuals of every size can improve their physical fitness.

In ten years of reasearch on 25,000 men and 8,000 women, scientists at the Cooper Institute for Aerobics Research in Dallas, Texas, have found that heavier individuals can be just as healthy and physically fit as their leaner counterparts. In their studies, obese people who exercised moderately (30 minutes of daily walking at three or four miles per hour) had half the death rate of those who were slimmer but more sedentary. Low cardiorespiratory fitness, regardless of an individual's weight, is as great a risk factor for dying of heart disease or other causes such as diabetes, high blood pressure, and other well-recognized threats.

Nonetheless, fitness doesn't completely reverse the increased risks associated with excess weight. If you're obese, even a high level of physical activity does not protect you from premature death. And if you're sedentary, being thin does not cancel out the dangers of inactivity. In the long-term Nurses Health Study, which has followed more than 100,000 women for decades, women who were both obese and inactive were most likely to die. Those who were fit but fat and those who were thin but sedentary also had higher death rates than others.

The Psychology of Losing Weight

Diets change what you eat. Exercise changes body composition, stamina, and strength. But changing your food-related thoughts and behaviors can be the key to lasting weight loss. If you think that you can shed pounds, if you think that you can control what you put in your mouth, if you think that there is a form of exercise that you could enjoy, then you are on your way to reaching your weight loss goals.

Who's in Charge?

As discussed in Chapter 1, if you see yourself as having control over your destiny, you have an internal locus of control. Your sense of self-efficacy is the belief in your ability to change and to reach a goal. Feeling in control and self-efficacy go hand in hand. The stronger your faith in yourself, the more energy and persistence you can put into making a change. The opposite is also true, especially for health behaviors.

How do you rate on locus of control and self-efficacy? Read the following statements, and jot down true or false:

1. I am overweight because I eat too much.
2. Weight problems run in my family.
3. Diet pills are my best hope for losing weight.
4. I would keep weight off if I exercised regularly.

5. I wouldn't overeat if I didn't have to cook for my family.
6. Some people are born thin and never have to diet.
7. I lose weight when I eat only diet shakes or prepared foods.
8. I could make time for exercise if I really wanted to.
9. My doctor will make sure I'm at a healthy weight.
10. I'm determined to lose weight, and I know I will.

"True" answers to numbers 1, 4, 8, and 10 indicate that you take responsibility for and see yourself in control of your weight. "True" answers to numbers 2, 3, 5, 6, 7, and 9 suggest that you credit or blame others for your weight. The more that you see external forces as being in charge, the more difficult you will find it to make changes and lose weight permanently.[24]

Reach Out for Support–Real and Virtual

Behind most successful dieters is a friend, spouse, coach, mentor, colleague, support group, or online community. In various studies, dieters with supportive "buddies" were more likely to stick to their diet and workout program and lost more weight.

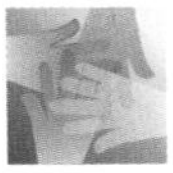

If you decide to diet with a roommate, friend, parent, spouse, or coworker, decide on a plan. You might walk or work out together or check in with each other every evening when you're most prone to overeating. Another alternative is to join a weight loss group, either one that is part of a commercial program or a more informal group that meets on campus or at a church or community center. Support has proved one of the most critical factors in weight management for African-American women.

Every month, an estimated five million Americans log on to commercial websites targeted to dieters. Online dieting is convenient, anonymous, and available around the clock. Some dieters post their weekly weights or before-and-after photos of the way (and weight) they were and how far they've come. Others find support in various blogs and chat groups, where they can commiserate, exchange tales of setbacks and successes, and encourage each other to stay the course. Simply reading diet blogs can help you feel less lonely in your quest.

YOUR LIFE COACH

Get a Grip on Emotional Eating

Occasionally all of us seek comfort at the tip of a spoon. However, many people use food as a way of coping with anger, frustration, stress, boredom, or fatigue. Whatever its motivation, emotional eating always involves eating for reasons other than physiological hunger. If you're not sure whether you do this, ask yourself the following questions:

- Do you eat when you're not hungry?
- Do you eat or continue eating even if the food doesn't taste good?
- Do you eat when you can't think of anything else to do?
- Do you eat when you're emotionally vulnerable—tired, frustrated, or worried?
- Do you eat after an argument or stressful situation to calm down?
- Do you eat as one of your favorite ways of enjoying yourself?
- Do you eat to reward yourself?
- Do you keep eating even after you're full?

If you answer yes to more than three of these, you're eating in response to what you feel, not what you need. Diets may work for you, but the extra weight will inevitably creep back unless you confront your hidden motives for overeating. Since neither emotions nor food ever go away, you have to learn to deal with both for as long as you live.

To get a grip on your emotional eating, try this three-step plan:

Step 1: Know Your Triggers

Whatever its specific motivation, emotional eating always involves eating for reasons other than physiological hunger. The key to getting it under control is awareness.

What are the feelings that set off an eating binge?

- **Anger?** Many people, especially women, swallow their anger by eating because they're afraid of what might happen if they express it.
- **Guilt?** Some people eat because they feel they're always falling short as children, partners, or parents.
- **Rebellion?** Eating may be the only way some people give themselves permission to take a break from being dutiful.
- **Deprivation?** At the end of a long day, a person may justify turning to food as a well-deserved reward, maybe the first nice thing done for herself or himself all day.

Did any of these possibilities hit home? If so, train yourself to take a step back and ask yourself a series of questions before you take a bite: Are you hungry? If not, what are you feeling? Stressed, tired, bored, anxious, sad, happy? Once you identify your true feeling, push deeper and ask why

nonexercise activity thermogenesis (NEAT) Nonvolitional movement that can be an effective way of burning calories.

you feel this way. Try writing down your answers in a notebook. This is an even more effective way to help make sure that every bite you take is a conscious one.

Step 2: Put Your Body, Not Your Emotions, In Charge of What You Eat

To keep mind and body on an even keel, avoid getting so hungry and feeling so deprived that you become desperate and panicky. If you're facing an emotionally intense period—exam week or a visit from an ornery relative—plan your meals and snacks in advance and try, as much as you can, to stick with your program. Rather than swearing off sweets forever, work indulgences into your weekly routine. If you plan to have a brownie for dessert on Friday night, you can look forward to it all week and not waste calories on a candy bar that won't taste as good.

Step 3: Focus on Your Feelings

Let yourself feel how you're feeling without eating. Breathe deeply for a minute or two. Focus on the places in your body that feel tense. Rate the intensity of the emotion on a scale from ten (life or death) to one (truly trivial). Ask yourself: What's the worst-case scenario of feeling this way? Is food going to make it better in any way? Will it make it worse?

When you're tempted to eat but aren't hungry, write down the circumstances and try to discern the underlying reasons. If you eat cookies at night, ask, What does it get me? The answer might be that it relaxes you. Once you realize that the cookies are a means to an end, you can figure out something else you can do to get the same emotional benefits.

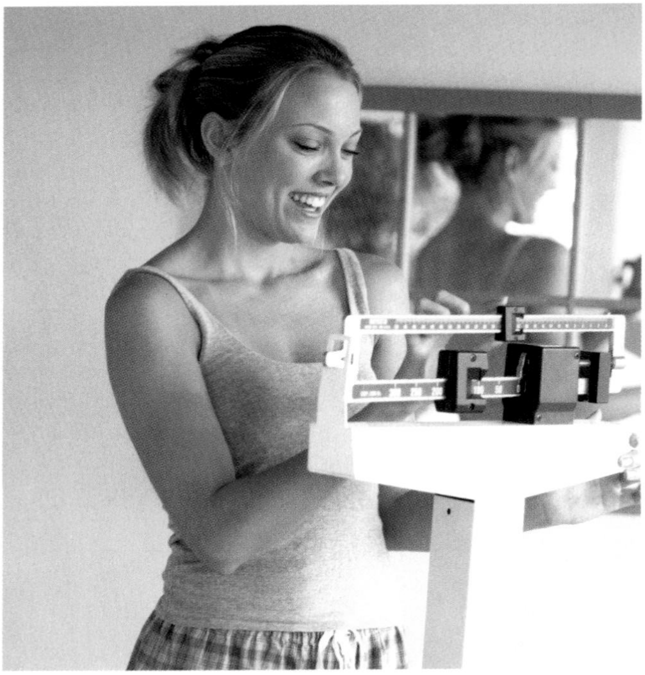

Vigilance helps keep weight off. If the number on the scale creeps upward, take action.

Maintaining Weight Loss

Surveys of people who lost significant amounts of weight and kept it off for several years show that most did so on their own—without medication, meal substitutes, or membership in an organized weight loss group. When a National Institutes of Health panel reviewed 48 separate weight loss trials, they found that participants lost about 8 percent of their body weight on average and kept it off.

Rather than focusing on why dieters fail, the creators of the National Weight Control Registry study the habits and lifestyles of those who've maintained a weight loss of at least 30 pounds for at least a year. The nearly 4,000 people in the registry have averaged a weight loss of 66 pounds, which they've kept off for 5.5 years.[25]

No one diet or commercial weight loss program helped all these formerly fat individuals. Many, through years of trial and error, eventually came up with a permanent exercise and eating program that worked for them. Despite the immense variety, their customized approaches share certain characteristics:

- **Personal responsibility for change.** Weight loss winners develop an internal locus of control. Rather than blaming others for their weight problem or relying on a doctor or trainer to fix it, they believe that the keys to a healthy weight lie within themselves.
- **Exercise.** Registry members report an hour of moderate physical activity almost every day. Their favorite exercise? Three in four say walking, followed by cycling, weight lifting, aerobics, running, and stair climbing. On average, they burn about 2,545 calories per week through physical activity.
- **Monitoring.** About 44 percent of registry members count calories, and almost all keep track of their food intake in some way, written or not.
- **Vigilance.** Rather than avoiding the scale or telling themselves their jeans shrunk in the wash, successful losers keep tabs on their weight and size. About a third check the scale every week. If the scale notches upward or their waistbands start to pinch, they take action.
- **Breakfast.** Your mother probably told you that breakfast is the most important meal of the day, and

40 years of breakfast-related studies, as well as the experience of registry members, have proved her right. A morning meal improves concentration and problem-solving ability, boosts energy levels, and helps control weight. Regular breakfast skippers are four times more likely to be obese than those who eat a morning meal.

Treating Severe Obesity

The biggest Americans are getting bigger. The prevalence of severe or "morbid" obesity is increasing faster than obesity itself. The number of extremely obese adults—those at least 100 pounds overweight with BMIs over 40—has quadrupled in the last two decades from 1 in 200 to about 1 in every 50 men and women. The number with BMIs greater than 50 has jumped from 1 in 2,000 in the 1980s to 1 in 400.

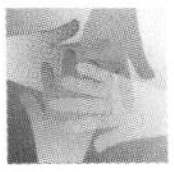

Extreme obesity poses extreme danger to health and survival and undermines quality of life. White women report more impairment than men or African-American women, even when they have lower BMIs. Severe obesity also has a profound effect on every aspect of an adolescent's life.

Drug Therapy

Obesity medications are recommended only for patients with BMIs equal to or greater than 30 or those with a BMI equal to or greater than 27 with risk factors (like high blood pressure) that increase their risk of disease. Researchers are experimenting with other medications, such as rimonabant and the epilepsy drug zonisamide, to enhance weight loss.[26] Currently, only two weight loss drugs are FDA approved.

Xenical (orlistat) blocks fat absorption by the gut but also inhibits absorption of water and vitamins in some patients and may cause cramping and diarrhea. It produces a weight loss of 2 to 3 percent of initial weight beyond the weight lost by dieting over the course of a year.

Meridia (sibutramine) is in the same chemical class as amphetamines and works by suppressing appetite. It also may increase blood pressure, heart rate, or both. Other side effects include headache, insomnia, dry mouth, and constipation. Patients taking these drugs generally lose less than 10 percent of their body weight, and many regain weight after they stop treatment.

Obesity Surgery

Gastric, or bariatric, surgery is recommended only for individuals whose BMIs are higher than 40 or who have BMIs of 35 along with severe health complications. The most common operation uses bands or staples to section off a small portion of the stomach. A small outlet, about the size of a pencil eraser, is left at the bottom of the stomach pouch. Since the outlet is small, food stays in the pouch longer so people feel full for a longer time.

The number of Americans having weight loss surgery has more than quadrupled since 1998.[27] About 80 percent of patients lose some weight; 30 percent reach a normal BMI. The long-term weight loss success rate is 40 to 63 percent of excess body weight over a three-year period and 50 to 60 percent after five years.[28] Besides weight loss, bariatric surgery also eliminates or improves diabetes, high blood pressure, high cholesterol, and obstructive sleep apnea.

Possible complications include leaking of stomach juices into the abdomen, injury to the spleen, slippage or erosion of the band, breakdown of the staple line, and the stomach pouch stretching from overeating. Up to 25 percent of patients may require reoperation within five years. Serious infection or death has been reported in fewer than 1 percent of patients.

Unhealthy Eating Behavior

Unhealthy eating behavior takes many forms, ranging from not eating enough to eating too much too quickly. Its roots are complex. In addition to media and external pressures, family history can play a role. Researchers have linked specific genes to some cases of anorexia nervosa and binge eating, but most believe that a variety of factors, including stress and culture, combine to cause disordered eating.

Sooner or later many people don't eat the way they should. They may skip meals, thereby increasing the likelihood that they'll end up with more body fat, a higher weight, and a higher blood cholesterol level. They may live on diet foods, but consume so much of them that they gain weight anyway. Some even engage in more extreme eating behavior: Dissatisfied with almost all aspects of their appearance, they continuously go on and off diets, eat compulsively, or binge on high-fat treats. Such behaviors can be warning signs of potentially serious eating disorders that should not be ignored.

Disordered Eating in College Students

College students—particularly women, including varsity athletes—are at risk for unhealthy eating behaviors. While some college students have full-blown eating disorders, many others develop "partial syndromes" and experience symptoms that are not severe or numerous enough for a diagnosis of anorexia nervosa or bulimia nervosa. Distress over body image increases the risk of all forms of disordered eating in college women.

In a survey at a large, public, rural university in the mid-Atlantic states, 17 percent of the women were struggling with disordered eating. Younger women (ages 18 to 21) were more likely than older students to have an eating disorder. In this study, eating disorders did not discriminate, equally affecting women of different races (white, Asian, African-American, Native American, and Hispanic), religions, athletic involvement, and living arrangements (on or off campus; with roommates, boyfriends, or family). Although the students viewed eating disorders as both mental and physical problems and felt that individual therapy would be most helpful, all said that they would first turn to a friend for help. Women in sororities are at slightly increased risk of an eating disorder compared with those in dormitories.

Extreme Dieting

About half of girls attempt to control their weight by dieting. In a year-long study of teenagers, both parents and the media had the most influence on the development of weight concerns and weight control practices, including dieting, among adolescents and preadolescents.

Extreme dieters go beyond cutting back on calories or increasing physical activity. They become preoccupied with what they eat and weigh. Although their weight never falls below 85 percent of normal, their weight loss is severe enough to cause uncomfortable physical consequences, such as weakness and sensitivity to cold. Technically, these dieters do not have anorexia nervosa (discussed later in the chapter), but they are at increased risk for it.

Extreme dieters may think they know a great deal about nutrition, yet many of their beliefs about food and weight are misconceptions or myths. For instance, they may eat only protein because they believe complex carbohydrates, including fruits and breads, are fattening.

Sometimes nutritional education alone can help change these eating patterns. However, many avid dieters who deny that they have a problem with food may need counseling (which they usually agree to only at their family's insistence) to correct dangerous eating behavior and prevent further complications.

Compulsive Overeating

People who eat compulsively cannot stop putting food in their mouths. They eat fast and they eat a lot. They eat even when they're full. They may eat around the clock rather than at set meal times, often in private because of embarrassment over how much they consume.

Some mental health professionals describe compulsive eating as a food addiction that is much more likely to develop in women. According to Overeaters Anonymous (OA), an international 12-step program, many women who eat compulsively view food as a source of comfort against feelings of inner emptiness, low self-esteem, and fear of abandonment.

The following behaviors may signal a potential problem with compulsive overeating:

- **Turning to food** when depressed or lonely, when feeling rejected, or as a reward.
- **A history of failed diets** and anxiety when dieting.
- **Thinking about food** throughout the day.
- **Eating quickly** and without pleasure.
- **Continuing to eat** even when you're no longer hungry.
- **Frequently talking about food** or refusing to talk about food.
- **Fear of not being able to stop** eating once you start.

Recovery from compulsive eating can be challenging because people with this problem cannot give up entirely the substance they abuse. Like everyone else, they must eat. However, they can learn new eating habits and ways of dealing with underlying emotional problems. An OA survey found that most of its members joined to lose weight but later felt the most important effect was their improved emotional, mental, and physical health. As one woman put it, "I came for vanity but stayed for sanity."

Binge Eating

Binge eating—the rapid consumption of an abnormally large amount of food in a relatively short time—often occurs in compulsive eaters. The 25 million Americans with a binge-eating disorder typically eat a larger than ordinary amount of food during a relatively brief period, feel a lack of control over eating, and binge at least twice a week for at least a six-month period.[29] During most of these episodes, binge eaters experience at least three of the following:

- **Eating much more rapidly** than usual.
- **Eating until they feel uncomfortably full.**
- **Eating large amounts of food** when not feeling physically hungry.
- **Eating large amounts of food** throughout the day with no planned mealtimes.
- **Eating alone** because they are embarrassed by how much they eat and by their eating habits.

Binge eaters may spend up to several hours eating, and consume 2,000 or more calories worth of food in a single binge—more than many people eat in a day.

After such binges, they usually do not do anything to control weight, but simply get fatter. As their weight climbs, they become depressed, anxious, or troubled by other psychological symptoms to a much greater extent than others of comparable weight.

Binge eating is probably the most common eating disorder. An estimated 8 to 19 percent of obese patients in weight loss programs are binge eaters.

Eating Disorders

According to the American Psychiatric Association, patients with **eating disorders** display a broad range of symptoms that occur along a continuum between those of anorexia nervosa and those of bulimia nervosa.

As many as 10 percent of teenage girls develop symptoms of or full-blown eating disorders. Among the factors that increase the risk are preoccupation with a thin body; social pressure; and childhood traits such as perfectionism and excessive cautiousness, which can reflect an obsessive-compulsive personality. Teenage girls who diet and have four specific risk factors—a high BMI, menarche (first menstruation) before sixth grade, extreme concern with weight or shape, and teasing by peers—are most likely to have an eating disorder.[30]

The best known eating disorders are anorexia nervosa, which affects fewer than 1 percent of adolescent women, and bulimia nervosa, which strikes 2 to 3 percent. The American Psychiatric Association has developed practice guidelines for the treatment of patients with eating disorders, which include medical, psychological, and behavioral approaches. One of the most scientifically supported is cognitive-behavioral therapy.

If you occasionally go on eating binges, use the behavioral technique called *habit reversal,* and replace your bingeing with a competing behavior. For example, every time you're tempted to binge, immediately do something—text-message a friend, play solitaire, check your e-mail—that keeps food out of your mouth.

If you binge twice a week or more for at least a six-month period, you may have binge-eating disorder, which can require professional help. Treatment usually consists of cognitive-behavioral therapy, either individually or in a group setting. As chronic binge eaters recognize their unhealthy behavior and confront the underlying issues, they usually are able to stop bingeing and resume normal eating patterns.

? FAQ Who Develops Eating Disorders?

Eating disorders affect an estimated 5 to 10 million women and 1 million men. Despite past evidence that eating disorders were primarily problems for white women, they are increasing among men and members of different ethnic and racial groups.

In the few studies of eating disorders in minority college students that have been completed, African-American female undergraduates had a slightly lower prevalence of eating disorders than whites. Asian Americans reported fewer symptoms of eating disorders but more body dissatisfaction, concerns about shape, and more intense efforts to lose weight.

In a survey of health-care professionals at the country's largest colleges and universities, 69 percent have professionals on staff who specialize in diagnosing and treating eating disorders. Of all the hurdles to helping students with eating disorders, 39 percent said denial is the biggest, while 24 percent felt it was unwillingness to seek

binge eating The rapid consumption of an abnormally large amount of food in a relatively short time.

eating disorders Bizarre, often dangerous patterns of food consumption, including anorexia nervosa and bulimia nervosa.

Strategies for Prevention: Do You Have an Eating Disorder?

Physicians have developed a simple screening test for eating disorders, consisting of the following questions:

- Do you make yourself sick because you feel uncomfortably full?
- Do you worry you have lost control over how much you eat?
- Have you recently lost more than 14 pounds in a three-month period?
- Do you believe yourself to be fat when others say you are too thin?
- Would you say that food dominates your life?

Score one point for every "yes." A score of two or more is a likely indication of anorexia nervosa or bulimia nervosa.

Source: Miller, Karl. "Treatment Guideline for Eating Disorders." *American Family Physician*, Vol. 62, No. 1, July 1, 2000.

treatment, and 20 percent blamed pressure from peers and the media to stay thin.

Eating disorders affect every aspect of college students' lives, including dating. Both men and women tend to avoid dating individuals with eating disorders, but men are far less accepting of obesity than women.

Male and female athletes are vulnerable to eating disorders, either because of the pressure to maintain ideal body weight or to achieve a weight that might enhance their performance.

Female college athletes are at especially high risk of disordered eating. According to various studies, 15 to 62 percent may develop some form of disordered eating, compared to only 0.5 to 3 percent of nonathletes.[31] Disordered eating, along with amenorrhea (lack of menstruation) and osteoporosis, is part of the triad of health problems called the *female athlete triad*. Psychosocial factors, such as perfectionism and pressure from parents and coaches, may increase the risk for women in competitive sports.

If someone you know has an eating disorder, let your friend know you're concerned and that you care. Don't criticize or make fun of his or her eating habits. Encourage your friend to talk about other problems and feelings, and suggest that he or she talk to the school counselor or someone at the mental health center, the family doctor, or another trusted adult. Offer to go along if you think that will make a difference.

Anorexia Nervosa

Although *anorexia* means "loss of appetite," most individuals with **anorexia nervosa** are, in fact, hungry all the time. For them, food is an enemy—a threat to their sense of self, identity, and autonomy. In the distorted mirror of their mind's eye, they see themselves as fat or flabby even at a normal or below-normal body weight. Some simply feel fat; others think that they are thin in some places and too fat in others, such as the abdomen, buttocks, or thighs.

The characteristics of anorexia nervosa include:

- A refusal to maintain normal body weight (weight loss leading to body weight of less than 85 percent of that expected for age and height).
- An intense fear of gaining weight or becoming fat, even though underweight.
- A distorted body image so that the person feels fat even when emaciated.
- In women, the absence of at least three menstrual cycles.

The incidence of anorexia nervosa has increased in the last three decades in most developed countries. The peak ages for its onset are 14½ and 18 years. According to the American Psychiatric Association's Work Group on Eating Disorders, cases are increasing among males, minorities, women of all ages, and possibly preteens. About 1 percent of American women develop anorexia.

In the *restricting* type of anorexia, individuals lose weight by avoiding any fatty foods, and by dieting, fasting, and exercising. Some start smoking as a way of controlling their weight. In the *binge-eating/purging* type, they engage in binge eating, purging (through self-induced vomiting, laxatives, diuretics, or enemas), or both. Obsessed with an intense fear of fatness, they may weigh themselves several times a day, measure various parts of their body, check mirrors to see if they look fat, and try on different items of clothing to see if they feel tight. Figure 6-8 shows the serious medical complications.

Bulimia Nervosa

Individuals with **bulimia nervosa** go on repeated eating binges and rapidly consume large amounts of food, usually sweets, stopping only because of severe abdominal pain or sleep, or because they are interrupted. Those with *purging* bulimia induce vomiting or take large doses of laxatives to relieve guilt and control their weight. In *nonpurging* bulimia, individuals use other means, such as fasting or excessive exercise, to compensate for binges.

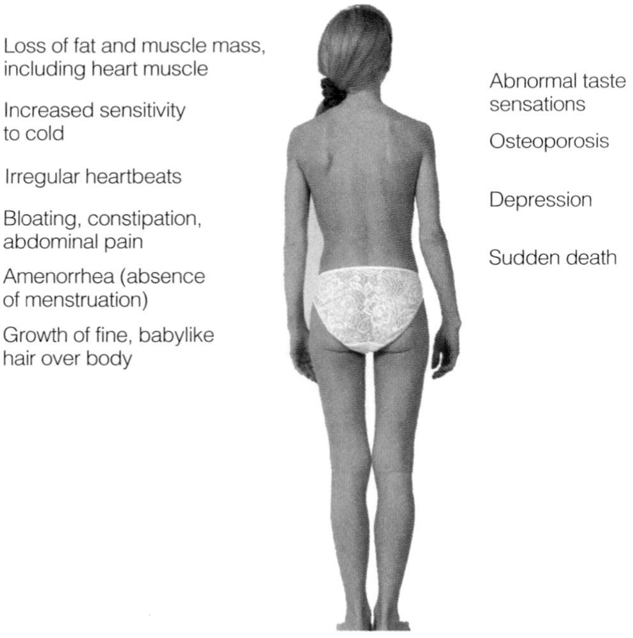

FIGURE 6-8 Medical Complications of Weight Loss from Anorexia Nervosa

The characteristics of bulimia nervosa include:

- Repeated binge eating.
- A feeling of lack of control over eating behavior.
- Regular reliance on self-induced vomiting, laxatives, or diuretics.
- Strict dieting or fasting, or vigorous exercise, to prevent weight gain.
- A minimum average of two bingeing episodes a week for at least three months.
- A preoccupation with body shape and weight.

An estimated 1 to 3 percent of adolescent and young American women develop bulimia. Some experiment with bingeing and purging for a few months and then stop when they change their social or living situation. Others develop longer-term bulimia. Among males, this disorder is about one-tenth as common. The average age for developing bulimia is 18.

LEARN IT / LIVE IT

Managing Your Weight

No diet—high-protein, low-fat, or high-carbohydrate—can produce permanent weight loss. Successful weight management, the American Dietetic Association has concluded, "requires a lifelong commitment to healthful lifestyle behaviors emphasizing sustainable and enjoyable eating practices and daily physical activity." Studies have shown that successful dieters are highly motivated, monitor their food intake, increase their activity, set realistic goals, and receive social support from others. Another key to long-term success is tailoring any weight loss program to an individual's gender, lifestyle, and cultural, racial, and ethnic values.

Here are some practical guidelines.

- **Be realistic.** Trying to shrink to an impossibly low weight dooms you to defeat. Start off slowly and make steady progress. If your weight creeps up 5 pounds, go back to the basics of your program. Take into account normal fluctuations, but watch out for an upward trend. If you let your weight continue to creep up, it may not stop until you have a serious weight problem—again.
- **Recognize that there are no quick fixes.** Ultimately, quick-loss diets are very damaging physically and psychologically because when you stop dieting and put the pounds back on, you feel like a failure.
- **Note your progress.** Make a graph, with your initial weight as the base, to indicate your progress. View plateaus or occasional gains as temporary setbacks rather than disasters.
- **Adopt the 90 percent rule.** If you practice good eating habits 90 percent of the time, a few indiscretions won't make a difference. In effect, you should allow for occasional cheating, so that you don't have to feel guilty about it.
- **Look for joy and meaning beyond your food life.** Make your personal goals and your relationships your priorities, and treat food as the fuel that allows you to bring your best to both.
- **Try, try again.** Remember, dieters usually don't keep weight off on their first attempt. The people who eventually succeed try various methods until they find the plant that works for them.

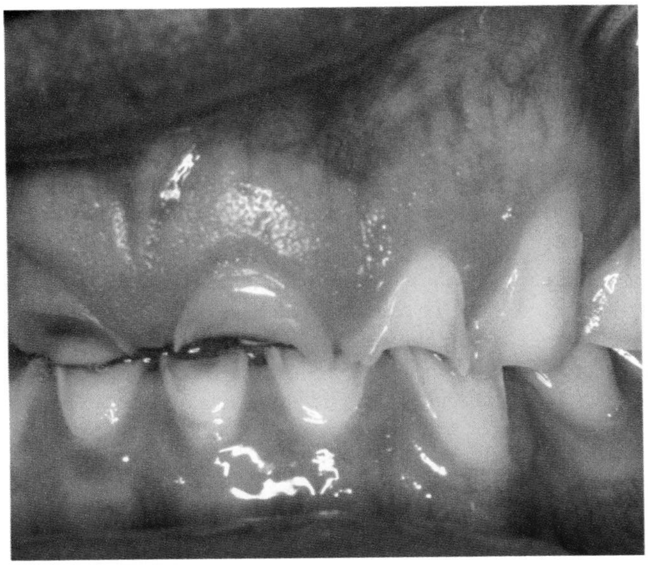

One of the health complications of purging is erosion and decay of dental enamel from the acid in vomit.

anorexia nervosa A psychological disorder in which refusal to eat and/or an extreme loss of appetite leads to malnutrition, severe weight loss, and possibly death.

bulimia nervosa Episodic binge eating, often followed by forced vomiting or laxative abuse, and accompanied by a persistent preoccupation with body shape and weight.

6 Making This Chapter Work for You

Review Questions

1. Which of the following statements is true?
   a. Obesity is a problem only in industrialized countries.
   b. Obesity is a problem that starts in middle age.
   c. The southern states have the highest percentage of people who are obese.
   d. If you were heavy as child, you will always be obese.
2. People gain weight when
   a. their basal metabolic rate increases.
   b. they consume more calories than they use up in daily activity.
   c. they eat fast food more than two times a week.
   d. they watch two hours of television a day.
3. The health dangers of excess weight include all of the following *except*
   a. increased risk of type 2 diabetes, heart disease, and cancer.
   b. increased risk of impaired immunity.
   c. increased risk of auto accidents.
   d. increased risk of dying prematurely.
4. If you have gone online to check out weight reduction support groups in your area, which stage of readiness for weight behavior change are you in?
   a. precontemplation stage
   b. contemplation stage
   c. preparation stage
   d. action stage
5. Which of the following statements is *incorrect?*
   a. I can lose weight successfully on a low-carbohydrate diet.
   b. I can lose weight successfully on a low-fat diet.
   c. I can lose weight successfully on a low-calorie diet.
   d. I can lose weight successfully by working out once a week.
6. Successful weight management strategies include which of the following?
   a. Learn to distinguish between actual and emotional hunger.
   b. Ask friends for recommendations for methods that helped them to lose weight quickly.
   c. Practice good eating habits 50 percent of the time so that you can balance your cravings with healthy food.
   d. Look at celebrity photos and pick one for a model.
7. Which of the following statements is true?
   a. Very low-calorie diets increase metabolism, which helps burn calories more quickly.
   b. An individual eating low-calorie or fat-free foods can increase the serving sizes.
   c. Low-carbohydrate diets have been shown safe over the short term but long-term studies have not been completed.
   d. Yo-yo dieting works best for long-term weight loss.
8. Which of the following eating behaviors may be a warning sign of a serious eating disorder?
   a. vegetarianism
   b. compulsive food washing
   c. binge eating
   d. weight gain during the first year of college
9. Individuals with anorexia nervosa
   a. believe they are overweight even if they are extremely thin.
   b. typically feel full all the time, which limits their food intake.
   c. usually look overweight, even though their body mass index is normal.
   d. have a reduced risk for heart-related abnormalities.
10. Bulimia nervosa is
    a. characterized by excessive sleeping followed by periods of insomnia.
    b. found primarily in older women who are concerned with the aging process.
    c. associated with the use of laxatives or excessive exercise to control weight.
    d. does not have serious health consequences.

Answers to these questions can be found on page **xxx**

Critical Thinking

1. Visualize the body you would like to have—where did the image come from? From television, movies, magazines? Name five influences on your concept of your body image. Examine the validity of each influence. How much are you swayed by media presentations?
2. Do you think you have a weight problem? If so, what makes you think so? Is your perception based on your actual BMI measurement or on how you believe you look? If you found out that your BMI was within the ideal range, would that change your opinion about your body? Why or why not?
3. Suppose one of your roommates appears to have symptoms of an eating disorder. You have told him or her of your concerns, but your roommate has denied having a problem and brushed off your fears. What can you do to help this individual? Should you contact his or her parent? Why or why not?

Media Menu

ThomsonNOW™ Go to the ThomsonNOW website at **http://www.thomsonedu.com** that will:
- Help you evaluate your knowledge of the material.
- Allow you to take an exam-prep quiz.

LACC Extra Credit Assignment

6. Standing naked and relaxed in front of a mirror, without sucking in your stomach, write what you see and what you need to do about it. Include diet and more importantly exercise.

24 Hour · Sep 1st
cancel Cora membership
11:00 – 12:00
← Nicole →

SOUTHERN CALIFORNIA GAS CO.

***** PAYMENT RECEIPT ******
4/24/2009 2:55:09 PM
TPRAL 0911455003 0220
5505 POMONA

ENERGY PAYMENT
1010168356 $80.00
JOHN SCOTT
2230 MARQUETTE AVE
POMONA CA 91766-6426

TOTAL $80.00

CASH TENDER $100.00

CHANGE $20.00

BALANCE $84.41

TYPE OFFICE

THANK YOU

****

TIME WARNER CABLE

www.TimeWarnerCable.com/SoCal/Customer
1-888-TW-CABLE

DATE 7-23-09

8448300700593343

Customer Account Number

NAME Cora Scott

ADDRESS 2230 Marquette **APT. #**

CITY Pomona **ZIP**

Tech# 3763 **Job#** 193-811

Time Warner Representative Bell

Customer Signature

Important Subscriber Information

The Digital Phone voice-enabled cable modem is electronically powered and in the event of a power outage or Time Warner Cable network failure, Enhanced 9-1-1 services will not be available. The Digital Phone Terms of Service prohibit moving the voice-enabled modem to a new address. If you do so, Enhanced 9-1-1 services will not work properly as emergency operators will be unable to accurately identify the caller's address in an emergency. If you would like to establish service at a new address you must call Time Warner Cable.

Payment Receipt

EMF- 077584

$ ____ . __ Amount

Payment Type

☐ M/O ☐ Credit Card ☐ Check ☐ Other

Notes: GI1851TBK663

C.C. Authorization #

Equipment:

I Issue **R** Return

Transaction		Serial #
I	Item #1	GI1518TC[illegible]
I	Item #2	GI1438TC[illegible]
I	Item #3	
I	Item #4	GI1513TC[illegible]
I	Item #5	GI1802T[illegible]979
I	Item #6	GI1845TC8379

My signature on this work order indicates that I have received and agreed to the terms of the Time Warner Cable Residential Services Subscriber Agreement, separately provided to me by Time Warner Cable, including Section 14 of the Time Warner Cable Residential Services Subscriber Agreement, which provides that the parties desire to resolve disputes relating to those Agreements through arbitration. I acknowledge that by agreeing to arbitration, I am giving up various rights including the right to a trial by jury. The terms of the Time Warner Cable Residential Services Subscriber Agreement, including the sections specified herein, are incorporated into this work order by reference as if set out in full herein.

INITIALS

- Provide a Personalized Learning Plan targeting resources that address areas you should study.
- Coach you through identifying target goals for behavioral change and creating and monitoring your personal change plan throughout the semester.

INTERNET CONNECTIONS

American Obesity Association
www.obesity.org

The American Obesity Association is the leading organization for advocacy and education on the nation's obesity epidemic. This comprehensive website features statistics on overweight and obesity in the United States, research articles, consumer protection links, prevention topics, library resources, fact sheets on a variety of weight management topics, and more.

Weight Control Information Network
http://win.niddk.nih.gov/index.htm

This government-sponsored website features a variety of publications in English and Spanish on nutrition, physical activity, and weight control for the general public and for health-care professionals. In addition, there are links for research, a newsletter, statistical data, and a bibliographic collection of journal articles on various aspects of weight management and obesity.

Something Fishy, A Website on Eating Disorders
www.something-fishy.org

This very comprehensive and popular site features the latest news on eating disorders, as well as links regarding signs to watch for, "Recovery Reach-out," treatment finders, doctors and patients, cultural issues, and a support chat.

- InfoTrac College Edition Activities Log on, insert **weight control** into the Keyword search box, and limit your search to the past year. When you get the results, Mark articles to review, then Select one to read. Summarize three or four key points from the article.

You can find additional readings related to personal health with InfoTrac College Edition, an online library of more than 900 journals and publications. Follow the instructions for accessing InfoTrac College Edition that were packaged with your textbook; then search for articles using a keyword search.

For additional links, resources, and suggested readings on the InfoTrac College Edition, visit our Health and Wellness Resource Center at **http://health.wadsworth.com.**

Key Terms

The terms listed are used on the page indicated. Definitions of the terms are in the Glossary at the end of the book.

anorexia nervosa 158
appetite 146
binge eating 156
bulimia nervosa 158
eating disorders 157
hunger 146
NEAT (nonexercise activity thermogenesis) 152
obesity 143
overweight 143
satiety 147

7 Relationships and Sexuality

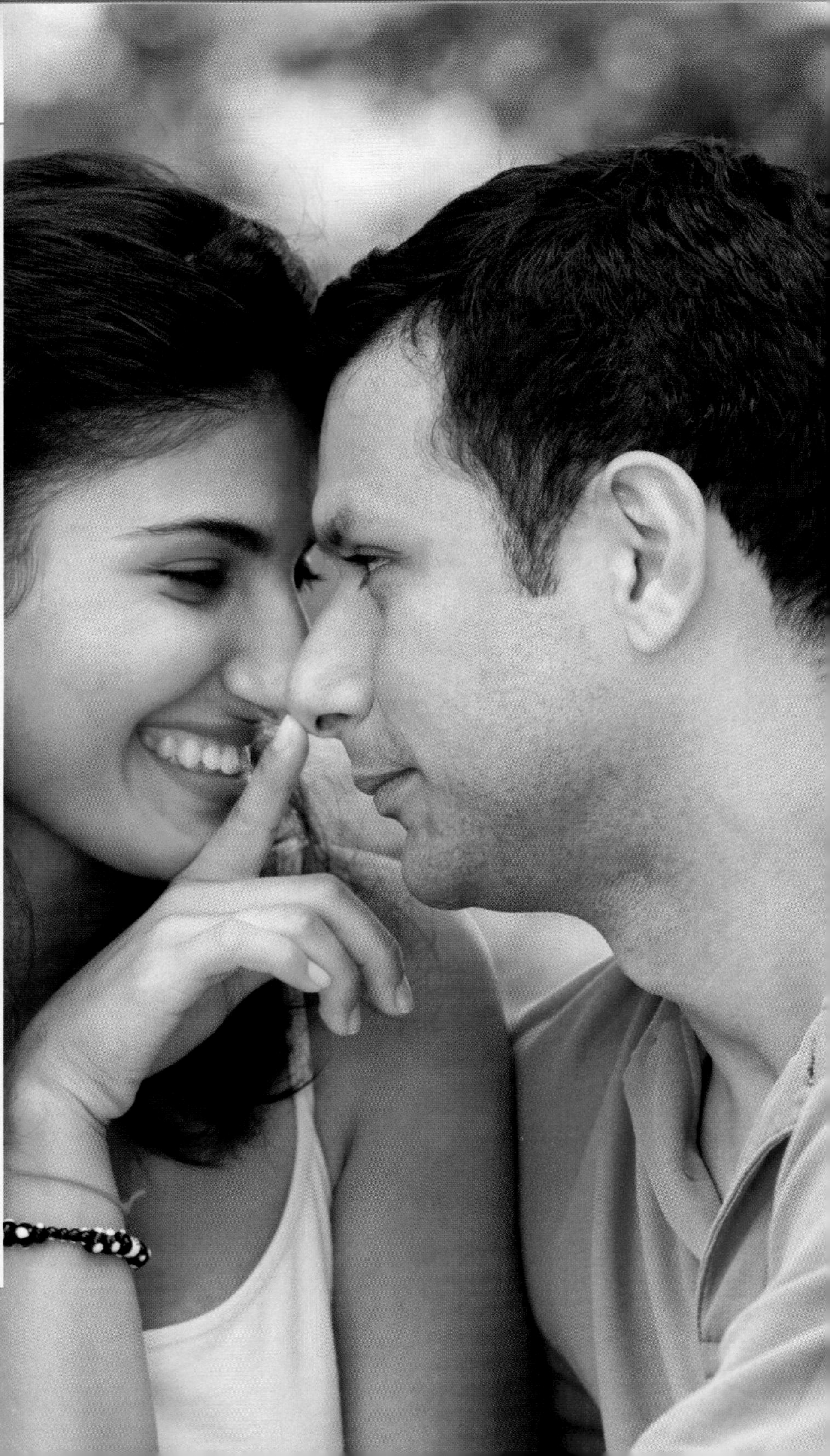

REAL HEALTH

Carson, several years older than the typical college freshman, usually doesn't think much about the age difference—until the conversation turns to sex. He understands his younger classmates' seemingly endless fascination with sex, but his perspective is different. As a teenager, he had plunged recklessly into dangerous territory of every type. Sex—casual and sometimes unprotected—was one of them. Looking back, he feels lucky that he didn't, as he puts it, "end up a statistic." But he still regrets the irresponsible ways he acted.

Carson enlisted in the military when he was 20 in part to finance the rest of his college education. Two years of war changed the way he thought about many things in life, including relationships. When he returned to the United States, Carson craved real commitment and intimacy. He found it with a woman named Tracy, whom he first met online.

At 25, Carson is a married man and an expectant father. His enjoyment of sex hasn't faded—in many ways, it's deepened. He now realizes that there is no such thing as casual sex, that sexual choices have effects on one's own life and on other people. These are the lessons he hopes someday to pass on to his own children.

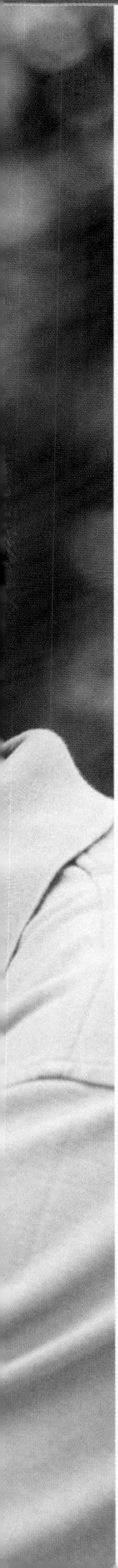

© Creatas Images/Jupiter

We are born social. From our first days of life, we reach out to others, struggle to express ourselves, strive to forge connections. People make us smile, laugh, cry, hope, dream, pray. The fabric of our personalities and lives becomes richer as others weave through it the threads of their experiences.

We are also innately sexual, Our biological maleness or femaleness is an integral part of who we are, how we see ourselves, and how we relate to others. Among all of our involvements with others, sexual intimacy, or physical closeness, can be the most rewarding. Although sexual expression and experience can provide intense joy, they also can involve great emotional turmoil.

You are ultimately responsible for your sexual health and behavior. You make decisions that affect how you express your sexuality, how you respond sexually, and how you give and receive sexual pleasure. Yet most sexual activity involves another person. Therefore, your decisions about sex—more so than those you make about nutrition, drugs, or exercise—affect other people. Recognizing this fact is the key to responsible sexuality.

Sexual responsibility means learning about your relationships, your body, your partner's body, your sexual development and preferences, and the health risks associated with sexual activity. This chapter, an introduction to your social and sexual self, is an exploration of relationships and sexual issues in today's world. It provides the information and insight you can use in making decisions and choosing behaviors that are responsible for all concerned.

? FAQ Frequently Asked Questions

- What is emotional abuse? *p. 168*
- What attracts two people to each other? *p. 169*
- What is the current divorce rate? *p. 173*
- How sexually active are college students? *p. 183*
- Why don't college students practice safer sex? *p. 183*
- What does it mean to abstain? *p. 186*

After studying the material in this chapter, you should be able to:

- **Discuss** the behavior and emotional expectations for friendship, dating, and intimate relationships.
- **Describe** at least three ways to improve a relationship.
- **Identify** the behaviors that may result in dysfunctional relationships.
- **Describe** the male and female reproductive systems and the functions of the individual structures of each system.
- **Describe** conditions or issues unique to women's and men's sexual health.
- **Define** sexual orientation and **give examples** of sexual diversity.
- **List** the range of sexual behaviors practiced by adults.

ThomsonNOW™ Log on to ThomsonNOW at **www.thomsonedu.com/thomsonnow** to find your Behavior Change Planner and to explore self-assessments, interactive tutorials, and practice quizzes.

Personal Communication

Getting to know someone is one of life's greatest challenges and pleasures. When you find another person intriguing—as a friend, as a teacher, as a colleague, as a possible partner—you want to find out as much as you can about him or her and to share more and more information about yourself. Roommates may talk for endless hours. Friends may spend years getting to know each other. Partners in committed relationships may delight in learning new things about each other.

Communication stems from a desire to know and a decision to tell. Each of us chooses what information about ourselves we want to disclose and what we want to conceal or keep private. But in opening up to others, we increase our own self-knowledge and understanding.

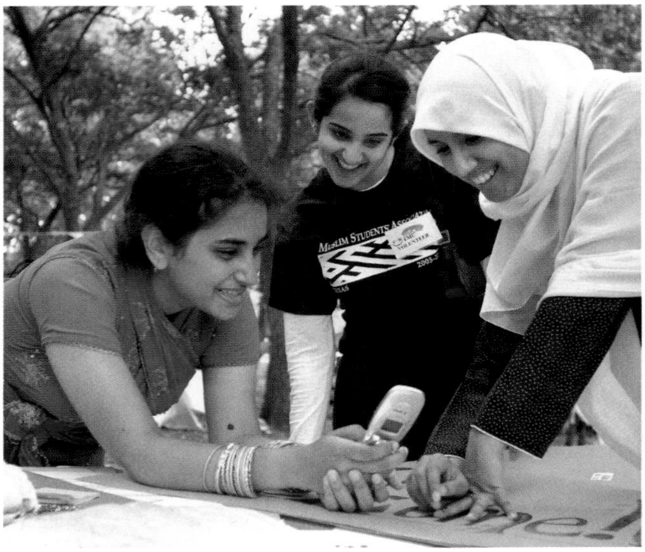
© Bob Daemmrich/The Image Works

Good communication is essential to healthy relationships.

Communicating Feelings

A great deal of daily communication focuses on facts: on the who, what, where, when, and how. Information is easy to convey and comprehend. Emotions are not. Some people have great difficulty saying "I appreciate you" or "I care about you," even though they are genuinely appreciative and caring. Others find it hard to know what to say in response and how to accept such expressions of affection. Men and women vary in their communication styles.

Some people feel that relationships shouldn't require any effort, that there's no need to talk of responsibility between people who care about each other. Yet responsibility is implicit in our dealings with anyone or anything we value—and what can be more valuable than those with whom we share our lives? Friendships and other intimate relationships always demand an emotional investment, but the rewards they yield are great.

Sometimes people convey strong emotions with a kiss or a hug, a pat or a punch, but such actions aren't precise enough to communicate exact thoughts. Stalking out of a room and slamming the door may be clear signs of anger, but they don't explain what caused the anger or suggest what to do about it. You must learn how to communicate all feelings clearly and appropriately if you hope to become truly close to another person.

As two people build a relationship, they must sharpen their communication skills so that they can discuss all the issues they may confront. They must learn how to communicate anger as well as affection, hurt as well as joy—and they must listen as carefully as they speak.

Listening involves more than waiting for the other person to stop talking. Listening is an active process of trying to understand the other person's feelings and motivation. Effective listeners ask questions when they're not sure they understand the other person and prompt the other person to continue.

More than 90 percent of communication may be nonverbal. While we speak with our vocal cords, we communicate with our facial expressions, tone of voice, hands, shoulders, legs, torsos, posture. Body language is the building block upon which more advanced verbal forms of communication rest.

Forming Relationships

We first learn how to relate in our families as children. Our relationships with parents and siblings change dramatically as we grow toward independence. Relationships between friends also change as they move or develop different interests; between lovers, as they come to know more about each other; between spouses, as they pass through life together; and between parents and children, as youngsters develop and mature. But throughout life, close relationships, tested and strengthened by time, allow us to explore the depths of our souls and the heights of our emotions. (See the Self-Survey: "How Strong Are the Communication and Affection in Your Relationship?" in the Self-Assessment Booklet.)

I, Myself, and Me

The way each of us perceives himself or herself affects all the ways we reach out and relate to others. If we feel unworthy of love, others may share that opinion. Self-esteem (discussed in Chapter 2) provides a positive foundation for our relationships with others. Self-esteem doesn't mean vanity or preoccupation with our own needs; rather, it is a genuine concern and respect for ourselves so that we remain true to our own feelings and beliefs. We can't know or love or accept others until we know and love and accept ourselves, however imperfect we may be.

Partners with low self-esteem may feel responsible for a partner's unhappiness. In studies of college students, those who scored low on measures of self-esteem were far more likely to feel rejected or hostile if their partners seemed distraught. Regardless of the reason for the distress, insecure, self-doubting individuals may read nonexistent meaning into their partners' ambiguous cues. As a result, they may unwittingly sabotage their relationships. This misreading of cues occurs not just in dating couples, but among long-married partners who still fear that their spouses love them less than they actually do.

Friendship

Friendship has been described as "the most holy bond of society." Every culture has prized the ties of respect, tolerance, and loyalty that friendship builds and nurtures. An anonymous writer put it well:

> A friend is one who knows you as you are,
> Understands where you've been,
> Accepts who you've become,
> And still gently invites you to grow.

Friends can be a basic source of happiness, a connection to a larger world, a source of solace in times of trouble. Although we have different friends throughout life, often the friendships of adolescence and young adulthood are the closest we ever form. They ease the normal break from parents and the transition from childhood to independence.

In the past, many people believed that men and women couldn't become close friends without getting romantically involved. But as the genders have worked together and come to share more interests, this belief has changed. Yet unique obstacles arise in male-female friendships, such as distinguishing between friendship and romantic attraction and dealing with sexual tension. However, men and women who overcome such barriers and become friends benefit from their relationship—but in different ways. For men, a friendship with a woman offers support and nurturance. What they report liking most is talking and relating to women, something they don't do with their male buddies. Women view their friendships with men as more light-hearted and casual, with more joking and less fear of hurt feelings. They especially like getting insight into what guys really think.

Friendship transcends all boundaries of distance and differences and enhances feelings of warmth, trust, love, and affection between two people. It is a common denominator of human existence that cuts across major social categories: In every country, culture, and language, human beings make friends. Friendship is both a universal and a deeply satisfying experience.

Dating

A date is any occasion during which two people share their time. It can be a Friday night dance, a bicycle ride, a dinner for two, or a walk in the park. Friends and lovers go on dates; so do complete strangers. Some men date other men; some women date other women. We don't expect to love, or even like, everyone we date. Yet the people you date reveal something about the sort of person you are. Dating peaks among young adults. Nearly 50 percent of 18-year-olds go out at least once a week. By age 32, only about 25 percent date that often.

With more people remaining single longer, the search for a good date has become more complex. Singles bars have become less popular because of the dangers of excessive drinking and casual sex. Cafés, laundromats, health clubs, and bookstores have become more acceptable as places to meet new people. Cyberspace has become a popular alternative way to meet potential dates.

Dating can do more than help you meet people. By dating, you can learn how to make conversation, get to know more about others as well as yourself, and share feelings, opinions, and interests. In adolescence and young adulthood, dating also provides an opportunity for exploring your sexual identity. Some people date for months and never share more than a good-night kiss. Others may fall into bed together before they fall in love or even "like."

Separating your emotional feelings about someone you're dating from your sexual desire is often difficult. The first step to making responsible sexual decisions is respecting your sexual values and those of your partner. If you care about the other person—not just his or her body—and the relationship you're creating, sex will be an important, but not the all-important, factor while you're dating.

Dating has potential dangers. As discussed in Chapter 13, approximately one in five female teens is physically and/or sexually abused by a dating partner, though in some cases girls are the aggressors.

Should You Keep Dating?

You've met someone, gone out a few times, and enjoyed yourself. Is it infatuation, "like," or love? Should you keep seeing each other? Here are some positive indications of a relationship worth continuing:

- You feel at ease with your new partner.
- You feel good about your new partner when you're together and when you're not.
- Your partner is open with you about his or her life—past, present, and future.

Strategies for Prevention — Do's and Don'ts of Online Dating

E-mail flirtations can be fun, but they also entail some risks, particularly if you decide to go off-line and meet in person. Here are some guidelines:

- Be careful of what you type. Anything you put on the Internet can end up almost anywhere. To avoid embarrassment, don't say anything you wouldn't want to see in a newspaper.
- Don't give out your address, telephone number, or any other identifying information.
- Don't "date" on an office or university computer. You could end up supplying your professors, classmates, or coworkers with unintentional entertainment.
- Remember that you have no way of verifying if a correspondent is telling the truth about anything—sex, age, occupation, marital status.
- If you do decide to meet, make your first face-to-face encounter a double or group date and make it somewhere public, like a cafe or museum.
- Make sure you tell a friend or family member your plans and have your own way of getting home.
- Don't rely on the Internet as your only method of meeting people. Continue to get out in the real world and meet potential dates the old-fashioned way: live and in-person.

- You can say no to each other without feeling guilty.
- You feel cared for, appreciated, and accepted as you are.
- Your partner really listens to what you have to say.

Following are some reasons to rethink your relationship:

- You don't feel comfortable together.
- You feel angry or let down when you're together or apart.
- Your partner is very secretive about his or her life.
- You feel your partner isn't attentive to you.
- You don't feel cared for and appreciated.

Hooking Up

Hooking up refers to a sexual encounter between two people who usually are not seriously dating and who may or may not know each other well. College students use the term to describe a variety of sexual interactions, including petting below the waist, oral sex, and sexual intercourse.

Alcohol often plays a role in hooking up. Under its influence, individuals may engage in sexual activities, including unsafe sex, that they normally would avoid with someone they usually would not choose. Most students surveyed believe that hooking up is more common than it may in fact be and that their peers—particularly men—are more comfortable with hooking up than they are.

Some young people also engage in sexual activities with friends with whom they are not romantically involved. Many "friends with benefits" may have had a sexual relationship in the past. Others have no expectation of any serious involvement.

YOUR LIFE COACH

Building Healthy Relationships

Healthy relationships are built on mutual respect, trust, and consideration. People who've grown up in dysfunctional families or who have had abusive relationships may not have a clear idea of what a healthy relationship is. Here are some of the characteristics to look and strive for:

- **Emotional support and sensitivity.**
- **Mutual good will.**
- **Respectful asking rather than ordering.**
- **Encouragement.**
- **Being listened and responded to with courtesy.**
- **Acknowledgement and appreciation of your feelings.**
- **The right to express your own point of view.**
- **Freedom from accusations, blame, criticism, and judgment.**
- **Respect for your work and interests.**
- **No rage, outbursts of anger, or emotional or physical threats.**
- **Sincere apologies for comments or jokes you find offensive.**

A healthy relationship requires empathy, the ability to appreciate what another person is experiencing. You

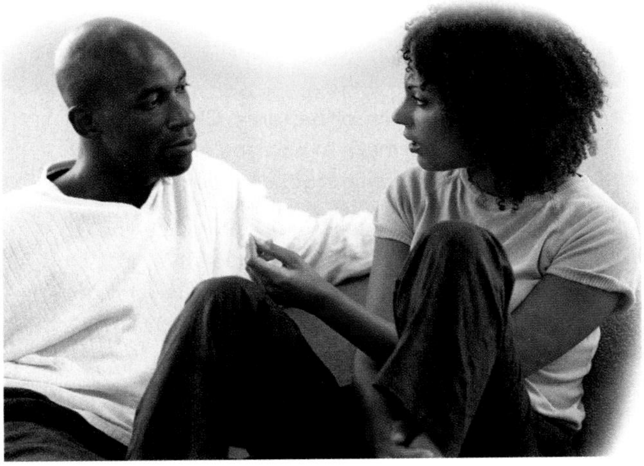

Talking about your feelings and listening intently move a relationship to a deeper and more meaningful level.

may not agree with your roommate's political opinions or your sibling's wardrobe choices, yet you respect their rights to think and dress as the individuals they are.

In an intimate relationship, empathy becomes even more important. You can develop your capacity for empathy by pulling back periodically, particularly in moments of stress or conflict, and asking yourself: What is my partner or spouse feeling right now? What does he or she need?

Assessing A Relationship

How do you know if you're in a healthy relationship? Ask yourself the following questions:

- **Do you have a clear sense of who you are,** what you believe and value, the goals you want? Such self-knowledge is critical for forming any mature relationship.
- **Do you feel that you can be yourself** when you're with this person? Do you feel good about yourself? Do you get—and give—compliments, support, and praise?
- **Do you share interests and values?** When you have things in common, you have a foundation to expand and build your relationship.
- **Do you respect the other person** and feel respected in return?
- **Do you have differences in values,** politics, religion, age, or race? Can you accept them?
- **Do you still feel like a unique, strong individual** within this relationship?

Improving Your Relationship

Being in a relationship should be an opportunity for fun, personal growth, and mutual support, never an excuse for hurting or controlling someone else. The following guidelines can help keep a relationship healthy:

- **Be willing to open up.** The more you share, the deeper the bond between you and your friend will become.
- **Be sensitive to your friend's or partner's feelings.** Keep in mind that, like you, he or she has unique needs, desires, and dreams.
- **Express appreciation.** Be generous with your compliments. Let your friends and family know you recognize their kindnesses.
- **Know that people will disappoint you from time to time.** We are only human. Accept your loved ones as they are. Admitting their faults need not reduce your respect for them.
- **Talk about your relationship.** If you have any gripes or frustrations, air them.
- **Recognize that both people in the relationship have the right to be accepted** as they are, to be treated with respect, to feel safe, to ask for what they want, to say no without feeling guilty, to express themselves, to give and receive affection, and to make some mistakes and be forgiven.
- **Remember that no one in a relationship has the right to force the other to do anything,** to tell the other where or when to speak up or go out, to humiliate the other in public or private, to isolate the other from friends and family, to read personal material without permission, to pressure the other to give up goals or interests, or to abuse the other person verbally or physically.

Dysfunctional Relationships

Although they enrich and fulfill us in many ways, our relationships with friends, siblings, parents, or colleagues can also sabotage our health. Mental health professionals define a "toxic" relationship as one in which either person is made to feel worthless or incompetent.

Relationships that don't promote healthy communication, honesty, and intimacy are sometimes called **dysfunctional.**

Often partners have magical, unrealistic expectations (e.g., they expect that a relationship with the right person will make their life okay), and one person uses the other

dysfunctional Characterized by negative and destructive patterns of behavior between partners or between parents and children.

Strategies for Change — Coping with an Unhealthy Relationship

- **Start a dialogue.** Focus on communication, not confrontation. Start with a positive statement, for instance, saying what you really value in the relationship. Volunteer what you might do to make it better, and state what you need from the other person.
- **Distance yourself.** Take a vacation from a toxic friendship. Skip the family reunion or Thanksgiving dinner. When forced into proximity, be polite. If you refuse to engage—not arguing, not getting angry, not trying to make things better—toxic people give up trying to get under your skin.
- **Consult a professional.** A therapist or minister can help people recognize and change toxic behavior patterns. Changes you make in how you act and react can trigger changes in others.
- **Save yourself.** If you can never get what you need in a relationship, you may need to let it go.

almost as if he or she were a mood-altering drug. The partners may compulsively try to get the other to act the way they want. Both persons may not trust or may deceive each other. Often they isolate themselves from others, thus trapping themselves in a recurring cycle of pain.

? FAQ What Is Emotional Abuse?

Abuse consists of any behavior that uses fear, humiliation, or verbal or physical assaults to control and subjugate another human being. Rather than being physical, emotional abuse often takes the form of constant berating, belittling, and criticism. Aggressive verbal abuse includes calling names, blaming, threatening, accusing, demeaning, and judging. Trivializing, minimizing, or denying what a person says or feels is a more subtle but equally destructive type of abuse. Even if done for the sake of "teaching" or "helping," emotional abuse wears away at self-confidence, sense of self-worth, and trust and belief in one's self. Because it is more than skin deep, emotional abuse can leave deeper, longer-lasting scars.

More than 15 percent of undergraduates in the National College Health Assessment said they had been in an abusive relationship. As Figure 7-1 shows, most reported emotional abuse.[1]

Among the signs of emotional abuse are:

- **Attempting to control various aspects of your life,** such as what you say or wear.
- **Frequently humiliating you** or making you feel badly about yourself.
- **Making you feel as if you are to blame** for what your partner does.
- **Wanting to know where you are** and whom you're with at all times.
- **Becoming jealous or angry** when you spend time with friends.
- **Threatening to harm you** if you break up.
- **Trying to coerce you** into unwanted sexual activity with statements such as, "If you loved me, you would. . . ."

If you can never get what you need or if you're afraid, you need to get out of the relationship. Take whatever steps necessary to ensure your safety. Find a trusted adult who can help. Don't isolate yourself from family and friends. This is the time when you need their support and often the support of a counselor, minister, or doctor as well.

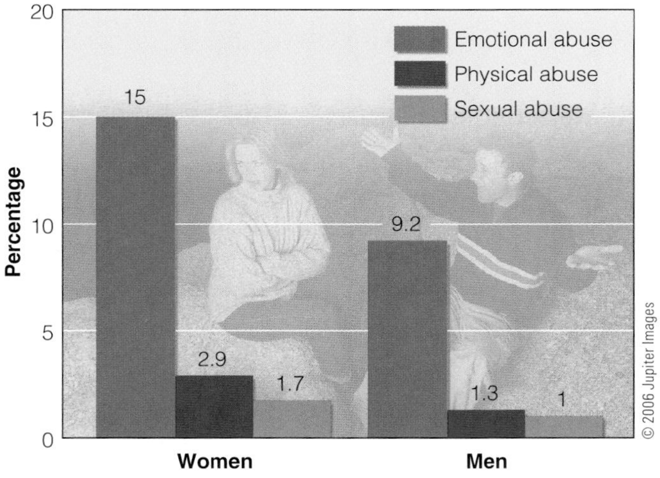

FIGURE 7-1 Abusive Relationships on Campus
Percentage of college students reporting abusive relationships in the last school year.

Source: American College Health Association. "American College Health Association-National College Health Assessment (ACHA-NCHA) Spring 2004 Reference Group Data Report (abridged)." *Journal of American College Health*, Vol. 54, No. 4, January-February 2006, p. 201.

Intimate Relationships

The term **intimacy**—the open, trusting sharing of close, confidential thoughts and feelings—comes from the Latin word for *within*.Intimacy doesn't happen at first sight, or in a day or a week or a number of weeks. Intimacy requires time and nurturing; it is a process of revealing rather than hiding, of wanting to know another and to be known by that other. Although intimacy doesn't require sex, an intimate relationship often includes a sexual relationship, heterosexual or homosexual.

? FAQ What Attracts Two People to Each Other?

What draws two people to each other and keeps them together: chemistry or fate, survival instincts or sexual longings? "Probably it's a host of different things," reports sociologist Edward Laumann, coauthor of *Sex in America,* a landmark survey of 3,432 men and women conducted by the National Opinion Research Center at the University of Chicago.[2] "But what's remarkable is that most of us end up with partners much like ourselves—in age, race, ethnicity, socioeconomic class, education."

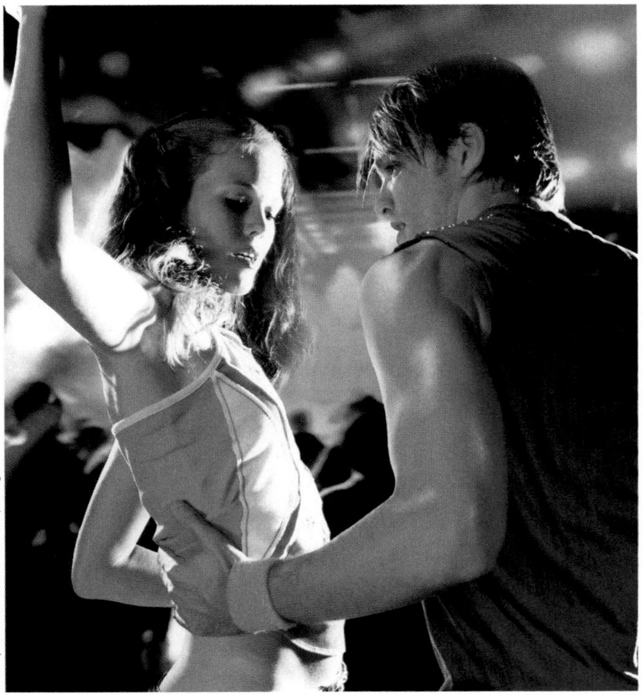

© Daly & Newton/Stone/Getty Images

Many factors, including chemistry and sexual attraction, draw two people together.

Why? "You've got to get close for sexual chemistry to occur," says Laumann. "Sparks may fly when you see someone across a crowded room, but you only see a pre-selected group of people—people enough like you to be in the same room in the first place. This makes sense because initiating a sexual relationship is very uncertain. We all have such trepidations about being too fat, too ugly, too undesirable. We try to lower the risk of rejection by looking for people more or less like us."

Scientists have tried to analyze the combination of factors that attracts two people to each other. In several studies of college students, four predictors ranked as the most important reasons for attraction: warmth and kindness, desirable personality, something specific about the person, and reciprocal liking.

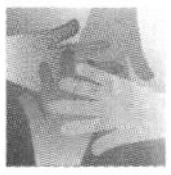

In his cross-cultural research, psychologist David Buss, author of *The Evolution of Desire,* found that men in 37 sample groups drawn from Africa, Asia, Europe, North and South America, Australia, and New Zealand rated youth and attractiveness as more important in a possible mate than did women. Women placed greater value on potential mates who were somewhat older, had good financial prospects, and were dependable and hardworking.[3]

Attractive women in different cultures, including the United States, use different mating strategies than less attractive ones, including more "attractiveness enhancement tactics" (such as wearing makeup), flirting with other men to make a date jealous, and acting possessively. Attractive women also may have more opportunities for "trial liaisons" in selecting long-term partners and for replacing a mate who fails to live up to expectations.

Romantic Love

According to psychologist Robert Sternberg, love can be viewed as a triangle with three faces: passion, intimacy, and commitment (Figure 7-2). Each person brings his or her own triangle to a relationship. If they match well, their relationship is likely to be satisfying.

Sternberg also identified six types of love:

- **Liking,** the intimacy friends share.
- **Infatuation,** the passion that stems from physical and emotional attraction.
- **Romantic love,** a combination of intimacy and passion.
- **Companionate love,** a deep emotional bond in a relationship that may have had romantic components.
- **Fatuous love,** a combination of passion and

intimacy A state of closeness between two people, characterized by the desire and ability to share one's innermost thoughts and feelings with each other either verbally or nonverbally.

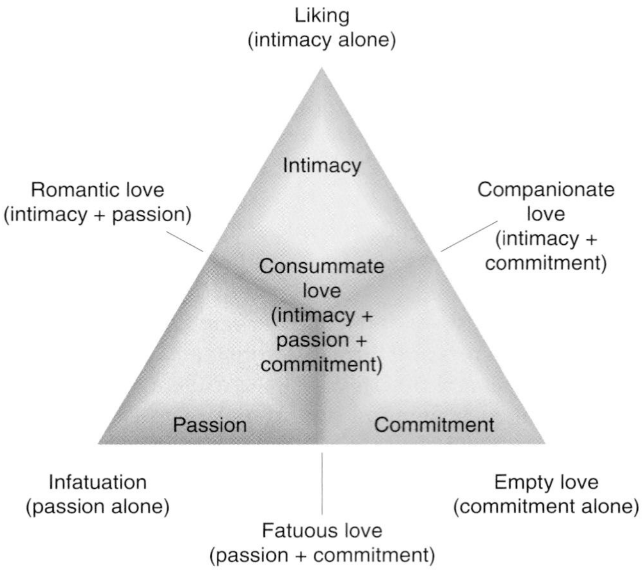

FIGURE 7-2 Sternberg's Love Triangle
The three components of love are intimacy, passion, and commitment. The various kinds of love are composed of different combinations of the three components.

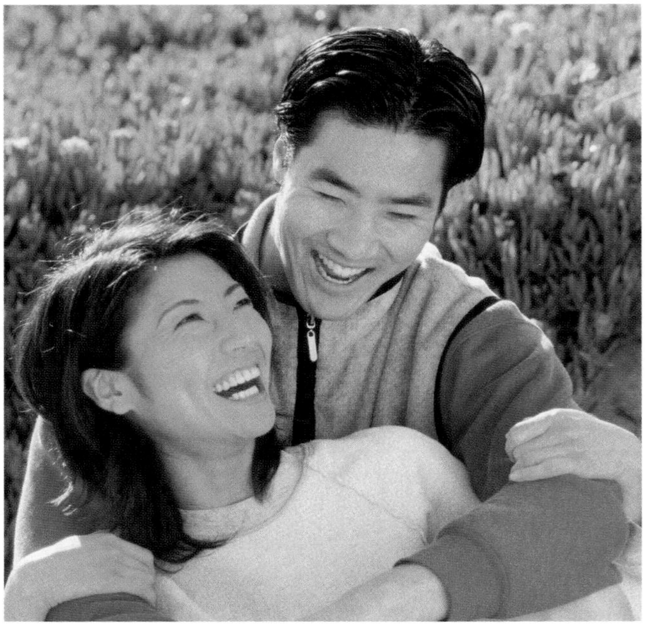
© Comstock/PictureQuest

Romantic love is a combination of intimacy and passion.

commitment in two people who lack a deep emotional intimacy.

- **Consummate love,** which combines passion, intimacy, and commitment over time.

Mature Love

Social scientists have distinguished between *passionate love* (characterized by intense feelings of elation, sexual desire, and ecstasy) and *companionate love* (characterized by friendly affection and deep attachment). Often relationships begin with passionate love and evolve into a more companionate love. Sometimes the opposite happens and two people who know each other well discover that their friendship has "caught fire" and the sparks have flamed an unexpected passion.

Mature love is a complex combination of sexual excitement, tenderness, commitment, and—most of all—an overriding passion that sets it apart from all other love relationships in one's life. This passion isn't simply a matter of orgasm but also entails a crossing of the psychological boundaries between oneself and one's lover. You feel as if you're becoming one with your partner while simultaneously retaining a sense of yourself.

When Love Ends

Breaking up is indeed hard to do. Sometimes two people grow apart gradually, and both of them realize that they must go their separate ways. More often, one person falls out of love first. It hurts to be rejected; it also hurts to inflict pain on someone who once meant a great deal to you.

In surveys, college students say it's more difficult to initiate a breakup than to be rejected. Those who decided to end a relationship reported greater feelings of guilt, uncertainty, discomfort, and awkwardness than those with whom they broke up. However, students with high levels of jealousy are likely to feel a desire for vengeance that can lead to aggressive behavior.

Research suggests that people do not end their relationships because of the disappearance of love. Rather a sense of dissatisfaction or unhappiness develops, which may then cause love to stop growing. The fact that love does not dissipate completely may be one of the reasons why breakups are so painful. While the pain does ease over time, it can help both parties if they end their relationship in a way that shows kindness and respect.

Your basic guideline should be to think of how you would like to be treated if someone were breaking up with you. Would it hurt more to find out from someone else? Would it be more painful if the person you cared for lied to you or deceived you, rather than admitted the truth? Saying "I don't feel the way I once did about you; I don't want to continue our relationship" is hard, but it's also honest and direct.

Cohabitation

Although couples have always shared homes in informal relationships without any official ties, "living together," or **cohabitation,** has become more common. Some five million couples are cohabiting in the United States;

Strategies for Change — Dealing with Rejection

- Remind yourself of your own worth. You are no less attractive, intelligent, interesting, or lovable because someone ends his or her relationship with you.
- Accept the rejection as a statement of the other person's preference rather than trying to debate or defend yourself.
- Think of other people who value or have valued you, who accept and even see as appealing the same characteristics the rejecting person viewed as undesirable.
- Don't withdraw from others. Although you may not want to risk further rejection, it's worth the gamble to get involved again. The only individuals who've never been rejected are those who've never reached out to connect with another.

the vast majority are heterosexual; 40 percent have children.[4]

About a quarter of unmarried women ages 25 to 39 are currently living with a partner; an additional quarter lived with a partner in the past. Couples live together before more than half of all marriages, a practice that was practically unknown 50 years ago.[5]

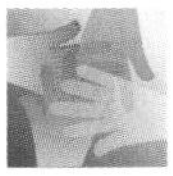

Asians and non-Hispanic white couples are the least likely to cohabit. A higher percentage of Native American, black, and Hispanic couples are unmarried. "Cohabiters" tend to have lower income and education levels. They also are younger—on average, some 12 years younger than married men and women.

Cohabitation can be a prelude to marriage, an alternative to living alone, or an alternative to marriage. Does living together help couples to find out if they get along and avoid a bad marriage? That does not seem to be the case. About half of men and women living together get married within five years; 40 percent break up; 10 percent continue to cohabit for a longer period. Among women cohabiting with a man, one in four says she doesn't ever expect to marry him.

A substantial body of evidence indicates that couples who live together before marriage are more likely to break up after marriage. It's not clear if something about the partners themselves or the actual experience of cohabitation jeopardizes a subsequent marriage.

Committed Relationships

Even though men and women today may have more sexual partners than in the past, most still yearn for an intense, supportive, exclusive relationship, based on mutual commitment and enduring over time. In our society, most such relationships take the form of heterosexual marriages, but partners of the same sex or heterosexual partners who never marry also may sustain long-lasting, deeply committed relationships. These couples are much like married people: They make a home, handle daily chores, cope with problems, celebrate special occasions, plan for the future—all the while knowing that they are not alone, that they are part of a pair that adds up to far more than just the sum of two individual souls.

Domestic Partners

Committed couples, both heterosexual and homosexual, can register as domestic partners in certain areas. This may enable them to qualify for benefits such as health insurance. Employers may require that the couple has lived together for a specified period (generally, at least six months) and are responsible for each other's financial welfare. Recent court rulings have placed domestic partners on the same legal footing as married couples in dealings with businesses.

Long-Term Same-Sex Relationships

Contrary to the stereotype that same-sex relationships tend to be brief, researchers have studied couples who have been together for more than 20 years. Like heterosexual couples, same-sex relationships progress through various stages. The first, blending, is a time of intense passion and romantic love. Gradually the couples move through nesting (starting a home together), to building trust and dependability, to merging assets, to establishing a strong sense of partnership.

Because there are no social norms for same-sex unions, researchers describe these relationships as more egalitarian. Each partner tends to be more self-reliant, and homosexual men and women tend to be more willing to communicate and experiment in terms of sexual behaviors.

Recent studies show that gay and lesbian relationships are comparable to straight relationships in many ways. But same-sex couples have to deal with every day ups and downs

cohabitation Two people living together as a couple, without official ties such as marriage.

in a social context of isolation from family, workplace prejudice, and other social barriers. However, gay and lesbian couples are more upbeat in the face of conflict. Compared to straight couples, they use more affection and humor when they bring up a disagreement and remain more positive after a disagreement. They also display less belligerence, domineering, and fear with each other than straight couples do. When they argue, they are better able to soothe each other so they show fewer signs of physiological arousal, such as an elevated heart rate or sweaty palms, than heterosexual couples.

Marriage

> Like everything which is not the involuntary result of fleeting emotion but the creation of time and will, any marriage, happy or unhappy, is infinitely more interesting and significant than any romance, however passionate.
>
> **W. H. Auden**

Contemporary marriage has been described as an institution that everyone on the outside wants to enter and everyone on the inside wants to leave. According to the Census Bureau, nine in ten people marry, but about half of first marriages end in divorce after an average of seven or eight years.

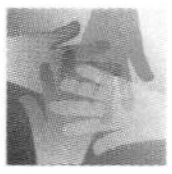

Not too long ago, marriage was often a business deal, a contract made by parents for economic or political reasons when the spouses-to-be were still very young. Today, in some countries, it is still culturally acceptable to arrange marriages in this manner. Even in America, certain ethnic groups, such as Asians who have recently immigrated to the United States, plan marriages for their children. In such arrangements, the marriage partners are likely to have similar values and expectations. However, the newlyweds also start out as strangers who may not even know whether they like—let alone love—each other. Sometimes arranged marriages do lead to loving unions; sometimes they trap both partners in loneliness and longing.

Most of today's marriages aren't arranged. Most people say they marry for one far-from-simple reason: love.

Preparing for Marriage

With more than half of all marriages ending in divorce, there's little doubt that modern marriages aren't made in heaven. Are some couples doomed to divorce even before they swap "I do's"? Could counseling before a marriage increase its odds of success? According to recent research findings, the answer to both questions is yes.

There have been government attempts to set requirements for couples who want to marry. Some states, such as Arizona and Louisiana, have established "covenant" marriages in which engaged couples are required to get premarital counseling. Utah allows counties to require counseling before issuing marriage licenses to minors and people who have been divorced. Florida requires high school students to take marriage education classes.

Finding Mr. or Ms. Right

Generally, men and women marry people from the geographical area they grew up in and from the same social background. Differences in religion and race can add to the pressures of marriage, but they also can enrich the relationship if they aren't viewed as obstacles. In our culturally diverse society, interracial and cross-cultural marriages are becoming more common and widely accepted, although the odds are much greater for partners of the same race to live together or marry.

Some of the traits that appeal to us in a date become less important when we select a mate; others become key ingredients in the emotional cement holding two people together. According to psychologist Robert

Strategies for Prevention — Think Twice About Getting Married If:

- You or your partner are constantly asking the other such questions as, "Are you sure you love me?"
- You spend most of your time together disagreeing and quarreling.
- You're both still very young (under the age of 20).
- Your boyfriend or girlfriend has behaviors (such as nonstop talking), traits (such as bossiness), or problems (such as drinking too much) that really bother you and that you're hoping will change after you're married.
- Your partner wants you to stop seeing your friends, quit a job you enjoy, or change your life in some other way that diminishes your overall satisfaction.

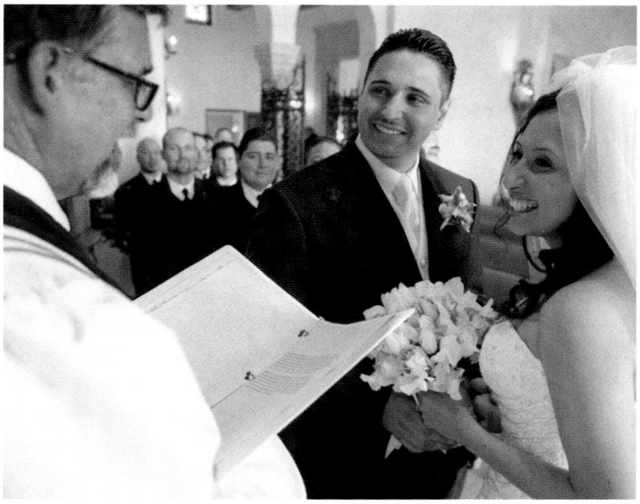

Marriage is a formal, legal, lifetime commitment to another person—and a great occasion for celebration!

Sternberg of Yale University, the crucial ingredients for commitment are the following:

- **Shared values.**
- **A willingness to change in response to each other.**
- **A willingness to tolerate flaws.**
- **A match in religious beliefs.**
- **The ability to communicate effectively.**

The single best predictor of how satisfied one will be in a relationship, according to Sternberg, is not how one feels toward a lover, but the difference between how one would like the lover to feel and how the lover actually feels. Feeling that the partner you've chosen loves too little or too much is, as he puts it, "the best predictor of failure."[6]

Premarital Assessments

There are scientific ways of predicting marital happiness. Some premarital assessment inventories identify strengths and weaknesses in many aspects of a relationship: realistic expectations, personality issues, communication, conflict resolution, financial management, leisure activities, sex, children, family and friends, egalitarian roles, and religious orientation. Couples who become aware of potential conflicts by means of such inventories may be able to resolve them through professional counseling. In some cases, they may want to reconsider or postpone their wedding.

Other common predictors of marital discord, unhappiness, and separation are:

- **A high level of arousal during a discussion.**
- **Defensive behaviors** such as making excuses and denying responsibility for disagreements.
- **A wife's expressions of contempt.**
- **A husband's stonewalling** (showing no response when a wife expresses her concerns).

By looking for such behaviors, researchers have been able to predict with better than 90 percent accuracy whether a couple will separate within the first few years of marriage.

Same-Sex Marriage

In recent years, gay and lesbian couples have formalized their unions by registering as domestic partners in places where allowed and in commitment celebrations.

Same-sex marriage has been legalized in several countries, including Spain and Canada. In the United States, advocates have been working for years to change laws to allow gay and lesbian couples to marry. One state, Massachusetts, currently recognizes same-sex marriages.

Legalizing marriage between same-sex partners, as other countries have done, has triggered intense controversy and political debate in the United States. Some contend that marriage can only be a union between a man and a woman. Others argue that same-sex couples should have equal economic and civil rights as heterosexual couples and these are only guaranteed by a legally recognized marriage. Should marriage be restricted to heterosexual couples? Or should homosexual couples have the same recognition?

You Decide

? FAQ What Is the Current Divorce Rate?

Like marriage rates, the divorce rate also has fallen—to 3.7 per 1,000 people.[7] Your risk of divorce depends on many factors. Simply having some college education improves your odds of a happy marriage. Other factors that do the same are an income higher than $50,000, marrying at age 25 or older, not having a baby during the first seven months after the wedding, coming from an intact family, and having some religious affiliation.

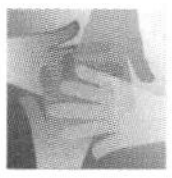

Race also influences marriage and divorce rates. African-American couples are more likely to break up than white couples, and black divorcées are less likely to marry again. Researchers have found that African Americans place an equally high value on marriage. However, there is a smaller "marriageable pool" of black men for a variety of reasons, including a higher mortality rate.

Children whose parents divorced are less likely to marry and to stay married. However, their adult relationships aren't doomed to fail. "Divorce isn't in the genes," says a child psychologist who has studied divorced families for thirty years. "Divorce is an avoidable human error."

Family Ties

Children have become the exception rather than the rule in American households. By 2010, only 28 percent of households will contain children under age 18.

While many traditionally viewed having children as the primary purpose for getting married, nearly 70 percent of Americans now cite another reason. When young adults—ages 18 to 34—react to the statement, "Those who want children should get married," only about half of men and even fewer women agree.

Fertility has declined in the United States since 1960. At that time, the average woman had about three and one-half children over the course of her life. Today's woman has an average of about two children, which is lower than the "replacement level" of 2.1 children per woman. This is the level at which the population would be replaced by births alone. In most European and several Asian countries, fertility has dropped even lower.

Diversity Within Families

The all-American **family**—as portrayed on television and in movies—is typically white and middle-class. But families of different cultures—Italian to Indian to Indonesian—reflect different traditions, beliefs, and values. Within African-American families, for instance, traditional gender roles are often reversed, with women serving as head of the household, a kinship bond uniting several households, and a strong religious commitment or orientation. In Chinese-American families, both spouses may work and see themselves as breadwinners, but the wife may not have an equal role in decision making. In Hispanic families, wives and mothers are acknowledged and respected as healers and dispensers of wisdom. At the same time, they are expected to defer to their husbands, who see themselves as the strong, protective, dominant head of the family. As time passes and families from different cultures become more integrated into American life, traditional gender roles and decision-making patterns often change, particularly among the youngest family members.

American families are diverse in other ways. *Multigenerational families,* with children, parents, and grandparents, make up 3.7 percent of households. They occur most often in areas where new immigrants live with relatives, where housing shortages or high costs force families to double up their living arrangements, or where high rates of out-of-wedlock childbearing force unwed mothers to live with their children in their parents' home.

Three of every ten households consist of *blended families,* formed when one or both of the partners bring children from a previous union. In the future, social scientists predict, American families will become even more diverse, or pluralistic. But as norms or expectations about the configurations of families have changed, values or ideas about the intents and purposes of families have not. American families of every type still support each other and strive toward values such as commitment and caring.

Working Parents

The traditional family with a breadwinner and a homemaker has been replaced by what some call "the juggler family." Two working parents or an unmarried working parent head 70 percent of American families with children. As a result, American parents have fewer hours to spend with their children. Women, balancing multiple roles as parents, spouses, caregivers, and employees often give their own personal needs the lowest priority.

The Family and Work Institute of New York calculates that American husbands put in 75 percent as much time as wives on workday chores—a dramatic rise from 30 percent in 1977. In actual clocktime, the gender difference in domestic "scutwork" amounts to just 45 minutes a day.

Plenty of sociologists—and lots of weary women still doing the lioness share of chores—doubt whether all men in all income groups are doing as much. However, the trend toward greater husbandly involvement is real—and likely to continue.

Personal Sexuality

You are ultimately responsible for your **sexual health** as well as your sexual behavior. Learning about your sexual anatomy and physiology deepens your understanding of how your body works and prepares you to protect your sexual health throughout your life.

Women's Sexual Health

A woman's decisions about sexual activity, birth control (discussed in Chapter 8), and family planning can affect her life in profound ways. Making good decisions depends on knowledge and understanding of sexual anatomy and reproductive processes as well as regular medical checkups. Yet less than two-thirds of college women report having had a routine gynecological examination in the last year.[8]

Female Sexual Anatomy

As illustrated in Figure 7-3a, the **mons pubis** is the rounded, fleshy area over the junction of the pubic bones. The folds of skin that form the outer lips of a woman's genital area are called the **labia majora**. They cover soft flaps of skin (inner lips) called the **labia minora.** The inner lips join at the top to form a hood over the **clitoris,** a small elongated erectile organ and the most sensitive spot in the entire female genital area. Below the clitoris is the **urethral opening,** the outer opening of the thin tube that carries urine from the bladder. Below that is a larger opening, the mouth of the **vagina,** the canal that leads to the primary internal organs of reproduction. The **perineum** is the area between the vagina and the anus (the opening to the rectum and large intestine).

At the back of the vagina is the **cervix,** the opening to the womb, or **uterus** (see Figure 7-3b). The uterine walls are lined by a layer of tissue called the **endometrium.** The **ovaries,** about the size and shape of almonds, are located on either side of the uterus and contain egg cells called **ova** (singular, **ovum**). Extending outward and back from the upper uterus are the **fallopian tubes,** the canals that transport ova from the ovaries to the uterus. When an egg is released from an ovary, the fingerlike ends of the adjacent fallopian tube "catch" the egg and direct it into the tube.

Discharge and changes in odor normally occur in a healthy vagina. They typically fluctuate through the menstrual cycle, depending on hormone level. In the past, many women practiced douching, the introduction of a liquid into the vagina, to cleanse the vagina. However, douching may increase the risk of pelvic inflammatory disease (discussed in Chapter 9) and ectopic or out-of-uterus pregnancy, particularly if done frequently. Despite the potential dangers, according to data from a southern university, four in ten female students had douched in the past; half currently douche. African-American women were encouraged to douche by their mothers; white women were more influenced by television advertisements. When advised to stop douching by a doctor or nurse, most students do so.

The Menstrual Cycle

Scientists have discovered that the menstrual cycle actually begins in the brain with the production of gonadotropin-releasing hormone (GnRH). Each month a surge of GnRH sets into motion the sequence of steps that lead to ovulation, the potential for conception, and if conception doesn't occur, menstruation. The hypothalamus monitors hormone levels in the blood and sends messages to the pituitary gland to release follicle-stimulating hormone (FSH) and luteinizing hormone (LH).

As shown in Figure 7-4, in the ovaries, these hormones stimulate the growth of a few of the immature eggs, or ova, stored in follicles in every woman's body. Usually, only one ovum matures completely during each monthly cycle. As it does, it increases its production of the female sex hormone estrogen, which in turn triggers the release of a larger surge of LH.

At midcycle, the increased LH hormone levels trigger **ovulation,** the release of the egg cell, or ovum, from the follicle. Estrogen levels drop, and the remaining cells of the follicle then enlarge, change character, and form the **corpus luteum,** or yellow body. In the second half of the menstrual cycle, the corpus luteum secretes estrogen and larger amounts of progesterone. The endometrium (uterine lining) is stimulated by progesterone to thicken and become more engorged with blood in preparation for nourishing an implanted, fertilized ovum.

If the ovum is not fertilized, the corpus luteum disintegrates. As the level of progesterone drops, **menstruation** occurs; the uterine lining is shed during the

family A group of people united by marriage, blood, or adoption; residing in the same household; maintaining a common culture; and interacting with one another on the basis of their roles within the group.

sexual health The integration of the physical, emotional, intellectual, and social aspects of sexual being in ways that are positively enriching and that enhance personality, communication, and love.

mons pubis The rounded, fleshy area over the junction of the female pubic bones.

labia majora The fleshy outer folds that border the female genital area.

labia minora The fleshy inner folds that border the female genital area.

clitoris A small erectile structure on the female, corresponding to the penis on the male.

urethral opening The outer opening of the thin tube that carries urine from the bladder.

vagina The canal leading from the exterior opening in the female genital area to the uterus.

perineum The area between the anus and vagina in the female and between the anus and scrotum in the male.

cervix The narrow, lower end of the uterus that opens into the vagina.

uterus The female organ that houses the developing fetus until birth.

endometrium The mucous membrane lining the uterus.

ovary The female sex organ that produces egg cells, estrogen, and progesterone.

ovum (plural, **ova**) The female gamete (egg cell).

fallopian tubes The pair of channels that transport ova from the ovaries to the uterus; the usual site of fertilization.

ovulation The release of a mature ovum from an ovary approximately 14 days prior to the onset of menstruation.

corpus luteum A yellowish mass of tissue that is formed, immediately after ovulation, from the remaining cells of the follicle; it secretes estrogen and progesterone for the remainder of the menstrual cycle.

menstruation Discharge of blood from the vagina as a result of the shedding of the uterine lining at the end of the menstrual cycle.

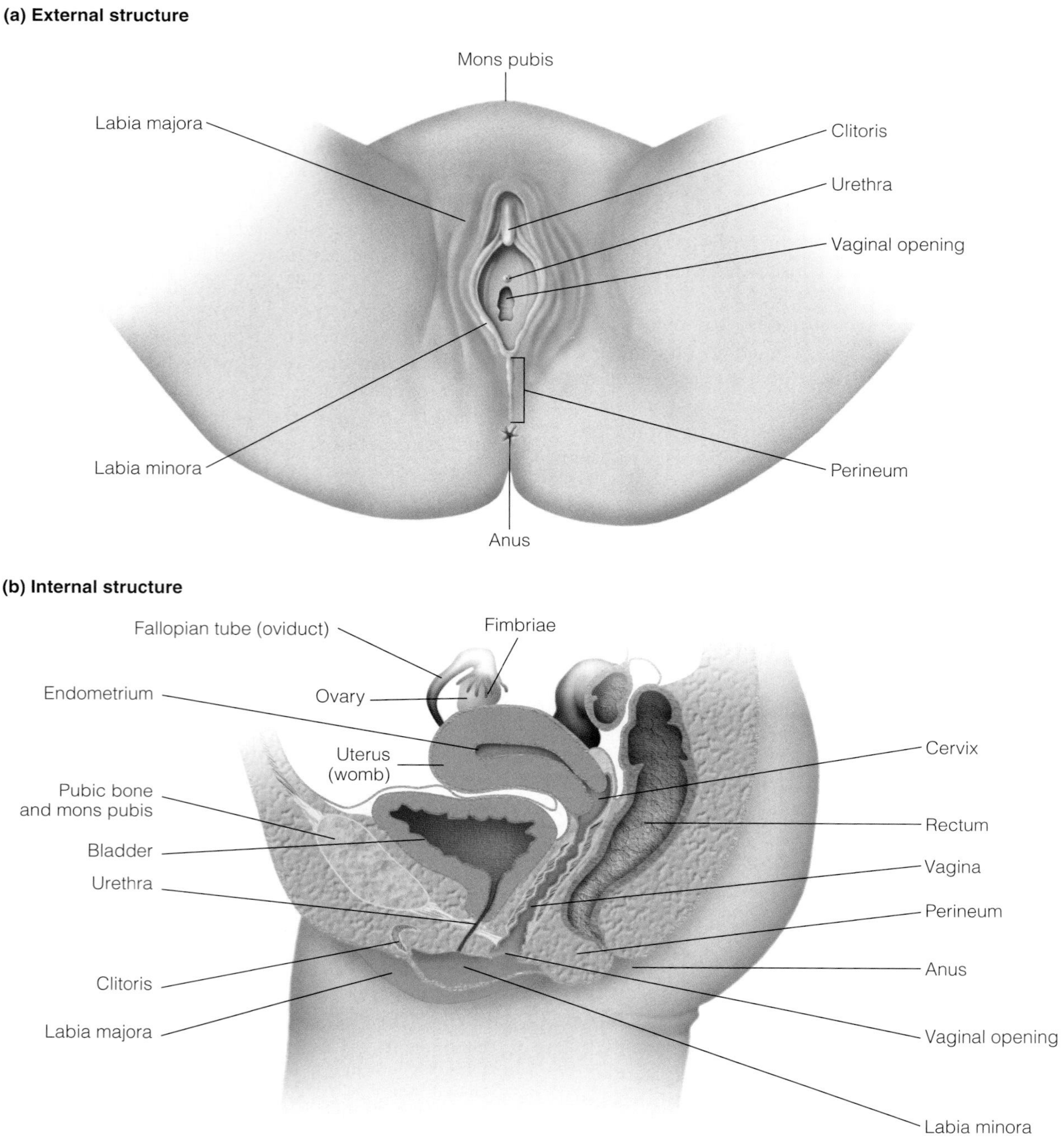

FIGURE 7-3 The Female Sex Organs and Reproductive Structures

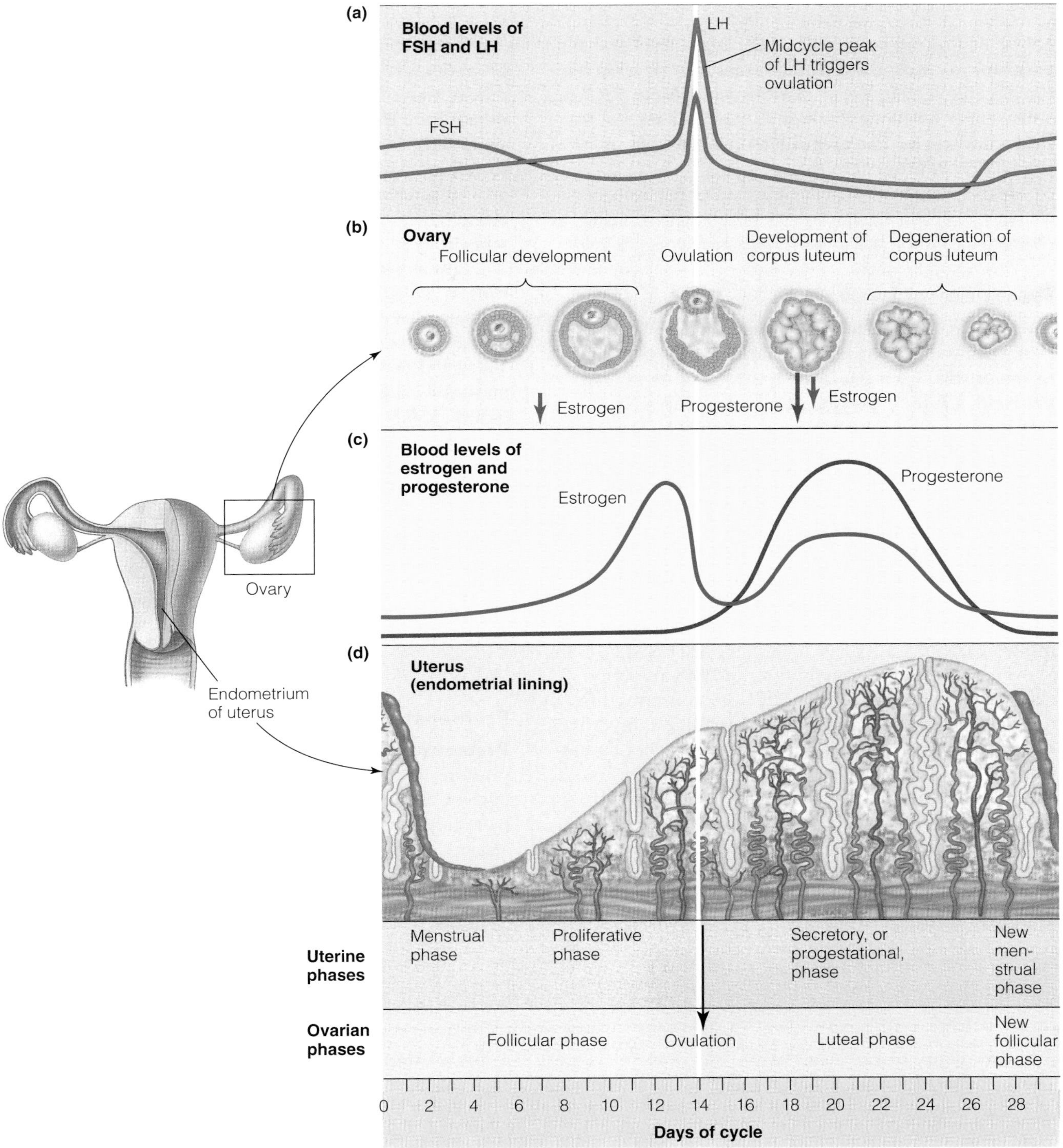

FIGURE 7-4 Menstrual Cycle

(a) In response to the hypothalamus, the pituitary gland releases the gonadotropins FSH and LH. Levels of FSH and LH stimulate the cycle (and in turn are affected by production of estrogen and progesterone).

(b) FSH does what its name says—it stimulates follicle development in the ovary. The follicle matures and ruptures, releasing an ovum (egg) into the fallopian tube.

(c) The follicle produces estrogen, and the corpus luteum produces estrogen and progesterone. The high level of estrogen at the middle of the cycle produces a surge of LH, which triggers ovulation.

(d) Estrogen and progesterone stimulate the endometrium, which becomes thicker and prepares to receive an implanted, fertilized egg.

If a fertilized egg is deposited in the uterus, pregnancy begins. If the egg is not fertilized, progesterone production decreases, and the endometrium is shed (menstruation). At this point, both estrogen and progesterone levels have dropped, so the pituitary responds by producing FSH, and the cycle begins again.

course of a menstrual period. If the egg is fertilized and pregnancy occurs, the cells that eventually develop into the placenta secrete *human chorionic gonadotropin (HCG)*, a messenger hormone that signals the pituitary not to start a new cycle. The corpus luteum then steps up its production of progesterone.

Many women experience physical or psychological changes, or both, during their monthly cycles. Usually the changes are minor, but more serious problems can occur.

Premenstrual Syndrome

Women with **premenstrual syndrome (PMS)** experience bodily discomfort and emotional distress for up to two weeks, from ovulation until the onset of menstruation. Up to 75 percent of menstruating women report one or more premenstrual symptoms; 3 to 9 percent experience disabling, incapacitating symptoms.

Once dismissed as a psychological problem, PMS has been recognized as a very real physiological disorder that may be caused by a hormonal deficiency; abnormal levels of thyroid hormone; an imbalance of estrogen and progesterone; or social and environmental factors, particularly stress. Recent studies indicate that changes in brain receptors during the ovarian cycle may be responsible.

The most common symptoms of PMS are mood changes, anxiety, irritability, difficulty concentrating, forgetfulness, impaired judgment, tearfulness, digestive symptoms (diarrhea, bloating, constipation), hot flashes, palpitations, dizziness, headache, fatigue, changes in appetite, cravings (usually for sweets or salt), water retention, breast tenderness, and insomnia. For a diagnosis to be made, women—using a self-rating symptom scale or calendar—must report troubling premenstrual symptoms in the period before menstruation in at least two successive menstrual cycles.

Treatments for PMS depend on specific symptoms. Diuretics (drugs that speed up fluid elimination) can relieve water retention and bloating. Relaxation techniques have led to a 60 percent reduction in anxiety symptoms. Sleep deprivation, or the use of bright light to adjust a woman's circadian or daily rhythm, also has proved beneficial. Behavioral approaches, such as exercise or charting cycles, help by letting women know when they're vulnerable.

Low doses of medications known as *selective serotonin-reuptake inhibitors*(SSRIs), such as fluoxetine (marketed as Prozac, Sarafem, and in generic forms) provide relief for symptoms such as tension, depression, irritability, and mood swings, even when taken only during the premenstrual phase rather than daily throughout the month. SSRIs are not effective in all women with PMS, and other factors, including a genetic susceptibility, may play a role. Oral contraceptives, though widely prescribed for PMS, have not been shown to be consistently effective.

A diet rich in calcium and vitamin D reduces the risk of PMS. Other treatments with some reported success include calcium supplements; vitamins; exercise; less caffeine, alcohol, salt, and sugar; acupuncture; and stress management techniques such as meditation or relaxation training.

Premenstrual Dysphoric Disorder (PMDD)

Premenstrual dysphoric disorder (PMDD), which is not related to PMS, occurs in an estimated 3 to 5 percent of all menstruating women. It is characterized by regular symptoms of depression (depressed mood, anxiety, mood swings, diminished interest or pleasure) during the last week of the menstrual cycle. Women with PMDD cannot function as usual at work, school, or home. They feel better a few days after menstruation

Strategies for Prevention — Reducing Premenstrual Problems

- **Get plenty of exercise.** Physically fit women usually have fewer problems both before and during their periods.
- **Eat frequently and nutritiously.** In the week before your period, your body doesn't regulate the levels of sugar, or glucose, in your blood as well as it usually does.
- **Swear off salt.** If you stop using salt at the table and while cooking, you may gain less weight premenstrually, feel less bloated, and suffer less from headaches and irritability.
- **Cut back on caffeine.** Coffee, colas, diet colas, chocolate, and tea can increase breast tenderness and other symptoms.
- **Don't drink or smoke.** Some women become so sensitive to alcohol's effects before their periods that a glass of wine hits with the impact of several stiff drinks. Nicotine worsens low blood sugar problems.
- **Watch out for sweets.** Premenstrual cravings for sweets are common, but try to resist. Sugar may pick you up, but later you'll feel worse than before.
- **Add more low-fat dairy products to your diet.** They can lower your risk of problems.

begins. SSRIs, which are used to treat PMS, also are effective in relieving symptoms of PMDD.

Menstrual Cramps

Dysmenorrhea is the medical name for the discomforts—abdominal cramps and pain, back and leg pain, diarrhea, tension, water retention, fatigue, and depression—that can occur during menstruation. About half of all menstruating women suffer from dysmenorrhea. The cause seems to be an overproduction of bodily substances called *prostaglandins,* which typically rise during menstruation. Medications that inhibit prostaglandins can reduce menstrual pain, and exercise can also relieve cramps.

Amenorrhea

Women may stop menstruating—a condition called **amenorrhea**—for a variety of reasons, including a hormonal disorder, drastic weight loss, strenuous exercise, or a change in environment. "Boarding-school amenorrhea" is common among young women who leave home for school. Distance running and strenuous exercise also can lead to amenorrhea. The reason may be a drop in body fat from the normal range of 18 to 22 percent to a range of 9 to 12 percent. To be considered amenorrheic, a woman's menstrual cycle is typically absent for three or more consecutive months. Prolonged amenorrhea can have serious health consequences, including a loss of bone density that may lead to stress fractures or osteoporosis.

Toxic Shock Syndrome

This rare, potentially deadly bacterial infection primarily strikes menstruating women under the age of 30 who use tampons. Both *Staphylococcus aureus* and group A *Streptococcus pyogenes* can produce **toxic shock syndrome (TSS).** Symptoms include a high fever; a rash that leads to peeling of the skin on the fingers, toes, palms, and soles; dizziness; dangerously low blood pressure; and abnormalities in several organ systems (the digestive tract and the kidneys) and in the muscles and blood. Treatment usually consists of antibiotics and intense supportive care; intravenous administration of immunoglobulins that attack the toxins produced by these bacteria also may be beneficial.

Men's Sexual Health

Because the male reproductive system is simpler in many ways than the female, it's often ignored—especially by healthy young men. However, men should make regular self-exams (including checking their penises and testes, as described in Chapter 10) part of their routine.

Male Sexual Anatomy

The visible parts of the male sexual anatomy are the **penis** and the **scrotum,** the pouch that contains the **testes** (Figure 7-5). The testes manufacture testosterone, the hormone that stimulates the development of a male's secondary sex characteristics, and **sperm,** the male reproductive cells. Immature sperm are stored in the **epididymis,** a collection of coiled tubes adjacent to each testis.

The penis contains three hollow cylinders loosely covered with skin. The two major cylinders, the *corpora cavernosa,* extend side by side through the length of the penis. The third cylinder, the *corpus spongiosum,* surrounds the **urethra,** the channel for both seminal fluid and urine; see Figure 7-5.

When hanging down loosely, the average penis is about 3¾ inches long. During erection, its internal cylinders fill with so much blood that they become rigid, and the penis stretches to an average length of 6¼ inches. About 90 percent of all men have erect penises measuring between 5 and 7 inches in length. There is no relation, however, between penis size and female sexual satisfaction: A woman's vagina naturally adjusts during intercourse to the size of her partner's penis.

Inside the body are several structures involved in the production of seminal fluid, or **semen,** the liquid in

premenstrual syndrome (PMS) A disorder that causes physical discomfort and psychological distress prior to a woman's menstrual period.

premenstrual dysphoric disorder (PMDD) A disorder that causes symptoms of psychological depression during the last week of the menstrual cycle.

dysmenorrhea Painful menstruation.

amenorrhea The absence or suppression of menstruation.

toxic shock syndrome (TSS) A disease characterized by fever, vomiting, diarrhea, and often shock, caused by a bacterium that releases toxic waste products into the bloodstream.

penis The male organ of sex and urination.

scrotum The external sac or pouch that holds the testes.

testes (singular, **testis**) The male sex organs that produce sperm and testosterone.

sperm The male gamete produced by the testes and transported outside the body through ejaculation.

epididymis That portion of the male duct system in which sperm mature.

urethra The canal through which urine from the bladder leaves the body; in the male, also serves as the channel for seminal fluid.

semen The viscous, whitish fluid that is the complete male ejaculate; a combination of sperm and secretions from the prostate gland, seminal vesicles, and other glands.

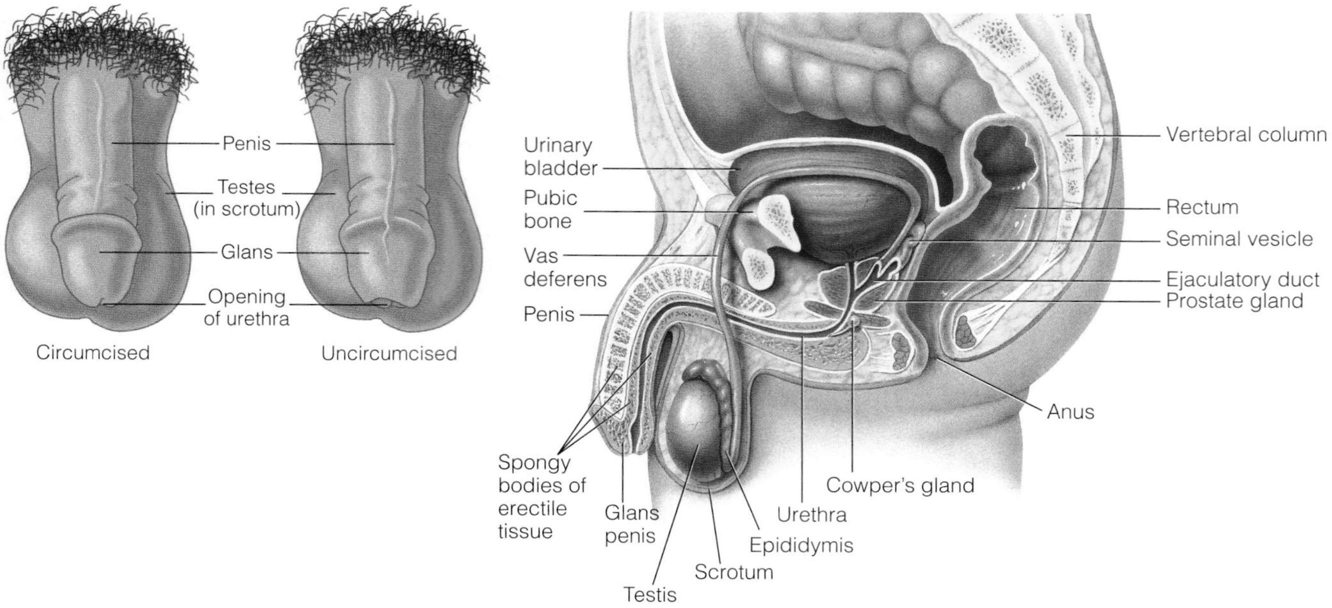

FIGURE 7-5 Male Sex Organs and Reproductive Structures

which sperm cells are carried out of the body during ejaculation. The **vas deferens** are two tubes that carry sperm from the epididymis into the urethra. The **seminal vesicles,** which make some of the seminal fluid, join with the vas deferens to form the **ejaculatory ducts.** The **prostate gland** produces some of the seminal fluid, which it secretes into the urethra during ejaculation. The **Cowper's glands** are two pea-sized structures on either side of the urethra (just below where it emerges from the prostate gland) and connected to it via tiny ducts. When a man is sexually aroused, the Cowper's glands often secrete a fluid that appears as a droplet at the tip of the penis. This fluid is not semen, although it occasionally contains sperm.

Circumcision

In its natural state, the tip of the penis is covered by a fold of skin called the *foreskin.* About 60 percent of baby boys in the United States undergo **circumcision,** the surgical removal of the foreskin.

An estimated 1.2 million newborn males are circumcised in the United States annually for reasons that vary from religious traditions to preventive health measures. Until the last half century, scientific evidence to support or repudiate routine circumcision was limited. The American Academy of Pediatrics (AAP) reviewed 40 years of data and concluded that although there are potential medical benefits, the data were not strong enough to recommend routine neonatal circumcision.[9] However, since this statement, many studies have been published on circumcision and the risks of HIV transmission as well as other diseases.

According to a review of recent scientific evidence, circumcision decreases the incidence of childhood urinary tract infections, the sexual transmission of human papilloma virus (HPV) and HIV, and invasive penile cancer. Studies from sub-Saharan Africa, where rates of HIV infection are extremely high, found that circumcision decreased the risk of acquiring HIV by more than half. Male circumcision may help to prevent the spread of HIV in part because the cells on the foreskin of the penis are more susceptible to HIV infection. Circumcision does not protect against herpes, syphilis, or gonorrhea, suggesting a biological rather than a behavioral explanation for the protective effect of circumcision against HIV.

Boys who are not circumcised are four times as likely to develop urinary tract infections in their first year; however, such infections develop in only 1 percent of circumcised boys. Uncircumcised men are three times as likely to develop penile cancer, but the absolute risk is low. (Only about nine in every million American men ever gets cancer of the penis.)

The drawbacks of circumcision include the risk of complications (which tend to be uncommon and minor) and pain. The AAP recommends that when circumcision is performed, analgesic creams or anesthetic shots be used to minimize discomfort. There is little consensus on what impact the presence or absence of a foreskin has on sexual functioning or satisfaction.

Responsible Sexuality

The World Health Organization defines *sexual health* as "the integration of the physical, emotional, intellectual, and social aspects of sexual being in ways that are positively enriching, and that enhance personality, communication, and love. . . . Every person has a right to receive sexual information and to consider sexual relationships for pleasure as well as for procreation."

Sexuality education is a lifelong process. Your own knowledge about sex may not be as extensive as you might assume. Most people grow up with a lot of myths and misconceptions about sex. (See Self-Survey: "How Much Do You Know About Sex?" in the Self-Assessment Booklet.). Rather than relying on what peers say or what you've always thought was true, find out the facts. This textbook is a good place to start. The student health center and the library can provide additional materials on sexual identity, orientation, behavior, and health, as well as on options for reducing your risk of acquiring sexually transmitted infections (discussed in Chapter 9) or becoming pregnant.

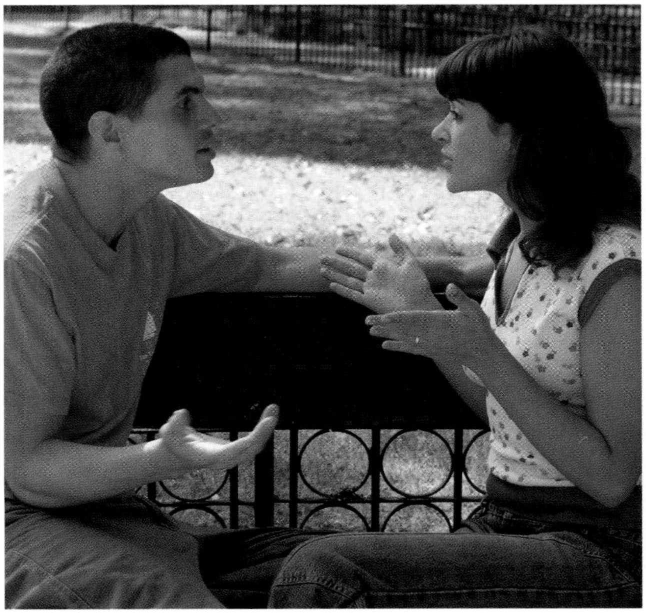

© T. Ozonas/Masterfile

Talking about sex means talking about values, trust, commitment, and responsibility.

Sexual Decision Making

Sexual decision making always takes place within the context of an individual's values and perceptions of right and wrong behavior. Making sexually responsible decisions means considering all the possible consequences of sexual behavior for both yourself and your partner. It must always take into account, not just personal preferences and desires, but the very real risks of unwanted pregnancy, sexually transmitted infections (STIs), and long-term medical consequences (such as impaired fertility). You also must consider the emotional consequences of a sexual relationship—not just for yourself but also for your partner.

Talking About Sex

Prior to any sexual activity that involves a risk of sexually transmitted infection or pregnancy, both partners should talk about their prior sexual histories (including number of partners and exposure to STIs) and other high-risk behavior, such as the use of injection drugs. They should also discuss the issue of birth control and which methods might be best for them to use. If you know someone well enough to consider having sex with that person, you should be able to talk about such sensitive subjects. If a potential partner is unwilling to talk or hedges on crucial questions, you shouldn't be engaging in sex.

Styles of communicating vary among white Americans, African Americans, Hispanic Americans, and Asian Americans. While whites and African Americans may openly discuss sex with partners, Hispanic-American couples generally do not discuss their sexual relationship. Asian Americans also are less inclined to discuss sex and to value nonverbal, indirect, and intuitive communication over explicit verbal interaction.

Here are some questions to consider as you think and talk about the significance of becoming sexually intimate with a partner:

- **What role do we want relationships and sex to have in our life at this time?**
- **What are my values and my potential partner's values as they pertain to sexual relationships?** Does each of us believe that intercourse should be reserved for a permanent partnership or committed relationship?

vas deferens Two tubes that carry sperm from the epididymis into the urethra.

seminal vesicles Glands in the male reproductive system that produce the major portion of the fluid of semen.

ejaculatory duct The canal connecting the seminal vesicles and vas deferens.

prostate gland A structure surrounding the male urethra that produces a secretion that helps liquefy the semen from the testes.

Cowper's glands Two small glands that discharge into the male urethra, also called bulbourethral glands.

circumcision The surgical removal of the foreskin of the penis.

- **Will a decision to engage in sex enhance my positive feelings about myself or my partner?** Does either of us have questions about sexual orientation or the kinds of people we are attracted to?
- **Do I and my partner both want to have sex?** Is my partner pressuring me in any way? Am I pressuring my partner? Am I making this decision for myself or my partner?
- **Have my partner and I discussed our sexual histories and risk factors?** Have I spoken honestly about any STIs I've had in the past? Am I sure that neither my partner nor I have a sexually transmitted infection?
- **Have we taken precautions against unwanted pregnancy and STIs?**

Saying No to Sex

Whether couples are on a first date or have been married for years, each partner always has the right not to have sex. Unfortunately, "no" sometimes seems to mean different things to men and women.

The following strategies can help you assert yourself when saying no to sex:

- **First of all, recognize** your own values and feelings. If you believe that sex is something to be shared only by people who've already become close in other ways, be true to that belief.
- **Be direct.** Look the person in the eyes, keep your head up, and speak clearly and firmly.
- **Just say no.** Make it clear you're rejecting the offer, not the person. You don't owe anyone an explanation for what you want, but if you want to expand on your reasons, you might say, "I enjoy your company, and I'd like to do something together, but no," or "Thank you. I appreciate your interest, but no."
- **If you're still at a loss for words,** try these responses: "I like you a lot, but I'm not ready to have sex." "You're a great person, but sex isn't something I do to prove I like someone." "I'd like to wait until I'm married to have sex."
- **If you're feeling pressured,** let your date know that you're uncomfortable. Be simple and direct. Watch out for emotional blackmail. If your date says, "If you really like me, you'd want to make love," point out that if he or she really likes you, he or she wouldn't try to force you to do something you don't want to do.
- **If you're a woman, monitor your sexual signals.** Men impute more sexual meaning to gestures (such as casual touching) that women perceive as friendly and innocent.
- **Communicate your feelings** to your date sooner rather than later. It's far easier to say, "I don't want to go to your apartment" than to fight off unwelcome advances once you're there.
- **Remember that if saying no to sex** puts an end to a relationship, it wasn't much of a relationship in the first place.

Improving a Sexual Relationship

A sexually healthy relationship, as defined by the Sexuality Information and Education Council of the United States (SIECUS), is based on shared values and has five characteristics: It is consensual, nonexploitative, honest, mutually pleasurable, and protected against unintended pregnancy and sexually transmitted infections. All individuals also have sexual rights, which include the right to the information, education, skills, support, and services they need to make responsible decisions about their sexuality consistent with their own values, as well as the right to express their sexual orientation without violence or discrimination.

Communication is vital in a sexually healthy relationship, even though these discussions can be awkward. Yet if you have a need or a problem that relates to your partner, it is your responsibility to bring it up. Choose an appropriate time and place for an intimate discussion. In a new relationship, talking in a public place, such as a park bench or a quiet table at a coffee house, can seem safer. If you're in an established relationship, choose a time when you can give each other complete attention and a setting in which you can both relax.

Here are some specific suggestions that can help:

- **Ask open-ended questions** that encourage a dialogue, for instance, "How do you feel about . . . ?" or "What are your thoughts about . . . ?"
- **Listen actively** rather than passively when your partner speaks. Show that you're paying attention by nodding, smiling, and leaning forward. Paraphrase what he or she says to show you understand it fully.
- **Use "I" statements,** such as "I really enjoy making love, but I'm so tired right now that I won't be a responsive partner. Why don't we get the kids to bed early tomorrow so we can enjoy ourselves a little earlier?"
- **Speak up** if something hurts during sex. Be specific.
- **If you would like to try something different, say so.** Practice saying the words first if they embarrass you. If your partner feels uncomfortable, don't force the issue, but do try talking it through.
- **If you want to request changes** or tackle a touchy topic, start with positive statements. Let your partner know how much you enjoy having sex, and then express your desire to enjoy lovemaking more often or in different ways.
- **Encourage small changes.** If you want your partner to be less inhibited, start slowly, perhaps by suggesting sex in a different room or place.

? FAQ How Sexually Active Are College Students?

According to federal statistics, about two-thirds of never-married 18- to 19-year-olds—69 percent of women and 64 percent of men—have had intercourse. In a study of sex, drug use, and binge drinking on campus, more than a third of students reported no sexual intercourse in the previous 12 months.

Three in four students surveyed in the National College Health Assessment report having had one or no sexual partners in the past school year. However, undergraduates consistently think that their peers have had more partners and more frequent sex.[10] (See Student Snapshot Sex an Campus). In a recent study at a large university in the Northeast, students showed the same tendency to overestimate the sexual experiences of their classmates. For example, the mean number of sexual partners the students reported was 2.6, but they believed that the typical student had had 4.8 partners in the previous year.[11]

Sexual behavior on campus has changed dramatically in the last 25 years. Surveys conducted in the United States and in Canada since 1980 reveal a steady increase in the number of students who have had intercourse and an increase in safer sex practices among sexually active students. Today's undergraduates are more likely to question potential partners about their past, use condoms with a new partner, and maintain fairly long-term monogamous relationships.

College students see sexual activity as normal behavior for their peer group. When researchers at Pennsylvania State University conducted focus groups with undergraduates, most agreed that the majority of college students (80 to 90 percent, in their estimate) are sexually active and that alcohol and drug use make sexual activity more likely.

College students who binge drink or participate in drinking games, which often involve physical skills (such as bouncing a coin into a glass) or word play, increase their odds of sexually risky behavior. Both men and women report being taken advantage of sexually, including someone having sex with them when they were too drunk to give consent, after such games.

Annual spring breaks provide what researchers describe as "ideal conditions for the potentially lethal interaction between alcohol, drugs, and sexual risk-taking." Students typically engage in binge drinking, illicit drug use, and unsafe sexual practices. The likelihood of casual sex depends on several factors, including peer influences, prior experiences with casual sex, alcohol consumption prior to sex, and impulsivity.

As with other aspects of health, cultural, religious, and personal values affect students' sexual behaviors. Young Latina women have the highest teen birth rate in the United States (twice the national rate) and are at greater risk of sexually transmitted infections. Although Latinas represent about 10 percent of women over age 21, they account for 20 percent of female AIDS cases. Among college students and other populations, Latinas are more likely to engage in unprotected intercourse than women from other ethnic groups. Sexually active Latina college students also are less likely to use condoms than their peers from other ethnic groups.[12]

Acculturation—the process of adaptation that occurs when immigrants enter a new country—also affects sexual behavior. As Latina immigrants become more acculturated in the United States, some aspects of their sexual behavior become more Americanized; for instance, they become more likely to engage in nonmarital sexual activity and to have multiple partners. In a study of Cuban-American college women, older, less religious, and U.S.-born Latinas were more likely to be sexually active and to engage in risky sexual behavior than other Latinas.[13]

Student Snapshot

Sex on Campus

Number of Sexual Partners in the Last 12 Months vs. Perceived Number of Sexual Partners

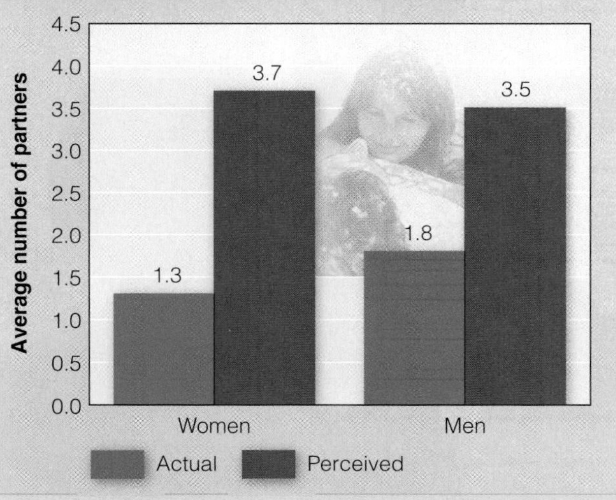

© Justin Pumfrey/Taxi/Getty Images

NCHA Fall 2005
Context area: Sexual Health Students self-reported data (n = 16,832)
Source: American College Health Association. American College Health Association-National College Health Assessment (ACHA-NCHA) Web Summary. Updated April 2006. Available at www.acha.org/projects_programs/ncha_sampledata.cfm.

? FAQ Why Don't College Students Practice Safer Sex?

Decades of education about sexual risks have had an impact. Most young Americans between the ages of 18 and 24 agree that "it's smart to carry condoms," according to a recent national survey. However, their words and actions often differ. Although nine in ten say they take personal responsibility for their sexual health, only half ask potential partners about sexually transmitted infections. Fewer than half always or often use a condom during sexual activity.

Researchers explain that the college environment "provides students with a sense of new independence, self-determination, and strong peer pressure to experiment with a variety of sexual behaviors." Yet by engaging in sex with multiple partners and not regularly using condoms, college students put themselves at high risk of contracting HIV and other sexual infections.

Providing information on sexual health does not influence condom use, nor does teaching specific communication skills. In one experiment, 106 heterosexual college students in sexually active relationships were taught specifically how to make direct requests for condom use and how to counter refusals from a partner. Nonetheless, the students did not change their subsequent communication or use condoms more consistently.

Trust is another issue that affects safer sex practices. Men tend to trust a woman as safe and healthy on the basis of the way she looks. Women trust a man because they believe they are in a monogamous relationship after a period of time (one month on average) or number of encounters (twelve). Neither men nor women base their feelings of trust on a discussion with a partner. They simply assume that a partner can be trusted and that condoms are not necessary.

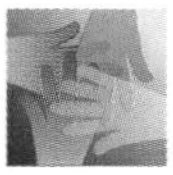

Race and ethnicity affect risk in the young. Young African-American men, who are more likely to be sexually active and to have more partners than young white men, also have higher STI infection rates. While the chlamydia rate for Hispanics is almost three times that of whites, the rate for blacks is ten times that of whites. The gonorrhea rate for African-American males aged 20 to 24 is 40 times that of whites. Although HIV infection rates have declined for all men, they are falling at a slower rate for African-American men.

As noted in Chapter 6, weight may affect risky sexual behaviors among college students. In a study of almost 1,000 undergraduates, sexually active women with the highest BMIs were more likely to have sex with a casual partner, to have multiple same-sex partners, and to recall being intoxicated at the time of their most recent sexual intercourse. There was no correlation between men's weight and their sexual behavior.[14]

The Sex Life of American Adults

The scientific study of Americans' sexual behavior began in 1938, when Alfred Kinsey, Ph.D., a professor of biology at the University of Indiana, and his colleagues asked 5,300 white men and 5,940 white women about their sexual practices. In his landmark studies—*Sexual Behavior in the Human Male,* published in 1948, and *Sexual Behavior in the Human Female,*published in 1953—Kinsey reported that 73 percent of men and 20 percent of women had premarital intercourse by age 20, and 37 percent of men and 17 percent of women had some homosexual experience in their lifetime.

The Janus Report on Sexual Behavior, published in 1993, was based on a survey of 2,765 individuals across the United States. A larger survey, conducted by researchers at the University of Chicago, was based on face-to-face interviews with 3,432 Americans, aged 18 to 59. It became the basis for two books published in 1994: *Sex in America,* aimed at a lay audience, and *The Social Organization of Sexuality,* a more scholarly work. Since then, the researcher's General Social Survey (GSS) database on sexual activity has grown to nearly 10,000 respondents.

The average American adult reports having sex about once a week. However, 1 in 5 Americans has been celibate for at least a year, and 1 in 20 engages in sex at least every other day. Men report more sexual frequency than women—not because men are more boastful about their prowess, the researchers contend, but because the sample of women includes many widows and older women without partners. Among married people, the frequency reports of husbands and wives (not in the same couples) are within one episode per year—58.6 for married men and 57.9 for married women. And if other differences between men and women are statistically controlled (such as sexual preference, age, and educational attainment), married women actually report a slightly higher frequency than men.

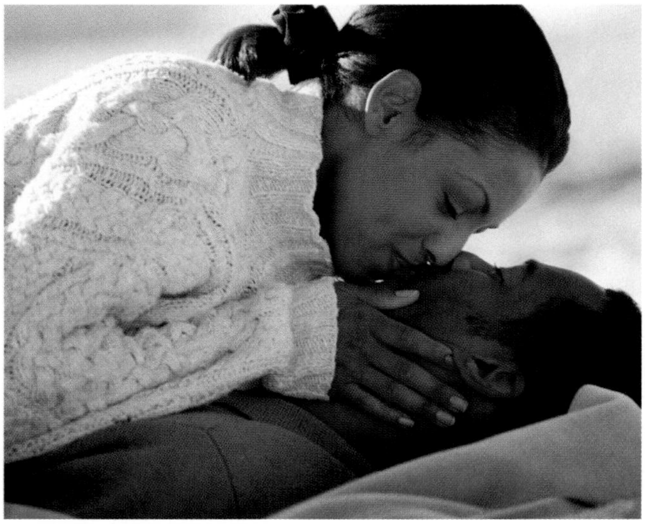

Thinkstock/Getty Images

In a loving, committed relationship, sex serves as an intimate form of communication.

Sexual frequency peaks among those with some college education, then decreases among four-year college graduates, and declines even further among those with professional degrees. Americans who have attended graduate school are the least sexually active educational group in the population. These respondents may be more honest than others in reporting sexual activity, or they may be more precise in their definition of what counts as sex.

Sexual Diversity

Human beings are diverse in all ways—including sexual preferences and practices. Physiological, psychological, and social factors determine whether we are attracted to members of the same sex or the other sex. This attraction is our **sexual orientation.** Sigmund Freud argued that we all start off **bisexual,** or attracted to both sexes. But by the time we reach adulthood, most males prefer female sexual partners, and most females prefer male partners. **Heterosexual** is the term used for individuals whose primary orientation is toward members of the other sex. In virtually all cultures, some men and women are **homosexuals,** preferring partners of their own sex.

In our society, we tend to view heterosexuality and homosexuality as very different. In reality, these orientations are opposite ends of a spectrum. Sex researcher Alfred Kinsey devised a seven-point continuum representing sexual orientation in American society. At one end of the continuum are those exclusively attracted to members of the other sex; at the opposite end are people exclusively attracted to members of the same sex. In between are varying degrees of homosexual, bisexual, and heterosexual orientation.

According to Kinsey's original data, 4 percent of men and 2 percent of women are exclusively homosexual. More recent studies have found lower numbers. For instance, in the University of Chicago's national survey, 2.8 percent of men and 1.4 percent of women defined themselves as homosexual. However, when asked if they'd had sex with a person of the same gender since age 18, about 5 percent of men and 4 percent of women said yes. When asked if they found members of the same gender sexually attractive, 6 percent of men and 5.5 percent of women said yes.

Most lesbian and bisexual women report that their first sexual experience occurred with a man (at the median age of 18) and that sex with a woman followed a few years later (at median age 21). Their most frequently reported sexual activities with men were mutual masturbation and vaginal penetration with penis or fingers. Their most common sex practices with women were oral sex, vaginal penetration with fingers, and mutual masturbation.

Bisexuality

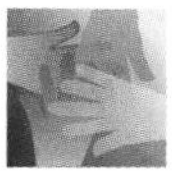

Bisexuality—sexual attraction to both males and females—can develop at any point in one's life. In some cultures, bisexual activity is considered part of normal sexual experimentation. Among the Sambia Highlanders in Papua New Guinea, for instance, boys perform oral sex on one another as part of the rites of passage into manhood.

Some people identify themselves as bisexual even if they don't behave bisexually. Some are *serial* bisexuals—that is, they are sexually involved with same-sex partners for a while and then with partners of the other sex, or vice versa. An estimated 7 to 9 million men, about twice the number thought to be exclusively homosexual, could be described as bisexual during some extended period of their lives. The largest group are married, rarely have sexual relations with women other than their wives, and have secret sexual involvements with men.

Fear of HIV infection has sparked great concern about bisexuality, particularly among heterosexual women who worry about becoming involved with a bisexual man. About 20 to 30 percent of women with AIDS were infected by bisexual partners, and health officials fear that bisexual men who hide their homosexual affairs could transmit HIV to many more women.

Homosexuality

Homosexuality—social, emotional, and sexual attraction to members of the same sex—exists in almost all cultures. Men and women homosexuals are commonly referred to as *gay;* women homosexuals are also called *lesbians.*

Homosexuality threatens and upsets many people, perhaps because homosexuals are viewed as different, or perhaps because no one understands why some people are heterosexual and others homosexual. *Homophobia* has led to an increase in *gay bashing* (attacking homosexuals) in many communities, including college campuses. Some blame the emergence of AIDS as a societal danger. However, researchers have found that fear of AIDS has not created new hostility but has simply given bigots an excuse to act out their hatred.

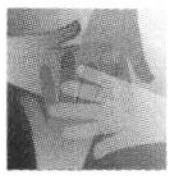

Different ethnic groups respond to homosexuality in different ways. To a greater extent than white homosexuals, gays and lesbians from

sexual orientation The direction of an individual's sexual interest, either to members of the opposite sex or to members of the same sex.

bisexual Sexually oriented toward both sexes.

heterosexual Primary sexual orientation toward members of the other sex.

homosexual Primary sexual orientation toward members of the same sex.

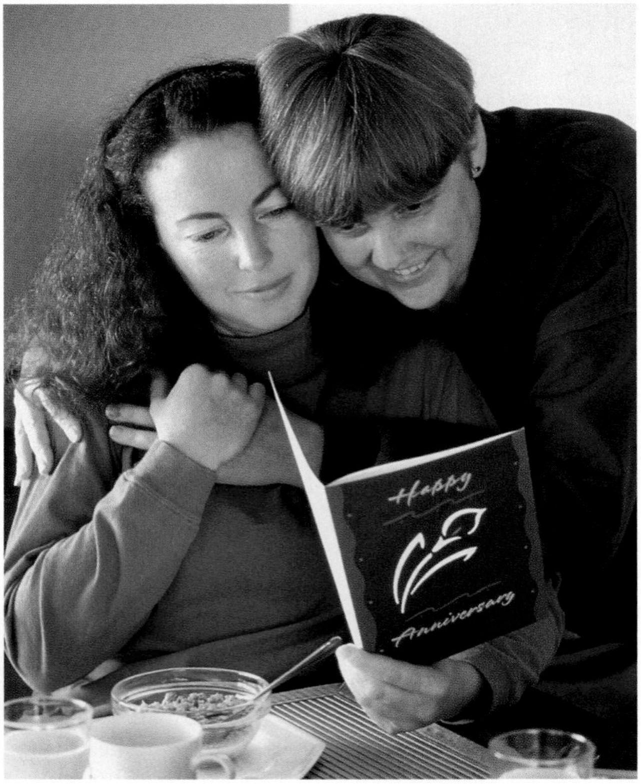

© Deborah Davis/PhotoEdit

Close-couple homosexual relationships are similar to stable heterosexual relationships.

ethnic groups tend to stay in the closet longer rather than risk alienation from their families and communities. Often they feel forced to choose between their gay and their ethnic identities.

In general, the African-American community has stronger negative views of homosexuals than whites, possibly because of the influence of strong fundamentalist Christian beliefs. Hispanic culture, with its emphasis on machismo, also has a very negative view of male homosexuality. Asian cultures, which tend to view an individual as a representative of his or her family, tend to view open declarations of sexual orientation as shaming the family and challenging their reputation and future.

Roots of Homosexuality

Most mental health experts agree that nobody knows what causes a person's sexual orientation. Research has discredited theories tracing homosexuality to troubled childhoods or abnormal psychological development. Sexual orientation probably emerges from a complex interaction that includes biological and environmental factors.

Homosexuality on Campus

In a study of almost 700 heterosexual students at six small liberal arts colleges, attitudes toward homosexuals and homosexuality varied, depending on students' membership in fraternities or sororities, sex role attitudes, religion and religiosity, and contact with and knowledge of gays, lesbians, and bisexuals. The students most likely to be accepting were women and those who had less traditional sex-role attitudes, were less religious, attended colleges that did not have Greek social clubs, and had gay, lesbian, and/or bisexual friends.

Transgenderism

The term **transgender** is used as an umbrella term to describe people who have gender identities, expressions, or behaviors not traditionally associated with their birth sex. Male-to-female transgenders have been assigned a male gender at birth, but identify their gender as female. Female-to-male transgenders at birth, but identify their gender as male.

Transgender individuals face varied health risks, including unprotected sex, sexually transmitted diseases, and HIV infection. Violence, including rape, sexual abuse, physical abuse, and suicide, is a major public health issue. In one study the majority of the transgender individuals reported being afraid for their life or physical safety at some point during their lives.

Sexual Activity

Part of learning about your own sexuality is having a clear understanding of human sexual behaviors. Understanding frees us from fear and anxiety so that we can accept ourselves and others as the natural sexual beings we all are.

Celibacy

A celibate person does not engage in sexual activity. Complete **celibacy** means that the person doesn't masturbate (stimulate himself or herself sexually) or engage in sexual activity with a partner. In partial celibacy, the person masturbates but doesn't have sexual contact with others. Many people decide to be celibate at certain times of their lives. Some don't have sex because of concerns about pregnancy or STIs; others haven't found a partner for a permanent, monogamous relationship. Many simply have other priorities, such as finishing school or starting a career, and realize that sex outside of a committed relationship is a threat to their physical and psychological well-being.

? FAQ What Does It Mean to Abstain?

The CDC defines **abstinence** as "refraining from sexual activities which involve vaginal, anal, and oral intercourse." The definition of abstinence remains a subject of debate and controversy, with some emphasizing positive choices and others avoidance of specific behaviors. In reality abstinence means different things to different people, cultures, and religious groups.

Increasing numbers of adolescents and young adults are choosing to remain virgins and abstain from sexual intercourse until they enter a permanent, committed, monogamous relationship. About 2.5 million teens have taken pledges to abstain from sex. According to a major study, teens who do so are 34 percent less likely to have premarital sex than others and are far older when they finally engage in intercourse. The federal government, which has promoted abstinence as a means of preventing pregnancy and sexually transmitted infections, funded abstinence education programs for two decades.

Although abstinence represents a healthy choice, major health organizations, such as the Society for Adolescent Medicine, have concluded that "abstinence-only education programs provide incomplete and/or misleading information about contraceptives, or none at all, and are often insensitive to sexually active teenagers." Although abstinence remains an important option for teenagers, the Society for Adolescent Medicine, among others, is urging that abstinence-only programs be abandoned.[15]

Many people who were sexually active in the past also are choosing abstinence because the risk of medical complications associated with STIs increases with the number of sexual partners a person has. Abstinence is the safest, healthiest option for many. However, there is confusion about what it means to abstain, and individuals who think they are abstaining may still be engaging in behaviors that put them at risk for HIV and STIs. (See Chapter 8 for more on abstinence as a form of birth control.)

Why abstain? Among the reasons students give are:

- **Remaining a virgin until** you meet someone you love and see as a life partner.
- **Being true to your religious and moral values.**
- **Getting to know a partner better.**
- **If you're heterosexual, to avoid pregnancy.**
- **To be sure you're safe from sexually transmitted infections.**

Fantasy

The mind is the most powerful sex organ in the body, and erotic mental images can be sexually stimulating. Sexual fantasies can accompany sexual activity or be pleasurable in themselves. Fantasies generally enhance sexual arousal, reduce anxiety, and boost sexual desire. They're also a way to anticipate and rehearse new sexual experiences, as well as to bolster a person's self-image and feelings of desirability. Part of what makes fantasies exciting is that they provide an opportunity for expressing forbidden desires, such as sex with a different partner or with a past lover.

Men and women have different types of sexy thoughts, with men's fantasies containing more explicit genital images and culminating in sexual acts more quickly than women's. In women's fantasies, emotional feelings play a greater role, and there is more kissing and caressing rather than genital contact. For many women, fantasy helps in reaching orgasm during intercourse; a loss of fantasy often is a sign of low sexual desire.

Masturbation

Not everybody masturbates, but most people do. Kinsey estimated that 7 out of 10 women and 19 out of 20 men masturbate (and admit they do). Their reason is simple: It feels good. Masturbation produces the same physical responses as sexual activity with a partner and can be an enjoyable form of sexual release.

Masturbation has been described as immature; unsocial; tiring; frustrating; and a cause of hairy palms, warts, blemishes, and blindness. None of these myths is true. Sex educators recommend masturbation to adolescents as a means of releasing tension and becoming familiar with their sexual organs. Throughout adulthood, masturbation often is the primary sexual activity of individuals not involved in a sexual relationship and can be particularly useful when illness, absence, divorce, or death deprives a person of a partner.

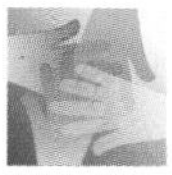

White men and women have a higher incidence of masturbation than African-American men and women. Latina women have the lowest rate of masturbation, compared with Latino men, white men and women, and black men and women. Individuals with a higher level of education are more likely to masturbate than those with less schooling, and people living with sexual partners masturbate more than those who live alone.

Nonpenetrative Sexual Activity (Outercourse)

Various pleasurable behaviors can lead to orgasm with little risk of pregnancy or sexually transmitted infection. The options for "outercourse" include kissing and hugging but do not involve genital-to-genital, mouth-to-genital, or insertive anal sexual contact.

A kiss is a universal sign of affection. A kiss can be just a kiss—a quick press of the lips—or it can lead to much more. Usually kissing is the first sexual activity that couples engage in, and even after years of sexual experimentation and sharing, it remains an enduring pleasure for partners.

transgender Having a gender identity opposite to one's biological sex.

celibacy Abstention from sexual activity; can be partial or complete, permanent or temporary.

abstinence Voluntary refrainment from sexual intercourse.

Touching is a silent form of communication between friends and lovers. Although a touch to any part of the body can be thrilling, some areas, such as the breasts and genitals, are especially sensitive. Stimulating these **erogenous** regions can lead to orgasm in both men and women. Though such forms of stimulation often accompany intercourse, more couples are gaining an appreciation of these activities as primary sources of sexual fulfillment—and as safer alternatives to intercourse.

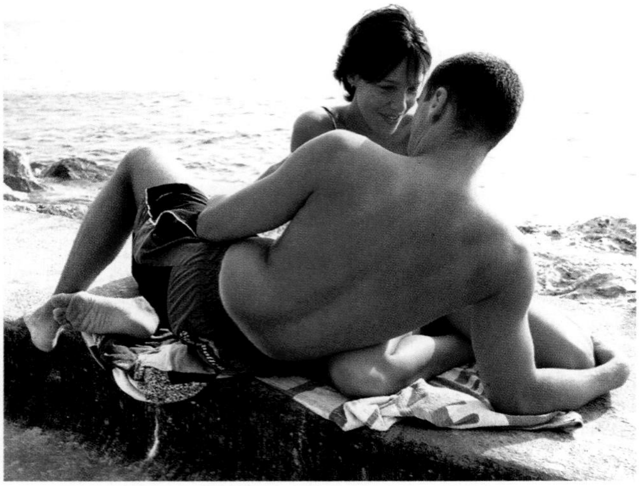

Touch—thrilling, soothing, stimulating—is a powerful way to communicate affection and sexual pleasure.

Intercourse

Vaginal **intercourse,** or coitus, refers to the penetration of the vagina by the penis (Figure 7-6). This is the preferred form of sexual intimacy for most heterosexual couples, who may use a wide variety of positions. The most familiar position for intercourse in our society is the so-called missionary position, with the man on top, facing the woman. An alternative is the woman on top, either lying down or sitting upright. Other positions include lying side by side (either face to face or with the man behind the woman, his penis entering her vagina from the rear); lying with the man on top of the woman in a rear-entry position; and kneeling or standing (again, in either a face-to-face or rear-entry position). Many couples move into several different positions for intercourse during a single episode of lovemaking; others may have a personal favorite or may choose different positions at different times.

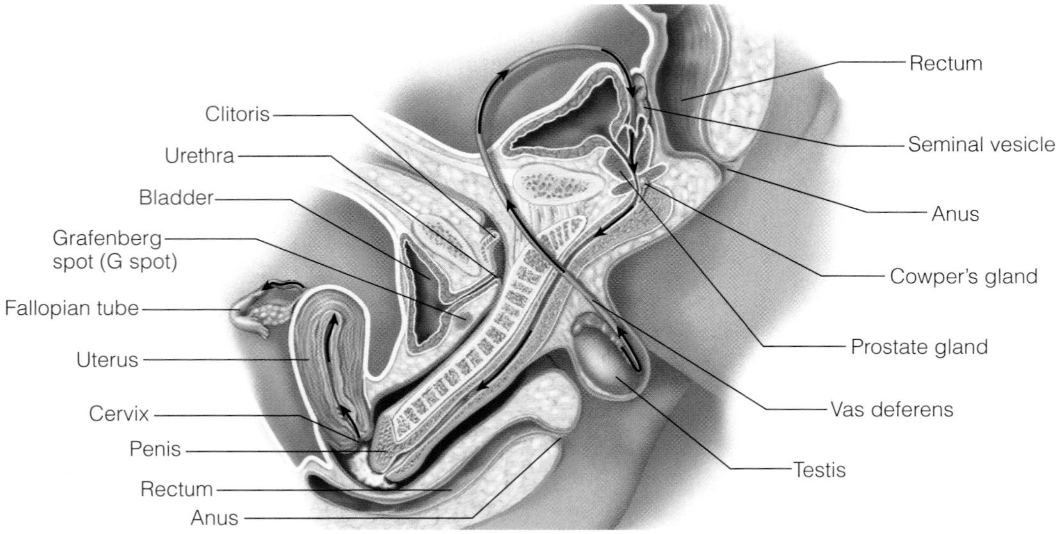

FIGURE 7-6 A Cross-Sectional View of Sexual Intercourse

Sperm are formed in each of the testes and stored in the epididymis. When a man ejaculates, sperm traveling in semen travel up the vas deferens. (The prostate gland and seminal vesicles contribute components of the semen.) The semen is expelled from the penis through the urethra and deposited in the vagina, near the cervix. During sexual excitement and orgasm in a woman, the upper end of the vagina enlarges and the uterus elevates. After orgasm, these organs return to their normal states, and the cervix descends into the pool of semen.

SAVVY CONSUMER

X-Rated Websites

Sex is the number-one word searched for online. About 15 percent of Americans logging onto the Internet visit sexually oriented sites. Men are the largest consumers of sexually explicit material and outnumber women by a ratio of six to one. However, while men look for visual erotica, women are more likely to visit chat rooms, which offer more interactions. Most people who check out sex sites on the Internet do not suffer any negative impact, but psychologists warn of some potential risks, including the following:

- **Dependence.** Individuals who spend 11 hours or more a week online in sexual pursuits show signs of psychological distress and admit that their behavior interferes with some areas of their lives.
- **Interference with work and study.** While most individuals use their home computers when surfing the Internet for sex-related sites, one in ten has used a school computer. Some universities have strict policies barring such practices and may take punitive actions against employees who violate the rules.
- **Sexual compulsivity.** A small but significant number of users are at risk of a serious problem as a result of their heavy Internet use.
- **Dishonesty.** Most Internet surfers admit that they occasionally "pretend" about their age on the Internet. Most keep secret how much time they spend on sexual pursuits in cyberspace.

Sexual activity, including intercourse, is possible throughout a woman's menstrual cycle. However, some women prefer to avoid sex while menstruating because of uncomfortable physical symptoms, such as cramps, or concern about bleeding or messiness. Others use a diaphragm or cervical cap (see Chapter 8) to hold back menstrual flow. Since different cultures have different views on intercourse during a woman's period, partners should discuss their own feelings and try to respect each other's views. If they choose not to have intercourse, there are other gratifying forms of sexual activity.

Vaginal intercourse, like other forms of sexual activity involving an exchange of bodily fluids, carries a risk of sexually transmitted infections, including HIV infection. In many other parts of the world, in fact, heterosexual intercourse is the most common means of HIV transmission (see Chapter 9.)

Oral Sex

Our mouths and genitals give us some of our most intense pleasures. Though it might seem logical to combine the two, some people are very uncomfortable with it. Some people consider oral-genital sex a perversion; it is against the law in some states and a sin in some religions. However, others find it normal and acceptable.

The formal terms for oral sex are **cunnilingus,** which refers to oral stimulation of the woman's genitals, and **fellatio,** oral stimulation of the man's genitals. For many couples, oral sex is a regular part of their lovemaking. For others, it's an occasional experiment. Oral sex with a partner carrying a sexually transmitted infection, such as herpes or HIV infection, can lead to infection, so a condom should be used (with cunnilingus, a condom cut in half to lay flat can be used).

Anal Stimulation and Intercourse

Because the anus has many nerve endings, it can produce intense erotic responses. Stimulation of the anus by the fingers or mouth can be a source of sexual arousal;

erogenous Sexually sensitive.

intercourse Sexual stimulation by means of entry of the penis into the vagina; coitus.

cunnilingus Sexual stimulation of a woman's genitals by means of oral manipulation.

fellatio Sexual stimulation of a man's genitals by means of oral manipulation.

anal intercourse involves penile penetration of the anus. An estimated 25 percent of adults have experienced anal intercourse at least once. However, anal sex involves important health risks, such as damage to sensitive rectal tissues and the transmission of various intestinal infections, hepatitis, and STIs, including HIV.

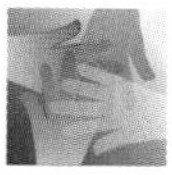

Cultural Variations

While the biological mechanisms underlying human sexual arousal and response are essentially universal, the particular sexual stimuli or behaviors that people find arousing are greatly influenced by cultural conditioning. For example, in Western societies, where the emphasis during sexual activity tends to be heavily weighted toward achieving orgasm, genitally focused activities are frequently defined as optimally arousing. In contrast, devotees to Eastern Tantric traditions (where spirituality is interwoven with sexuality) often achieve optimal pleasure by emphasizing the sensual and spiritual aspects of shared intimacy rather than orgasmic release.

Kissing on the mouth, a universal source of sexual arousal in Western society, may be rare or absent in many other parts of the world. Certain North American Eskimo people and inhabitants of the Trobriand Islands would rather rub noses than lips, and among the Thonga of South Africa, kissing is viewed as odious behavior. The Hindu people of India are also disinclined to kiss because they believe such contact symbolically contaminates the act of sexual intercourse. One survey of 190 societies found that mouth kissing was acknowledged in only 21 societies and practiced as a prelude or accompaniment to coitus in only 13.

Oral sex (both cunnilingus and fellatio) is a common source of sexual arousal among island societies of the South Pacific, in industrialized nations of Asia, and in much of the Western world. In contrast, in Africa (with the exception of northern regions), such practices are likely to be viewed as unnatural or disgusting behavior.

Foreplay in general, whether it be oral sex, sensual touching, or passionate kissing, is subject to wide cultural variation. In some societies, most notably those with Eastern traditions, couples may strive to prolong intense states of sexual arousal for several hours. While varied patterns of foreplay are common in Western cultures, these activities often are of short duration as lovers move rapidly toward the "main event" of coitus. In still other societies, foreplay is either sharply curtailed or absent altogether. For example, the Lepcha farmers of the southeastern Himalayas limit foreplay to men briefly caressing their partners' breasts, and among the Irish inhabitants of Inis Beag, precoital sexual activity is reported to be limited to mouth kissing and rough fondling of the woman's lower body by her partner.

LEARN IT / LIVE IT

Being Sexually Responsible

We remain sexual beings throughout life. At different ages and stages, sexuality can take on different meanings. As you forge relationships and explore your sexuality, you may encounter difficult situations and unfamiliar feelings. But sex is never just about hormones and body parts. People describe the brain as the sexiest of our organs. Using your brain to make responsible sexual decisions leads to both a smarter and a more fulfilling sex life.

- **Communicate openly.** If you or your partner cannot talk openly and honestly about your sexual histories and contraception, you should avoid having sex. For the sake of protecting your sexual health, you have to be willing to ask—and answer—questions that may seem embarrassing.
- **Share responsibility in a sexual relationship.** Both partners should be involved in protecting themselves and each other from STIs and, if heterosexual, unwanted pregnancy.
- **Respect sexual privacy.** Revealing sexual activities violates the trust between two partners. Bragging about a sexual conquest demeans everyone involved.
- **Do not sexually harass others.** Pinches, pats, sexual comments or jokes, and suggestive gestures are offensive and disrespectful.
- **Be considerate.** A public display of sexual affection can be extremely embarrassing to others. Roommates, in particular, should be sensitive and discrete in their sexual behavior.
- **Be prepared.** If there's any possibility that you may be engaging in sex, be sure you have the means to protect yourself against unwanted pregnancy and sexually transmitted infections.
- **In sexual situations, always think ahead.** For the sake of safety, think about potential dangers—parking in an isolated area, going into a bedroom with someone you hardly know, and the like—and options to protect yourself.
- **Be aware of your own and your partner's alcohol and drug intake.** The use of such substances impairs judgment and reduces the ability to say no. While under their influence, you may engage in sexual behavior you'll later regret.
- **Be sure sexual activity is consensual.** Coercion can take many forms: physical, emotional, and verbal. All cause psychological damage and

undermine trust and respect. At any point in a relationship, whether the couple is dating or married, either individual has the right to say no.

Source: Adapted from Hatcher, Robert, et al. *Sexual Etiquette 101 and More.* Atlanta, GA: Emory University School of Medicine, 2002.

7 Making This Chapter Work for You

Review Questions

1. In friendships and other intimate relationships, which of the following is *not* true?
   a. Friends can communicate feelings as well as facts.
   b. Listening is just as important as talking.
   c. Emotional investment is required but the rewards are great.
   d. There is no need to pay attention to nonverbal communication.
2. The characteristics of a good relationship include which of the following?
   a. trust
   b. financial stability
   c. identical interests
   d. physical attractiveness
3. Which of the following is more likely a sign of a dysfunctional relationship?
   a. The partners have frequent disagreements about money.
   b. One partner makes all the decisions for the couple and the other partner.
   c. Each partner has a demanding career.
   d. One partner is much older than the other partner.
4. Partners in successful marital relationships
   a. are generally from the same social and ethnic background.
   b. usually lived together before marrying.
   c. were usually very young at the time of their marriage.
   d. have premarital agreements.
5. Which of the following statements about the menstrual cycle is true?
   a. The pituitary gland releases estrogen and progesterone.
   b. Ovulation occurs at the end of the menstrual cycle.
   c. Premenstrual syndrome is a physiological disorder that usually results in amenorrhea.
   d. The endometrium becomes thicker during the cycle and is shed during menstruation.
6. Which statement about male anatomy is *incorrect?*
   a. The testes manufacture testosterone and sperm.
   b. Sperm cells are carried in the liquid semen.
   c. Cowper's glands secrete semen.
   d. Circumcision is the surgical removal of the foreskin of the penis.
7. Which of the following behaviors is most likely to be a characteristic of sexually healthy and responsible adults?
   a. engages in frequent sexual encounters with many partners
   b. avoids the use of condoms in order to heighten sexual enjoyment for both partners
   c. uses alcohol sparingly and only to help loosen the inhibitions of a resistant partner
   d. engages in sex that is unquestionably consensual
8. Which of the following statements is true about sexual orientation?
   a. Most individuals who identify themselves as bisexual are really homosexual.
   b. Homosexuality is caused by a poor family environment.
   c. Homosexual behavior is found only in affluent and well-educated cultures.
   d. The African-American, Hispanic, and Asian cultures tend to be less accepting of homosexuality than the white community.
9. According to the Centers for Disease Control, abstinence is defined as
   a. refraining from all sexual behaviors that result in arousal.
   b. refraining from all sexual activities that involve vaginal, anal, and oral intercourse.
   c. having sexual intercourse with only one partner exclusively.
   d. refraining from drinking alcohol before sexual activity.
10. Which statement about college students is *not* true?
   a. They consider sexual activity as normal for their peer group.
   b. Most take sex and monogamy seriously.
   c. More than 40 percent do not use condoms.
   d. Women trust a man as safe and healthy on the basis of the way he looks.

Answers to these questions can be found on page 422.

Critical Thinking

1. Bill has told his girlfriend, Anita, that he has never taken any sexual risks. But when she suggested that they get tested for STIs, he became furious and refused. Now Anita says she doesn't know what to believe. Could Bill be telling the truth, or is he hiding something? If he is telling the truth, why is Bill so upset? Anita doesn't want to take any risks, but she doesn't want to lose him either.

What would you advise her to say or do? What would you advise Bill to say or do?

2. While our society has become more tolerant, marriages between people of different religious and racial groups still face special pressures. What issues might arise if a Christian marries a Jew or Muslim? What about the issues facing partners of different races? How could these issues be resolved? What are your own feelings about mixed marriages? Would you date someone of a different religion or race? Why or why not?
3. What are your personal criteria for a successful relationship? Develop a brief list of factors you consider important, and support your choices with examples or experiences from your own life.

Media Menu

ThomsonNOW™ Go to the ThomsonNOW website at **http://www.thomsonedu.com** that will:

- Help you evaluate your knowledge of the material.
- Allow you to take an exam-prep quiz.
- Provide a Personalized Learning Plan targeting resources that address areas you should study.
- Coach you through identifying target goals for behavioral change and creating and monitoring your personal change plan throughout the semester.

INTERNET CONNECTIONS

The Sexuality Information and Education Council of the United States (SIECUS)
www.siecus.org

This website is sponsored by SIECUS, a national nonprofit organization that promotes comprehensive education about sexuality and advocates the right of all individuals of all sexual orientations to make responsible sexual choices. The site features a library of fact sheets and articles designed for educators, adults, teens, parents, media, international audiences, and religious organizations on a variety of sexuality topics and STIs.

Youth.org
www.youth.org

This website provides information on gay, lesbian, bisexual, and questioning youth and provides young people with a safe space online to be themselves, to know they are not alone, and to interact with others who have already accepted their sexuality.

Family and relationship articles from the APA
www.apahelpcenter.org/articles/topic.php?id=2

The American Psychological Association provides a wealth of articles and information on sustaining healthy relationships.

Go Ask Alice
www.goaskalice.columbia.edu/index.html

Sponsored by the health education and wellness program of the Columbia University Health Service, this site features educators' answers to questions on a wide variety of topics of concern to young people, including those related to sexual orientation and healthy sexuality.

- InfoTrac College Edition Activities Log on, insert **safe sex** into the Keyword search box, and limit your search to the past year. When you get the results, Mark articles to review, then Select one to read. Summarize three or four key points from the article.

You can find additional readings related to personal health with InfoTrac College Edition, an online library of more than 900 journals and publications. Follow the instructions for accessing InfoTrac College Edition that were packaged with your textbook; then search for articles using a keyword search.

For additional links, resources, and suggested readings on InfoTrac College Edition, visit our Health and Wellness Resource Center at **http://health.wadsworth.com.**

Key Terms

The terms listed are used on the page indicated. Definitions of the terms are in the Glossary at the end of this book.

abstinence 186
amenorrhea 179
bisexual 185
celibacy 186
cervix 175
circumcision 180
clitoris 175
cohabitation 170
corpus luteum 175
Cowper's glands 180
cunnilingus 189
dysfunctional 167
dysmenorrhea 179
ejaculatory ducts 180
endometrium 175
epididymis 179
erogenous 188
fallopian tubes 175
family 174
fellatio 189
heterosexual 185
homosexual 185
intercourse 188
intimacy 169
labia majora 175
labia minora 175
menstruation 175
mons pubis 175
ovum (ova) 175
ovaries 175
ovulation 175
penis 179
perineum 175
premenstrual dysphoric disorder (PMDD) 178
premenstrual syndrome (PMS) 178

LACC Extra Credit Assignment

7. Discuss what attributes are personally necessary for a long term relationship if its death till you part.

prostate gland 180
scrotum 179
semen 179
seminal vesicles 180
sexual health 175
sexual orientation 185
sperm 179
testes 179
toxic shock syndrome (TSS) 179
transgender 186
urethra 179
urethral opening 175
uterus 175
vagina 175
vas deferens 180

8 Reproductive Choices

REAL HEALTH

Jess and Sara, juniors at the same community college, can't remember a time when safe sex wasn't a concern of every sexually active individual. Yet even though they were aware of the risks, neither used contraception during every single sexual encounter. Then one of Jess's partners had a pregnancy scare. He decided never again to engage in unprotected sex. Sara had a different reality check: At her regular physical, she learned that she had contracted chlamydia, the most common sexually transmitted infection in the United States.

When Jess and Sara started dating, they decided to take every step toward intimacy slowly. Both talked about their personal priorities and concerns. Even though it was awkward, they also discussed their own sexual histories and underwent tests for STIs.

Looking toward a continuing committed relationship, they decided on not one but two forms of contraception: the birth control pill and a condom. In the future, they realized that they might switch to other forms of birth control—and might well consider different options, including both marriage and parenthood.

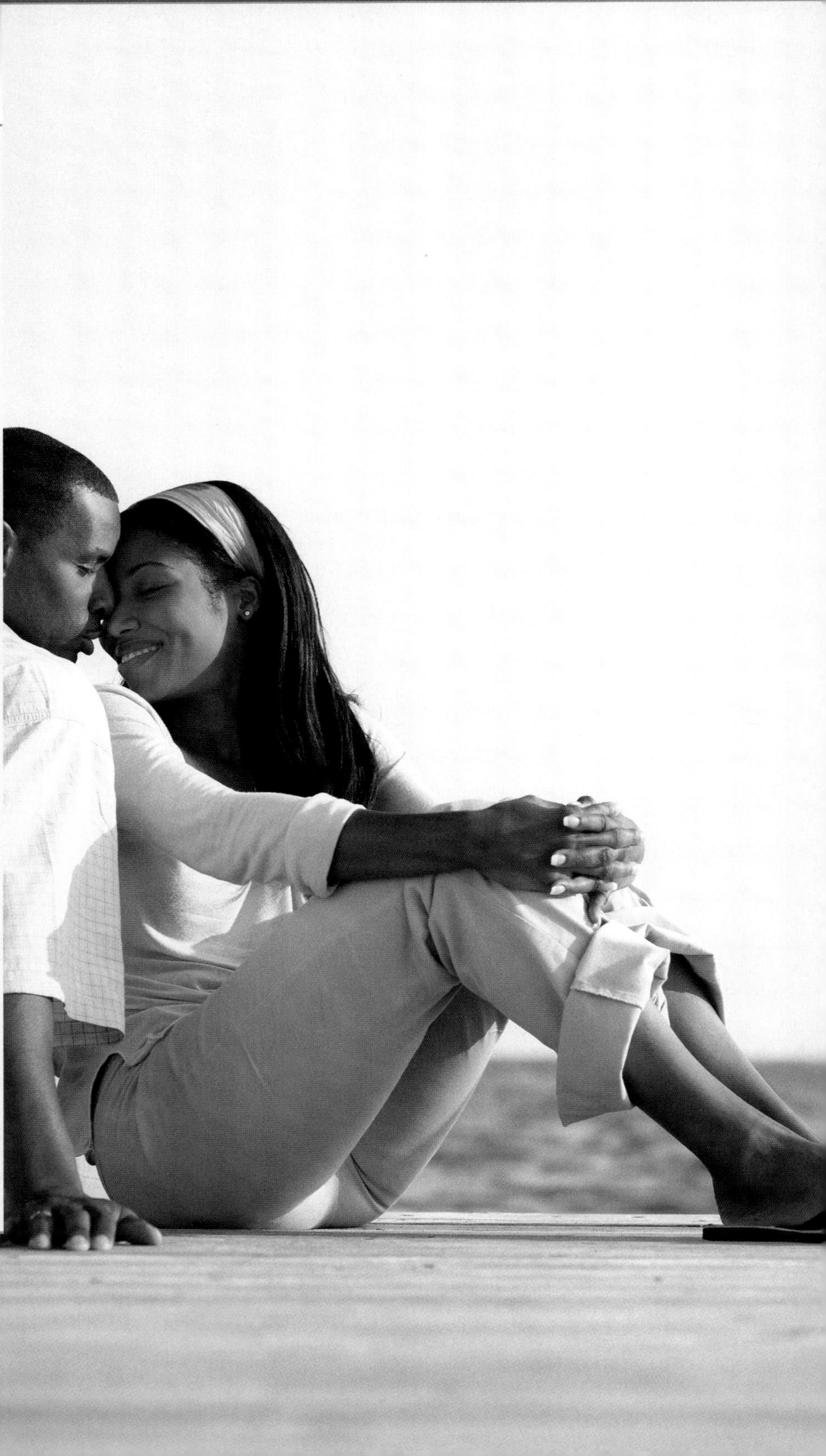

As human beings, we have a unique power: the ability to choose to conceive or not to conceive. No other species on Earth can separate sexual activity and pleasure from reproduction. However, simply not wanting to get pregnant is never enough to prevent conception; nor is wanting to have a child always enough to get pregnant. Both desires require individual decisions and actions.

Anyone who engages in vaginal intercourse must be willing to accept the consequences of that activity—the possibility of pregnancy and responsibility for the child who might be conceived—or take action to avoid those consequences. Although many people are concerned about the risks associated with contraception, using birth control is safer and healthier than not using it. According to the Population Reference Bureau, the use of contraceptives, including oral contraceptives, saves millions of lives each year. Some forms of contraception also reduce the risk of sexually transmitted infections.

This chapter provides information on conception, birth control, abortion, infertility, pregnancy, and the processes by which a new human life develops and enters the world.

? FAQ Frequently Asked Questions

- Do men and women use condoms for different reasons? *p. 209*
- What is emergency contraception? *p. 212*
- What is the psychological impact of abortion? *p. 216*
- What is childbirth like? *p. 221*
- What are the options for infertile couples? *p. 223*

After studying the material in this chapter, you should be able to:

- **List** the major options available for contraception, and **identify** the advantages and disadvantages of each.
- **Describe** the commonly used abortion methods.
- **Discuss** the physiological effects of pregnancy on a woman and **describe** fetal development.
- **Describe** the three stages of labor and the birth process.

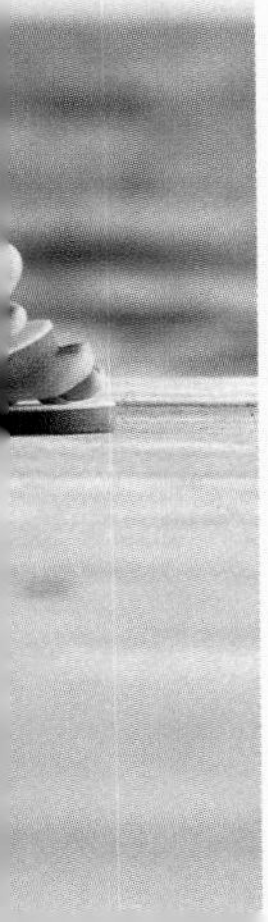

© LWA/Dann Tardif/Jupiter

ThomsonNOW™ Log on to ThomsonNOW at **www.thomsonedu.com/thomsonnow** to find your Behavior Change Planner and to explore self-assessments, interactive tutorials, and practice quizzes.

Conception

The equation for making a baby is quite simple: One sperm plus one egg equals one fertilized egg, which can develop into an infant. But the processes that affect or permit **conception** are quite complicated. The creation of sperm, or **spermatogenesis,** starts in the male at puberty, and the production of sperm is regulated by hormones. Sperm cells form in the seminiferous tubules of the testes and are passed into the epididymis, where they are stored until ejaculation (Figure 8-1); a single male ejaculation may contain 500 million sperm. Each sperm released into the vagina during intercourse moves on its own, propelling itself toward its target, an ovum.

To reach its goal, the sperm must move through the acidic secretions of the vagina, enter the uterus, travel up the fallopian tube containing the ovum, then fuse with the nucleus of the egg (**fertilization**). Just about every sperm produced by a man in his lifetime fails to accomplish its mission.

There are far fewer human egg cells than there are sperm cells. Each woman is born with her lifetime supply of ova, and between 300 and 500 eggs eventually mature and leave her ovaries during ovulation. As discussed in Chapter 7, every month, one or the other of the woman's ovaries releases an ovum to the nearby fallopian tube. It travels through the fallopian tube until it reaches the uterus, a journey that takes three to four days. An unfertilized egg lives for about 24 to 36 hours, disintegrates, and during menstruation is expelled along with the uterine lining.

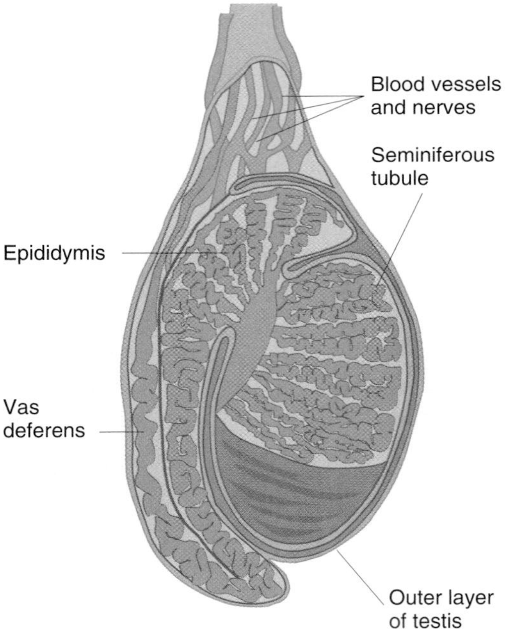

FIGURE 8-1 The Testes

Spermatogenesis takes place in the testes. Sperm cells form in the seminiferous tubules and are stored in the coils of the epididymis. Eventually, the sperm drain into the vas deferens, ready for ejaculation.

Even if a sperm, which can survive in the female reproductive tract for two to five days, meets a ripe egg in a fallopian tube, its success is not assured. A mature ovum releases the chemical allurin, which attracts the sperm. A sperm is able to penetrate the ovum's outer membrane because of a protein called fertilin. The egg then pulls the sperm inside toward its nucleus (Figure 8-2). The fertilized egg travels down the fallopian tube, dividing to form a tiny clump of cells called a **zygote.** When it reaches the uterus, about a week after fertilization, it burrows into the endometrium, the lining of the uterus. This process is called **implantation.**

Conception can be prevented by **contraception.** Some contraceptive methods prevent ovulation or implantation, and others block the sperm from reaching the egg. Some methods are temporary; others permanently alter one's fertility.

Birth Control Basics

Most sexually active women use some form of birth control. According to the Centers for Disease Control and Prevention, more than 98 percent of women between the ages of 15 and 44 who have ever had intercourse have used at least one contraceptive method. Most of the women not using any form of contraception are pregnant, trying to get pregnant, unable to conceive, or not having intercourse.

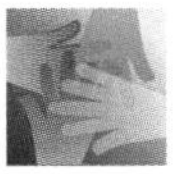

The use of contraception has declined in recent years, particularly among poor women. As a result, they are more likely to get pregnant unintentionally and to have abortions. An estimated 11 percent of sexually active women, including white, Hispanic, and black women who are not trying to get pregnant do not use birth control, up from 7 percent in 1994. The rate of unintended births also has risen. About half of the three million pregnancies that occur every year in the United States are unintended. Half of these are carried to term. About 14,000 women who continue their pregnancies put the children up for adoption; 1.3 million women have abortions.[1] Among sexually active students, 2 percent of women and 2 percent of men report having become pregnant or having gotten someone pregnant unintentionally in the past year.[2]

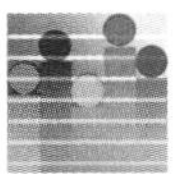

If you are engaging in sexual activity that could lead to conception, you have to be realistic about your situation. This may mean assuming full responsibility for your reproductive ability, whether you're a man or a woman. The more you know about contraception, the more likely you are to use birth control.

You also have to recognize the risks associated with various methods of contraception. If you're a woman, the risks are chiefly yours. Various methods of birth control

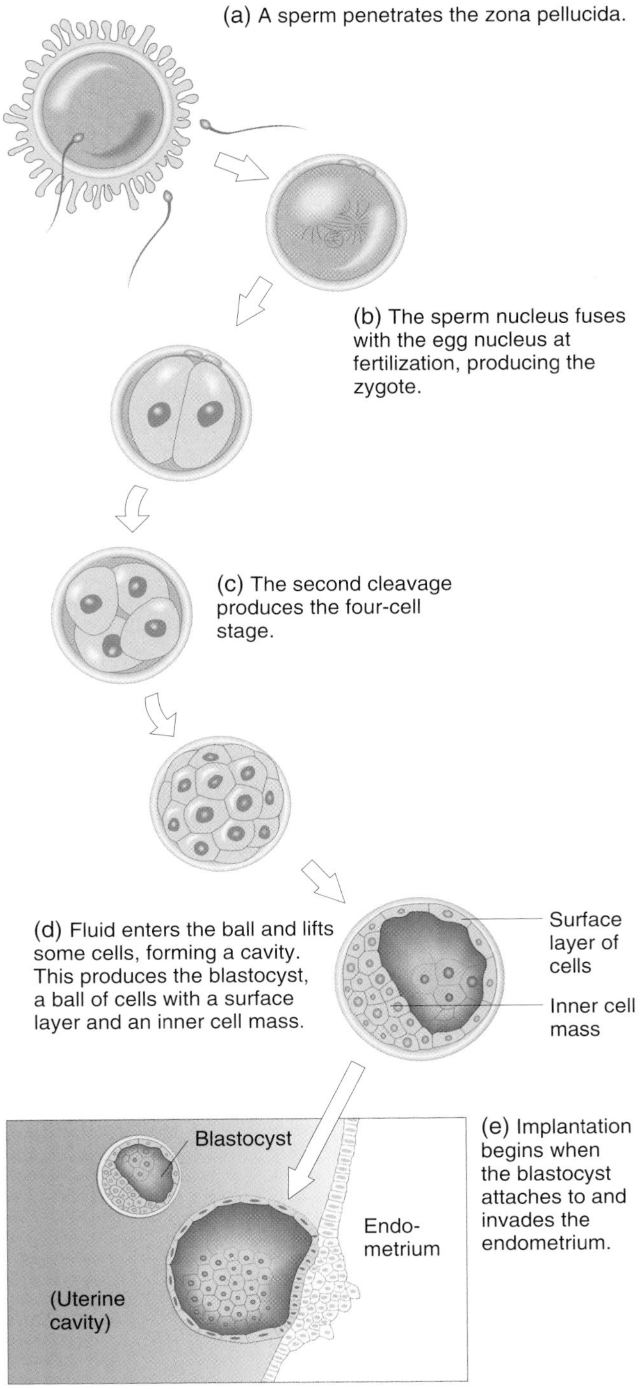

(a) A sperm penetrates the zona pellucida.
(b) The sperm nucleus fuses with the egg nucleus at fertilization, producing the zygote.
(c) The second cleavage produces the four-cell stage.
(d) Fluid enters the ball and lifts some cells, forming a cavity. This produces the blastocyst, a ball of cells with a surface layer and an inner cell mass.
Surface layer of cells
Inner cell mass
Blastocyst
Endo-metrium
(Uterine cavity)
(e) Implantation begins when the blastocyst attaches to and invades the endometrium.

FIGURE 8-2 Fertilization

(a) The efforts of hundreds of sperm may allow one to penetrate the ovum's corona radiata, an outer layer of cells, and then the zona pellucida, a thick inner membrane. (b) The nuclei of the sperm and the egg cells merge, and the male and female chromosomes in the nuclei come together, forming a zygote. (c) The zygote divides into two cells, then four cells, and so on. (d) As fluid enters the ball, cells form a ball of cells called a blastocyst. (e) The blastocyst implants itself in the endometrium.

have side effects, but pregnancy and childbirth account for much higher rates of medical complications and deaths than any contraceptive. Although most women never experience any serious complications, it's important to be aware of the potential for long-term risks. Risks that are acceptable to others may not be acceptable to you.

YOUR LIFE COACH

Choosing a Birth Control Method

When it comes to deciding which form of birth control to use, there's no one "right" decision. Good decisions are based on sound information. You should consult a physician or family-planning counselor if you have questions or want to know how certain methods might affect existing or familial medical conditions, such as high blood pressure or diabetes.

Table 8-1 presents your contraceptive choices. As the table indicates, contraception doesn't always work. When you evaluate any contraceptive, always consider its *effectiveness* (the likelihood that it will indeed prevent pregnancy). The **failure rate** refers to the number of pregnancies that occur per year for every 100 women using a particular method of birth control.

The reliability of contraceptives in actual, real-life use is much lower than those reported in national surveys or clinical trials. In general, failure rates are highest among cohabiting and other unmarried women, very poor families, black and Hispanic women, adolescents, and women in their twenties.

Some couples use withdrawal or **coitus interruptus,** removal of the penis from the vagina before ejaculation, to prevent pregnancy, even though this is not a reliable form of birth control. About half the men who have tried coitus interruptus find it unsatisfactory, either because they don't know when they're going to ejaculate or because they can't withdraw quickly enough. Also, the Cowper's glands, two pea-sized structures located on each side of the urethra, often produce a fluid that appears as drops at the tip of the penis any time from arousal and erection to orgasm. This fluid can contain active sperm and, in infected men, human immunodeficiency virus (HIV).

conception The merging of a sperm and an ovum.

spermatogenesis The process by which sperm cells are produced.

fertilization The fusion of sperm and egg nucleus.

zygote A fertilized egg.

implantation The embedding of the fertilized ovum in the uterine lining.

contraception The prevention of conception; birth control.

failure rate The number of pregnancies that occur per year for every 100 women using a particular method of birth control.

coitus interruptus The removal of the penis from the vagina before ejaculation.

TABLE 8-1 Overview of Contraceptive Options

Method	Failure Rate—Number of Unintended Pregnancies Within First Year of Use (per 100 women)	Frequency of Use	Protection Against STIs	Cost
None	85	–	–	–
Spermicide	20–50	Each time	No	$0.35 to 12
Withdrawal	27	Each time	No	None
Periodic abstinence	20	Each month	No	None
Sponge*	14–28	Each time	No	$2.50–3 a sponge
Cervical cap* (FemCap) (women who have not had children)	23	Each time	No	$30 to 40
Diaphragm*	17	Each time	No	$30 to 40
Female condom	21	Each time	Yes	$2 to 3 each
Male condom	11	Each time	Yes	$0.50 to 2 each
The pill (combination)	1–2	Taken daily	No	$20 to 50 per cycle
Contraceptive patch	1–2	Applied weekly	No	$36 per month
NuvaRing	1–2	Inserted every 4 weeks	No	$43 per month
Seasonale	1–2	Taken daily for 3 months	No	$160–200 for 91 pills
Progestin-only pill	2	Given every 12 weeks	No	$30 to 35 every 3 months
Copper-containing IUD	<1	Inserted every 10 years	No	$250 to 300 every 10 years
Mirena	0.1	Inserted every 5 years	No	$300 to 400 every 5 years
Female sterilization	<1	Done once	No	$1,200 to 2,500
Male sterilization	<1	Done once	No	$250 to 1,000

STI, sexually transmitted infection; IUD, intrauterine device.
*Used with spermicide.
Source: Food and Drug Administration, www.fda.gov.

Many unintentional pregnancies are the result of contraceptive failure, either from problems with the drug or device itself or from improper use. Partners can lower the risk of unwanted pregnancy by using backup methods—that is, more than one form of contraception simultaneously. Emergency or after-intercourse contraception (discussed later in this chapter) could prevent as many as 1.7 million unwanted pregnancies each year.[3]

Even college students aware of the risks associated with unprotected sexual intercourse often do not practice safe-sex behaviors. There are many reasons, ranging from the influence of sex and alcohol to embarrassment about buying condoms. Generally, the ability to talk about a desire to use condoms has been found to be associated with a greater use of condoms.

The bottom line is that it takes two people to conceive a baby, and two people should be involved in deciding not to conceive a baby. In the process, they can also enhance their skills in communication, critical thinking, and negotiating.

Abstinence and Nonpenetrative Sexual Activity

The contraceptive methods discussed in this chapter are designed to prevent pregnancy as a consequence of vaginal intercourse. Couples who choose abstinence make a very different decision—to abstain from vaginal intercourse and forms of nonpenetrative sexual activity that could result in conception (any in which ejaculation occurs near the vaginal opening).

For many individuals, abstinence represents a deliberate choice regarding their bodies, minds, spirits, and

Strategies for Prevention: Choosing a Contraceptive

Your contraceptive needs may change throughout your life. To decide which method to use now, you need to know:

- How well will it fit into your lifestyle?
- How convenient will it be?
- How effective will it be?
- How safe will it be?
- How affordable will it be?
- How reversible will it be?
- Will it protect against sexually transmitted infections?

Source: "Facts About Birth Control," www.plannedparenthood.org.

sexuality. People choose abstinence for various reasons, including waiting until they are ready for a sexual relationship or until they find the "right" partner, respecting religious or moral values, enjoying friendships without sexual involvement, recovering from a breakup, or preventing pregnancy and sexually transmitted infection (see Chapter 9).

Abstinence is the only form of birth control that is 100 percent effective and risk-free. It is also an important, increasingly valued lifestyle choice. A growing number of individuals, including some who have been sexually active in the past, are choosing abstinence until they establish a relationship with a long-term partner.

Abstinence offers special health benefits for women. Those who abstain until their twenties and engage in sex with fewer partners during their lifetime are less likely to get sexually transmitted infections, to suffer infertility, or to develop cervical cancer. However, some people find it difficult to abstain for long periods of time. There also is a risk that people will abruptly end their abstinence without being prepared to protect themselves against pregnancy or infection.

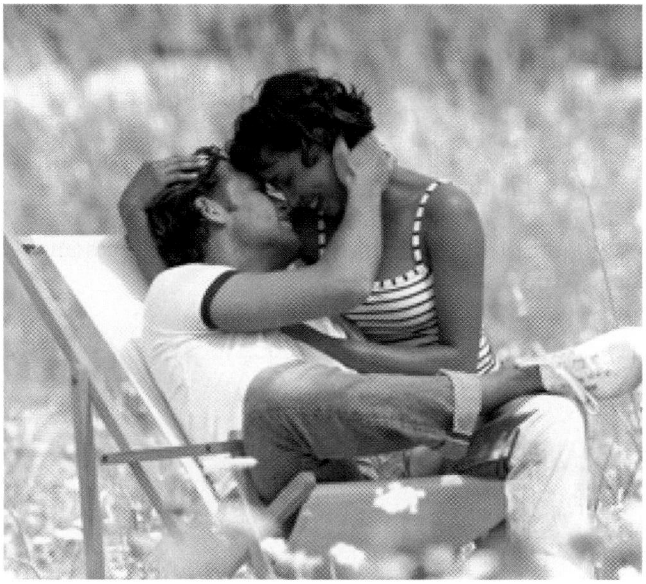

© Royalty-Free/CORBIS

Some couples refrain from intercourse but engage in "outercourse," or intimacy that includes kissing and hugging.

Individuals who choose abstinence from vaginal intercourse often engage in activities sometimes called *outercourse,* such as kissing, hugging, sensual touching, and mutual masturbation. Outercourse is nearly 100 percent effective as a contraceptive measure, but pregnancy is possible if there is genital contact. If the man ejaculates near the vaginal opening, sperm can swim up into the vagina and fallopian tubes to fertilize an egg. Except for oral-genital sex, outercourse also may lower the risk of contracting sexually transmitted infections. It is an effective form of safe sex as long as no body fluids are exchanged.

Some couples routinely restrict themselves to outercourse; others temporarily choose such sexual activities when it is inadvisable for them to have vaginal intercourse, for example, after childbirth. Other benefits: Outercourse has no medical or hormonal side effects; it may prolong sex play and enhance orgasm, and it can be used when no other birth control methods are available.

Hormonal Contraceptives

In recent years, birth control methods made with synthetic hormones have become available in a variety of forms. Oral contraceptives have been available for decades, and the birth control pill is one of the most well-researched medications. Other options for hormonal birth control include a skin patch, a vaginal ring, and a monthly or quarterly injection. All are extremely effective when used consistently and conscientiously.

Hormonal contraceptives do not protect against HIV infection and other STIs, so condoms and spermicides should also be used if you need protection against infections.

Student Snapshot

Contraception on Campus

Method	Percentage of Students
Birth control pills	40
Condoms (male or female)	39.2
Withdrawal	14.4
Spermicide	2.9
Fertility awareness	2.8
Depo Provera	1.8
Nothing	3.7
Have not had vaginal intercourse	21.5

Based on responses to the question, "If you have had vaginal intercourse, what method did you or your partner use to prevent pregnancy the last time?"
Source: American College Health Association. "American College Health Association National College Health Assessment (ACHA-NCHA) Spring 2005 Reference Group Data Report (abridged)." *Journal of American College Health,* Vol. 55, No. 1, 2006, pp. 5–16.

Oral Contraceptives

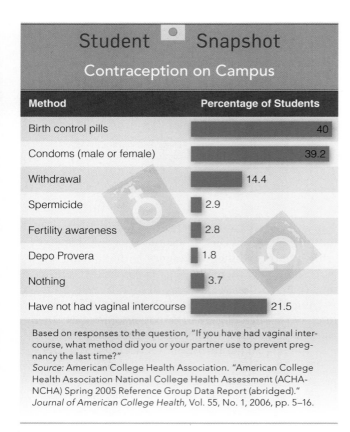

The pill—the popular term for **oral contraceptives**—is the method of birth control preferred by unmarried women and by those under age 30, including college students (see Student Snapshot: Contraception on Campus). Women 18 to 24 years old are most likely to choose oral contraceptives. In use for 40 years, the pill is one of the most researched, tested, and carefully followed medications in medical history—and one of the most controversial.

Although many women incorrectly think that the risks of the pill are greater than those of pregnancy and childbirth, long-term studies show that oral contraceptive use does not increase mortality rates. Combination oral contraceptives significantly reduce the risk of ovarian and endometrial cancer and produce no increase in breast cancer, diabetes, multiple sclerosis, rheumatoid arthritis, and liver disease.

Although research is limited, the use of common antibiotics, including many prescribed for dental procedures or skin conditions, may lower the effectiveness of oral contraceptives, particularly low-dose birth control pills. Always ask a dentist or doctor who prescribes an antibiotic about its potential effect on your oral contraceptive, and check with your gynecologist or primary physician about using an additional nonhormonal means of contraception (such as a condom) to ensure protection against an unwanted pregnancy.

Combination Pills

These pills consist of two hormones, synthetic estrogen and progestin, which play important roles in controlling ovulation and the menstrual cycle. The doses in today's oral contraceptives are much lower—less than one-fourth the amount of estrogen and one-twentieth the progestin in the original pill. This means fewer side effects and lower risk of heart disease and stroke. Stroke risk among women taking newer, low-dose formulations of oral contraceptive pills may be extremely low.

Monophasic pills release a constant dose of estrogen and progestin throughout a woman's menstrual cycle. **Multiphasic pills** mimic normal hormonal fluctuations of the natural menstrual cycle by providing different levels of estrogen and progesterone at different times of the month. Multiphasic pills reduce total hormonal dose and side effects. Both monophasic and multiphasic pills block the release of hormones that would stimulate the process leading to ovulation. They also thicken and alter the cervical mucus, making it more hostile to sperm, and they make implantation of a fertilized egg in the uterine lining more difficult.

One combination pill, Yasmin, contains a unique progestin that works like a mild diuretic and prevents fluid retention. Researchers have found that it lessens

Strategies for Prevention: Is Abstinence the Right Choice for You?

- Think about your values, goals, and priorities. Would abstinence support them?
- Realize that drugs and alcohol could affect your ability to make sexual decisions. Are you prepared to avoid their use to be sure to maintain your abstinence?
- Talk about your feelings before a relationship gets sexual. Can you put your thoughts and feelings about abstinence into words?
- Abstinence does not mean an end to all sexual experiences. What behaviors would you consider acceptable? What limits would you set?

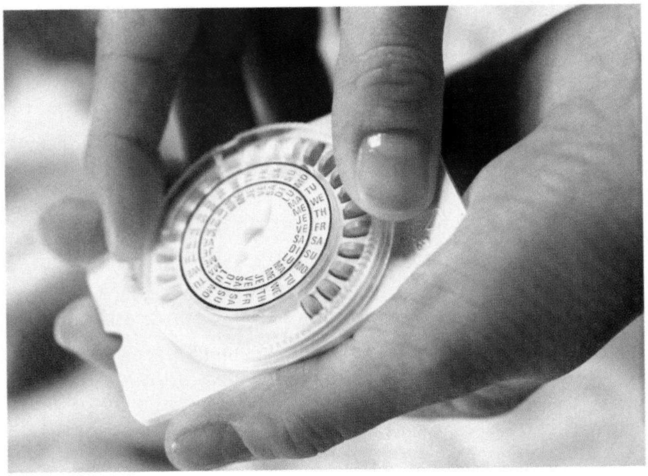

Various types of birth control pills contain different hormones and combinations of hormones.

symptoms of premenstrual problems. Women who are taking potassium supplements, daily anti-inflammatory drugs, or heparin, a blood-thinner, should not take Yasmin because of potentially dangerous drug interactions. Other pills offer different benefits, such as clearer skin and reduced facial hair.

Progestin-Only Pills

Progestin-only **"minipills"** contain only a small amount of progestin and no estrogen. They work somewhat differently than combination pills. Women taking **progestin-only pills** probably ovulate, at least occasionally. In those cycles, the pills prevent pregnancy by thickening cervical mucus, making it hard for sperm to penetrate, and by interfering with implantation of a fertilized egg.

The risk of heart disease and stroke is lower with progestin-only pills than with any combination pill. For this reason, they are a good choice for women over age 35 and others who cannot take estrogen-containing pills because of high blood pressure, diabetes, or clotting disorders. Because they do not affect the quality or quantity of breast milk, progestin-only pills often are recommended for nursing mothers, and they are recommended for smokers. Because progestin can affect mood and worsen the symptoms of depression, progestin-only pills are not recommended for women with a history of depression. Anti-seizure medications, such as Dilantin, which accelerate liver metabolism, may make the minipill less effective.

Users of progestin-only pills have to be conscientious about taking these pills, not just every day, but at the same time every day. If you take a progestin-only pill three or more hours later than usual, use a back-up method of contraception, such as a condom, for two days after you resume taking the pill.

Advantages of Oral Contraceptives

- Extremely effective when taken consistently.
- Convenient.
- Moderately priced.
- Do not interrupt sexual activity.
- Reversible within three months of stopping the pill.
- Reduce the risk of benign breast lumps, ovarian cysts, iron-deficiency anemia, pelvic inflammatory disease, endometrial and ovarian cancer.
- May relieve painful menstruation.

Disadvantages of Oral Contraceptives

- Require a prescription.
- Increased risk of cardiovascular problems, primarily for women over age 35 who smoke and those with high blood pressure or other health problems.
- Side effects vary with different brands but include spotting between periods, weight gain or loss, nausea and vomiting, breast tenderness, and decreased sex drive.
- Must be taken at the same time every day (especially critical with low-dose estrogen and progestin-only pills).
- No protection against STIs.
- Must use a secondary form of birth control for the initial seven days of use.

Before Using Oral Contraceptives Before starting on the pill, you should undergo a thorough physical examination that includes the following tests:

- Routine blood pressure test.
- Pelvic exam, including a Pap smear.
- Breast exam.
- Blood test.
- Urine sample.

Let your doctor know about any personal or family incidence of high blood pressure or heart disease, diabetes, liver dysfunction, hepatitis, unusual menstrual history, severe depression, sickle-cell anemia, cancer of the

oral contraceptives Preparations of synthetic hormones that inhibit ovulation; also referred to as birth control pills or simply the pill.

monophasic pill An oral contraceptive that releases synthetic estrogen and progestin at constant levels throughout the menstrual cycle.

multiphasic pill An oral contraceptive that releases different levels of estrogen and progestin to mimic the hormonal fluctuations of the natural menstrual cycle.

minipill, progestin-only pill An oral contraceptive containing a small amount of progestin and no estrogen, which prevents contraception by making the mucus in the cervix so thick that sperm cannot enter the uterus.

SAVVY CONSUMER

Evaluating the Risks of Contraceptives

For individuals with certain medical conditions, specific types of birth control can pose a health risk. To be safe, follow these guidelines:

- **High blood pressure** (180/110 mmHg or higher): Avoid birth control pills or injectables containing estrogen, which may increase your risk of a heart attack or stroke.
- **Episodes of depression:** Avoid products that contain progestin, such as Depo-Provera, contraceptive implants, and the minipill. In some women with depression, progestin may worsen depressive symptoms. Also, check with your doctor if you are taking an antidepressant medication; it may affect or be affected by oral contraceptives and you may require a different dose.
- **Seizure disorder:** Avoid low-dose birth control pills. Some antiseizure medications, such as Dilantin, accelerate liver metabolism of all substances, including oral contraceptives, and make them less effective.
- **Ectopic pregnancy:** Avoid IUDs. Although IUDs do not cause ectopic pregnancies, if your fallopian tubes have been scarred by a previous ectopic gestation, you're more likely to have another ectopic if you use an IUD.
- **Hepatitis:** Avoid birth control pills or injectables containing estrogen, which is metabolized in the liver—an organ damaged by hepatitis.

breast, ovaries, or uterus, high cholesterol levels, or migraine headaches. (See Savvy Consumer: "Evaluating the Risks of Contraceptives.")

How to Use Oral Contraceptives The pill usually comes in 28-day packets: 21 of the pills contain the hormones, and 7 are "blanks," included so that the woman can take a pill every day, even during her menstrual period. If a woman forgets to take one pill, she should take it as soon as she remembers. However, if she forgets during the first week of her cycle or misses more than one pill, she should rely on another form of birth control until her next menstrual period.

Even if you experience no discomfort or side effects while on the pill, see a physician at least once a year for an examination, which should include a blood pressure test, a pelvic, and a breast exam. Notify your doctor at once if you develop severe abdominal pain, chest pain, coughing, shortness of breath, pain or tenderness in the calf or thigh, severe headaches, dizziness, faintness, muscle weakness or numbness, speech disturbance, blurred vision, a sensation of flashing lights, a breast lump, severe depression, or yellowing of your skin.

Generally, when a woman stops taking the pill, her menstrual cycle resumes the next month, but it may be irregular for the next couple of months. However, 2 to 4 percent of pill users experience prolonged delays. Women who become pregnant during the first or second cycle after discontinuing use of the pill may be at greater risk of miscarriage; they also are more likely to conceive twins. Most physicians advise women who want to conceive to change to another method of contraception for three months after they stop taking the pill.

Extended-Use Oral Contraceptives

For years physicians have prescribed prolonged use of birth control pills to lessen the number of menstrual cycles for women with asthma, migraines, rashes, or other conditions that flare up during their periods. Eliminating periods eliminates symptoms, and having fewer cycles also may lower a woman's long-term risk of ovarian cancer. A new package of standard combination birth control pills, called Seasonale, provides pills for 84 days of continuous use so women have four periods a year rather than twelve.

The Patch (Ortho Evra)

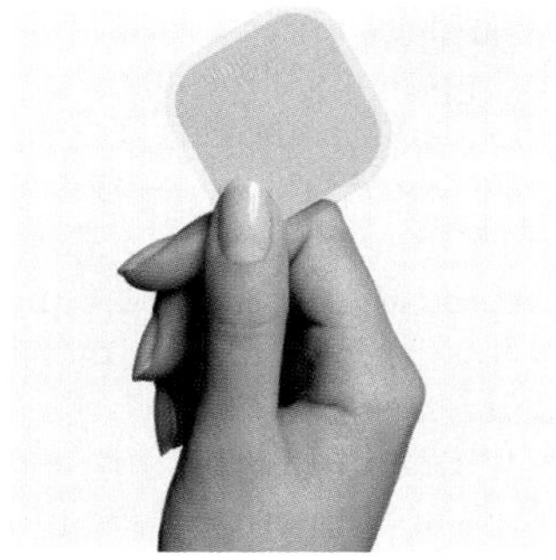
Ortho-McNeil Pharmaceutical

The Ortho Evra birth control patch, the first transdermal (through the skin) contraceptive, works like a combination pill but looks like a band-aid. Embedded in its adhesive layer are two hormones, a low-dose estrogen and a progestin. It prevents pregnancy by delivering continuous levels of estrogen and progestin through the skin directly into the bloodstream so women are exposed to higher overall levels of estrogen, which may increase their risk of blood clots.[4] The patch is waterproof and stays on in the shower, swimming pools, or hot tubs.

Advantages of the Patch

- Good alternative for women who can't remember, don't like, or have problems swallowing daily pills.
- Highly effective when used correctly.
- Does not interrupt sexual activity.
- Fewer side effects, such as nausea, breakthrough bleeding, and mood swings, than pills.
- Fertility returns quickly after you stop using it.

Disadvantages of the Patch

- Must apply a new patch every week.
- Requires a prescription.
- No protection against STIs.
- Increased risk of blood clots, heart attack, and stroke, particularly for women who smoke or have certain health conditions. The risk of dying or suffering a survivable blood clot while using the patch is estimated to be about three times higher than while using birth control pills.[5]
- Less effective in women who weigh more than 198 pounds.
- Some women report breast tenderness, headaches, upper respiratory infections, or self-consciousness wearing the patch.
- Contact lens wearers may experience vision changes.
- 5 percent of women report that at least one patch slipped off; 2 percent report skin irritation.
- Must use another form of birth control for the initial seven days of use.

How to Use the Patch A woman applies the 1¾ inch square to her back, upper arm, lower abdomen, or buttocks and changes it every seven days for three weeks. During the patch-free week, she experiences menstrual bleeding. A user should check every day to make sure the patch is still in place. If you don't replace a detached patch within 24 hours, use a backup method of contraception until your next period.

The NuvaRing

The silver-dollar-sized NuvaRing, a 2-inch ring made of flexible, transparent plastic, slowly emits the same hormones as oral contraceptives through the vaginal tissues (Figure 8-3). Smaller than the smallest diaphragm, it contains less estrogen than any pill. As effective as the pill, it provides a steady dose of hormones and causes fewer side effects.

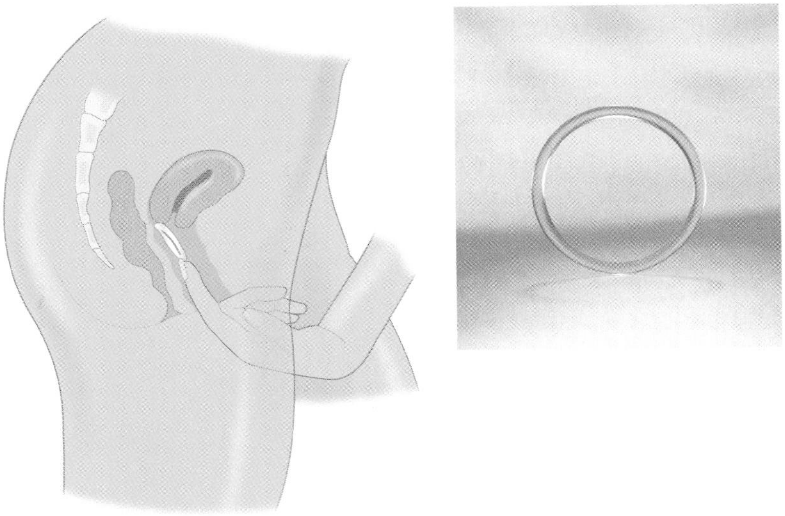

FIGURE 8-3 NuvaRing
The NuvaRing releases estrogen and progestin, preventing ovulation. The exact position of NuvaRing in the vagina is not critical.

Advantages of NuvaRing

- Under medical supervision, may be safer than birth control pills for women with mild hypertension or diabetes.
- Less likelihood of pill-related side effects, such as nausea, mood swings, spotting, and cramping.
- No need to remember a daily pill or weekly patch.
- Fertility returns quickly when ring is removed.

Disadvantages of NuvaRing

- Some women do not feel comfortable placing and removing something inside their vaginas.
- Possible side effects include vaginal discharge, irritation, and infection.
- Cannot use oil-based vaginal medications for yeast infections while ring is in place.
- No protection against STIs.

How to Use the Ring Unlike a diaphragm, the NuvaRing does not have to be exactly positioned within the vagina or used with a spermicide (sperm-killing foam or jelly). The flexible, plastic 2-inch ring compresses so a woman can easily insert it. Each ring stays in place for three weeks, then is removed for the fourth week of the menstrual cycle.

If a NuvaRing pops out (uncommon but possible), it should be washed, dried, and replaced within three hours. If a longer time passes, users should rely on a backup form of birth control until the ring has been reinserted for a week and the medications have risen to protective levels again.

Contraceptive Injectables

Two different hormonal contraceptives are available in the form of "shots" or injections. Lunelle, which consists of the same hormones as combination birth control pills, is administered monthly. Depo-Provera, which contains only progestin, must be given every 12 weeks. Injectable contraceptives provide no protection against HIV and other STIs.

Lunelle

Lunelle is a contraceptive injection of estrogen and progestin, given each month by a health professional (doctor, nurse, or in some places, pharmacist) into the arm, thigh, or buttocks during the first five days of a woman's menstrual cycle. It is considered 99.5 percent effective in preventing pregnancy.

Advantages of Lunelle

- No risk of user error.
- No worry about buying, storing, or using contraceptives.
- No need to think about contraception for four weeks at a time.

Disadvantages of Lunelle

- Must visit a doctor's office or clinic every month for an injection.
- Weight gain (average is 4 pounds, but some women gain 10 to 20 pounds).
- Side effects include nausea, breakthrough bleeding, acne, headache, change in sexual desire, depression, and breast tenderness, particularly during the first few months of use.
- No protection against STIs.

Depo-Provera

One injection of Depo-Provera, a synthetic version of the natural hormone progesterone, provides three months of contraceptive protection. This long-acting hormonal contraceptive raises levels of progesterone, thereby simulating pregnancy. The pituitary gland doesn't produce FSH and LH, which normally cause egg ripening and release. The endometrial lining of the uterus thins, preventing implantation of a fertilized egg.

Advantages of Depo-Provera

- Because it contains only progestin, it is safe for women who cannot take combination birth control pills.
- No risk of user error.
- No worry about buying, storing, or using contraceptives.
- No need to think about contraception for three months at a time.
- Possible protection against endometrial and ovarian cancer.

Disadvantages of Depo-Provera

- Must visit a doctor or clinic every three months for injection.
- Menstrual cycles become irregular or cease.
- Potential side effects include decreased libido, depression, headaches, dizziness, frequent urination, and allergic reactions.
- Increased weight gain, especially for obese women and teenage girls.[6]
- No protection against STIs.
- According to recent NIH study, appears to triple risk of acquiring chlamydia and gonorrhea compared to women not using a hormonal contraceptive. Scientists do not know the reason for this increased risk.
- Delayed return of fertility.
- Long-term use may significantly reduce bone density.

Contraceptive Implants

Hormonal implants, placed under the skin, deliver a constant low dose of progestin. They work primarily by suppressing ovulation, but they also thicken the cervical mucus (which inhibits sperm migration), inhibit the development and growth of the uterine lining, and limit secretion of progesterone during the second, or luteal, half of the menstrual cycle.

Norplant, consisting of six thin silicone rubber capsules containing a synthetic form of progestin, was the first such implant available in the United States. Approximately 9 million women used this method before it was taken off the market for reasons unrelated to its efficacy. Women with Norplant implants, who include many adolescents and young adults, should consult their doctors. They can safely leave the rods in place for the entire five-year period of contraceptive protection. However, they should discuss all options, including removal of the Norplant rods and switching to an alternative form of contraception.

A newer generation of implants may provide the benefits of long-term pregnancy protection with fewer complications. Implanon, a single Silastic rod that is simpler to insert and remove than Norplant, provides at least three years of contraception. Available in Europe and Australia, it uses a different type of progestin than Norplant and may cause fewer side effects like weight gain or acne. It should be available in the United States soon.

Intrauterine Contraceptives: Mirena

An **intrauterine device (IUD)** is a small piece of molded plastic, with a nylon string attached, that is inserted into the uterus through the cervix. It prevents pregnancy by interfering with implantation. Once widely used, IUDs became less popular after most brands were removed from the market because of serious complications such as pelvic infection and infertility.

A new option is the Mirena intrauterine system, which consists of a T-shaped device inserted in the uterus by a physician, that releases a continuous low dose of progestin and provides five years of protection from pregnancy. Used in Europe, Asia, and Latin America for years, it is 99 percent effective.

Mirena is increasingly being used, not just for contraception, but as an alternative to hysterectomy for extremely heavy menstrual bleeding and as a treatment for problems such as iron-deficiency anemia.

Advantages of Mirena

- Highly effective at preventing pregnancy.
- No need to think about contraception for five years.
- Allows sexual spontaneity; neither partner can feel it.
- Starts working immediately.
- New mothers can breast-feed while using it.
- Periods become shorter and lighter or stop altogether.
- Low incidence of side effects.
- Can be removed at any time.

Disadvantages of Mirena

- Spotting or breakthrough bleeding in first three to six months.
- No protection against STIs.
- Potential side effects include acne, headaches, nausea, breast tenderness, mood changes.
- Increased risk of benign ovarian cysts.
- May take up to a year for fertility to return after discontinuation.

How to Use the Mirena System A physician must insert the Mirena in a woman's uterus. In a five-year clinical trial, about 5 in every 100 women reported that the Mirena had slipped out of the uterus. Users should check for the string that extends from the device through the vagina at least once a month.

Barrier Contraceptives

As their name implies, **barrier contraceptives** block the meeting of egg and sperm by means of a physical barrier (a diaphragm, cervical cap, FemCap, or condom) or a chemical one (vaginal spermicide in jellies, foams, creams, suppositories, or film).

Prescription Barriers

The prescription barrier contraceptives are used by women: the diaphragm, cervical cap, and FemCap. They are placed in the vagina with a spermicide. They do not protect against HIV infection and most STIs.

Diaphragm

The **diaphragm** is a bowl-like rubber cup with a flexible rim that is inserted into the vagina to cover the cervix and prevent the passage of sperm into the uterus during sexual intercourse (Figure 8-4). When used with a spermicide, the diaphragm is both a physical and a chemical barrier to sperm. The effectiveness of the diaphragm in preventing pregnancy depends on strong motivation (to use it faithfully) and a precise understanding of its use. If diaphragms with spermicide are used consistently and carefully, they can be 95 to 98 percent effective. Without a spermicide, the diaphragm is not effective.

intrauterine device (IUD) A device inserted into the uterus through the cervix to prevent pregnancy by interfering with implantation.

barrier contraceptives Birth-control devices that block the meeting of egg and sperm, either by physical barriers, such as condoms, diaphragms, or cervical caps, or by chemical barriers, such as spermicide, or both.

diaphragm A bowl-like rubber cup with a flexible rim that is inserted into the vagina to cover the cervix and prevent the passage of sperm into the uterus during sexual intercourse; used with a spermicidal foam or jelly, it serves as both a chemical and a physical barrier to sperm.

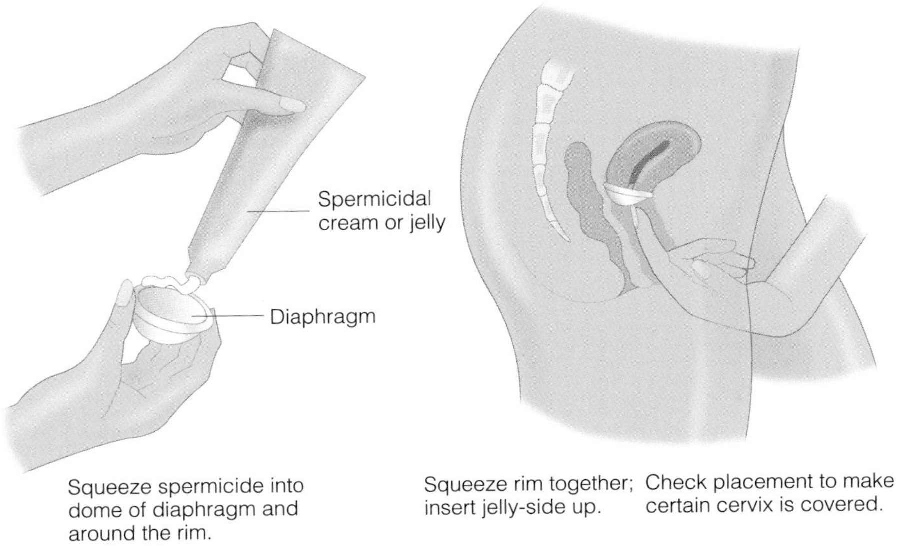
Spermicidal cream or jelly
Diaphragm
Squeeze spermicide into dome of diaphragm and around the rim.
Squeeze rim together; insert jelly-side up.
Check placement to make certain cervix is covered.

FIGURE 8-4 Diaphragm
When used correctly and consistently and with a spermicide, the diaphragm is effective in preventing pregnancy. It must be fitted by a health-care professional.

Cervical Cap

Like the diaphragm, the **cervical cap** combined with spermicide serves as both a chemical and physical barrier blocking the path of the sperm to the uterus. The rubber or plastic cap is smaller and thicker than a diaphragm. It resembles a large thimble that fits snugly around the cervix and may work better for some women. It is about as effective as a diaphragm (95 to 98 percent).

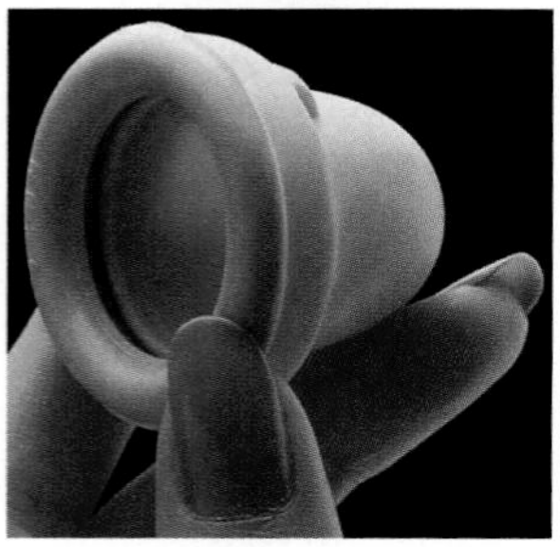

© Joel Gordon Photography

FemCap

The FemCap is a nonhormonal, latex-free barrier contraceptive that works with a spermicide (Figure 8-5). The FemCap, designed to conform to the anatomy of the cervix and vagina, comes in three sizes. The smallest usually best suits women who have never been pregnant; the medium size, for women who have been pregnant but have not had a vaginal delivery; the largest, for those who have delivered a full-term baby vaginally.

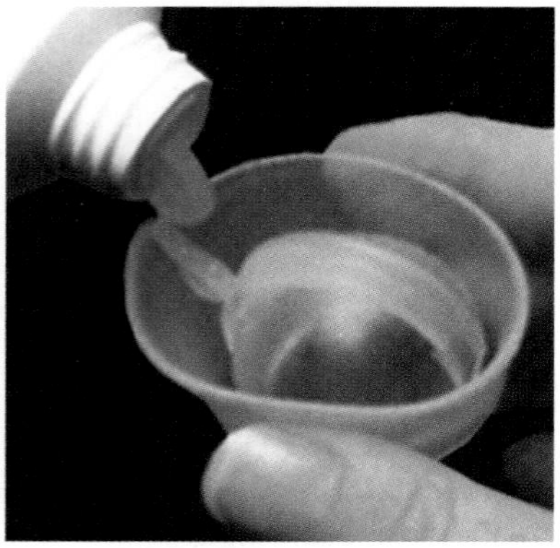

Courtesy of FemCap, Inc., and Alfred Shihata, MD

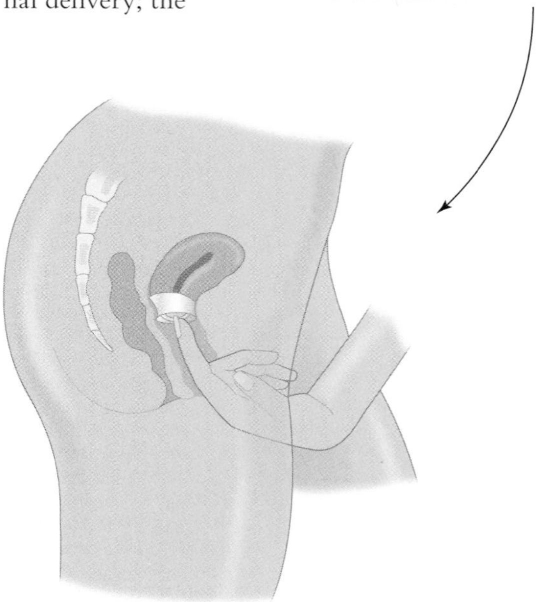

FIGURE 8-5 FemCap

The FemCap must be used with spermicide and correctly positioned to cover the cervix completely.

Source: Reproduced with permission from FemCap, Inc., and Alfred Shihata, M.D.

Advantages of Prescription Barriers

- Relatively inexpensive.
- Don't interrupt sexual activity; can be inserted hours ahead of time.
- Usually not felt by either partner.
- Can easily be carried in pocket or purse.
- No hormones or side effects.
- Cervical caps are an alternative for women who cannot use diaphragms or find them too messy.

Disadvantages of Prescription Barriers

- Less effective than hormonal contraceptives.
- Available by prescription only.
- Require advance planning or interruption of sexual activity to position the device before intercourse.
- May slip out of place during intercourse.
- May be uncomfortable for some women and their partners.
- Spermicidal foams, creams, and jellies may be messy, cause irritation, and detract from oral-genital sex.
- Some diaphragm users report bladder discomfort, urethral irritation, or recurrent cystitis.
- Some cap users find it difficult to insert and remove and uncomfortable to wear.

How to Use a Diaphragm Diaphragms are fitted and prescribed by a qualified health-care professional in diameter sizes ranging from 2 to 4 inches (50 to 105 millimeters). The diaphragm's main function is to serve as a container for a spermicidal (sperm-killing) foam or jelly, which is available at pharmacies without a prescription. A diaphragm should remain in the vagina for at least six hours after intercourse to ensure that all sperm are killed. If intercourse occurs again during this period, additional spermicide must be inserted with an applicator tube.

The key to proper use of the diaphragm is having it available. A sexually active woman should keep it in the most accessible place—her purse, bedroom, bathroom. Before every use, a diaphragm should be checked for tiny leaks (hold up to the light or place water in the dome). A health-care provider should check its fit and condition every year when the woman has her annual Pap smear. Oil-based lubricants will deteriorate the latex of the diaphragm and should not be used with one.

How to Use a Cervical Cap Like the diaphragm, the cervical cap is fitted by a qualified health-care professional. For use, the woman fills it one-third to two-thirds full with spermicide and inserts it by holding its edges together and sliding it into the vagina. The cup is then pressed onto the cervix. (Most women find it easiest to do so while squatting or in an upright sitting position.) The cap can be inserted up to 6 hours prior to intercourse and should not be removed for at least 6 hours afterward. It can be left in place up to 24 hours. Pulling on one side of the rim breaks the suction and allows easy removal. Oil-based lubricants should not be used with the cap because they can deteriorate the latex.

How to Use FemCap A prescription is required to purchase FemCap, and the woman selects the appropriate size. Apply spermicide to the bowl of the FemCap (which goes over the cervix), to the outer brim, and to the groove that will face into the vagina. Insert the squeezed, flattened cap into the vagina with the bowl facing upward. The FemCap must be pushed all the way in to cover the cervix completely and left in place at least six hours after intercourse.

Nonprescription Barriers

The nonprescription barrier contraceptives include the male and female condom, vaginal spermicides, the contraceptive sponge, and vaginal contraceptive film. Both condoms provide some protection against HIV infection and other STIs; spermicides, sponges, and films do not.

Male Condom

The male **condom** covers the erect penis and catches the ejaculate, thus preventing sperm from entering the woman's reproductive tract (Figure 8-6). Most are made of thin surgical latex or sheep membrane; a new type is made of polyurethane, which is thinner, stronger, more heat sensitive, and more comfortable than latex. In a study of 901 couples over six months, the polyurethane condom was not as effective as the latex condom for pregnancy prevention. Experts now advise against use of condoms with nonoxynol-9 (see discussion in Chapter 9).

Although the theoretical effectiveness rate for condoms is 97 percent, the actual rate is only 80 to 85 percent. The condom can be torn during the manufacturing process or during its use; testing by the manufacturer may not be as strenuous as it could or should be. Careless removal can also decrease the effectiveness of condoms. However, the major reason that condoms have such a low actual effectiveness rate is that couples don't use them each and every time they have sex. Users who have little experience with condoms—who are young, single, or childless, or who engage in risky behaviors—are more likely to have condoms break.

Condoms are second only to the pill in popularity among college-age adults. About half (53 percent) of sexually active students report using condoms the last time they had vaginal intercourse.[7] However, only 17 percent of students say they always used condoms during vaginal intercourse during the previous 30 days; 20 percent said they never used them (Figure 8-7).[8] Nearly one-third of students in one survey reported discomfort, such as a too-tight fit or loss of pleasurable sensation. These students were less likely to use condoms correctly and more likely to report condom breakage. Larger-sized condoms and/or vaginal lubricants can eliminate many complaints of discomfort.[9]

College men also may try to avoid condom use because of concern about erectile dysfunction (ED), the inability to maintain a penile erection sufficient for sexual relations. In an anonymous survey of 234 sexually active males between the ages of 18 to 25 on three university campuses, 25 percent reported ED with condom use.

cervical cap A thimble-sized rubber or plastic cap that is inserted into the vagina to fit over the cervix and prevent the passage of sperm into the uterus during sexual intercourse; used with a spermicidal foam or jelly, it serves as both a chemical and a physical barrier to sperm.

condom A latex sheath worn over the penis during sexual acts to prevent conception and/or the transmission of disease; the female condom lines the walls of the vagina.

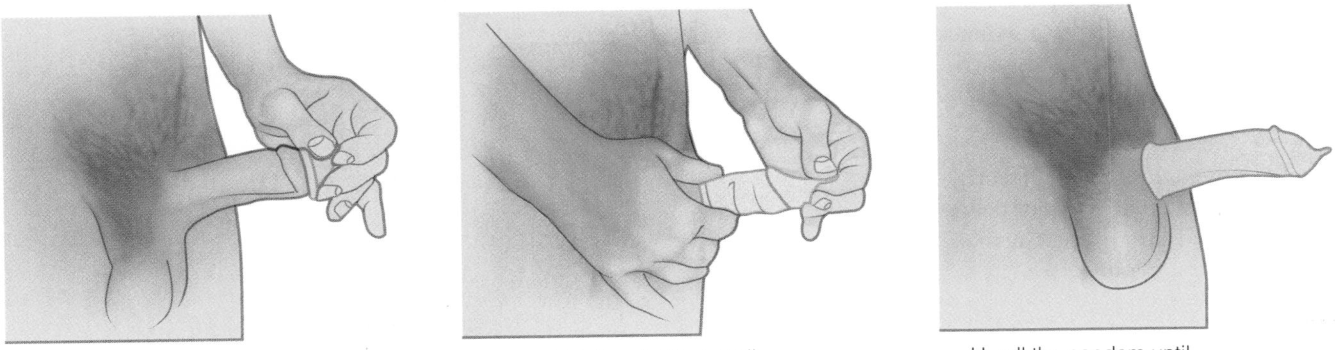

Pinch or twist the tip of the condom, leaving one-half inch at the tip to catch the semen.

Holding the tip, unroll the condom.

Unroll the condom until it reaches the pubic hairs.

FIGURE 8-6 Male Condom
Condoms effectively reduce the risk of pregnancy as well as STIs if used consistently and correctly.

Type of Sexual Activity	Total	Women	Men
	(%)	(%)	(%)
Oral intercourse	3.7	3.1	4.3
Vaginal intercourse	53.3	50.7	57.9
Anal intercourse	28.3	23.2	36.1

FIGURE 8-7 Condoms on Campus

Based on answers to the question, "If you are sexually active, did you use a condom the last time you had oral sex, vaginal intercourse, anal intercourse?"

Source: American College Health Association. "American College Health Association National College Health Assessment (ACHA-NCHA) Spring 2005 Reference Group Data Report (abridged)." *Journal of American College Health*, Vol. 55, No. 1, 2006, pp. 5–16.

These men were much more inconsistent in their use of condoms than other students. Six percent of all the students surveyed had taken ED medications, such as Viagra. Almost two-thirds mixed these medications with alcohol and drugs, such as ecstasy or methamphetamine.[10]

Female Condom

The female condom, made of polyurethane, consists of two rings and a polyurethane sheath, and is inserted into the vagina with a tamponlike applicator (Figure 8-8). Once in place, the device loosely lines the walls of the vagina. Internally, a thickened rubber ring keeps it anchored near the cervix. Externally, another rubber ring, 2 inches in diameter, rests on the labia and resists slippage.

Although not widely used in the West, the female condom is gaining acceptance in Africa, Asia, and Latin America. Properly used, it is believed to be as good or better than the male condom for preventing infections, including HIV, because it is stronger and covers a slightly larger area. However, it is slightly less effective at preventing pregnancy. The efficacy of female condoms does increase with a woman's experience in using them.

Advantages of Condoms

- Effective when used correctly.
- Lower a woman's risk of pelvic inflammatory disease (PID) and may protect against some urinary tract and genital infections.
- No side effects, unless you're allergic to latex.
- No prescription required.
- Inexpensive.
- The female condom gives women more control in reducing their risk of pregnancy and STIs and does not require a prescription or medical appointment.

Disadvantages of Condoms

- Requires consistent and diligent use.
- Not 100 percent effective in preventing pregnancy or STIs.
- Risk of manufacturing defects, such as pin-size holes, and breaking or slipping off during intercourse.
- May inhibit sexual spontaneity.

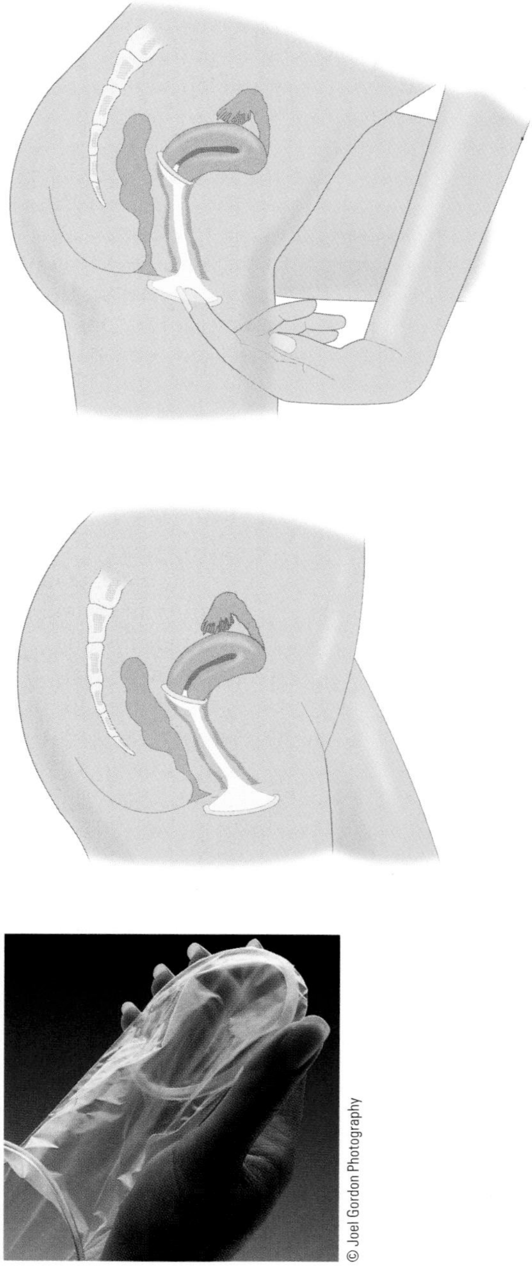

© Joel Gordon Photography

FIGURE 8-8 Female Condom

This device is less effective than the male condom for preventing pregnancy and STIs (since no spermicide is used). Like the male condom, this method does not require a prescription.

- Users or partners may complain about odor, lubrication (too much or too little), feel, taste, difficulty opening the packages, and disposal.
- Some men dislike reduced penile sensitivity or cannot sustain an erection while putting on a condom.
- Some women complain that the female condom is difficult to use, squeaks, and looks odd.

How to Use a Male Condom Most physicians recommend prelubricated, spermicide-treated, American-made latex or polyurethane condoms, not membrane condoms ("natural" or "sheepskin"). Before using a condom, check the expiration date and make sure it's soft and pliable. If it's yellow or sticky, throw it out. Don't check for leaks by blowing up a condom before using it; you may weaken or tear it.

The condom should be put on at the beginning of sexual activity, before genital contact occurs. There should be a little space left at the top of the condom to catch the semen (Figure 8-6). Wait until just before intercourse to apply spermicide. Any vaginal lubricant should be water-based. Petroleum-based creams or jellies (such as Vaseline, baby oil, massage oil, vegetable oils, or oil-based hand lotions) can deteriorate the latex. After ejaculation, the condom should be held firmly against the penis so that it doesn't slip off or leak during withdrawal. Couples engaging in anal intercourse should use a water-based lubricant as well as a condom, but should never assume the condom will provide 100 percent protection from HIV infection or other STIs.

How to Use a Female Condom As illustrated in Figure 8-8, a woman removes the condom and applicator from the wrapper and inserts the condom slowly by gently pushing the applicator toward the small of the back. When properly inserted, the outer ring should rest on the folds of skin around the vaginal opening, and the inner ring (the closed end) should fit against the cervix.

The female condom can be washed and reused several times and still meet the standards set by the FDA, according to the study conducted in South Africa in which a sample of women washed, dried, and relubricated female condoms up to seven times.

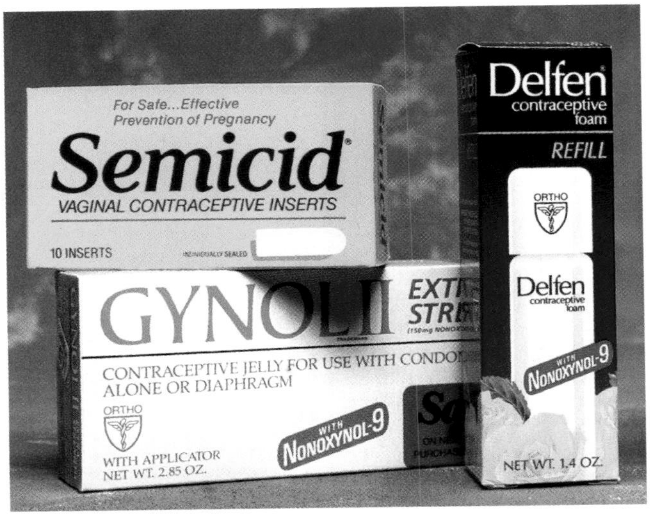

© Aaron Haupt/Photo Researchers, Inc.

Vaginal spermicides are available as creams, foams, and jellies. Spermicides are most effective in preventing pregnancy and STIs when used together with a male condom.

FAQ Do Men and Women Use Condoms for Different Reasons?

The genders have very different motives both for engaging in sex and for using condoms. In focus groups, young women say they engage in sexual relations because of a desire for physical intimacy and a committed relationship. They generally report having sex only with men they care for and deeply trust and expect that these men would be honest and forthright about their sexual history. This trust plays a significant role in their decision whether to insist on condom use.

In contrast, few young men say relationships are an important dimension of their sexual involvements. Their primary motivation is a desire for physical and sexual satisfaction. Most say they are not interested in commitment and view emotional expectations as a complication of becoming sexually involved with a woman. Young men also admit to making judgments about types of girls. To them, young women they didn't care about were "sluts" with whom they used a condom for their own protection.

Which partner determines whether a couple uses a condom? The answer is often the women—if they choose to do so. Regardless of race or ethnicity, many young women are adamant in demanding that their partners use condoms—and many young men say they would not challenge such a demand out of fear of losing the opportunity for sex. Men often expect potential partners to want to use condoms and describe themselves as "suspicious" of women who do not.

Both sexes name two primary reasons for using condoms: preventing pregnancy and protecting against sexually transmitted infections. Young women see an unwanted pregnancy as an occurrence that would be disruptive, expensive, and could "ruin" their lives and their parents' lives. Young men see condom use as a way of protecting themselves against emotional entanglements and paternity issues.

Vaginal Spermicide

The various forms of **vaginal spermicide** include chemical foams, creams,

vaginal spermicide A substance that kills or neutralizes sperm, inserted into the vagina in the form of a foam, cream, jelly, or suppository.

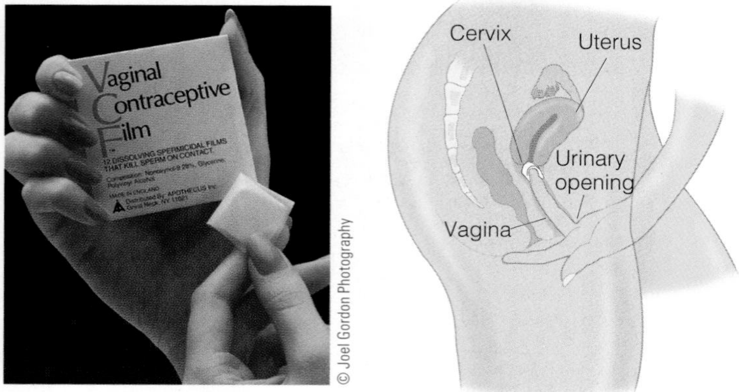

FIGURE 8-9 Vaginal Contraceptive Film (VCF)
The effectiveness of this thin film, laced with spermicide, is similar to other spermicides and greatest when used with a condom.

jellies, vaginal suppositories, and gels. Some creams and jellies are made for use with a diaphragm; others can be used alone. Several vaginal suppositories claim high effectiveness, but no American studies have confirmed these claims. In general, failure rates for vaginal suppositories are as high as 10 to 25 percent.

Advantages of Vaginal Spermicide

- Easy to use.
- Effective if used with another form of contraception, such as condoms.
- Reduces the risk of some vaginal infections, PID, and STIs.
- No effect on fertility.

Disadvantages of Vaginal Spermicide

- Insertion interrupts sexual spontaneity.
- May cause irritation.
- Some people cannot use them because of an allergic reaction.
- Some users complain that spermicides are messy or interfere with oral-genital contact.
- Spermicidal suppositories that do not dissolve completely can feel gritty.

How to Use a Vaginal Spermicide The various types of spermicide come with instructions that should be followed carefully for maximum protection. Contraceptive vaginal suppositories take about 20 minutes to dissolve and cover the vaginal walls. Foam, inserted with an applicator, goes into place much more rapidly. You must apply additional spermicide before each additional intercourse. After sex, women should shower rather than bathe to prevent the spermicide from being rinsed out of the vagina, and they should not douche for at least six hours.

Vaginal Contraceptive Film

Available from pharmacies without a prescription, the 2-inch-by-2-inch thin film known as **vaginal contraceptive film (VCF)** is laced with spermicide (Figure 8-9). Once folded and inserted into the vagina, it dissolves into a stay-in-place gel.

Advantages of VCF

- Easy to use.
- Can be used by people allergic to foams and jellies.
- Dissolves gradually and almost unnoticeably.
- As effective as most spermicides; almost 100 percent effective paired with a condom.
- No effect on fertility.

Disadvantages of VCF

- Insertion interrupts sexual spontaneity.
- Effective for only one hour and one act of intercourse.
- No protection against STIs.

How to Use Vaginal Contraceptive Film Fold one square of VCF in half; place it on your second or third finger; then insert high into the vagina, near the cervix. VCF is effective for one hour. One film should be used for each act of intercourse.

Contraceptive Sponge

The Today Sponge, which is made of soft polyurethane foam laced with spermicide was sold as an over-the-counter contraceptive in the United States from 1983 to 1995, when it was withdrawn because of contamination problems at the manufacturing plant. It is now available again.

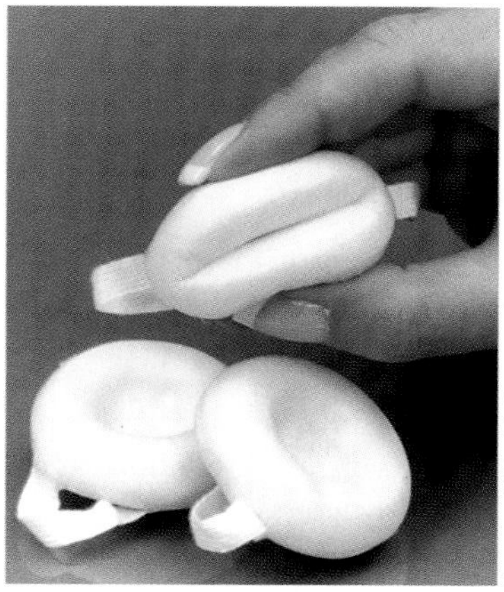

Courtesy of Allendale Pharmaceuticals

The contraceptive sponge works on the same principle as the diaphragm and cervical cap but is available without a prescription.

Advantages of the Contraceptive Sponge

- Easy to use.
- Can be inserted several hours before intercourse and left in place for 24 hours afterward.
- Effective immediately if used correctly.
- No effect on fertility.

Disadvantages of the Contraceptive Sponge

- May be difficult to remove.
- May be less effective in women who have had children.
- No reliable protection against STIs.
- Requires advance planning to place the sponge.
- Side effects include vaginal irritation and allergic reactions.
- Should not be used during menstruation.

Periodic Abstinence and Fertility Awareness Methods

Awareness of a woman's cyclic fertility can help in both conception and contraception. The different methods of birth control based on a woman's menstrual cycle are sometimes referred to as *natural family planning* or *fertility awareness methods.* They include the calendar method, the basal-body-temperature method, and the cervical mucus method. New fertility monitors that use saliva to determine time of ovulation can improve the accuracy of these methods.

Women's menstrual cycles vary greatly. To use one of the fertility awareness methods, a woman must know and understand her cycle. She should track her cycle for at least eight months—marking day one (the day bleeding begins) on a calendar and counting the length of each cycle. Figure 8-10 shows the days in a 28-day cycle when abstinence or other contraceptive methods would be necessary.

The calendar method, often called the **rhythm method,** is based on counting the woman's safe days based on her individual menstrual cycle. The basal-body-temperature method determines the safe days based on the woman's *Basel body temperature,* which rises after ovulation. The cervical mucus method, also called the *ovulation method,* is based on observation of changes in the consistency of the woman's vaginal mucus throughout her menstrual cycle. The period of maximum fertility occurs when the mucus is smooth and slippery.

Advantages of Fertility Awareness

- No expense.
- No side effects.

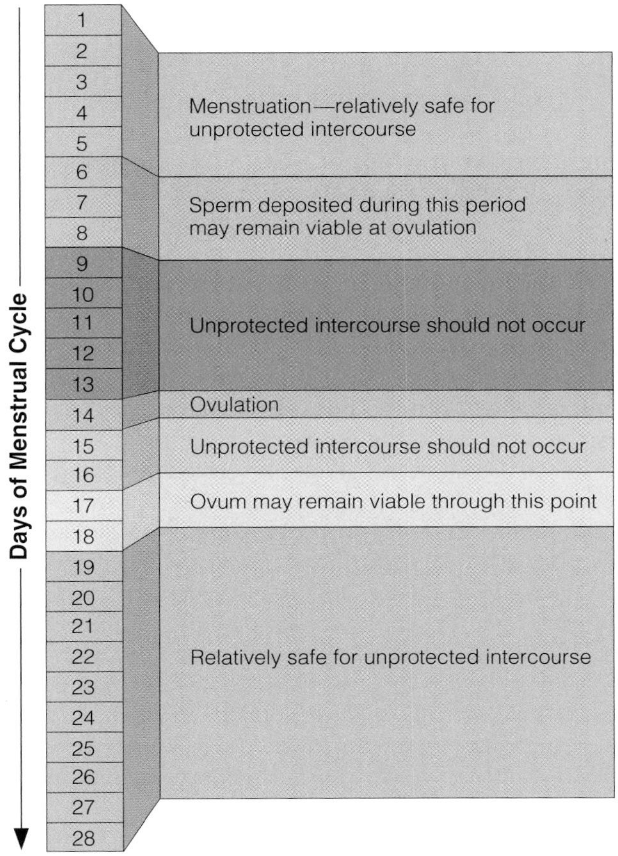

FIGURE 8-10 Safe and Unsafe Days
Events in the menstrual cycle determine the relatively safe days for unprotected intercourse.

- No need for a prescription, medical visit, or fittings.
- Nothing to insert, swallow, or check.
- No effect on fertility.
- Complies with the teachings of the Roman Catholic Church.

Disadvantages of Fertility Awareness

- Less reliable than other forms of birth control.
- Couples must abstain from vaginal intercourse eight to eleven days a month or use some form of contraception.
- Conscientious planning and scheduling is essential.
- May not work for women with irregular menstrual cycles.
- Some women find the mucus or temperature methods difficult to use.

vaginal contraceptive film (VCF) A small dissolvable sheet saturated with spermicide that can be inserted into the vagina and placed over the cervix.

rhythm method A birth-control method in which sexual intercourse is avoided during those days of the menstrual cycle in which fertilization is most likely to occur.

? FAQ What Is Emergency Contraception?

Emergency contraception (EC) is the use of a method of contraception to prevent unintended pregnancy after unprotected intercourse or the failure of another form of contraception, such as a condom breaking or slipping off. If emergency contraception were widely available and widely used, it would result in 800,000 fewer abortions and 1.7 million fewer unintended pregnancies.[11] EC has proved extremely safe in almost all women, as confirmed by numerous health organizations, including the World Health Organization and American College of Obstetricians and Gynecologists.[12]

Combination estrogen-progestin pills, progestin-only pills, and the copper-bearing intrauterine device (IUD) have been used as methods of emergency contraception for decades.[13] The progestin-only pills, referred to as Plan B, have proved more effective with fewer side effects than the combination pills. Originally Plan B consisted of two pills, but recent studies have shown that a single dose of 1.5 mg of the progestin levonorgestrel is as effective as two 0.75-mg doses, without increasing side effects.[14]

Emergency contraception pills (ECPs) stop pregnancy in the same way as other hormonal contraceptives: They delay or inhibit ovulation, inhibit fertilization, or block implantation of a fertilized egg, depending on a woman's phase of the menstrual cycle. They have no effect once a pregnancy has been established.

Most women can safely use ECPs, even if they cannot use birth control pills as their regular method of birth control. (Although ECPs use the same hormones as birth control pills, not all brands of birth control pills can be used for emergency contraception.) Some women may experience spotting or a full menstrual period a few days after taking ECPs, depending on where they were in their cycle when they began therapy. Most women have their next period at the expected time.[15]

Among sexually active college women, 11 percent report having used emergency contraception in the past year.[16] According to a national survey of colleges and universities, slightly more than half of student health centers offer emergency contraception.[17] The primary reasons for not dispensing EC are religious affiliation, insufficient staff, and lack of funding. None of the two-year colleges surveyed provide EC. More public institutions, rural schools, four-year institutions, and schools with enrollments smaller than 15,000 are offering EC than in the past.[18]

Many medical and health organizations have urged the FDA to make EC available without a physician's prescription as an over-the-counter product. As of this printing, the FDA has not done so. Some states are trying to make EC more accessible by mandating it for women who have been sexually assaulted, allowing pharmacists to dispense EC without a prescription, or requiring pharmacies that stock contraceptives to provide EC as well.[19]

Some health-care providers, including college health centers, have refused to provide emergency contraception to women because of religious or moral beliefs. Legislators have proposed laws that would require health professionals who dispense other forms of birth control to provide emergency contraception as well. Should a doctor or pharmacist have the right to withhold a legal, tested, effective form of contraception from a woman concerned about an unintentional pregnancy? Or should a woman have the right to decide whether to use emergency contraception?

Your Decide

Sterilization

The most popular method of birth control among married couples in the United States is **sterilization** (surgery to end a person's reproductive capability). Each year an estimated 1 million men and women in the United States undergo sterilization procedures. Fewer than 25 percent ever seek reversal.

Male Sterilization

In men, the cutting of the vas deferens, the tube that carries sperm from one of the testes into the urethra for ejaculation, is called **vasectomy.** During the 15- or 20-minute office procedure, done under a local anesthetic, the doctor makes small incisions in the scrotum, lifts up each vas deferens, cuts them, and ties off the ends to block the flow of sperm (Figure 8-11). Sperm continue to form, but they are broken down and absorbed by the body.

The man usually experiences some local pain, swelling, and discoloration for about a week after the procedure. More serious complications, including the formation of a blood clot in the scrotum (which usually disappears without treatment), infection, and an inflammatory reaction, occur in a small percentage of cases.

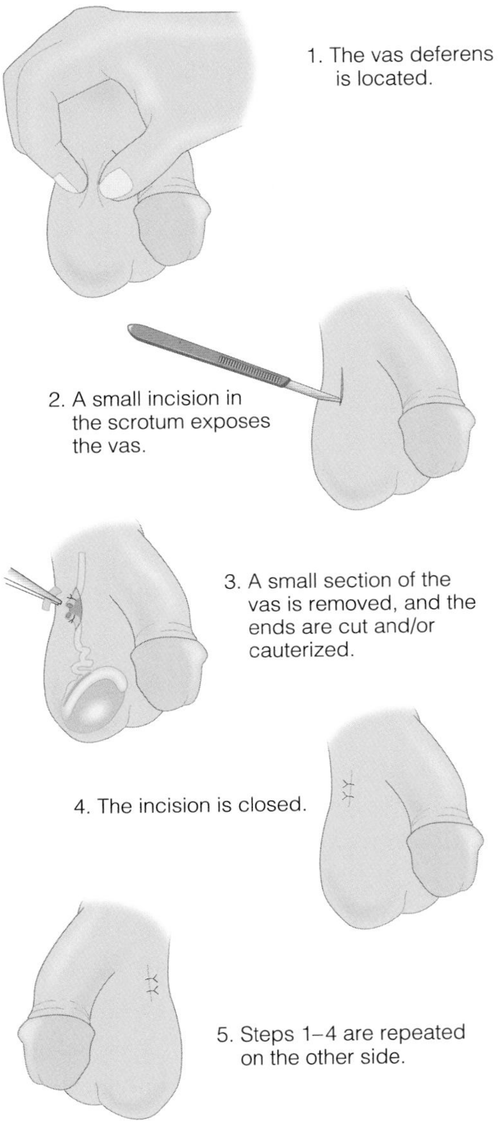

1. The vas deferens is located.
2. A small incision in the scrotum exposes the vas.
3. A small section of the vas is removed, and the ends are cut and/or cauterized.
4. The incision is closed.
5. Steps 1–4 are repeated on the other side.

FIGURE 8-11 Male Sterilization, or Vasectomy

Sometimes men want to reverse their vasectomies, usually because they want to have children with a new spouse. Although anyone who chooses to have a vasectomy should consider it permanent, surgical reversal (*vasovasostomy*) is sometimes successful. New microsurgical techniques have led to annual pregnancy rates for the wives of men having undergone vasovasostomies of about 50 percent, depending on such factors as the doctor's expertise and the time elapsed since the vasectomy.

Female Sterilization

Eleven million U.S. women ages 15 to 44 rely on tubal sterilization for contraception. An estimated 750,000 tubal sterilization procedures are performed each year in the United States. The average age of sterilization is about 30. Female sterilization procedures modify the fallopian tubes, which each month normally carry an egg from the ovaries to the uterus. The two terms used to describe female sterilization are **tubal ligation** (the cutting or tying of the fallopian tubes) and **tubal occlusion** (the blocking of the tubes). The tubes may be cut or sealed with thread, a clamp, or a clip, or by electrical coagulation to prevent the passage of eggs from the ovaries (Figure 8-12). They also can be blocked with bands of silicone.

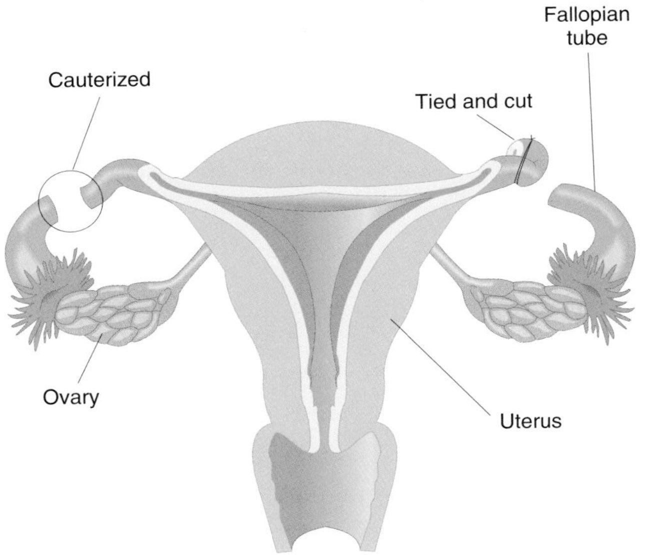

FIGURE 8-12 Female Sterilization, or Tubal Ligation

One of the common methods of tubal ligation or occlusion uses **laparoscopy,** commonly called *belly-button* or *band-aid surgery.* This procedure is done on an outpatient basis and takes 15 to 30 minutes. A lighted tube called a *laparoscope* is inserted through a half-inch incision made right below the navel, giving the doctor a view of the fallopian tubes. Using surgical instruments that may be inserted through the laparoscope

emergency contraception (CE) Types of oral contraceptive pills, usually taken within 72 hours after intercourse, that can prevent pregnancy.

sterilization A surgical procedure to end a person's reproductive capability.

vasectomy A surgical sterilization procedure in which each vas deferens is cut and tied shut to stop the passage of sperm to the urethra for ejaculation.

tubal ligation The suturing or tying shut of the fallopian tubes to prevent pregnancy.

tubal occlusion The blocking of the fallopian tubes to prevent pregnancy.

laparoscopy A surgical sterilization procedure in which the fallopian tubes are observed, with a laparoscope inserted through a small incision, and then cut or blocked.

or through other tiny incisions, the doctor then cuts or seals the tubes, most commonly by electrical coagulation.

The cumulative failure rate of tubal sterilization is about 1.85 percent during a 10-year period. Complications include problems with anesthesia, hemorrhage, organ damage, and mortality.

Essure

This new method for permanent sterilization involves placement of small, flexible microcoils into the fallopian tubes via the vagina by a physician. Unlike other methods, it does not require the risks of general anesthesia and surgery. The procedure itself does not require incisions and takes an average of about 35 minutes. Recovery occurs quickly. In clinical trials, about 90 percent of women returned to work within 24 hours. For the first three months after insertion, women should use another form of contraception. An X ray called a hysterosalpingogram must confirm that the inserts are correctly placed and the fallopian tubes are completely blocked.

Like traditional forms of tubal ligation, Essure cannot be reversed. It is recommended only for women who definitely do not want more children and especially for those with medical and health problems (such as diabetes, heart disease, or obesity) that make surgery and anesthesia more dangerous. There is a risk that the microinserts may not be placed correctly at the first attempt (this occurred in 14 percent of women in one study). Because the procedure is new, long-term data on the effectiveness of Essure are not yet available.

Advantages of Sterilization

- Offers permanent protection against unwanted pregnancy.
- No effect on sex drive in men or women. Many couples report greater sexual activity and pleasure because they no longer have to worry about pregnancy or deal with contraceptives.
- Vasectomy and tubal ligation are performed as outpatient procedures, with a quick recovery time.
- Use of Essure requires no incision, so there's less discomfort and very rapid recovery. Essure may be an option for women with chronic health conditions, such as obesity, diabetes, or heart disease.

Disadvantages of Sterilization

- All procedures should be considered permanent and used only if both partners are certain they want no more children.
- No protection against STIs.
- Must use another form of birth control for first three months.
- Many long-term risks remain unknown, but there is no evidence of any link between vasectomy and prostate cancer.

Abortion

More than half of unintended pregnancies end in induced abortions. Abortion rates vary greatly around the world. The U.S. abortion rate, which has declined, still remains higher than that of many Western countries, including Canada, Great Britain, the Netherlands, and Sweden. Although there is no one single or simple explanation for this difference, researchers focus on America's high rate of unintended pregnancies. In many nations with fewer unwanted pregnancies and lower abortion rates, contraceptives are generally easier and cheaper to obtain, and early sex education strongly emphasizes their importance.

No woman in any country ever elects to be in a situation where she has to consider abortion. But if faced with an unwanted pregnancy, many women consider *elective abortion* as an option.

After rising steadily through the 1970s, the number of legal abortions leveled off in the 1980s and declined in the 1990s. As fewer Americans have used contraception, the decline in abortion rates has halted. Although women of all backgrounds have abortions, abortion in the United States is most likely to occur among single women, racial or ethnic minorities, low-income women, and women who have had at least one child.

Claims that abortion increases the risk of breast cancer, based on retrospective studies that are less accurate because they rely on individuals' recall, have proved false. Research has found no correlation between the termination of a pregnancy, whether induced or spontaneous, and increased risk of breast cancer.[20]

Thinking Through the Options

A woman faced with an unwanted pregnancy—often alone, unwed, and desperate—can find it extremely difficult to decide what to do. The political debate over the right to life almost always is secondary to practical and emotional matters, such as the quality of her relationship with the baby's father, their capacity to provide for the child, the impact on any children she already has, and other important life issues.

Giving up her child for adoption is an option for women who do not feel abortion is right for them. Because the number of would-be adoptive parents greatly exceeds the number of available newborns, some women considering adoption may feel pressured by offers of money from couples eager to adopt. Others, particularly minority women, may feel cultural pressures to keep a child—regardless of their age, economic situation, or ability to care for an infant. Advocates of adoption reform are pressing for mandatory counseling for all pregnant women considering adoption (available now in agency-arranged, but not private, adoptions) and for extending the period of time during which a new mother can change her mind about giving up her child for adoption.

Medical Abortion

The term **medical abortion** describes the use of drugs, also called *abortifacients,* to terminate a pregnancy. In 2000, the abortion pill mifepristone (Mifeprex), formerly known as RU-486, became available for use in the United States. Mifepristone, which is 97 percent effective in inducing abortion, blocks progesterone, the hormone that prepares the uterine lining for pregnancy. Two days after taking this compound, a woman takes a prostaglandin to increase uterine contractions. The uterine lining is expelled along with the fertilized egg (Figure 8-13).

Women have compared the discomfort of this experience to severe menstrual cramps. Common side effects include excessive bleeding, nausea, fatigue, abdominal pain, and dizziness. About 1 woman in 100 requires a blood transfusion. The FDA has warned doctors about rare but deadly bloodstream infections in women using mifepristone. The rate of infection is about 1 in 100,000 uses, comparable to infection risks with surgical abortions and childbirth.

Although condemned by right-to-life advocates, abortion medications may in time lower the public profile of pregnancy termination. They are not painless, cheap, or equally available to all, but they do offer women a chance to carry through on their personal choice in greater privacy and safety.

Medical abortion does not require anesthesia and can be performed very early in pregnancy. However, women experience more cramping and bleeding during medical abortion than during surgical abortion, and bleeding lasts for a longer period.

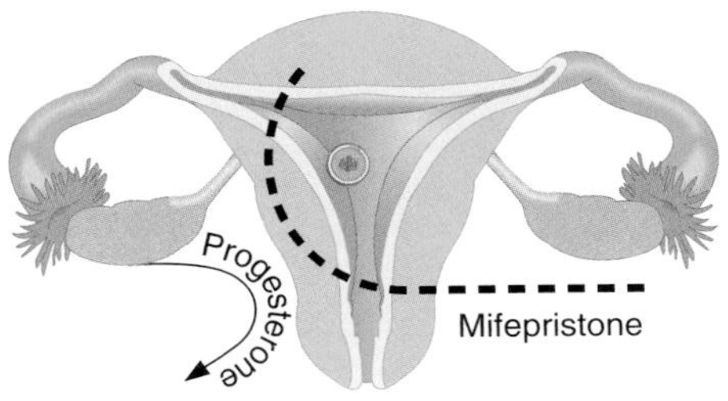

Step 1. Taken early in pregnancy, mifepristone blocks the action of progesterone and makes the body react as if it weren't pregnant.

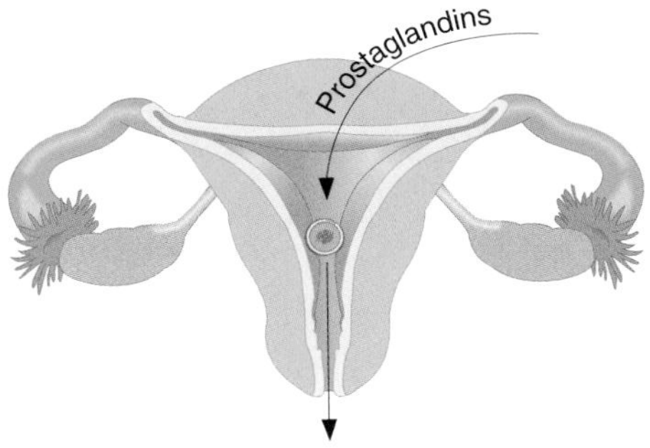

Step 2. Prostaglandins, taken two days later, cause the uterus to contract and the cervix to soften and dilate. As a result, the fertilized egg is expelled in 97 percent of cases.

FIGURE 8-13 Medical Abortion

Mifepristone works by blocking the action of progesterone, a hormone produced by the ovaries that is necessary for the implantation and development of a fertilized egg.

Other Abortion Methods

About half of all abortions (54 percent) are performed within the first 8 weeks of pregnancy. Only about 1 percent of abortions occur after 20 weeks. Medically, first-trimester abortion is less risky than childbirth. However, the likelihood of complications increases when abortions are performed in the second trimester (the second three-month period) of pregnancy.

The majority of abortions performed in the United States today are surgical. **Suction curettage,** usually done from 7 to 13 weeks after the last menstrual period, involves the gradual dilation (opening) of the cervix, often by inserting into the cervix one or more sticks of *laminaria* (a sterilized seaweed that absorbs moisture and expands, thus gradually stretching the cervix). Some women feel pressure or cramping with the laminaria in place. Occasionally, the laminaria itself starts to bring on a miscarriage.

At the time of abortion, the laminaria is removed, and dilators are used to further enlarge the cervical opening, if needed. The physician inserts a suction tip into the cervix, and the uterine contents are drawn out via a vacuum system (Figure 8-14). A *curette* (a spoon-shaped surgical instrument used for scraping) is used to check for complete removal of the contents of the uterus. With suction curettage, the risks of complication are low. Major complications, such as perforation of the uterus, occur in fewer than 1 in 100 cases.

For early second-trimester abortions, physicians generally use a technique called **dilation and evacuation (D and E),** in

medical abortion Method of ending a pregnancy within nine weeks of conception using hormonal medications that cause expulsion of the fertilized egg.

suction curettage A procedure in which the contents of the uterus are removed by means of suction and scraping.

dilation and evacuation (D and E) A medical procedure in which the contents of the uterus are removed through the use of instruments.

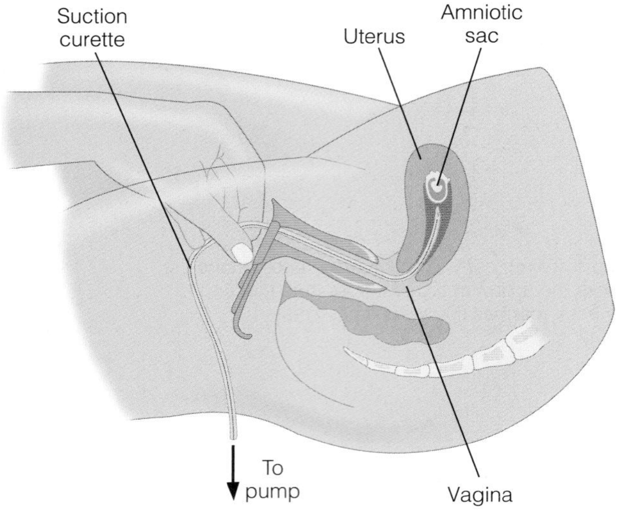

FIGURE 8-14 Suction Curettage
The contents of the uterus are extracted through the cervix with a vacuum apparatus.

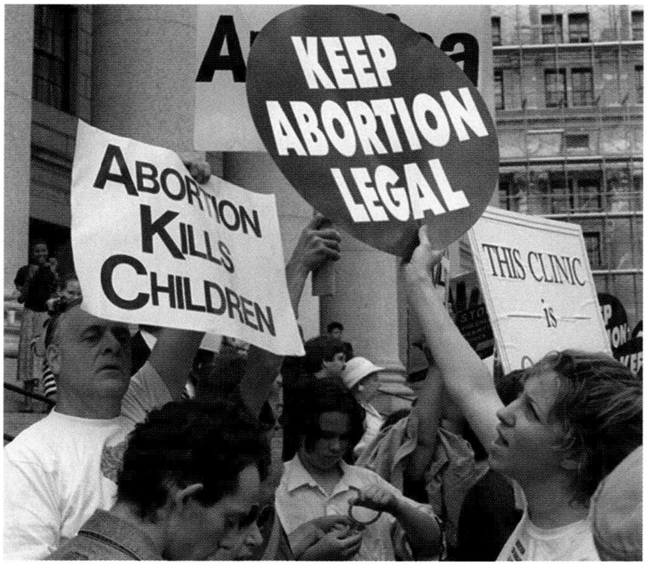

The controversy over abortion has resulted in countless demonstrations and encounters between pro-choice and pro-life supporters.

which they open the cervix and use medical instruments to remove the fetus from the uterus. D and E procedures are performed under local or general anesthesia.

To induce abortion from week 16 to week 20, prostaglandins (natural substances found in most body tissues) are administered as vaginal suppositories or injected into the amniotic sac by inserting a needle through the abdominal wall. They induce uterine contractions, and the fetus and placenta are expelled within 24 hours. Injecting saline or urea solutions into the amniotic sac also can terminate the pregnancy by triggering contractions that expel the fetus and placenta. Sometimes vaginal suppositories or drugs that help the uterus contract are used. Complications from abortion techniques that induce labor include nausea, vomiting, diarrhea, tearing of the cervix, excessive bleeding, and possible shock and death.

? FAQ What Is the Psychological Impact of Abortion?

Many assume that abortion must be psychologically devastating, that women who abort a fetus sooner or later develop what some have termed *postabortion trauma syndrome.* In her studies at the University of Chicago, psychiatrist Nada Stotland found that there is no such thing. The primary emotion of women who have just had an abortion, she discovered, is relief. Although many women also express feelings of sadness or guilt, their anxiety levels eventually drop until they are lower than they were immediately before the abortion.

Nonetheless, although psychologists consider the mental health risks minimal compared to those of bearing an unwanted child, this does not mean women who have abortions never have regrets. But a feeling—even one as painful as loss, sadness, or guilt—is not a syndrome, and a woman's responses to abortion often change with passing days, weeks, months, or years. Anniversaries—of conception, of the date a woman found out she was pregnant, of the abortion, of the delivery date—can trigger memories and a sense of loss, but most women deal with these and move on with their lives.

The best predictor of psychological well-being after abortion is a woman's emotional well-being prior to pregnancy. At highest risk are women who have had a psychiatric illness, such as an anxiety disorder or clinical depression, prior to an abortion, and those whose abortions occurred among complicated circumstances (such as a rape, or coercion by parents or a partner). The vast majority of women manage to put the abortion into perspective as one of many life events.

Politics of Abortion

Abortion is one of the most controversial political, religious, and ethical issues of our time. The issues of when life begins, a woman's right to choose, and an unborn child's right to survival are among the most divisive Americans face. Abortions were legal in the United States until the 1860s. For decades after that, women who decided to terminate unwanted pregnancies did so by attempting to abort on their own or by obtaining illegal abortions—often performed by untrained individuals using unsanitary and unsafe procedures. In the late 1960s, some states changed their laws to make abortions legal. In 1973, the U.S. Supreme Court, following a 1970 ruling on the case of *Roe v. Wade* by the New York Supreme Court, said that an abortion in the first trimester of pregnancy was a decision between a woman and her physician and was protected by privacy laws. The Court further ruled that abortion during the second trimester could be performed on the basis of health risks and that abortion during the final trimester could be performed only for the sake of the mother's health.

The debate over abortion continues to stir passionate emotions, with pro-life supporters arguing that life begins at conception and that abortion is therefore immoral, and pro-choice advocates countering that an individual woman should have the right to make decisions about her body and health. The controversy over abortion has at times become violent: Physicians who perform abortions have been shot and killed; abortion clinics have been bombed, wounding and killing patients and staff members. Although the majority of Americans continue to support abortion, many feel that it should be more restricted and difficult to obtain.

Congress has banned partial birth abortion, which is performed in the later stages of pregnancy and involves collapsing the skull to allow a fetus to slip easily from the birth canal. Courts in several states have challenged the ban as "unconstitutional" because it does not provide a "health" exception.

In a controversial move, South Dakota has banned abortion except in cases where the mother's life is in danger. It prohibits administering, prescribing, procuring, or selling any substance that terminates a pregnancy, although it does allow the sale of contraceptives that can be administered before a pregnancy "could be determined through conventional medical testing."[21]

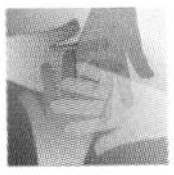

A Cross-Cultural Perspective

Throughout the world an estimated 10 to 20 million illegal abortions are performed each year. About 1 in 100 women dies as a result. Women who survive illegal abortions may suffer chronic health problems related to the lack of adequate medical care.

In other countries, abortion laws vary greatly. In Eastern Europe, where abortions were once legal and common, the collapse of communism has led to new restrictions on abortion. By contrast, Spain's supreme court has relaxed legal restrictions on abortions performed on social grounds. In Pakistan, new, more liberal rules on abortion state that abortion is no longer a crime if carried out to provide "necessary treatment." In Latin America, where anti-abortion laws are very strict, Cuba is the only country in which abortion on request is legal in early pregnancy. In other nations of Central and South America, women obtaining abortions and those performing them face criminal penalties, including imprisonment.

Childfree by Choice

More women and men are deliberately choosing to remain "childfree." According to the limited data available, single childfree women tend to be better educated, more cosmopolitan, less religious, and more professional than those in the general population. In general, childfree women are high achievers, often in demanding careers, who describe their work as exciting and satisfying. Childless couples are predominantly urban, well-educated, and upper middle class, with egalitarian and long-running marriages.

Their reasons for not having children are diverse: a desire to maintain their freedom, more time with their partners, career ambitions, concern about overpopulation and the fate of the Earth. Some women cite the hostile work environment for mothers and the inadequacy of day care. Others say they're disillusioned with the have-it-all hopes of baby boomers and believe in a have-most-of-it philosophy.

Pregnancy

In the last half century, pregnancy rates have generally declined. The average age of mothers in the United States has risen, but about 70 percent of babies are still born to women in their twenties. Mothers are now averaging about two children each.

The number of never-married, college-educated, career women who are becoming single parents has risen dramatically. They want children—with or without an ongoing relationship with a man—and may feel that, because of their age, they can't delay getting pregnant any longer.

Preconception Care

The time *before* a child is conceived can be crucial in assuring that an infant is born healthy, full-size, and full-term. Women who smoke, drink alcohol, take drugs, eat poorly, are too thin or too heavy, suffer from unrecognized infections or illnesses, or are exposed to toxins at work or home may start pregnancy with one or more strikes against them and their unborn babies. The best chance for lowering the infant mortality rate and preventing birth defects is before pregnancy. **Preconception care**—the enhancement of a woman's health and well-being prior to conception in order to ensure a healthy pregnancy and baby—includes risk assessment (evaluation of medical, genetic, and lifestyle risks), health promotion (such as teaching good

preconception care Health care to prepare for pregnancy.

nutrition), and interventions to reduce risk (such as treatment of infections and other diseases, and assistance in quitting smoking or drug use).

Home Pregnancy Tests

The sooner a woman realizes she is pregnant, the more she can do to take care of herself and her child. Home pregnancy tests detect the presence of human chorionic gonadotropin (hCG), which is secreted as the fertilized egg implants in the uterus. If the concentration of hCG is high enough, a woman will test positive for pregnancy. If the test is done too early, the result will be a false negative. A follow-up test a week later can usually confirm a pregnancy. Although home pregnancy tests are 85 to 95 percent accurate, medical laboratory tests provide definitive confirmation of a pregnancy.

How a Woman's Body Changes During Pregnancy

The 40 weeks of pregnancy transform a woman's body. At the beginning of pregnancy, the woman's uterus becomes slightly larger, and the cervix becomes softer and bluish due to increased blood flow. Progesterone and estrogen trigger changes in the milk glands and ducts in the breasts, which increase in size and feel somewhat tender. The pressure of the growing uterus against the bladder causes a more frequent need to urinate. As the pregnancy progresses, the woman's skin stretches as her body shape changes, her center of gravity changes as her abdomen protrudes, and her internal organs shift as the baby grows (Figure 8-15). Pregnancy is typically divided into three-month periods called trimesters.

How a Baby Grows

Silently and invisibly, over a nine-month period, a fertilized egg develops into a human being. When the zygote reaches the uterus, it's still smaller than the head of a pin. Once nestled into the spongy uterine lining, it becomes an **embryo.** The embryo takes on an elongated shape, rounded at one end. A sac called the **amnion** envelops it (see photo on page **220**). As water and other small molecules cross the amniotic membrane, the embryo floats freely in the absorbed fluid, cushioned from shocks and bumps. At nine weeks the embryo is called a **fetus.**

A special organ, the **placenta,** forms. Attached to the embryo by the umbilical cord, it supplies the growing baby with fluid and nutrients from the maternal bloodstream and carries waste back to the mother's body for disposal (Figure 8-16).

Complications of Pregnancy

In about 10 to 15 percent of all pregnancies, there is increased risk of some problem, such as a baby's failure to grow normally. *Perinatology,* or maternal-fetal medicine, focuses on the special needs of high-risk mothers and their unborn babies. Perinatal centers, with state-of-the-art equipment and 24-hour staffs of specialists in this field, have been set up around the country. Several of the most frequent potential complications of pregnancy are discussed next.

Ectopic Pregnancy

Any woman who is of childbearing age, has had intercourse, and feels abdominal pain with no reasonable cause may have an **ectopic pregnancy.** In this type of pregnancy, the fertilized egg remains in the fallopian tube instead of traveling to the uterus. Ectopic, or tubal, pregnancies have increased dramatically in recent years, now accounting for 2 percent of all reported pregnancies. STIs, particularly chlamydia infections (discussed in Chapter 9), have become a major cause of ectopic pregnancy. Other risk factors include previous pelvic surgery, particularly involving the fallopian tubes; pelvic inflammatory disease; infertility; and use of an IUD.

Miscarriage

About 10 to 20 percent of pregnancies end in **miscarriage,** or spontaneous abortion, before the 20th week of gestation. Major genetic disorders may be responsible for 33 to 50 percent of pregnancy losses. The most common cause is an abnormal number of chromosomes. About 0.5 to 1 percent of women suffer three or more miscarriages, possibly because of genetic, anatomic, hormonal, infectious, or autoimmune factors. An estimated 70 to 90 percent of women who miscarry eventually become pregnant again.

Infections

The infectious disease most clearly linked to birth defects is **rubella** (German measles). All women should be vaccinated against this disease at least three months prior to conception, to protect themselves and any children they may bear. (See Chapter 9 for more on immunization.) The most common prenatal infection today is *cytomegalovirus.* This infection produces mild flulike symptoms in adults but can cause brain damage, retardation, liver disease, cerebral palsy, hearing problems, and other malformations in unborn babies.

STIs, such as syphilis, gonorrhea, and genital herpes, can be particularly dangerous during pregnancy if not recognized and treated. If a woman has a herpes

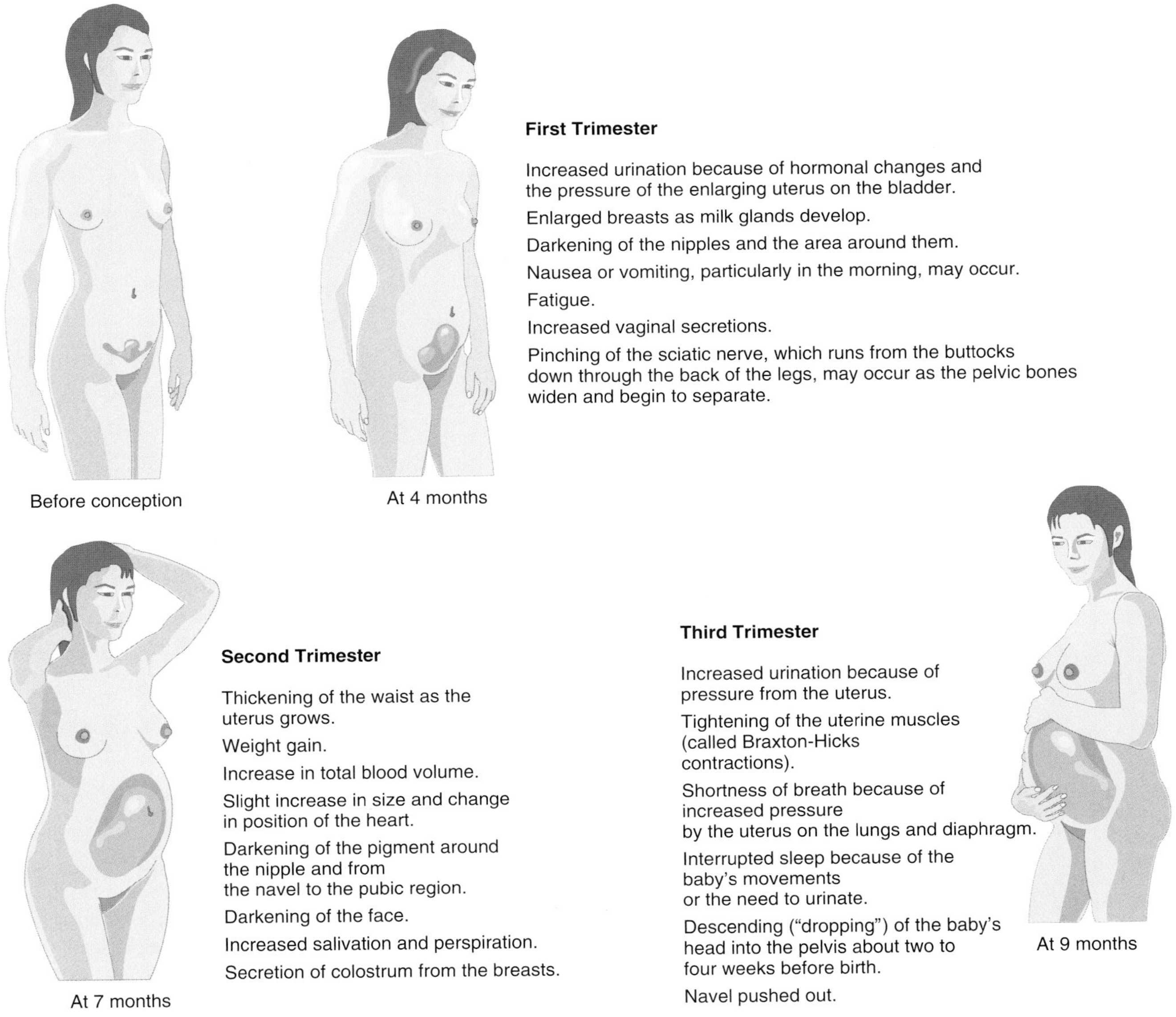

First Trimester
Increased urination because of hormonal changes and the pressure of the enlarging uterus on the bladder.
Enlarged breasts as milk glands develop.
Darkening of the nipples and the area around them.
Nausea or vomiting, particularly in the morning, may occur.
Fatigue.
Increased vaginal secretions.
Pinching of the sciatic nerve, which runs from the buttocks down through the back of the legs, may occur as the pelvic bones widen and begin to separate.
Before conception
At 4 months
Second Trimester
Thickening of the waist as the uterus grows.
Weight gain.
Increase in total blood volume.
Slight increase in size and change in position of the heart.
Darkening of the pigment around the nipple and from the navel to the pubic region.
Darkening of the face.
Increased salivation and perspiration.
Secretion of colostrum from the breasts.
At 7 months
Third Trimester
Increased urination because of pressure from the uterus.
Tightening of the uterine muscles (called Braxton-Hicks contractions).
Shortness of breath because of increased pressure by the uterus on the lungs and diaphragm.
Interrupted sleep because of the baby's movements or the need to urinate.
Descending ("dropping") of the baby's head into the pelvis about two to four weeks before birth.
Navel pushed out.
At 9 months

FIGURE 8-15 Physiological Changes of Pregnancy

outbreak around the date her baby is due, her physician will deliver the baby by caesarean section to prevent infecting the baby. HIV infection endangers both a pregnant woman and her unborn baby, and all pregnant women and new mothers should be aware of the HIV epidemic, the risks to them and their babies, and the availability of anonymous testing.

Genetic Disorders

In some sense, each of us is a carrier of a genetic problem. Every individual has an estimated four to six defective genes, but the chances of passing them on to a child are slim. Almost all are recessive, which means they are "masked" by a more influential dominant gene. The

embryo An organism in its early stage of development; in humans, the embryonic period lasts from the second to the eighth week of pregnancy.

amnion The innermost membrane of the sac enclosing the embryo or fetus.

fetus The human organism developing in the uterus from the ninth week until birth.

placenta An organ that develops after implantation and to which the embryo attaches, via the umbilical cord, for nourishment and waste removal.

ectopic pregnancy A pregnancy in which the fertilized egg has implanted itself outside the uterine cavity, usually in the fallopian tube.

miscarriage A pregnancy that terminates before the twentieth week of gestation; also called spontaneous abortion.

rubella An infectious disease that may cause birth defects if contracted by a pregnant woman; also called German measles.

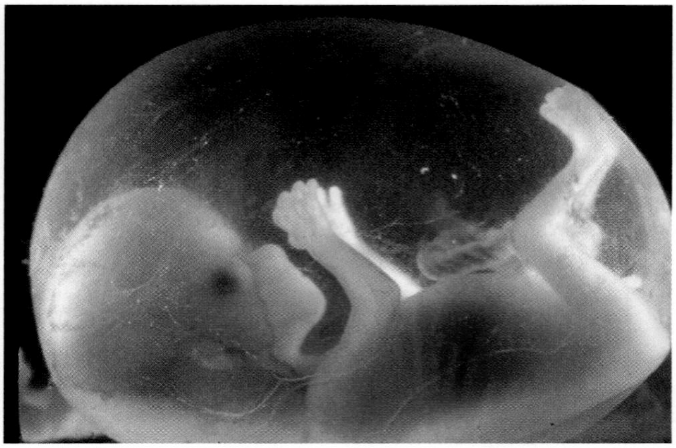

Embryo within the amnion.

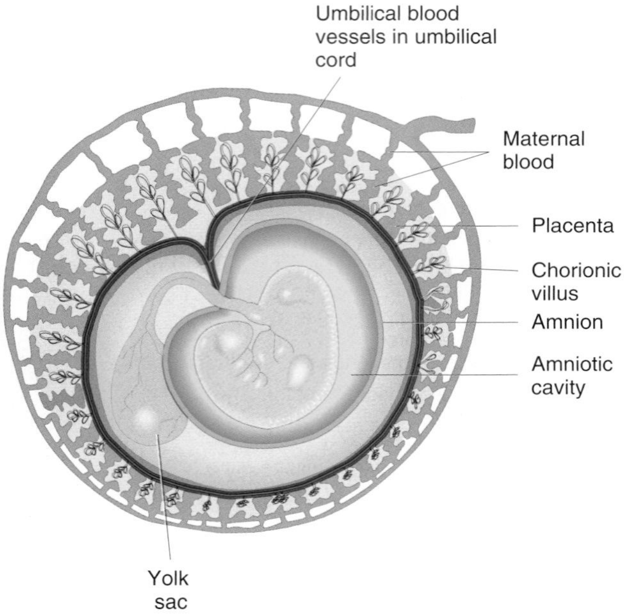

FIGURE 8-16 The Placenta

The placenta supplies the growing embryo with fluid and nutrients from the maternal bloodstream and carries waste back for disposal.

likelihood of a child inheriting the same faulty recessive gene from both parents is remote—unless the parents are so closely related that they have very similar genetic makeup.

The child of a parent with an abnormal dominant gene has a 50 percent likelihood of inheriting it. The most common of such defects are minor, such as the growth of an extra finger or toe. However, some single-gene defects can be fatal. Huntington's chorea, for example, is a degenerative disease that in the past was usually not diagnosed until midlife.

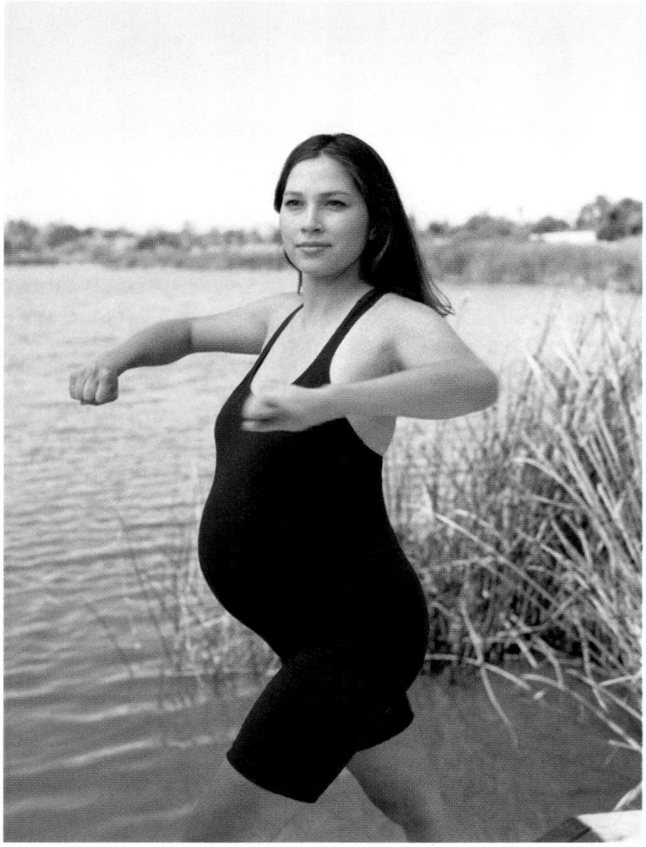

Most pregnant women benefit from regular moderate exercise.

Genetic tests can identify "carriers" of abnormal recessive genes for diseases such as sickle-cell anemia (the most common genetic disorder among African Americans), beta-thalassemia (found in families of Mediterranean origin), and Tay-Sachs (found in Jews of Eastern European origin). Two carriers of the same abnormal recessive genes can pass such problems on to their children.

Premature Labor

Approximately 10 percent of all babies are born too soon (before the 37th week of pregnancy). According to researchers, prematurity is the main underlying cause of stillbirth and infant deaths within the first few weeks after birth. Bed rest, close monitoring, and, if necessary, medications for at-risk women can buy more time in the womb for their babies. But women must recognize the warning signs of **premature labor**—dull, low backache; a feeling of tightness or pressure on the lower abdomen; and intestinal cramps, sometimes with diarrhea. Low-birthweight premature babies face the highest risks, but comprehensive, enriched programs can reduce developmental and health problems.

Strategies for Prevention — A Mother-to-Be's Guide to a Healthy Pregnancy

- The American College of Obstetricians and Gynecologists (ACOG) recommends consuming about 300 more calories a day than before pregnancy and concentrating on eating the right foods, not on watching your weight. Never diet during pregnancy. Don't restrict salt intake either, unless specifically directed to by your doctor.
- Drink six to eight glasses of liquids each day, including water, fruit and vegetable juices, and milk.
- Don't exercise strenuously for more than 15 minutes, ACOG advises. Avoid vigorous exercise in hot, humid weather. Never let your body temperature rise above 100°F or your heart rate climb above 140 beats per minute.
- Stretch and flex carefully because the joints and connective tissue soften and loosen during pregnancy. After the fourth month of pregnancy, don't do any exercises while lying on your back, as this could impair blood flow to the placenta.
- Walk, swim, and jog in moderation; play tennis only if you played before pregnancy. Ski only if you're experienced, and stick to low altitudes and safe slopes. Do not water-ski, surf, or ride a horse.

Childbirth

A generation ago, delivering a baby was something a doctor did in a hospital. Today parents can choose from many birthing options, including a birth attendant, who can be a physician or a nurse-midwife, and a birthing center, hospital, or home birth.

Preparing for Childbirth

The most widespread method of childbirth preparation is the **Lamaze method** (*psychoprophylaxis*). Fernand Lamaze, a French doctor, instructed women to respond to labor contractions with prelearned, controlled breathing techniques. As the intensity of each contraction increases, the laboring woman concentrates on increasing her breathing rate in a prescribed way. Her partner coaches her during each contraction and helps her cope with discomfort.

Women who attend prenatal classes are less likely to undergo Caesarean deliveries and more likely to breast feed. They also tend to have fewer complications and require fewer medications. However, painkillers or anesthesia are always an option if labor is longer or more painful than expected. The lower body can be numbed with an *epidural block,* which involves injecting an anesthetic into the membrane around the spinal cord, or a *spinal block,* in which the injection goes directly into the spinal canal. General anesthesia is usually used only for emergency caesarean births.

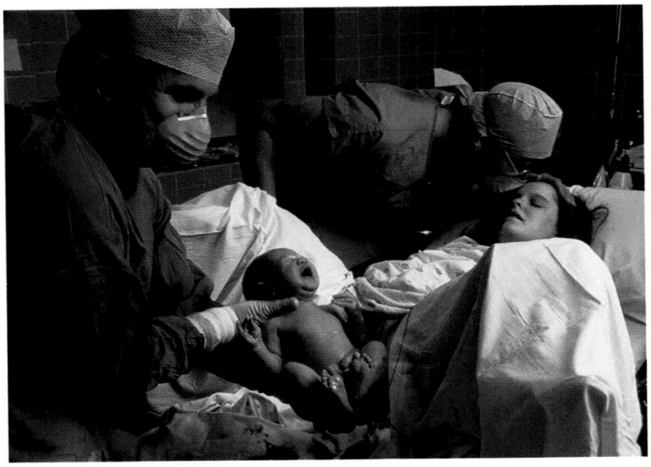

© SIU/Peter Arnold, Inc.

Today's fathers are active participants at the birth of their children.

? FAQ What Is Childbirth Like?

There are three stages of **labor.** The first starts with *effacement* (thinning) and *dilation* (opening up) of the cervix. Effacement is measured in percentages, and dilation in centimeters or finger-widths. Around this time, the amniotic sac of fluids usually breaks, a sign that the woman should call her doctor or midwife.

The first contractions of the early, or *latent,* phase of labor are usually not

premature labor Labor that occurs after the twentieth week but before the thirty-seventh week of pregnancy.

Lamaze method A method of childbirth preparation taught to expectant parents to help the woman cope with the discomfort of labor; combines breathing and psychological techniques.

labor The process leading up to birth: effacement and dilation of the cervix; the movement of the baby into and through the birth canal, accompanied by strong contractions; and contraction of the uterus and expulsion of the placenta after the birth.

uncomfortable; they last 15 to 30 seconds, occur every 15 to 30 minutes, and gradually increase in intensity and frequency. The most difficult contractions come after the cervix is dilated to about 8 centimeters, as the woman feels greater pressure from the fetus. The first stage ends when the cervix is completely dilated to a diameter of 10 centimeters (or five finger-widths) and the baby is ready to come down the birth canal (Figure 8-17). For women having their first baby, this first stage of labor averages 12 to 13 hours. Women having another child often experience shorter first-stage labor.

When the cervix is completely dilated, the second stage of labor occurs, during which the baby moves into the vagina, or birth canal, and out of the mother's body. As this stage begins, women who have gone through childbirth preparation training often feel a sense of relief from the acute pain of the transition phase and at the prospect of giving birth.

This second stage can take up to an hour or more. Strong contractions may last 60 to 90 seconds and occur every two to three minutes. As the baby's head descends, the mother feels an urge to push. By bearing down, she helps the baby complete its passage to the outside.

As the baby's head appears, or *crowns,* the doctor may perform an *episiotomy*—an incision from the lower end of the vagina toward the anus to enlarge the vaginal opening. The purpose of the episiotomy is to prevent the baby's head from causing an irregular tear in the vagina, but routine episiotomies have been criticized as unnecessary. Women may be able to avoid this procedure by trying different birthing positions or having an attendant massage the perineal tissue.

Usually the baby's head emerges first, then its shoulders, then its body. With each contraction, a new part is born. However, the baby can be in a more difficult position, facing up rather than down, or with the feet or

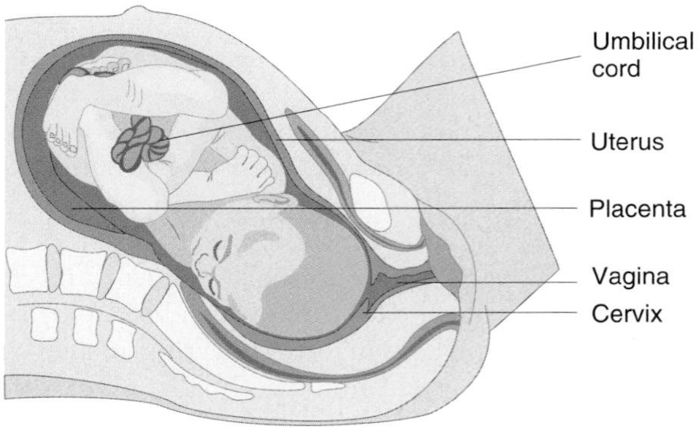

(a) The cervix is partially dilated, and the baby's head enters the birth canal.

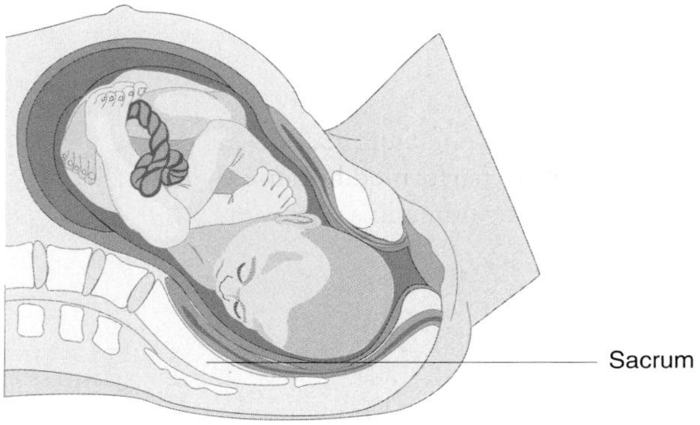

(b) The cervix is nearly completely dilated. The baby's head rotates so that it can move through the birth canal.

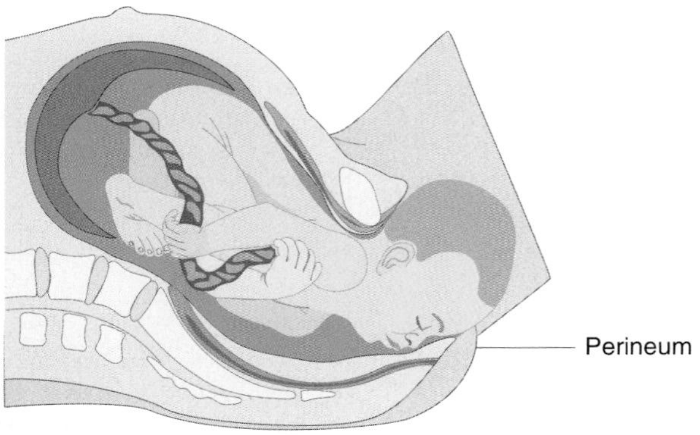

(c) The baby's head extends as it reaches the vaginal opening, and the head and the rest of the body pass through the birth canal.

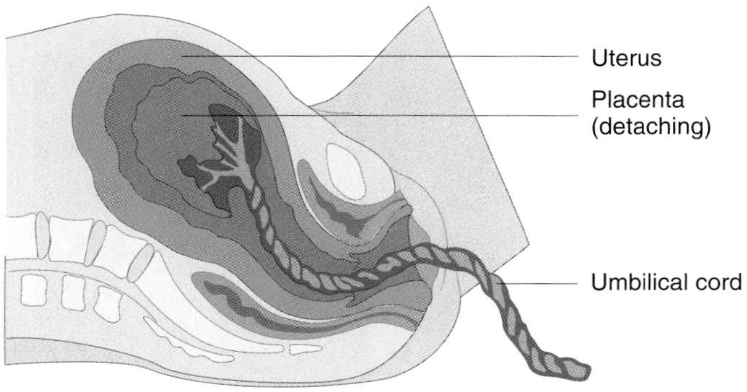

(d) After the baby is born, the placenta detaches from the uterus and is expelled from the woman's body.

FIGURE 8-17 Birth

buttocks first (a *breech birth*), and a cesarean birth may then be necessary.

In the third stage of labor, the uterus contracts firmly after the birth of the baby and, usually within five minutes, the placenta separates from the uterine wall. The woman may bear down to help expel the placenta, or the doctor may exert gentle external pressure. If an episiotomy has been performed, the doctor sews up the incision. To help the uterus contract and return to its normal size, it may be massaged manually, or the baby may be put to the mother's breast to stimulate contraction of the uterus.

Caesarean Birth

In a **caesarean delivery** (also referred to as a *caesarean section*), the doctor lifts the baby out of the woman's body through an incision made in the lower abdomen and uterus. The most common reason for caesarean birth is *failure to progress,* a vague term indicating that labor has gone on too long and may put the baby or mother at risk. Other reasons include the baby's position (if feet or buttocks are first) and signs that the fetus is in danger.

Thirty years ago, only 5 percent of babies born in America were delivered by caesarean birth; the current rate is 22.6 percent, substantially higher than in most other industrialized countries. About 36 percent of caesarean sections are performed because the woman has had a previous caesarean birth. However, four of every five women who have had caesarean births can have successful vaginal deliveries in subsequent pregnancies.

Caesarean birth involves abdominal surgery, so many women feel more physical discomfort after a caesarean than a vaginal birth, including nausea, pain, and abdominal gas. Women who have had a caesarean section must refrain from strenuous activity, such as heavy lifting, for several weeks.

Infertility

The World Health Organization defines **infertility** as the failure to conceive after one year of unprotected intercourse. Infertility affects one in seven couples. Women between ages 35 and 44 are about twice as likely to have fertility problems as women ages 30 to 34.

Infertility is a problem of the couple, not of the individual man or woman. In 40 percent of cases, infertility is caused by female problems, in 40 percent by male problems, in 10 percent by a combination of male and female problems, and in 10 percent by unexplained causes. A thorough diagnostic workup can reveal a cause for infertility in 90 percent of cases.

In women, the most common causes of subfertility or infertility are age, abnormal menstrual patterns, suppression of ovulation, and blocked fallopian tubes. A woman's fertility peaks between ages 20 and 30 and then drops quickly: by 20 percent after 30, by 50 percent after 35, and by 95 percent after 40.

Male subfertility or infertility is usually linked to either the quantity or the quality of sperm, which may be inactive, misshapen, or insufficient (less than 20 million sperm per milliliter of semen in an ejaculation of 3 to 5 milliliters). Sometimes the problem is hormonal or a blockage of a sperm duct. Some men suffer from the inability to ejaculate normally, or from retrograde ejaculation, in which some of the semen travels in the wrong direction, back into the body of the male.

Infertility can have an enormous emotional impact. Many women long to experience pregnancy and childbirth and feel great loss if they cannot conceive. Women in their thirties and forties fear that their biological clock is running out of time. Men may be confused and surprised by the intensity of their partner's emotions.

? FAQ What Are the Options for Infertile Couples?

The treatment of infertility has become a $2 billion a year enterprise in the United States. The odds of successful pregnancy range from 30 to 70 percent, depending on the specific cause of infertility. One result of successful infertility treatments has been a boom in multiple births, including quintuplets and sextuplets. Multiple births are associated with greater risk, both to the babies—including prematurity, low birthweight, neonatal death, and lifelong disability—and to the mothers, including caesarean section and hemorrhage.

Artificial Insemination

Since the 1960s, **artificial insemination**—the introduction of viable sperm into the vagina by artificial means—has led to an estimated 250,000 births in the

caesarean delivery The surgical procedure in which an infant is delivered through an incision made in the abdominal wall and uterus.

infertility The inability to conceive a child.

artificial insemination The introduction of viable sperm into the vagina by artificial means for the purpose of inducing conception.

United States, primarily in couples in which the husband was infertile. Some states do not recognize such children as legitimate; others do, but only if the woman's husband gave consent for the insemination.

Assisted Reproductive Technology

New approaches to infertility include microsurgery, sometimes with lasers, to open destroyed or blocked egg and sperm ducts; new hormone preparations to induce ovulation; and the use of balloons, inserted through the cervix and inflated, to open blocked fallopian tubes (a procedure called *balloon tuboplasty*). More than 35,000 babies are born each year as a result of assisted reproductive technology (ART).

The most common ART procedure is *in vitro fertilization (IVF),* which removes the ova from a woman's ovary and placing the woman's egg and her mate's sperm in a laboratory dish for fertilization. If the fertilized egg cell shows signs of development, within several days it is returned to the woman's uterus, the egg cell implants itself in the lining of the uterus, and the pregnancy continues as normal. The success rate varies but is generally about 25 percent, and the costs are high.

Adoption

Men and women who cannot conceive children biologically can still become parents. **Adoption** matches would-be parents yearning for youngsters to love with infants or children who need loving. Couples interested in adoption can work with either public agencies or private counselors who contact obstetricians directly. Or they can contact organizations that arrange adoptions of children in need from other countries.

There are no reliable statistics on the annual number of adoptions in the United States, but census records indicate there are currently 1.5 million adopted children in the United States. Each year some 50,000 U.S. children become available for adoption—far fewer than the number of would-be parents looking for youngsters to adopt. By some estimates, only 1 in 30 couples receive a child—and they spend about two years and as much as $100,000 on the adoption process.

adoption The legal process for becoming the parent to a child of other biological parents.

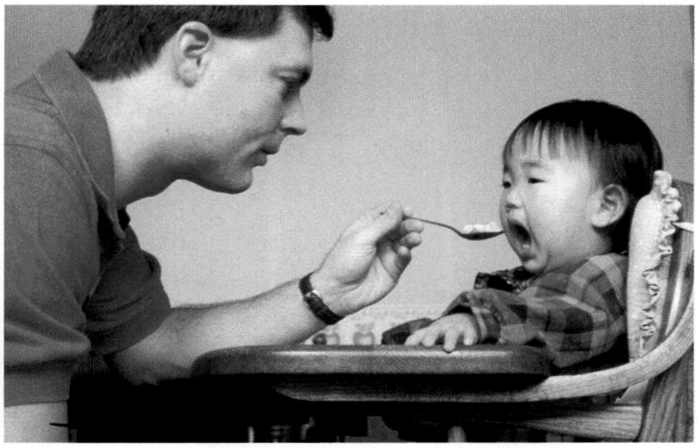

Mike Greenlar/The Image Works

Adoption matches would-be parents yearning for youngsters to love with infants or children who need loving homes.

LEARN IT / LIVE IT

Protecting Your Reproductive Health

The decisions you make about birth control can affect your reproductive health—and your partner's. Here are guidelines that can help prevent pregnancy and protect your reproductive well-being.

- **Abstain.** The only 100 percent safe and effective way to avoid unwanted pregnancy is not to engage in heterosexual intercourse.
- **Limit sexual activity to "outercourse."** You can engage in many sexual activities—kissing, hugging, touching, massage, oral-genital sex—without risking pregnancy.
- **Talk about birth control with any potential sex partner.** If you are considering sexual intimacy with a person, you should feel comfortable enough to talk about contraception.
- **Know what doesn't work—and don't rely on it.** There are many misconceptions about ways to avoid getting pregnant, such as having sex in a standing position or during menstruation. Only the methods described in this chapter are reliable forms of birth control.
- **Talk with a health-care professional.** A great deal of information and advice is available—in writing, from family planning counselors, from physicians on the Internet. Check it out.
- **Choose a contraceptive method that matches your personal habits and preferences.** If you can't remember to take a pill every day, oral contraceptives aren't for you. If you're constantly forgetting where you put things, a diaphragm might not be a good choice.
- **Consider long-term implications.** Since you may well wish to have children in the future, find out about the reversibility of various methods and possible effects on future fertility.

- **Resist having sex without contraceptive protection "just this once."** It only takes once—even the very first time—to get pregnant. Be wary of drugs and alcohol. They can impair your judgment and make you less conscientious about using birth control—or using it properly.
- **Use backup methods.** If there's a possibility that a contraceptive method might not offer adequate protection (for instance, if it's been almost three months since your last injection of Depo-Provera), use an additional form of birth control.
- **Inform yourself about emergency contraception.** Just in case a condom breaks or a diaphragm slips, find out about the availability of forms of after-intercourse contraception.

8 Making This Chapter Work for You

Review Questions

1. Conception occurs
   a. when a fertilized egg implants in the lining of the uterus.
   b. when sperm is blocked from reaching the egg.
   c. when a sperm fertilizes the egg.
   d. after the uterine lining is discharged during the menstrual cycle.
2. Factors to consider when choosing a contraceptive method include all of the following *except*
   a. cost.
   b. failure rate.
   c. effectiveness in preventing sexually transmitted infections.
   d. preferred sexual position.
3. When used correctly, which is the most effective nonhormonal contraceptive method?
   a. male condom
   b. female condom
   c. spermicide
   d. diaphragm
4. Which of the following contraceptive choices offers the best protection against STIs?
   a. condom alone
   b. condom plus spermicide
   c. abstinence
   d. withdrawal plus spermicide
5. Which statement about prescription contraceptives is *not* true?
   a. Prescription contraceptives do not offer protection against STIs.
   b. Some prescription contraceptives contain estrogen and progestin, and some contain only progestin.
   c. The contraceptive ring must be changed every week.
   d. IUDs prevent pregnancy by preventing or interfering with implantation.
6. Which of the following statements is true about sterilization?
   a. In women, the most frequently performed sterilization technique is Essure.
   b. Many couples experience an increase in sexual encounters after sterilization.
   c. Vasectomies are easily reversed with surgery.
   d. Sterilization is recommended for single men and women who are unsure about whether they want children.
7. Which statement about abortion is *false?*
   a. The abortion rate in the United States started declining in the 1990s.
   b. The U.S. abortion rate is higher than the rate in Canada and England.
   c. Most women are traumatized by an abortion.
   d. Mifepristone is 97 percent effective in inducing abortion.
8. In the third trimester of pregnancy,
   a. the woman experiences shortness of breath as the enlarged uterus presses on the lungs and diaphragm.
   b. the embryo is now called a fetus.
   c. the woman should begin regular prenatal checkups.
   d. the woman should increase her activity level to ensure that she is fit for childbirth.
9. During childbirth,
   a. breech birth can be prevented by practicing the Lamaze method.
   b. the cervix thins and dilates so that the baby can exit the uterus.
   c. the intensity of contractions decreases during the second stage of labor.
   d. the placenta is expelled immediately before the baby's head appears.
10. Which of the following statements is true about infertility?
    a. Infertility is most often caused by female problems.
    b. In men, infertility is usually caused by a combination of excess sperm production and an ejaculation problem.
    c. In vitro fertilization involves introducing sperm into the vagina with a long needle.
    d. In some cases of infertility, no cause can be demonstrated.

Answers to these questions can be found on page 422.

Critical Thinking

1. After reading about the various methods of contraception, which do you think would be most effective for you? What factors enter into your decision (convenience, risks, effectiveness, etc.)?
2. In Wyoming, a pregnant woman went to the police station to report that her husband had beaten her. Instead of charges being brought against him, she was arrested for intoxication and charged with abusing her fetus by drinking. Across the country, other women who use hard drugs or alcohol while pregnant or whose newborns test positive for drugs have been arrested and put on trial for abusing their unborn children. Prosecutors argue that they are defending the innocent victims of substance abuse. Some health officials, on the other hand, argue that addicted women need help, not punishment. What do you think? Why?
3. Suppose that you and your partner were told that your only chance of having a child is by using fertility drugs. After taking the drugs, you and your partner are informed that there are seven fetuses. Would you carry them all to term? What if you knew that the chances of them all surviving were very slim and that eliminating some of them would improve the odds for the others? What ethical issues do cases like this raise?

Media Menu

ThomsonNOW™ Go to the ThomsonNOW website at **http://www.thomsonedu.com** that will:

- Help you evaluate your knowledge of the material.
- Allow you to take an exam-prep quiz.
- Provide a Personalized Learning Plan targeting resources that address areas you should study.
- Coach you through identifying target goals for behavioral change and creating and monitoring your personal change plan throughout the semester.

INTERNET CONNECTIONS

The Alan Guttmacher Institute
www.agi-usa.org

This site offers excellent resources on teen pregnancy rates and sexual health for teens and young adults, including discussions on contraceptives versus abstinence.

Association of Reproductive Health Professionals
www.arhp.org

ARHP calls their website "the ultimate resource offering comprehensive information and education on all reproductive health topics to healthcare professionals, policymakers, the media, and the public."

National Abortion Rights Action League
www.naral.org

The website of this national organization provides information on the politics of the pro-choice movement.

National Right to Life Committee
www.nrlc.org

The website of this national organization provides information on the politics of the pro-life movement.

Planned Parenthood
www.plannedparenthood.org

The website for the Planned Parenthood Federation of America offers a wealth of information on sexual and reproductive health, reproductive choices, methods of contraception, and reproductive policy.

InfoTrac College Edition Activities Log on, insert **birth control** into the Keyword search box, and limit your search to the past year. When you get the results, Mark articles to review, then Select one to read. Summarize three or four key points from the article.

You can find additional readings related to personal health with InfoTrac College Edition, an online library of more than 900 journals and publications. Follow the instructions for accessing InfoTrac College Edition that were packaged with your textbook; then search for articles using a keyword search.

For additional links, resources, and suggested readings on the InfoTrac College Edition, visit our Health and Wellness Resource Center at **http://health.wadsworth.com.**

Key Terms

The terms listed are used on the page indicated. Definitions of the terms are in the Glossary at the end of this book.

adoption 224
amnion 218
artificial insemination 223
barrier contraceptives 205
caesarean delivery 223
cervical cap 206
coitus interruptus 197
conception 196
condom 207
contraception 196
diaphragm 205
dilation and evacuation (D and E) 215
ectopic pregnancy 218
embryo 218
emergency contraception (EC) 212
failure rate 197
fertilization 196
fetus 218
implantation 196
infertility 223
intrauterine device (IUD) 204
labor 221
Lamaze method 221
laparoscopy 213
medical abortion 215

LACC Extra Credit Assignment

8. Discuss why some people may not utilize contraceptive methods.

minipills 201
miscarriage 218
monophasic pills 200
multiphasic pills 200
oral contraceptives 200
placenta 218
preconception care 217
premature labor 220
progestin-only pills 201
rhythm method 211
rubella 218
spermatogenesis 196
sterilization 212
suction curettage 215
tubal ligation 213
tubal occlusion 213
vaginal contraceptive film (VCF) 210
vaginal spermicide 209
vasectomy 212
zygote 196

9 Preventing Infectious Diseases

REAL HEALTH

"There's something I have to tell you." Anise knew, just by the sound of her boyfriend's voice, that the "something" wasn't good news.

"My herpes is back."

Stunned, Anise tried to absorb all the information packed into this short sentence: She'd had no idea that the man she'd been sleeping with for several months had a sexually transmitted infection. How did Clay get it? What else hadn't he told her about his past? What did he mean that it was "back"? Could she have caught it?

A mix of emotions—shock, fear, anger—washed over Anise. She had never believed in casual sex. Neither did Clay, or so she thought. When they first began sleeping together, she'd insisted that he use a condom, even though she was taking birth control pills. But Clay seemed such a gentleman—tender, respectful, trustworthy. When he argued that sex would be so much better for him without a condom, she felt that she couldn't keep insisting that he use one.

It never occurred to Anise to ask Clay about sexual diseases. Wouldn't anyone who really cared about her want to protect her? Too late Anise realized that when it comes to sexual responsibility, you can't take anything for granted.

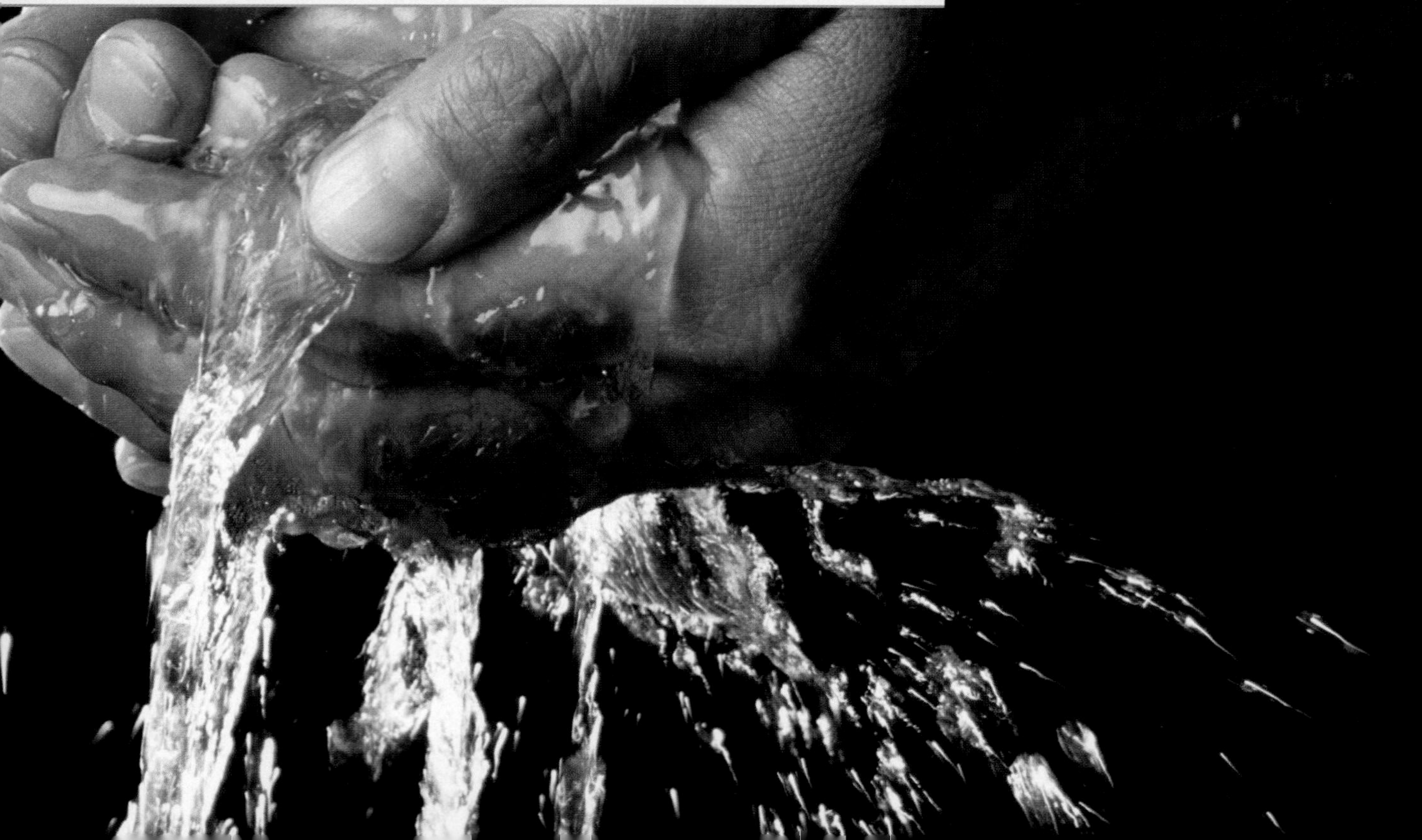

Throughout history, infectious diseases have claimed more lives than any military conflict or natural disaster. Although modern medicine has won many victories against the agents of infection, we remain vulnerable to a host of infectious illnesses. Drug-resistant strains of tuberculosis and *Staphylococcus* bacteria challenge current therapies. New infectious diseases, such as bird flu are emerging and traveling around the world. Scientists also warn that agents of infection can be used as weapons of war and terrorism.

Some of today's most common and dangerous infectious illnesses spread primarily through sexual contact, and their incidence has skyrocketed. The federal government estimates that 65 million Americans have a sexually transmitted infection (STI). These diseases cannot be prevented in the laboratory. Only you, by your behavior, can prevent and control them.

This chapter is a lesson in self-defense against all forms of infection. The information it provides can help you boost your defenses, recognize and avoid enemies, protect yourself from sexually transmitted infections, and realize when to seek help.

? FAQ Frequently Asked Questions

- How do you catch an infection? *p. 231*
- Which sex is more susceptible to infection? *p. 234*
- Who is at highest risk of infectious diseases? *p. 235*
- What is a pandemic? *p. 238*
- Am I at risk of getting bird flu? *p. 243*
- How common are STIs on campus? *p. 245*

After studying the material in this chapter, you should be able to:

- **Explain** how the different agents of infection spread disease.
- **Describe** how your body protects itself from infectious disease.
- **List** and **describe** some common infectious diseases.
- **Identify** the sexually transmitted infections and the symptoms and treatment for each.
- **List** the methods of STI transmission.
- **Define** HIV infection and **describe** its symptoms.
- **Explain** some practical methods for preventing HIV infection and other sexually transmitted infections.

ThomsonNOW™ Log on to ThomsonNOW at **www.thomsonedu.com/thomsonnow** to find your Behavior Change Planner and to explore self-assessments, interactive tutorials, and practice quizzes.

Understanding Infection

We live in a sea of microbes. Most of them don't threaten our health or survival; some, such as the bacteria that inhabit our intestines, are actually beneficial. Yet in the course of history, disease-causing microorganisms have claimed millions of lives. The twentieth century brought the conquest of infectious killers such as cholera and scarlet fever. Although modern science has won many victories against the agents of infection, infectious illnesses remain a serious health threat.

Infection is a complex process, triggered by various **pathogens** (disease-causing organisms) and countered by the body's own defenders. Physicians explain infection in terms of a **host** (either a person or a population) that contacts one or more agents in an environment. A **vector**—a biological or physical vehicle that carries the agent to the host—provides the means of transmission.

Agents of Infection

The types of microbes that can cause infection are viruses, bacteria, fungi, protozoa, and helminths (parasitic worms).

Viruses

The tiniest pathogens—**viruses**—are also the toughest; they consist of a bit of nucleic acid (DNA or RNA, but never both) within a protein coat. Unable to reproduce on its own, a virus takes over a body cell's reproductive machinery and instructs it to produce new viral particles, which are then released to enter other cells. The common cold, the flu, herpes, hepatitis, and AIDS are viral diseases.

The problem in fighting viruses is that it's difficult to find drugs that harm the virus and not the cell it has commandeered. **Antibiotics** (drugs that inhibit or kill bacteria) have no effect on viruses. **Antiviral drugs** don't completely eradicate a viral infection, although they can decrease its severity and duration. Because viruses multiply very quickly, antiviral drugs are most effective when taken before an infection develops or in its early stages.

Bacteria

Simple one-celled organisms, **bacteria** are the most plentiful microorganisms as well as the most pathogenic. Most kinds of bacteria don't cause disease; some, like certain strains of *Escherichia coli* that aid in digestion, play important roles within our bodies. Even friendly bacteria, however, can get out of hand and cause acne, urinary tract infections, vaginal infections, and other problems.

Bacteria harm the body by releasing either enzymes that digest body cells or toxins that produce the specific effects of such diseases as diphtheria or toxic shock syndrome. In self-defense, the body produces specific proteins (called *antibodies*) that attack and inactivate the invaders. Tuberculosis, tetanus, gonorrhea, scarlet fever, and diphtheria are examples of bacterial diseases.

Because bacteria are sufficiently different from the cells that make up our bodies, antibiotics can kill them without harming our cells. Antibiotics work only against specific types of bacteria. If your doctor thinks you have a bacterial infection, tests of your blood, pus, sputum, urine, or stool can identify the particular bacterial strain.

Fungi

Single-celled or multicelled organisms, **fungi** consist of threadlike fibers and reproductive spores. Fungi lack chlorophyll and must obtain their food from organic material, which may include human tissue. Fungi release enzymes that digest cells and are most likely to attack hair-covered areas of the body, including the scalp, beard, groin, and external ear canals. They also cause athlete's foot. Treatment consists of antifungal drugs.

Protozoa

These single-celled, microscopic animals release enzymes and toxins that destroy cells or interfere with their function. Diseases caused by **protozoa** are not a major health problem in this country, primarily because of public health measures. Around the world, however, some 2.24 billion people (more than 40 percent of the world's population) are at risk for acquiring malaria—a protozoan-caused disease. Up to 3 million die from this disease annually. Many more come down with amoebic dysentery. Treatment for protozoa-caused diseases consists of general medical care to relieve the symptoms, replacement of lost blood or fluids, and drugs that kill the specific protozoan.

The most common disease caused by protozoa in the United States is *giardiasis,* an intestinal infection caused by microorganisms in human and animal feces. It has become a threat at day-care centers, as well as among campers and hikers who drink contaminated water. Symptoms include nausea, lack of appetite, gas, diarrhea, fatigue, abdominal cramps, and bloating. Many people recover in a month or two without treatment. However, in some cases the microbe causes recurring attacks over many years. Giardiasis can be life-threatening in small children and the elderly, who are especially prone to severe dehydration from diarrhea. Treatment usually consists of antibiotics.

Helminths (Parasitic Worms)

Small parasitic worms that attack specific tissues or organs and compete with the host for nutrients are called **helminths.** One major worldwide health problem is *schistosomiasis,* a disease caused by a parasitic worm, the fluke, that burrows through the skin and enters the circulatory system. Infection with another helminth, the tapeworm, may be contracted from eating undercooked beef, pork, or fish containing larval forms of the tapeworm. Helminthic diseases are treated with appropriate medications.

? FAQ How Do You Catch an Infection?

The major vectors, or means of transmission, for infectious disease are animals and insects, people, food, and water.

Animals and Insects

Disease can be transmitted by house pets, livestock, birds, and wild animals. Insects also spread a variety of diseases. The housefly may spread dysentery, diarrhea, typhoid fever, or trachoma (an eye disease rare in the United States but common in other parts of the world). Other insects, including mosquitoes, ticks, mites, fleas, and lice, can transmit such diseases as malaria, yellow fever, encephalitis, dengue fever (a growing threat in Mexico), and Lyme disease.

New threats in the United States include West Nile virus (WNV), which can be spread to humans by mosquitoes that bite infected birds, and monkeypox virus, carried by various animals, including prairie dogs. Concern has grown about avian influenza, or bird flu, which has spread to wild and domestic birds around the world.[1] (These illnesses are discussed later in this chapter.)

People

The people you're closest to can transmit pathogens through the air, through touch, or through sexual contact. To avoid infection, stay out of range of anyone who's coughing, sniffling, or sneezing, and don't share food or dishes. Carefully wash your dishes, utensils, and hands, and abstain from sex or make self-protective decisions about sexual partners. (See "Your Life Coach: Safer, Smarter Sex" later in this chapter.)

Food

Every year foodborne illnesses strike millions of Americans, sometimes with fatal consequences. Bacteria account for two-thirds of foodborne infections, and thousands of suspected cases of infection with *Escherichia coli* bacteria in undercooked or inadequately washed food have been reported.

Every year as many as 4 million Americans have a bout with *Salmonella* bacteria, which have been found in about a third of all poultry sold in the United States. These infections can be serious enough to require hospitalization and can lead to arthritis, neurological problems, and even death. Consumers can greatly reduce the number of salmonella infections by proper handling, cooking, and refrigeration of poultry (see Chapter 5).

Water

Waterborne diseases, such as typhoid fever and cholera, are still widespread in less developed areas of the world. They have been rare in the United States, although outbreaks caused by inadequate water purification have occurred.

The Process of Infection

If someone infected with the flu sits next to you on a bus and coughs or sneezes, tiny viral particles may travel into your nose and mouth. Immediately, the virus finds or creates an opening in the wall of a cell, and the process of infection begins. During the **incubation period,** the time between invasion and the first symptom, you're unaware of the pathogen multiplying inside you. In some diseases, incubation may go on for months, even years; for most, it lasts several days or weeks.

The early stage of the battle between your body and the invaders is called the *prodromal period.* As infected cells die, they release chemicals that help block the invasion. Other chemicals, such as *histamines,* cause blood vessels to dilate, thus allowing more blood to reach the battleground. During all of this, you feel mild, generalized symptoms, such as headache, irritability, and discomfort. You're also highly contagious. At the height of the battle—the typical illness period—you cough, sneeze, sniffle, ache, feel feverish, and lose your appetite.

Recovery begins when the body's forces gain the advantage. With time, the body destroys the last of the

pathogen A microorganism that produces disease.

host A person or population that contracts one or more pathogenic agents in an environment.

vector A biological or physical vehicle that carries the agent of infection to the host.

virus A submicroscopic infectious agent; the most primitive form of life.

antibiotics Substances produced by micro-organisms, or synthetic agents, that are toxic to other types of microorganisms; in dilute solutions, used to treat infectious diseases.

antiviral drug A substance that decreases the severity and duration of a viral infection if taken prior to or soon after onset of the infection.

bacteria (singular, **bacterium**) One-celled microscopic organisms; the most plentiful pathogens.

fungi (singular, **fungus**) Organisms that reproduce by means of spores.

protozoa Microscopic animals made up of one cell or a group of similar cells.

helminth A parasitic roundworm or flatworm.

incubation period The time between a pathogen's entrance into the body and the first symptom.

invaders and heals itself. However, the body is not able to develop long-lasting immunity to certain viruses, such as colds, flu, or HIV.

How Your Body Protects Itself

Various parts of your body safeguard you against infectious diseases by providing **immunity,** or protection, from these health threats. Your skin, when unbroken, keeps out most potential invaders. Your tears, sweat, skin oils, saliva, and mucus contain chemicals that can kill bacteria. Cilia, the tiny hairs lining your respiratory passages, move mucus, which traps inhaled bacteria, viruses, dust, and foreign matter, to the back of the throat, where it is swallowed; the digestive system then destroys the invaders.

When these protective mechanisms can't keep you infection-free, your body's immune system, which is on constant alert for foreign substances that might threaten the body, swings into action. The immune system includes structures of the lymphatic system—the spleen, thymus gland, lymph nodes, and lymph vessels—that help filter impurities from the body (Figure 9-1). The **lymph nodes,** or glands, are small tissue masses in which some protective cells are stored. If pathogens

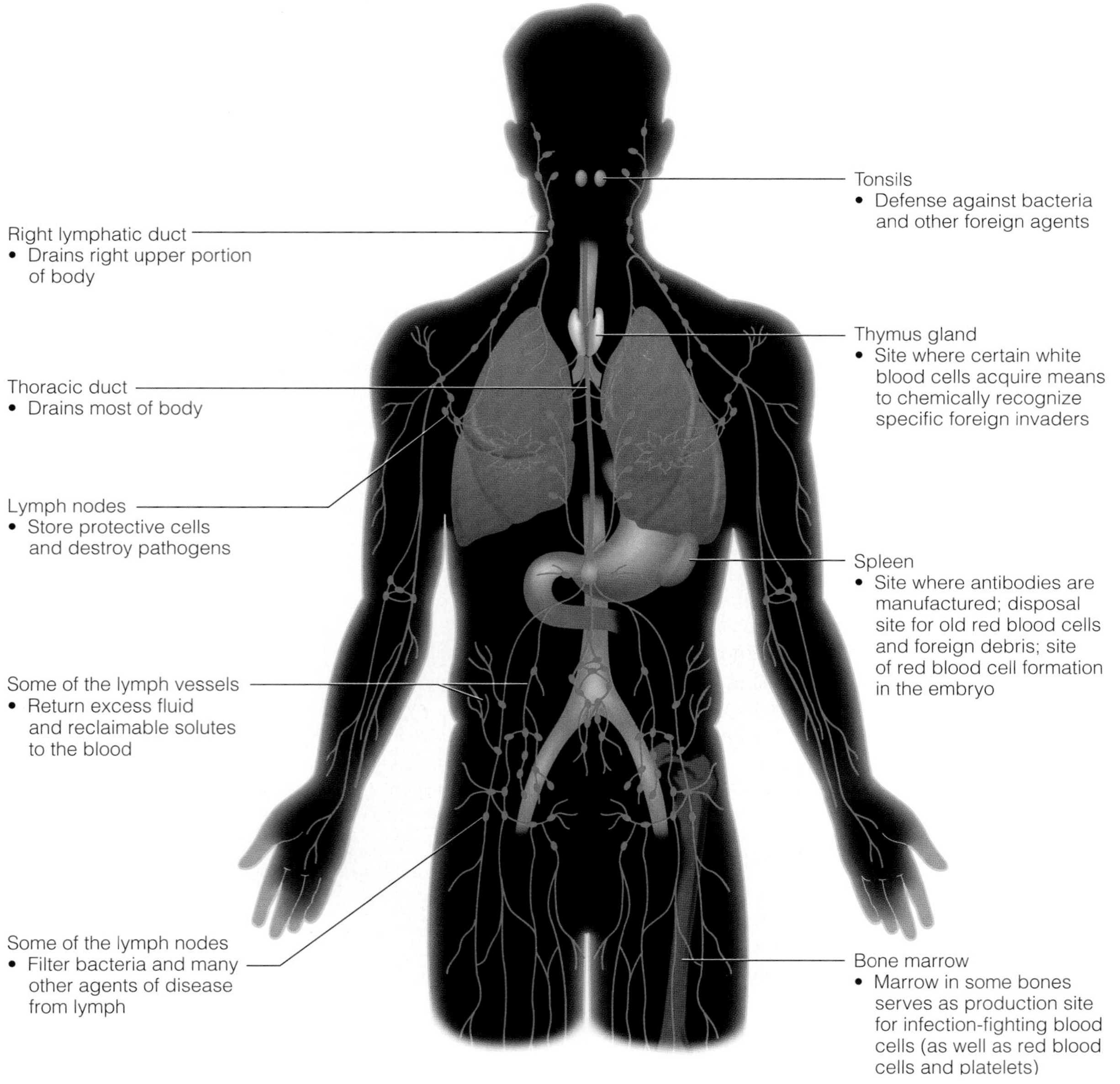
Tonsils
• Defense against bacteria and other foreign agents
Right lymphatic duct
• Drains right upper portion of body
Thymus gland
• Site where certain white blood cells acquire means to chemically recognize specific foreign invaders
Thoracic duct
• Drains most of body
Lymph nodes
• Store protective cells and destroy pathogens
Spleen
• Site where antibodies are manufactured; disposal site for old red blood cells and foreign debris; site of red blood cell formation in the embryo
Some of the lymph vessels
• Return excess fluid and reclaimable solutes to the blood
Some of the lymph nodes
• Filter bacteria and many other agents of disease from lymph
Bone marrow
• Marrow in some bones serves as production site for infection-fighting blood cells (as well as red blood cells and platelets)

FIGURE 9-1 The Human Lymphatic System and Its Functions
The lymphatic system helps filter impurities from the body.

invade your body, many of them are carried to the lymph nodes to be destroyed. This is why your lymph nodes often feel swollen when you have a cold or the flu.

More than a dozen different types of white blood cells (lymphocytes) are concentrated in the organs of the lymphatic system or patrol the entire body by way of the blood and lymph vessels. Some of these white blood cells are generalists and some are specialists. The generalists include *macrophages,* which are large scavenger cells with insatiable appetites for foreign cells, diseased and run-down red blood cells, and other biological debris (Figure 9-2). The specialists are the *B cells* and *T cells,* which respond to specific invaders.

An *antigen* is any substance the white blood cells recognize as foreign. B cells create antibodies, which are proteins that bind to antigens and mark them for destruction by other white blood cells. Antigens are specific to the pathogen, and the antibody to a particular antigen binds only to that antigen (Figure 9-2). Once the human body produces antibodies against a specific antigen—the mumps virus, for instance—you're protected against that antigen for life. If you're again exposed to mumps, the antibodies previously produced prevent another episode of the disease.

But you don't have to suffer through an illness to acquire immunity. Inoculation with a vaccine containing synthetic or weakened antigens can give you the same protection. The type of long-lasting immunity in which the body makes its own antibodies to a pathogen is called *active immunity.* Immunity produced by the injection of **gamma globulin,** the antibody-containing part of the blood from another person or animal that has developed antibodies to a disease, is called *passive immunity.*

Immune Response

Attacked by pathogens, the body musters its forces and fights. Sometimes the invasion is handled like a minor border skirmish; other times a full-scale battle is waged throughout the body. Together, the immune cells work like an internal police force. When an antigen enters the body, the T cells aided by macrophages engage in combat with the invader. Certain T cells (cytotoxic T cells) can destroy infected body cells or tumor cells by "touch-killing." Meanwhile, the B cells churn out antibodies, which rush to the scene and join in the fray. Also busy at surveillance are natural killer cells that, like the elite forces of a SWAT team, seek out and destroy viruses and cancer cells (Figure 9-2).

If the microbes establish a foothold, the blood supply to the area increases, bringing oxygen and nutrients to the fighting cells. Tissue fluids, as well as antibacterial and antitoxic proteins, accumulate. You may develop redness, swelling, local warmth, and

immunity Protection from infectious diseases.

lymph nodes Small tissue masses in which some immune cells are stored.

gamma globulin The antibody-containing portion of the blood fluid (plasma).

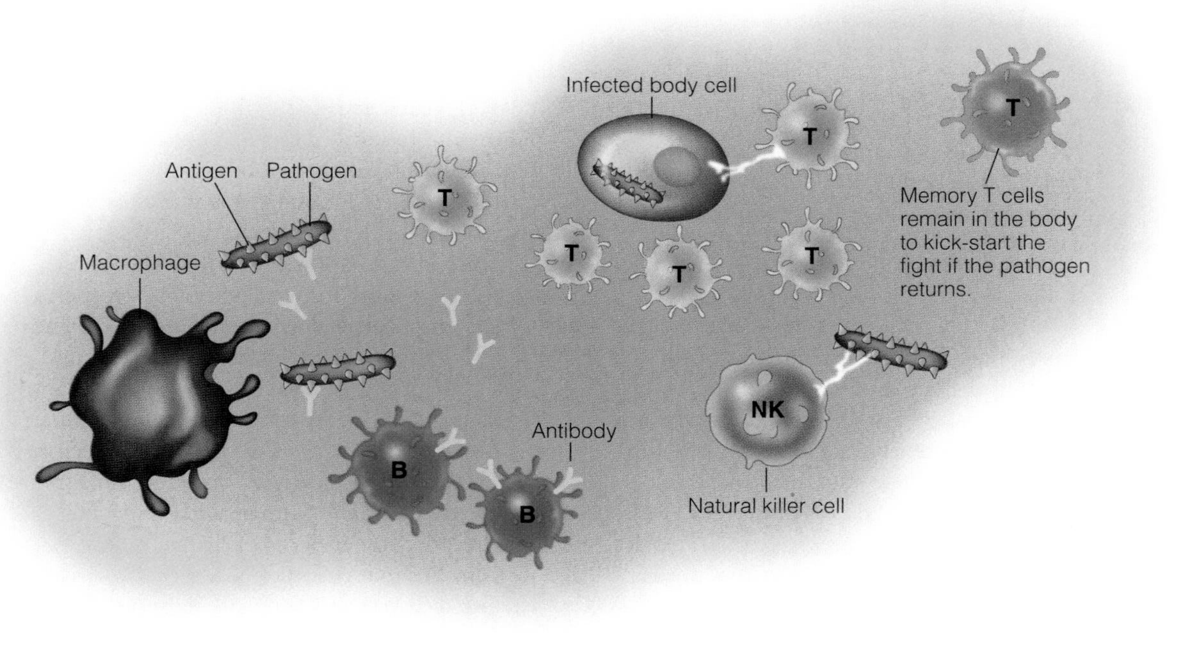

FIGURE 9-2 The Immune Response

Some T cells can kill infected body cells. B cells churn out antibodies to tag pathogens for destruction by macrophages and other white blood cells.

pain—the signs of **inflammation.** As more tissue is destroyed, a cavity, or **abscess,** forms and fills with fluid, battling cells, and dead white blood cells (pus). If the invaders aren't killed or inactivated, the pathogens are able to spread into the bloodstream and cause what is known as **systemic disease.**

Some people have an **immune deficiency**—either inborn or acquired. A very few children are born without an effective immune system; their lives can be endangered by any infection. Although still experimental, therapy to implant a missing or healthy gene may offer new hope for a normal life.

Immunity and Stress

Whenever we confront a crisis, large or small, our bodies produce powerful hormones that provide extra energy. However, this stress response dampens immunity, reducing the number of some key immune cells and the responsiveness of others.

Stress affects the body's immune system in different ways, depending on two factors: the controllability or uncontrollability of the stressor and the mental effort required to cope with the stress. An uncontrollable stressor that lasts longer than 15 minutes may interfere with cytokine interleukin-6, which plays an essential role in activating the immune defenses. Uncontrollable stressors also produce high levels of the hormone cortisol, which suppresses immune system functioning. The mental efforts required to cope with high-level stressors produce only brief immune changes that appear to have little consequence for health. However, stress has been shown to slow pro-inflammatory cytokine production, which is essential for wound healing.

Immune Disorders

Sometimes our immune system overreacts to certain substances, mistakes the body's own tissues for enemies, or doesn't react adequately. The result is an immune disorder such as allergies and autoimmune disorders.

Allergies

An **allergy** represents a hypersensitivity to a substance in our environment or diet. More than half of Americans between ages 6 and 59 are sensitive to one or more allergens. Allergies consistently rate as one of the top health problems among college students.[2]

Allergy sufferers run annual tabs of up to $2 billion in doctor visits, diagnostic tests, prescriptions, and decreased productivity. Every year allergies account for more than 10 million workdays missed; every day they keep 10,000 children out of school.

Thanks to treatment breakthroughs, allergy sufferers no longer have to choose between feeling better or feeling alert. Treatment options include nonsedating oral medications, nasal sprays, and **immunotherapy,** which consists of a series of injections of small but increasing doses of an allergen.

? FAQ Which Sex Is More Susceptible to Infection?

When the flu hits a household, the last one left standing is likely to be Mom. The female immune system responds more vigorously to common infections, offering extra protection against viruses, bacteria, and parasites. But this enhanced immunity doesn't apply to sexually transmitted infections (STIs). A woman who has unprotected sex with an infected man is more likely to contract an STI than a man who has sex with an infected woman. These infections can be transmitted through breaks in the mucous membranes, and women have more mucosal area exposed and experience more trauma to these tissues during sexual activity than men.[3] Symptoms of STIs also tend to be more "silent" in women, so they often go undetected and untreated, leading to potentially serious complications.

The genders also differ in their vulnerability to allergies and autoimmune disorders. Although both men and women frequently develop allergies, allergic women are twice as likely to experience potentially fatal anaphylactic shock. A woman's robust immune system also is more likely to overreact and turn on her own organs and tissues. On average, three of four people with autoimmune disorders, such as multiple sclerosis, Hashimoto's thyroiditis, and scleroderma, are women.

Why are there such large gender differences in susceptibility? Scientists believe that the sex hormones have a great impact on immunity. Through a woman's childbearing years, estrogen, which protects heart, bone, brain, and blood vessels, also bolsters the immune system's response to certain infectious agents. Women produce greater numbers of antibodies when exposed to an antigen.

In contrast, testosterone may suppress this response—possibly to prevent attacks on sperm cells, which might otherwise be mistaken as alien invaders. When the testes are removed from mice and guinea pigs, their immune systems become more active.

Pregnancy dampens a woman's immune response, probably to ensure that her natural protectors don't attack the fetus as a foreign invader. This impact is so great that pregnant women with transplanted kidneys may require lower doses of drugs to prevent organ rejection. Pregnant women with multiple sclerosis and rheumatoid arthritis typically experience decreased symptoms during the nine months of gestation, then return to their prepregnancy state after giving birth. Oral contraceptives also can diminish symptoms of multiple sclerosis and rheumatoid arthritis. Neither pregnancy nor birth control pills has such an impact on lupus.

Immunizations for Adults

One of the great success stories of modern medicine has been the development of vaccines that provide protection against many infectious diseases. Immunization has reduced cases of measles, mumps, tetanus, whooping cough, and other life-threatening illnesses by more than 95 percent.

Although many people think that vaccines are only for children, they remain an important part of protection throughout life (Figure 9-3). One increased risk for adults is pertussis, or whooping cough, which has been steadily increasing to as many as 600,000 cases a year. Because immunity typically wanes five to ten years after vaccination, adolescents and young adults are at risk. With the development of safer new vaccines, the CDC is recommending a "Tdap" (tetanus, diphtheria, and pertussis) booster vaccination every ten years for everyone aged 19 to 64.[4]

Infectious Diseases

Although infections can be unavoidable at times, the more you know about their causes, the more you can do to protect yourself.

? FAQ Who Is at Highest Risk of Infectious Diseases?

Like human bullies, the viruses responsible for the most common infectious illnesses tend to pick on those least capable of fighting back. Among the most vulnerable are the following groups:

- **Children and their families.** Youngsters get up to a dozen colds annually; adults average two a year. When a flu epidemic hits a community, about 40 percent of school-age boys and girls get sick, compared with only 5 to 10 percent of adults. But parents get up to six times as many colds as other adults.
- **The elderly.** Statistically, fewer older men and women are likely to catch a cold or flu, yet when they do, they face greater danger than the rest of

inflammation A localized response by the body to tissue injury, characterized by swelling and the dilation of the blood vessels.

abscess A localized accumulation of pus and disintegrating tissue.

systemic disease A pathologic condition that spreads throughout the body.

immune deficiency Partial or complete inability of the immune system to respond to pathogens.

allergy A hypersensitivity to a particular substance in one's environment or diet.

immunotherapy A series of injections of small but increasing doses of an allergen, used to treat allergies.

Vaccine	19–49 years	50–64 years	≥ 65 years
Tetanus, diphtheria, pertussis [Tdap]	1 dose booster every 10 years		
Measles, mumps, rubella	1 or 2 doses	1 dose	
Varicella (chicken pox)	2 doses (0, 4–8 weeks)	2 doses (0, 4–8 weeks)	
Influenza	1 dose annually	1 dose annually	
Pneumococcal (polysaccharide)	1–2 doses		1 dose
Hepatitis A	2 doses (0, 6–12 months, or 0, 6–18 months)		
Hepatitis B	3 doses (0, 1–2, 4–6 months)		
Meningococcal	1 or more doses		

For all persons who lack evidence of immunity

Recommended if some other risk factor is present (e.g., health-care workers for flu, measles, chicken pox; first year college students for measles, meningococcal)

FIGURE 9.3 Recommended Adult Immunization

Source: Centers for Disease Control and Prevention, www.cdc.gov.

the population. People over 65 who get the flu have a one in ten chance of being hospitalized for pneumonia or other respiratory problems, and a one in fifty chance of dying from the disease.

- **The chronically ill.** Lifelong diseases, such as diabetes, kidney disease, or sickle-cell anemia, decrease an individual's ability to fend off infections. Individuals taking medications that suppress the immune system, such as steroids, are more vulnerable to infections, as are those with medical conditions that impair immunity, such as infection with HIV.
- **Smokers and those with respiratory problems.** Smokers are a high-risk group for respiratory infections and serious complications, such as pneumonia. Chronic breathing disorders, such as asthma and emphysema, also greatly increase the risk of respiratory infections.
- **Those who live or work in close contact with someone sick.** Health-care workers who treat high-risk patients, nursing home residents, and others living in close quarters—such as students in dormitories—face greater odds of catching others' colds and flus.
- **Residents or workers in poorly ventilated buildings.** Building technology has helped spread certain airborne illnesses, such as tuberculosis, via recirculated air. Indoor air quality can be closely linked with disease transmission in winter, when people spend a great deal of time in tightly sealed rooms.

Common Cold

There are more than 200 distinct cold viruses. Although in a single season you may develop a temporary immunity to one or two, you may then be hit by a third. Americans come down with 1 billion colds annually.

Every year, about 25 million cold sufferers in the United States visit their family doctors with uncomplicated upper respiratory infections. The common cold results in about 20 million days of absence from work and 22 million days of absence from school.

Colds can strike in any season, but different cold viruses are more common at different times of years. *Rhinoviruses* cause most spring, summer, and early fall colds and tend to cause more symptoms above the neck (stuffy nose, headache, runny eyes). *Adenoviruses*, parainfluenza viruses, *coronaviruses*, influenza viruses, and others that strike in the winter are more likely to get into the trachea and bronchi (the breathing passages) and cause more fever and bronchitis.

Cold viruses spread by coughs, sneezes, and touch. Cold sufferers who sneeze and then touch a doorknob or countertop leave a trail of highly contagious viruses behind them. The best preventive tactics are frequent hand-washing, replacing toothbrushes regularly, exercising regularly, and avoiding stress overload. High levels of stress increase the risk of becoming infected by respiratory viruses and developing cold symptoms. People who feel unable to deal with everyday stresses have an exaggerated immune reaction that may intensify cold or flu symptoms once they've contracted a virus. Those with a positive emotional outlook are less vulnerable.

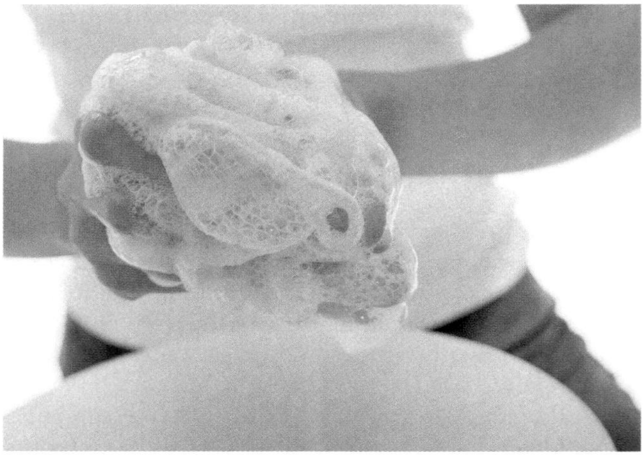

Washing your hands frequently is one of your best defenses against cold and flu viruses.

Until scientists develop truly effective treatments, experts advise against taking aspirin and acetaminophen (Tylenol), which may suppress the antibodies the body produces to fight cold viruses and increase symptoms such as nasal stuffiness. A better alternative for achiness is ibuprofen (brand names include Motrin, Advil, and Nuprin), which doesn't seem to affect immune response. Children, teenagers, and young adults should never take aspirin for a cold or flu because of the danger of Reye's syndrome, a potentially deadly disorder that can cause convulsions, coma, swelling of the brain, and kidney damage.

The main drawback of antihistamines, the most widely used cold remedy, is drowsiness, which can impair a person's ability to safely drive or operate machinery. Another common ingredient, pseudoephedrine, opens and drains sinus passages without drowsiness but can speed up heart rate and cause complications for individuals with high blood pressure, diabetes, heart disease, or thyroid disorders. Nasal sprays clear a stuffy nose, but they invariably cause a rebound effect.

In general, doctors recommend treating specific symptoms—headache, cough, chest congestion, sore throat—rather than taking a multisymptom medication. According to new practice guidelines for the management of cough, over-the-counter cough expectorants and suppressants do not relieve cough. Americans spend an estimated $3.6 billion on drugs that are ineffective against a cough caused by the common cold.[5]

Many Americans try alternative remedies for colds. Vitamin C and extracts of the plant *Echinacea* are widely used to prevent the common cold, but there is no conclusive evidence that they help. Echinacea tablets have proved no more effective than placebos in reducing the duration or severity of a cold. Zinc lozenges, another popular alternative treatment in recent years, also have not proved to be clearly beneficial.

Although colds and sore throats—a frequent cold symptom—are caused by viruses, many people seek treatment with antibiotics, which are effective only against bacteria. Unless you're coughing up green or foul yellow mucus (signs of a secondary bacterial infection), antibiotics won't help. They have no effect against viruses and may make your body more resistant to such medications when you develop a bacterial infection in the future. An estimated 5 to 17 percent of sore throats in adults are caused by bacteria (*Group A streptococci*).

Excess prescribing for antibiotics accounts for more than half of all prescriptions and costs $726 million a year. In addition to their costs, antibiotics may increase risks to users and their contacts. An increasing number of studies show that antibiotics foster the growth of one or more strains of antibiotic-resistant bacteria for at least two to six months inside the person taking the pills—who can pass on this drug-resistant bug to family, roommates, and others.

Your own immune system can do something modern science cannot: cure a cold. All it needs is time, rest, and plenty of fluids. Usually, cold symptoms last for one to two weeks, although chest colds (bronchitis) may last two or three weeks. Warmth is important because the aptly named "cold" viruses replicate at lower temperatures. Hot soups and drinks (particularly those with a touch of something pungent, like lemon or ginger) raise body temperature and help clear the nose. Tea may enhance the immune system. Even more important is getting off your feet. Taking it easy reduces demands on the body, which helps speed recovery.

Influenza

Although similar to a cold, **influenza**—or the flu—causes more severe symptoms that last longer. Every year 10 to 20 percent of Americans develop influenza, more than 200,000 are hospitalized, and 36,000 die.

Flu viruses, transmitted by coughs, sneezes, laughs, and even normal conversation, are extraordinarily contagious, particularly in the first three days of the disease. The usual incubation period is two days, but symptoms can hit hard and fast. Two varieties of viruses—influenza A and influenza B—cause most flus. In recent years, the deadliest flu epidemics have been caused by various forms of influenza A viruses.

The CDC has set priorities for individuals who should get a flu shot because they are at higher risk for flu complications, such as heart disease, diabetes, and asthma. They are:

- **Individuals aged 65 years and older,** with and without chronic health conditions.
- **Residents of long-term care facilities.**
- **Individuals aged 2 to 64 years** with chronic health conditions.
- **Children aged 6 to 23 months.**
- **Pregnant women.**
- **Health-care personnel** who provide direct patient care.
- **Household contacts and caregivers** of children under six months.

In older individuals, flu shots may offer significant protection against strokes and heart disease. The only individuals who should steer clear are those allergic to eggs, since the inactivated flu viruses are grown in chick embryos.

Vaccination with the live, nasal-spray flu vaccine (FluMist®) is an option for healthy people aged 5 to 49 years who are not pregnant. The aerosol vaccine significantly reduces flu severity, days lost from work, health-care visits, and the use of over-the-counter medication. The spray represents a particular advantage for children since more than 30 percent of youngsters get the flu, but most don't receive a flu shot.

For those who don't get vaccinated, antiviral drugs, which must be taken within 36 to 48 hours of the first flu symptom, have provided the next best line of defense. Two of the oldest of these medications, amantadine and rimantadine, which work only against the type A flu virus, are no longer effective, possibly because the flu virus has mutated and become resistant.[6] Two newer agents, Tamiflu (oseltamivir) and Relenza (zanamivir), which fight both type A and type B influenza, still work. Tamiflu is approved by the FDA to prevent as well as treat the flu, particularly when there is a serious outbreak in a community. The other three drugs can also be used preventively, but Relenza, which is inhaled rather than swallowed, can cause wheezing.

The Risk of Colds and Flus on Campus

College and university students are at increased risk for colds and influenza-like illnesses. In one study that followed more than 3,000 students from fall to spring, nine in ten had at least one cold or flu-like illness. These infections were responsible for 6,023 days in bed, 4,263 days of missed class, 3,175 days of missed work, and 45,219 days of illness.[7]

Flu shots are now advised for almost everyone, but the majority of college health centers report vaccinating fewer than 20 percent of their students. Those living in dormitories are at higher risk of influenza than those in nondormitory settings. The specific aspects of dormitory life that increase the risk of flu symptoms include the number of roommates and the presence/absence of carpeting. Students living in "triples," with three beds to a room; those sleeping in the same room with a

influenza Any type of fairly common, highly contagious viral diseases.

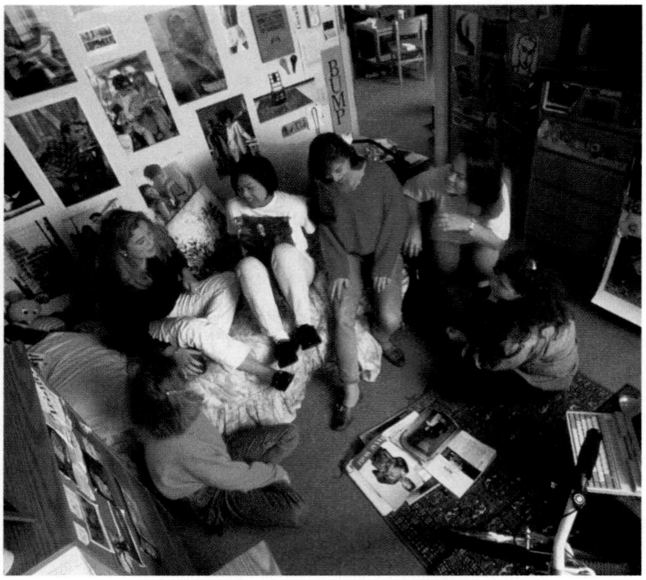

© Len Rubenstein/Index Stock Imagery

Students living in dormitories are more likely to catch the flu. The more roommates you have, the higher the risk.

roommate in a double; and those with uncarpeted floors have higher rates of flu symptoms, such as fever, sore throat, and fatigue.

? FAQ What Is a Pandemic?

Pandemic flu is a virulent human flu that causes a global outbreak, or pandemic, of serious illness. Influenza pandemics tend to occur when disease-causing organisms that typically affect only animals adapt and infect humans, then further adapt so they can pass easily from human to human. The flu pandemic of 1918–1919 claimed half a million lives.

Concern about the spread of avian or bird flu (discussed later in this chapter), which is caused by influenza viruses that occur naturally among wild birds, has spawned fears of a deadly new pandemic. The virus can be transmitted from birds to humans, and no vaccine is available. However, there have not been any cases of human-to-human transmission of avian flu.[8] Although experts disagree about the probability of an avian flu pandemic, a worldwide influenza epidemic may occur.[9]

Here are some ways you can protect yourself:

- **Stay informed.** Check reliable sources of information, such as the federal website www.pandemicflu.gov.
- **Get an annual flu shot.** It won't protect you from a pandemic flu virus, but it can prevent simultaneous infections.
- **See your doctor** within two days of developing flu symptoms.
- **Wash your hands frequently,** particularly after being in crowded public places.
- **Stay healthy.** Eating right, working out, and getting enough sleep keep your immune system strong.
- **Think carefully about travel in flu season,** when viruses are easily transmitted in confined spaces such as airplanes, trains, and buses, or to places with outbreaks of deadly viruses.

Meningitis

Meningitis, or invasive meningococcal disease, attacks the membranes around the brain and spinal cord and can result in hearing loss, kidney failure, and permanent brain damage. An estimated 2,400 to 3,000 cases occur every year; approximately 10 percent are fatal. One of the most common types is caused by the bacterium *Neisseria meningitidis,* which is spread through coughing; kissing; sharing drinks, eating utensils, or cigarettes; or prolonged exposure to infected individuals. Viral meningitis is typically less severe.

Most common in the first year of life, the incidence of bacterial meningitis rises in young people between ages 15 and 24. Adolescents and young adults account for nearly 30 percent of all cases of meningitis in the United States. Approximately 100 to 125 cases of meningococcal disease occur on college campuses each year, and 5 to 15 students will die as a result.

In a study of 15- to 19-year-olds in Great Britain, students were at greater risk than other adolescents. Certain behaviors multiply the chance of getting meningitis. Intimate kissing with multiple partners almost quadruples a teenager's risk of meningococcal disease.[10]

Symptoms may include fever, stiff neck, rash, nausea, and vomiting. The disease progresses very rapidly and can easily be misdiagnosed as the flu. Students should seek medical attention if any of these symptoms are present and unusually sudden or severe. If not treated early, meningitis can lead to death or permanent disabilities. One in five of those who survive will suffer from long-term side effects, such as brain damage, hearing loss, seizures, or limb amputation. Fatality rates are five times higher among 15- to 24-year-olds.

Protecting Yourself Against Meningitis

With the approval of a safer reformulated meningococcal vaccine that provides longer protection, the American College Health Association, as well as the CDC's Advisory Committee on Immunization Practices, has called for immunization of all incoming college freshmen living in dormitories or residence halls. Other college students under 25 years of age may choose to receive meningococcal vaccination to reduce their risk for the disease. Immunizing a large proportion of the student population is likely to protect even those who are not vaccinated.

At most schools, the cost of vaccination ranges from $50 to $75. Research into the success of meningococcal vaccination programs on college campuses has shown that women are more likely than men to be vaccinated and that vaccination rates for all nonwhite ethnic groups are somewhat lower than rates for whites. Students majoring in science-oriented fields have higher vaccination rates than those majoring in the humanities. More younger students living on campus than older ones get vaccinations, possibly because of greater parental influence or because they see themselves as being at higher risk.

Hepatitis

An estimated 500,000 Americans contract hepatitis each year. At least five different viruses, referred to as **hepatitis** A, B, C, Delta, and E, can cause this inflammation of the liver. Newly identified viruses also may be responsible for some cases of what is called "non-A, non-B" hepatitis.

All forms of hepatitis target the liver, the body's largest internal organ. Symptoms include headaches, fever, fatigue, stiff or aching joints, nausea, vomiting, and diarrhea. The liver becomes enlarged and tender to the touch; sometimes the yellowish tinge of jaundice develops. Treatment consists of rest, a high-protein diet, and the avoidance of alcohol and drugs that may stress the liver. Alpha interferon, a protein that boosts immunity and prevents viruses from replicating, may be used for some forms.

Most people begin to feel better after two or three weeks of rest, although fatigue and other symptoms can linger. As many as 10 percent of those infected with hepatitis B and up to two-thirds of those with hepatitis C become carriers of the virus for several years or even life. Some have persistent inflammation of the liver, which may cause mild or severe symptoms and increase the risk of liver cancer.

Hepatitis A

Hepatitis A, a less serious form, is generally transmitted by poor sanitation, primarily fecal contamination of food or water, and is less common in industrialized nations than in developing countries. As many as 30 percent of individuals in the United States show evidence of past infection with the virus. Among those at highest risk in the United States are children and staff at day-care centers, residents of institutions for the mentally handicapped, sanitation workers, and workers who handle primates such as monkeys. Gamma globulin can provide short-term immunity; vaccines against hepatitis A have been approved by the FDA. The CDC recommends routine immunization against hepatitis A in states with high rates, as well as for travelers to countries where hepatitis A is common, men who have sex with men, and persons who use illegal drugs.

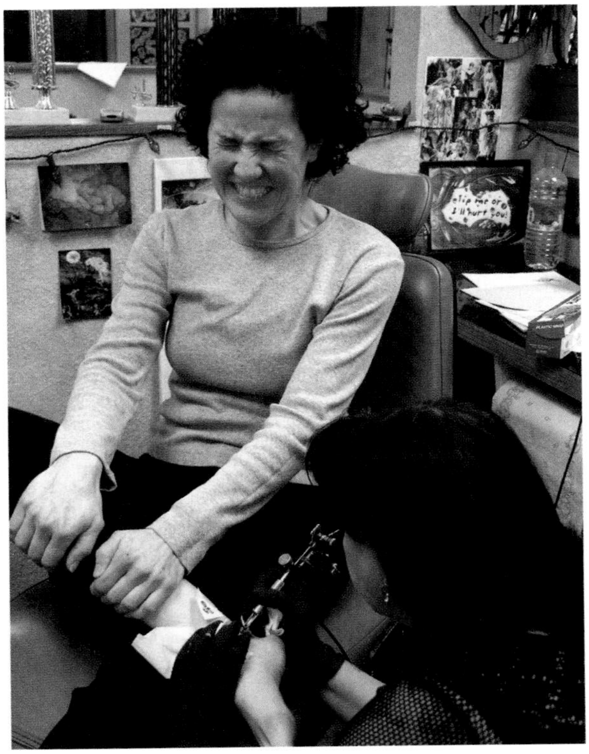

© Kent Meireis/The Image Works

Getting a tattoo or a piercing can pose health risks, including bacterial infection and hepatitis.

Hepatitis B

Hepatitis B, a potentially fatal disease transmitted through the blood and other bodily fluids, infects an estimated 400,000 people around the world each year. Once spread mainly by contaminated tattoo needles, needles shared by drug users, or transfusions of contaminated blood, hepatitis B is now transmitted mostly through sexual contact. It can cause chronic liver infection, cirrhosis, and liver cancer. Medications for hepatitis B often must be taken long-term, or the disease comes back even stronger.[11]

Hepatitis B is a particular threat to young people; 75 percent of new cases are diagnosed in those between ages 15 to 39. They usually contract hepatitis B through high-risk behaviors such as multiple sex partners and use of injected drugs. Individuals who have tattoos or body piercing may also be at risk if procedures are not done under regulated conditions. At highest risk are male

meningitis An extremely serious, potentially fatal illness that attacks the membranes around the brain and spinal cord; caused by the bacterium *Neisseria meningitis*.

hepatitis An inflammation and/or infection of the liver caused by a virus, often accompanied by jaundice.

SAVVY CONSUMER

Before You Get a Tattoo or Piercing

"Body art"—tattoos and piercings—may seem harmless, but health officials warn of hidden risks, including hepatitis B and C infection and transmission of HIV. In a survey of undergraduates at a university in New York, 51 percent reported body piercings, and 23 percent had gotten tattoos. Almost one in five of those with piercings reported medical complications. Bacterial infection was the most common, followed by bleeding and injury or tearing at the site.

With no state or federal regulations of "body artists," unsafe tattooing and piercing practices can put consumers in danger. In one survey of "skin-penetration operators," only half said that they followed governmental guidelines for infection control. Many were not knowledgeable about standard infection-control principles and practices.

Epidemiologists have identified tattooing as a strong, independent risk factor for testing positive for hepatitis C virus (HCV) but not with development of acute hepatitis. In other words, individuals with tattoos may acquire HCV but may not develop symptoms themselves. This does not mean that they will never become symptomatic or that they cannot transmit HCV to others.

Even so-called temporary tattooing with henna is not without risk. Dermatologists have reported an increasing number of skin reactions. The culprit is an ingredient in many henna preparations called paraphenylenediamine (PPD). Allergic reactions to henna itself can occur but are much rarer. Piercings of the tongue, lips, or cheeks present different dangers, including recessed gums; loose, chipped, or fractured teeth; pain; infection; inflammation; nerve damage; and tooth loss.

You may think you're safe if you go to a licensed tattoo or piercing salon. However, there are no formal schools, no certification requirements, and no diplomas for these practitioners. In many states it is possible to get a license without the benefit of any kind of training. Your best assurance of quality is making sure that basic safety principles are followed:

- **Ask to see certification that the autoclave, a high-temperature pressure cooker used for medical instruments, has been sterilized.** Ask to see the autoclave itself. Is it clean? More importantly, are the shop personnel happy to show it to you, or do they seem to have something to hide? Autoclaves need to be regularly tested to ensure that they are working properly. Ask to see the results of their latest spore test. Check the date. The results should be no more than two months old.
- **Make sure the artist is wearing standard medical latex gloves.** Check the fit. If the gloves are too big or too small, the artist runs the risk of either poking a hole in the gloves or tearing them. All it takes is a pinhole to run the risk of cross-contamination.
- **Find out if the artist is vaccinated for hepatitis B.** As this infection has spread, vaccination has become essential for a tattoo artist's own safety as well as that of clients. If artists claim to be vaccinated, never just take their word for it. Can they show you proof, such as a doctor's record, that they were vaccinated? If they tell you they don't remember if they've been vaccinated, they're probably lying. Most people vividly remember the vaccinations.
- **Make sure the artist uses only new sterile needles.** The needles should not be removed from the autoclave bag, the sort of pouch you see in dentists' offices, until you are ready for your tattoo. Ask to see the sterile confirmation logo on the bag itself. Usually the name of the company that made the bag will be visible on the front of the bag only when the equipment has been properly autoclaved. To determine if the needles are new and not just sterilized after previous use, check the color. They should be bright silver, not stained with ink or brownish looking.
- **Ask how the artist disposes of used needles.** They should be placed in a sharps container, a plastic container, usually red, with a biohazard symbol on the outside, and removed in a timely manner.
- **Always ask to see photos of the artist's finished work.** Examine the designs up close to check precision and skill. If you have the time, watch the artist work on another client before you go ahead with your tattoo.
- **If you require prophylactic antibiotics for dental cleanings or other procedures, do not get a tattoo.** Consumers with rheumatic heart disease and other conditions that increase their risk of infections have died as a result of bacterial infection contracted from a tattoo.

homosexuals, heterosexuals with multiple sex partners, health-care workers with frequent contact with blood, injection drug users, and infants born to infected mothers. Vaccination can prevent hepatitis B and is recommended for all newborns.

Hepatitis C

Hepatitis C virus (HCV) is four times as widespread as HIV, infecting about 2 percent of Americans. A simple blood test can show if you are infected with HCV. However, few of the estimated 3 to 4 million carriers in the United States realize they are infected. Of those infected with HCV, 80 percent have no symptoms.[12]

The risk factors for HCV infection are blood transfusion or organ transplant before 1992, exposure to infected blood, illegal drug use, tattoos, or body piercing. If you choose to have a body piercing, avoid piercing guns, and make certain that the piercing equipment has been sterilized (see Savvy Consumer: "Before You Get a Tattoo or Piercing"). Hepatitis C virus is not spread by casual contact, such as hugging, kissing, or sharing food utensils. There is controversy over whether HCV also can be transmitted sexually.

About three-quarters of those infected with HCV develop chronic or long-term hepatitis. About one-quarter develop progressive, irreversible liver damage, with scar tissue (cirrhosis) gradually replacing healthy liver tissue.

The most common treatment for Hepatitis C is a combination of interferon, which stops the virus from making copies of itself; and ribavirin, an antiviral medication. If the liver no longer functions adequately, a patient may require liver transplantation.

Mononucleosis

You can get **mononucleosis** through kissing—or any other form of close contact. "Mono" is a viral disease that targets people 15 to 24 years old. Its symptoms include a sore throat, headache, fever, nausea, and prolonged weakness. The spleen is swollen and the lymph nodes are enlarged. You may also develop jaundice or a skin rash similar to rubella (German measles).

The major symptoms usually disappear within two to three weeks, but weakness, fatigue, and often depression may linger for at least two more weeks. The greatest danger is from physical activity that might rupture the spleen, resulting in internal bleeding. The liver may also become inflamed. A blood test can determine whether you have mono. However, there's no specific treatment other than rest.

Chronic Fatigue Syndrome (CFS)

As many as 500,000 Americans have the array of symptoms known as **chronic fatigue syndrome (CFS).** Diagnosis of CFS remains difficult, although numerous studies have found significant immune abnormalities, such as high levels of certain immune cells (B lymphocytes and cytokines) that act as if they were constantly battling a viral infection. Researchers are working to develop a blood test that will definitively diagnose CFS.

Tuberculosis

A bacterial infection of the lungs that was once the nation's leading killer, **tuberculosis (TB)** still claims the lives of more people than any acute infectious disease other than pneumonia (Figure 9-4). About 30 percent of the world's population is infected with the TB organism, although not all develop active disease. In the United States, immigration from countries where TB is common, poverty, homelessness, alcoholism and drug abuse, the HIV/AIDS epidemic, and the emergence of resistant strains of TB account for most new cases of TB. Approximately 15 million Americans have the disease.

mononucleosis An infectious viral disease characterized by an excess of white blood cells in the blood, fever, bodily discomfort, a sore throat, and kidney and liver complications.

chronic fatigue syndrome (CFS) A cluster of symptoms whose cause is not yet known; a primary symptom is debilitating fatigue.

tuberculosis A highly infectious bacterial disease that primarily affects the lungs and is often fatal.

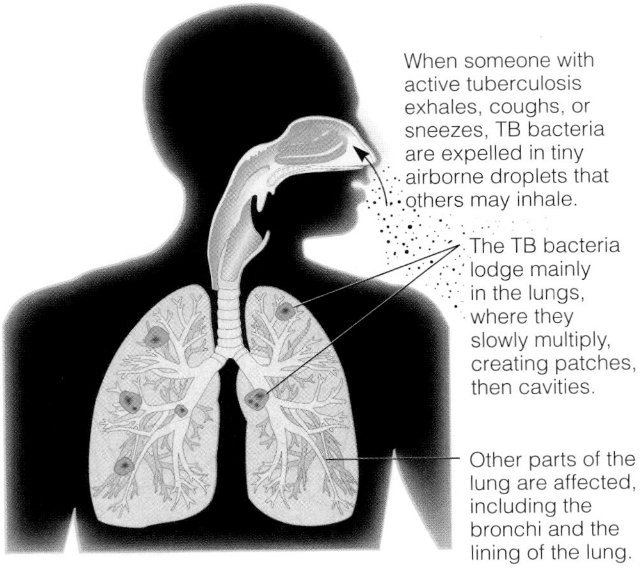

When someone with active tuberculosis exhales, coughs, or sneezes, TB bacteria are expelled in tiny airborne droplets that others may inhale.
The TB bacteria lodge mainly in the lungs, where they slowly multiply, creating patches, then cavities.
Other parts of the lung are affected, including the bronchi and the lining of the lung.
If untreated, TB can eventually spread to and damage the brain, bone, eyes, liver and kidneys, spine, and skin.

FIGURE 9-4 How Tuberculosis Spreads
If untreated, TB can eventually spread to and damage the brain, bone, eyes, liver, kidneys, spine, and skin.

Insect- and Animal-Borne Infections

Common insects and animals, including ticks and mosquitoes, can transmit dangerous infections. Lyme disease is the most widespread in the United States. Other threats include West Nile virus, monkeypox virus, and avian influenza, or bird flu.

Lyme Disease

Lyme disease, a bacterial infection, is spread by ticks carrying a particular bacterium—the spirochete *Borrelia burgdorferi*. An infected person may have various symptoms, including joint inflammation, heart arrhythmias, blinding headaches, and memory lapses. The disease can also cause miscarriages and birth defects. Lyme disease is by far the most commonly reported vector-borne infectious disease in the United States. The vast majority of all reported cases have occurred in just ten states, including New York, New Jersey, Connecticut, Pennsylvania, and Wisconsin.

The FDA has licensed a vaccine to prevent Lyme disease in individuals 15 to 70 years old. LYMErix, like most vaccines, stimulates the immune system to produce antibodies, in this case against the bacterium that causes Lyme disease. But the vaccine, administered in three doses over a one-year period, is not 100 percent effective and should not be considered a substitute for protective clothing and tick repellent.

The primary culprit in most cases of Lyme disease is the deer tick, although other ticks, including the western black-legged tick, the dog tick, and the Lone Star tick, also may transmit the bacterium that causes Lyme disease.

West Nile Virus

West Nile virus (WNV) is transmitted by a mosquito that feeds on an infected bird and then bites a human. The first cases in the United States occurred in 1999.

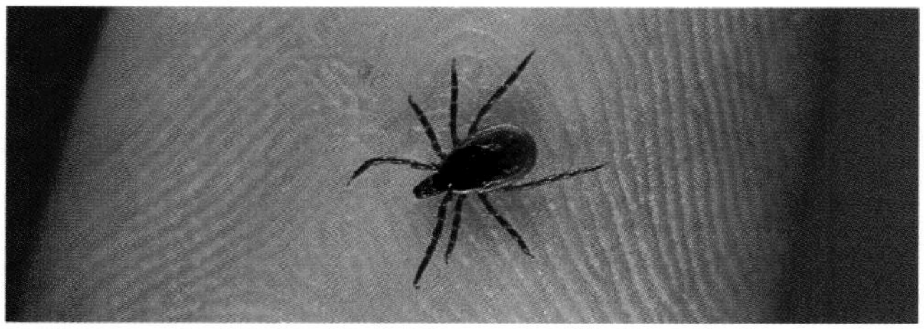

Ticks are responsible for the spread of Lyme disease. If you spot a tick, remove it as soon as possible with tweezers or small forceps. Put it in a plastic bag or sealed bottle and save it. If you develop a rash or other symptoms, take it with you to the doctor.

Experts now see WNV as a seasonal epidemic that flares up in the summer and continues into the fall. WNV also can be spread through blood transfusions, organ transplants, breast-feeding, and from mother to fetus during pregnancy.

WNV interferes with normal central nervous system functioning and causes inflammation of brain tissue. The risk of catching WNV is low. Relatively few mosquitoes carry WNV, and fewer than 1 percent of people who are bitten by mosquitoes experience any symptoms. Repellents that contain DEET, picaridin, and oil of lemon eucalyptus can protect against WNV.

There is no specific treatment for WNV infection. People with more severe cases usually require hospitalization and supportive treatment, including intravenous fluids and help with breathing. An antiviral drug, interferon, which might lessen the symptoms and duration of the illness in infected patients, is undergoing testing.

Monkeypox Virus

This rare viral disease occurs mainly in Africa, where it was first identified in monkeys. Researchers have since recovered monkeypox from other animals, including rats, mice, and rabbits, as well as humans.

Strategies for Prevention — Protecting Yourself from Insect-Borne Diseases

- Apply insect repellent containing DEET (N,N-diethyl-meta-toluamide), which provides the longest-lasting protection against bites, when you're outdoors.
- When possible, wear long-sleeved clothes and long pants treated with repellents containing permethrin or DEET since insects may bite through thin clothing. Do not apply repellents containing permethrin directly to exposed skin. If you spray your clothing, there is no need to spray repellent containing DEET on the skin under your clothing.
- Consider staying indoors at dawn, dusk, and in the early evening, which are peak mosquito-biting times.
- After spending time outdoors, examine yourself for ticks or bites every day. Check less obvious places, such as the scalp and behind the ears.
- If you do spot a tick, remove it right away. Using tweezers or forceps, grasp the tick firmly as close to its head and as near to your skin as possible. Gently pull backward, without squeezing the tick's body, until its hold is released. Wash your hands thoroughly. Treat the wound with rubbing alcohol.

The signs and symptoms of monkeypox are similar to those of smallpox but milder. People can catch monkeypox from an infected animal's bite, blood, or body fluids. It can spread from person to person during long periods of face-to-face contact or by touching the body fluids of a sick person or bedding or clothing contaminated with the virus. There is no specific treatment.

? FAQ Am I At Risk of Getting Bird Flu?

Avian influenza, or bird flu, is caused by viruses that occur naturally among wild birds. Most strains of bird flu virus cannot infect humans, but a few can, usually with great difficulty. Influenza viruses jumped from birds to humans three times in the twentieth century. In each case a mutation in the genes of the virus allowed it to infect humans. Then a further change allowed the virus to pass easily from one human to another, rapidly spreading around the world in a deadly pandemic.

A new threat emerged in Hong Kong in 1997, when a virus called H5N1, previously found only in birds, spread to domestic poultry and infected people who had worked closely with sick birds. Some died. Millions of poultry were killed in an attempt to contain the virus. However, several outbreaks again occurred in Hong Kong. The H5N1 virus spread to wild migratory birds in 2003, which have carried it to other countries and continents.[13]

The H5N1 virus has infected millions of wild and domestic birds and animals such as pigs and cats. The humans who have developed this strain of bird flu handled sick birds in the process of plucking or butchering them or were exposed to the birds' feces. The United States has banned the importation of all birds and bird products from countries known to have bird flu outbreaks.

So far the H5N1 virus has not mutated into a form that can easily infect humans or that humans can transmit to another person.[14] Experts disagree as to whether H5N1 will ever mutate in such a way as to cause a pandemic. Some worry because the virus has already evolved to infect cats, pigs, and humans.[15] Others note that the virus is unlikely to spread easily from one person to another because it clusters in the deepest branches of the respiratory tract and cannot be spread easily by coughs and sneezes.[16]

Bird flu can be very severe, and even healthy young adults who contracted it have died. However, others have developed only mild symptoms; some exposed to the virus developed no symptoms at all. The initial symptoms are similar to those of ordinary influenza, but people with bird flu are likely to have high fevers, more severe coughing, and muscle and joint pain; feel out of breath even when resting; become confused; and feel too weak to get out of bed.

Scientists are developing a vaccine from an inactivated H5N1 virus. In its experimental form, it requires two doses, each of which is six times stronger than a standard influenza shot. A French vaccine maker has produced another bird flu vaccine that boosts immune system response.[17] The United States has developed a bird flu response program, including plans for a worst-case scenario that would restrict travel and screen international visitors.[18]

New Infectious Threats

The twenty-first century has ushered in new agents of infection and new apprehension about the potential use of infectious diseases as instruments of terror and mass destruction.

Major outbreaks of severe acute respiratory syndrome (SARS) have occured in several Asian countries, including China and Hong Kong, and in Toronto. SARS is highly infectious and spreads when an infected person coughs or sneezes. Symptoms include high fever, coughing, headache, chills, muscle aches, and shortness of breath. Most of those infected develop pneumonia. There are no specific treatments. SARS could re-emerge as an infectious threat at any time.

Bioterror agents, such as anthrax and, potentially, smallpox have been added to the ranks of emerging infectious diseases. Anthrax, which is found naturally in wild and farm animals, can also be produced in a laboratory. The disease is spread through exposure to anthrax spores, not through exposure to an infected person.

Smallpox is a serious, contagious, and sometimes fatal infectious disease. Smallpox was eradicated decades ago after a successful worldwide vaccination program. The last case of smallpox in the United States was in 1949. The last naturally occurring case in the world was in Somalia in 1977. There is no treatment, and up to 30 percent of those infected with smallpox die. Because of fear that terrorists might use smallpox as a biological weapon, the U.S. government has stockpiled enough vaccine to inoculate everyone in the event of an emergency.

Lyme disease A disease caused by a bacterium carried by a tick; it may cause heart arrhythmias, neurological problems, and arthritis symptoms.

Reproductive and Urinary Tract Infections

Reproductive and urinary tract infections are very common. Many are not spread exclusively by sexual contact, so they are not classified as sexually transmitted infections.

Vaginal Infections

Vaginal complaints account for approximately 10 million medical office visits a year. The most common are trichomoniasis, candidiasis, and bacterial vaginosis (Table 9-1).

Protozoa (*Trichomonas vaginalis*) that live in the vagina can multiply rapidly, causing itching, burning, and discharge—all symptoms of **trichomoniasis.** Male carriers usually have no symptoms, although some may develop urethritis or an inflammation of the prostate and seminal vesicles. Anyone with this infection should be screened for syphilis, gonorrhea, chlamydia, and HIV. Sexual partners must be treated with oral medication (metronidazole, trade name Flagyl), even if they have no symptoms, to prevent reinfection.

Populations of a yeast called *Candida albicans*—normal inhabitants of the mouth, digestive tract, and vagina—are usually held in check. Under certain conditions, however (such as poor nutrition, stress, or antibiotic use), the microbes multiply, causing burning, itching, and a whitish discharge, and producing what is commonly known as a yeast infection. Common sites for **candidiasis,** which is also called *moniliasis,* are the vagina, vulva, penis, and mouth. The women most likely to test positive for candidiasis have never been pregnant, use condoms for birth control, have sexual intercourse more than four times a month, and have taken antibiotics in the previous 15 to 30 days. Vaginal medications, such as GyneLotrimin and Monistat, are nonprescription drugs that provide effective treatment. Male sexual partners may be advised to wear condoms during outbreaks of candidiasis. Women should keep the genital area dry and wear cotton underwear.

Bacterial vaginosis is characterized by alterations in the microorganisms that live in the vagina, including depletion of certain bacteria and overgrowth of others. It typically causes a white or gray vaginal discharge with a distinctive fishy odor similar to that of trichomoniasis. Its underlying cause is unknown, although it occurs most frequently in women with multiple sex partners. Long-term dangers include pelvic inflammatory disease (PID, discussed later in this chapter) and pregnancy complications. Metronidazole, either in the form of a pill or a vaginal gel, is the primary treatment. According to CDC guidelines, treatment for male sex partners appears to be of little benefit, but some health practitioners recommend treatment for both partners in cases of recurrent infections.

Urinary Tract Infections

A urinary tract infection (UTI) can be present in any of the three parts of the urinary tract: the urethra, the bladder, or the kidneys. An infection involving the urethra is known as **urethritis.** If the bladder is also infected, it's called **cystitis.** If it reaches the kidneys, it's called *pyelonephritis.*

An estimated 40 percent of women report having had a UTI at some point in their lives. Three times as many women as men develop UTIs, probably for anatomical reasons. A woman's urethra is only 1.5 inches long; a man's is 6 inches. Therefore, bacteria, the major cause of UTIs, have a shorter distance to travel to infect a woman's bladder and kidneys. About one-fourth to one-third of all women between ages 20 and 40 develop UTIs, and 80 percent of those who experience one infection develop recurrences.

Conditions that can set the stage for UTIs include irritation and swelling of the urethra or bladder as a result of pregnancy, bike riding, irritants (such as bubble bath, douches, or a diaphragm), urinary stones, enlargement of the prostate gland in men, vaginitis, and stress. Early diagnosis is critical because infection can spread to the kidneys and, if unchecked, result in kidney failure. Symptoms include frequent burning, painful urination, chills, fever, fatigue, and blood in the urine.

Recurrent UTIs, a frequent problem among young women, have been linked with a genetic predisposition, sexual intercourse, and the use of diaphragms.

TABLE 9-1 Common Reproductive Tract Infections

Infection	Transmission	Symptoms	Treatment
Bacterial vaginosis	Most common causative agent, *Gardnerella vaginalis* bacterium, sometimes transmitted through coitus	Women: Fishy- or musty-smelling, thin discharge, like flour paste in consistency and usually gray Men: Mostly asymptomatic	Metronidazole (Flagyl) by mouth or intravaginal applications of topical metronidazole gel or clindamycin cream
Candidiasis (yeast infection)	*Candida albicans* fungus may accelerate growth when the chemical balance of the vagina is disturbed; also transmitted through sexual interaction	Women: White, "cheesy" discharge; irritation of vaginal and vulval tissues	Vaginal suppositories or topical cream, such as clotrimazole (GyneLotrimin) and miconazole (Monistat), or oral fluconazole
Trichomoniasis	Protozoan parasite *Trichomonas vaginalis,* usually passed through genital sexual contact	Women: White or yellow vaginal discharge with an unpleasant odor; sore and irritated vulva Men: No symptoms	Metronidazole (Flagyl) for both women and men

Postintercourse treatment with antibiotics can lower the risk.

Sexually Transmitted Infections

Venereal diseases (from the Latin *venus,* meaning *love* or *lust*) are called **sexually transmitted infections (STIs),** or sexually transmitted diseases (STDs). Around the world, some 50 million cases of curable STIs occur each year (not including HIV and herpes). Almost 700,000 people are infected every day with one of the over 20 STIs tracked by world health officials. STIs are much more widespread in developing nations because of lack of adequate health standards, prevention practices, and access to treatment.

More Americans are infected with STIs now than at any other time in history. According to the Institute of Medicine, the odds of acquiring an STI during a lifetime are one in four. STIs are among the top ten most frequently reported diseases in the United States. The major cause of preventable sterility in America, STIs have tripled the rate of ectopic (tubal) pregnancies, which can be fatal if not detected early. STI complications, including miscarriage, premature delivery, and uterine infections after delivery, annually affect more than 100,000 women. Moreover, infection with an STI greatly increases the risk of HIV transmission (discussed later in this chapter). The incidence of STIs is highest in 16- to 24-year-olds, particularly older teenagers, and homosexual men. Others affected by STIs include unborn and newborn children who can "catch" potentially life-threatening infections in the womb or during birth.

Although each STI is a distinct disease, all STI pathogens like dark, warm, moist body surfaces, particularly the mucous membranes that line the reproductive organs; they hate light, cold, and dryness (Figure 9-5). It is possible to catch or have more than one STI at a time. Curing one doesn't necessarily cure another, and treatments don't prevent another bout with the same STI (Table 9-2).

Many STIs, including early HIV infection and gonorrhea in women, may not cause any symptoms. As a result, infected individuals may continue their usual sexual activity without realizing that they're jeopardizing others' well-being.

? FAQ How Common Are STIs on Campus?

Young people of college age account for about half of new cases of sexually transmitted infections (STIs). The college years are a prime time for contracting STIs. According to the American College Health Association, chlamydia and HPV have reached epidemic levels at many schools—although many of those infected aren't even aware of it.

According to the National College Health Assessment, infection with human papilloma virus (HPV) is the most commonly reported STI on campus. Chlamydia is ranked second, followed by genital herpes and pelvic inflammatory disease.[19] Sexually Transmitted infections/Diseases on Campus, (All of these infections are discussed in the following pages.) As noted in

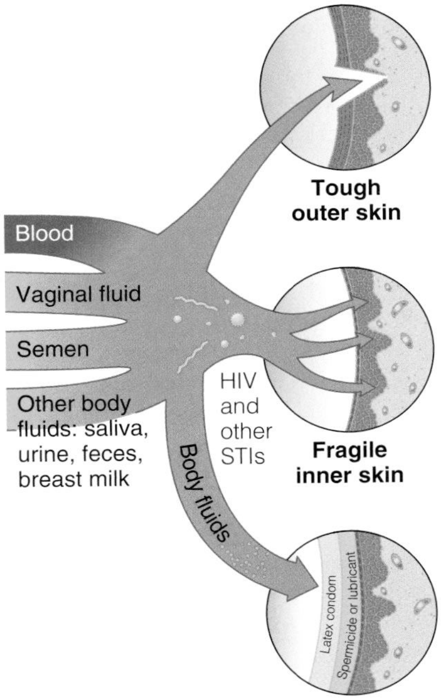
Blood
Vaginal fluid
Semen
Other body fluids: saliva, urine, feces, breast milk
Body fluids
HIV and other STIs
Tough outer skin
Fragile inner skin
Latex condom
Spermicide or lubricant
Tough outer skin covers the outside of your body, including hands and lips. Viruses and bacteria enter when skin is chapped or through a hangnail, cut, scrape, sore, or needle puncture.
Fragile inner skin lines the inside of your vagina or penis, anus, and mouth. Viruses and bacteria can enter when skin is torn during sexual contact that involves rubbing, stretching, or not enough lubrication (wetness).
Barrier protection made of latex helps prevent body fluids from entering your body. Latex condoms are recommended for intercourse. Spermicides help kill many STI microbes. They also reduce friction so latex condoms are less likely to break.

FIGURE 9-5 How HIV Infection and Other STIs Are Spread
Most STIs are spread by viruses or bacteria carried in certain body fluids.

trichomoniasis An infection of the protozoan *Trichomonas vaginalis;* females experience vaginal burning, itching, and discharge, but male carriers may be asymptomatic.

candidiasis An infection of the yeast *Candida albicans,* commonly occurring in the vagina, vulva, penis, and mouth and causing burning, itching, and a whitish discharge.

bacterial vaginosis A vaginal infection caused by overgrowth and depletion of various microorganisms living in the vagina, resulting in a malodorous white or gray vaginal discharge.

urethritis Infection of the urethra.

cystitis Inflammation of the urinary bladder.

sexually transmitted infections (STIs) Any of a number of diseases that are acquired through sexual contact.

TABLE 9-2 Common Sexually Transmitted Infections (STIs): Mode of Transmission, Symptoms, and Treatment

STI	Transmission	Signs and Symptoms	Treatment
Chlamydia (p. 249)	*Chlamydia trachomatis* bacterium transmitted primarily through sexual contact (can also be spread by fingers from one body site to another)	Men: Watery discharge; pain when urinating Women: Usually asymptomatic; sometimes a similar discharge to men's; leading cause of pelvic inflammatory disease (PID)	Antibiotics: doxycycline, azithromycin, ofloxacin, levofloxacin
Human papilloma virus (HPV) (genital warts) (p. 249)	Spread primarily through vaginal, anal, or oral-genital sexual interaction	Cauliflowerlike growths in genital and rectal areas	Removal of lesions by laser surgery or chemicals
Herpes simplex (p. 250)	Genital herpes virus (HSV-2) transmitted primarily by vaginal, anal, or oral-genital intercourse. Oral herpes virus (HSV-1) transmitted primarily by kissing	Small, painful red bumps (papules) in the genital region (genital herpes) or mouth (oral herpes). The papules become painful blisters that eventually rupture to form wet, open sores.	No known cure. Treatment may reduce symptoms; acyclovir, famcyclovir, or valacyclovir promote healing and suppress recurrent outbreaks
Gonorrhea ("clap") (p. 252)	*Neisseria gonorrhoeae* bacterium ("gonococcus") spread through genital, oral-genital, or genital-anal contact	Men: Pus discharge from urethra; burning during urination Women: Usually asymptomatic; can lead to PID and sterility in both men and women	Antibiotics: ceftriaxone, cefixime, or spectinomycin
Nongonococcal urethritis (NGU) (p. 253)	Bacteria, most commonly transmitted through sexual intercourse	Men: Discharge from the penis and irritation during urination Women: Mild discharge of pus from the vagina but often no symptoms	A single dose of azithromycin or doxycycline for seven days
Syphilis (p. 253)	*Treponema pallidum* bacterium ("spirochete") transmitted from open lesions during genital, oral-genital, or genital-anal contact	Primary: Chancre Secondary: Rash Latent: Asymptomatic Late: Irreversible damage to central nervous system, cardiovascular system	Penicillin or other antibiotic
Chancroid (p. 254)	*Haemophilus ducrevi* bacterium transmitted by sexual interaction	Men: Painful irregular chancre on penis Women: Chancre on labia	Tetracycline
Viral hepatitis (p. 239)	Hepatitis A primarily spread via the fecal-oral route, but oral-anal sexual contact a common mode. Hepatitis B virus transmitted by blood, semen, vaginal secretions, and saliva. Manual, oral, or penile stimulation of the anus strongly associated with the spread of this virus	Vary from nonexistent to mild, flulike symptoms to an incapacitating illness characterized by high fever, vomiting, and severe abdominal pain	Bed rest and adequate fluid intake; combination therapy with interferon and ribavarin possibly effective for hepatitis C infections
Pubic lice ("crabs") (p. 254)	*Phthirus pubis* spread easily through body contact or through shared clothing or bedding	Persistent itching; visible lice often located in pubic hair or other body hairs	1% permethrin cream for body areas; 1% lindane shampoo for hair
HIV/AIDS (p. 254)	HIV transmitted in blood and semen, primarily through sexual contact or needle sharing among injection drug users	Asymptomatic at first; opportunistic infections	Combination of three or more antiretroviral drugs (termed highly active antiretroviral therapies, or HAART) plus other specific treatment for opportunistic infections and tumors

Student Snapshot

Sexually Transmitted Infections/ Diseases on Campus

Type of STI or STD	Total	Women	Men
	(%)	(%)	(%)
HPV / Genital warts	2.2	2.7	1.3
Genital herpes	1.1	1.3	0.8
Chlamydia	0.7	0.8	0.6
Pelvic inflammatory disease	0.3	0.4	0.2
HIV	0.3	0.1	0.3
Gonorrhea	0.2	0.1	0.3

Based on the answers to the question, "Within the past school year, have you had any of the following?"
Source: American College Health Association, "American College Health Association-National College Health Assessment (ACHA-NCHA) Spring 2005 Reference Group Data Report (abridged)." *Journal of American College Health*, Vol. 55, No. 1, 2006, pp. 5–16.

Student Snapshot, about half of students used condoms the last time they had vaginal intercourse; a quarter used condoms for anal intercourse.[20]

Contracting STIs may increase the risk of being infected with HIV, and half of new HIV infections occur in people under age 25. Because college students have more opportunities to have different sexual partners and may use drugs and alcohol more often before sex, they are at greater risk. More than half of 13- to 24-year-old women with HIV are infected heterosexually.

Schools vary in the STI services, including screening, diagnosis, and treatment, that they offer. In a national survey, about half of colleges and universities made condoms available to students—some free in an open display, some free on request, and some for a fee or in vending machines. Larger schools, those with health centers, and those with on-campus housing are more likely to provide STI education and services.

Risk Factors and Risk Continuum

Various factors put young people at risk of STIs, including:

- **Feelings of invulnerability,** which lead to risk-taking behavior. Even when they are well informed of the risks, adolescents and young adults may remain unconvinced that anything bad can or will happen to them.
- **Multiple partners.** STI risks increase as relationships become less familiar and exclusive. In surveys of students, a significant minority report having had four or more sexual partners during their lifetime.
- **Failure to use condoms.** Among those who reported having had sexual intercourse in the previous three months, fewer than half reported condom use. Figure 9-6 shows the risk continuum for protected and nonprotected sexual behaviors. STI risks increase as sexual activities become unprotected and receptive. Students who'd had four or more sexual partners were significantly less likely to use condoms than those who'd had fewer partners.
- **Substance abuse.** Individuals who drink or use drugs are more likely to engage in sexually risky behaviors, including sex with partners whose health status and history they do not know, and unprotected intercourse.

Rate your own sexual health risk by taking the Self Survey "STI Quiz" in the Self-Assessment Booklet.

YOUR LIFE COACH

Safer, Smarter Sex

How can you tell if someone you're dating or hope to date has been exposed to an STI? The bad news is you can't. But the good news is it doesn't matter—as long as you avoid sexual activity that could put you at risk of infection. Ideally, before engaging in any such behavior, both of you should talk about your prior sexual history (including number of partners and sexually transmitted infections) and other high-risk behavior, such as the use of injection drugs. If you are considering having sex with a person, you should be able to talk about STIs. If the person is unwilling to talk, you shouldn't have sex. Here are some specific steps to lower your risk of STIs:

- **Abstain.** Abstinence from vaginal and anal intercourse is free, available to everyone, extremely effective at preventing both pregnancy and sexually transmitted infections, and has no medical or hormonal side effects. Even without vaginal or anal penetration, other sexual activity such as oral sex can expose you to STIs.
- **Practice monogamy.** For men and women who are sexually active, a mutually faithful sexual relationship with just one healthy partner is the safest option.
- **If you are sexually active and are not in a mutually monogamous relationship, protect yourself,** but keep in mind that no "protection" is 100 percent "safe." Condoms reduce the

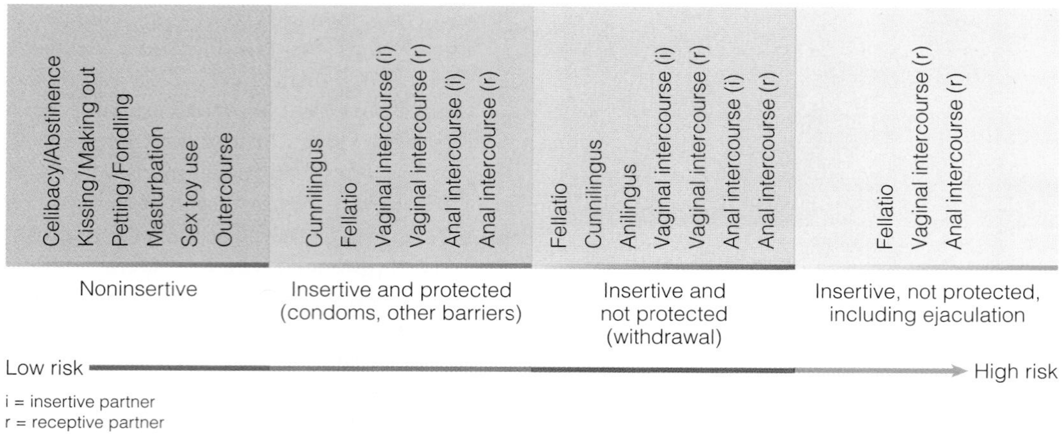

FIGURE 9-6 A Continuum of Risk for Sexual Behaviors
STI risks increase as sexual activities become unprotected and receptive.

risk of transmission of an STI by 50 to 80 percent—they are more effective against STIs transmitted by bodily fluids (chlamydia, gonorrhea, trichomoniasis, HIV) than those transmitted by skin-to-skin contact (herpes, HPV, chancroid, syphilis).

- **Use a new condom** each and every time you engage in any form of intercourse.
- **Do not use spermicide containing nonoxynol-9.** Contrary to past advice, experts now advise against choosing safer sex products with nonoxynol-9. According to recent research, nonoxynol-9 without condoms is ineffective against HIV transmission. Even with condoms, it does not protect women from the bacteria that cause gonorrhea and chlamydia.
- **If a condom fails** during vaginal or anal intercourse, remove it carefully. If you continue sexual activity, replace it with a new condom.
- **Make sure the package says that the condoms are meant to prevent disease.** If not, the condoms may not provide adequate protection, even though they may be the most expensive ones you can buy.
- Because bacteria can be transmitted by hand, **wash your hands with hot water** and antibacterial soap after sex.

- **If You Are A Woman:**
  - Keep in mind that your risk of getting an infection is greater than a man's because a woman's vagina and rectum are more easily infected than a man's penis.
  - Don't think you don't have to worry just because you have no symptoms. Because many sexual infections are "silent" in women, you are less likely to know if you are infected and may have pelvic inflammatory disease, which puts you at risk of infertility and ectopic pregnancy.
  - At your checkup talk to your doctor about whether you should be tested for sexually transmitted infections. You need to ask for these tests, or else they won't be done.
- **If You Are A Man:**
  - Use a new condom each and every time you engage in any form of intercourse. Try different brands to find the ones you like best.
  - After potential exposure to an STI, give yourself a little extra protection by urinating and washing your genitals with an antibacterial soap.
  - At your checkup talk to your doctor about whether you should be tested for sexually transmitted infections. You need to ask for these tests, or else they won't be done.
- **If you have oral sex,** make it safer by using effective barrier methods such as condoms or latex dental dams. In the absence of barrier methods, men should avoid ejaculating in their partners' mouths.
  - **Be aware of sores and discharge or unpleasant odors** from your partner's genitals. These are signs to avoid oral sex.
  - **Don't floss or brush teeth before oral sex.** It might tear the lining of the mouth, increasing exposure to viruses.
  - **Avoid aggressive and deep thrusting in oral sex,** which can damage throat tissues and

increase susceptibility for throat-based gonorrhea, herpes, and abrasions.

- **Remember that oral sex can transmit various STIs,** including herpes, gonorrhea, syphilis, and HIV.

About half of campuses in one national survey make condoms available to students—for free, on request, or in vending machines. Although condoms are one of the most effective forms of protection from sexually transmitted infections, some feel that providing condoms shows approval of casual sexual involvement. Should colleges encourage condom use by distributing them on campus? Or should condom use be a student's personal responsibility and choice?

You Decide

Chlamydia

The most widespread sexually transmitted bacterium in the United States is *Chlamydia trachomatis,* which causes an estimated 3 million cases of **chlamydia** each year. One in 25 young Americans is infected with chlamydia, according to a recent nationwide study. Chlamydia is six

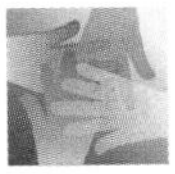

times more prevalent in young black adults than in young white adults, with almost 14 percent of young black women and more than 11 percent of black men testing positive. Chlamydial infections are more common in younger than in older women, and they also occur more often in both men and women with gonorrhea.

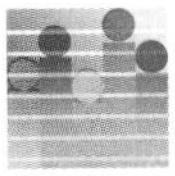

College freshmen under the age of 20 may be at a higher risk for chlamydia than students between 20 and 24 years of age. In a study at ten southern colleges, 13 percent of the freshmen women and 9.7 percent of older students tested positive for chlamydia.[21] Younger women also are at higher risk of being reinfected, probably by partners who are not diagnosed and treated.[22]

Those at greatest risk of chlamydial infection are individuals 25 years old or younger who engage in sex with more than one new partner within a two-month period and women who use birth control pills or other nonbarrier contraceptive methods. The U.S. Preventive Services Task Force recommend regular screening for chlamydia for all sexually active women under age 25 and for older women with multiple sexual partners, a history of STIs, or inconsistent use of condoms.

As many as 75 percent of women and 50 percent of men with chlamydia have no symptoms or symptoms so mild that they don't seek medical attention. Without treatment, up to 40 percent of cases of chlamydia can lead to pelvic inflammatory disease, a serious infection of the woman's fallopian tubes that also can damage the ovaries and uterus. Also, women infected with chlamydia may have three to five times the risk of getting infected with HIV if exposed. Babies exposed to chlamydia in the birth canal during delivery can be born with pneumonia or with an eye infection called conjunctivitis, both of which can be dangerous unless treated early with antibiotics. Symptomless women who are screened and treated for chlamydial infection are almost 60 percent less likely than unscreened women to develop pelvic inflammatory disease. Chlamydia may also be linked to cervical cancer.

The use of condoms with spermicide can reduce, but not eliminate, the risk of chlamydial infection. Sexual partners should be examined and treated if necessary. The CDC, in its most recent guidelines, recommends that all women with chlamydia be rescreened three to four months after treatment is completed. The reason is that re-infection, which often happens because a patient's sex partners were not treated, increases the risk of pelvic inflammatory disease and other complications. Immediately treating the partners of people infected with gonorrhea or chlamydia can reduce rates of recurrence of these infections.

chlamydia A sexually transmitted disease caused by the bacterium *Chlamydia trachomatis,* often asymptomatic in women, but sometimes characterized by urinary pain; if undetected and untreated, may result in pelvic inflammatory disease (PID).

human papilloma virus (HPV) A pathogen that causes genital warts and increases the risk of cervical cancer.

Human Papilloma Virus

Infection with **human papilloma virus (HPV),** a pathogen that can cause *genital warts,* is the most common viral STI. At least 15 percent of sexually active

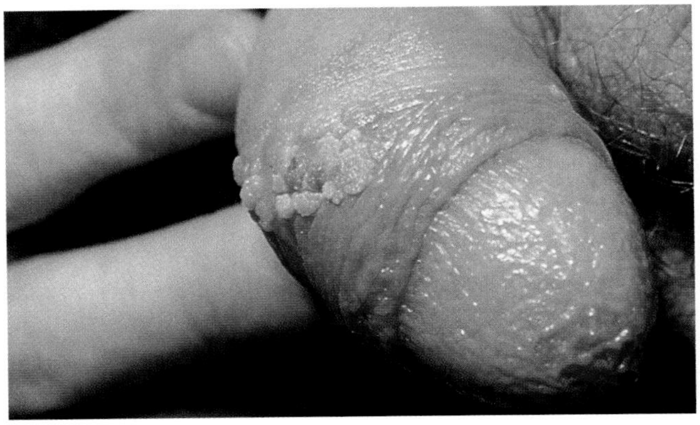

© Marazzi/Photo Researchers, Inc.

Human papilloma virus, which causes genital warts, is the most common viral STI.

adults in the United States have genital HPV infection. The highest rates of HPV infection occur in young adults between ages 18 and 28. Young women who engage in sexual intercourse at an early age are more likely than those with later sexual debuts to become infected with HPV. Their risk also increases if they have multiple sexual partners or a history of a sexually transmitted infection, use drugs, or have partners with multiple sexual partners. An estimated 9.2 million young adults have been infected with HPV and could spread the virus.

College-age women are among those at greatest risk of acquiring HPV infection. In various studies conducted in college health centers, 10 to 46 percent of female students (mean age 20 to 22) had a cervical HPV infection—and increased risk of precancerous cell changes. Risk factors include smoking, use of oral contraceptives, multiple sex partners, anal as well as vaginal intercourse, alcohol consumption at the time of engaging in vaginal intercourse, and sex partners with a history of HPV.

HPV infections in young women tend to be of short duration. In a three-year study, 60 percent of 608 college women became infected with the virus; the average duration of infection was eight months. According to the researchers, many young women who get HPV may not require treatment, because the condition often regresses on its own.

HPV is transmitted primarily through vaginal, anal, and oral-genital sex. More than half of HPV-infected individuals do not develop any symptoms. After contact with an infected individual, genital warts may appear from three weeks to eighteen months, with an average period of about three months. The warts are treated by freezing, cauterization, chemicals, or surgical removal. Recurrences are common because the virus remains in the body.

HPV infection may invade the urethra and cause urinary obstruction and bleeding. It greatly increases a woman's risk of developing a precancerous condition called cervical *intraepithelial neoplasia*, which can lead to cervical cancer. Scientists have developed a vaccine that blocks infection by the four virus types that cause most cervical cancers and genital warts and could reduce the annual number of new cervical cancers worldwide. The vaccine does not protect people already infected with HPV. There also is a strong association between HPV infections and cancer of the vagina, vulva, urethra, penis, and anus.

HPV may be the single most important risk factor in 95 percent of all cases of cervical cancer. Adolescent girls infected with HPV appear to be particularly vulnerable to developing cervical cancer. It is not known if HPV itself causes cancer or acts in conjunction with cofactors (such as other infections, smoking, or suppressed immunity).

Most HPV infections are asymptomatic in men, who may unwittingly increase their partners' risk. Men who test positive for HPV typically report significantly more sex partners than those who do not. A woman's risk of cervical cancer is strongly related to the number of her partner's current and lifetime female partners.[23] Women are five to eleven times as likely to get cervical cancer if their steady sexual partner has had 20 or more previous partners.

Women who have had an HPV infection should examine their genitals regularly and get an annual Pap smear. However, this standard diagnostic test that for cervical cancer doesn't identify HPV infection. A new laboratory test that can detect the presence of HPV, including the high-risk types associated with the development of cervical cancer, could help prevent as many as 80 to 90 percent of cervical cancers and deaths.[24] If left untreated, these changes can eventually lead to cancer in some women. Surgery or laser therapy can prevent further damage.

HPV may also cause genital warts in men and increase the risk of cancer of the penis. HPV-infected men, who may not develop any symptoms, can spread the infection to their partners. People with visible genital warts also may have asymptomatic or subclinical HPV infections that are extremely difficult to treat.

No form of therapy has been shown to completely eradicate HPV, nor has any single treatment been uniformly effective in removing warts or preventing their recurrence. CDC guidelines suggest treatments that focus on the removal of visible warts—cryotherapy (freezing) and topical applications of podofilox, podophyllin, or trichloroacetic acid—and then eradication of the virus. At least 20 to 30 percent of treated individuals experience recurrence. In experimental studies, interferon, a biologic substance produced by virus-infected cells that inhibits viral replication, has proved helpful.

Herpes

Herpes (from the Greek word that means *to creep*) collectively describes some of the most common viral infections in humans. Characteristically, **herpes simplex** causes blisters on the skin or mucous membranes. Herpes simplex exists in several varieties. *Herpes simplex virus 1 (HSV-1)* generally causes cold sores and fever blisters around the mouth. *Herpes simplex virus 2 (HSV-2)* may cause blisters on the penis, inside the vagina, on the cervix, in the pubic area, on the buttocks, or on the thighs. With the increase of oral-genital sex, some doctors report finding type 2 herpes lesions in the mouth and throat.

Genital herpes has skyrocketed during the last three decades, yet only a minority of infections with HSV-2 are recognized by those infected. About 40 percent of

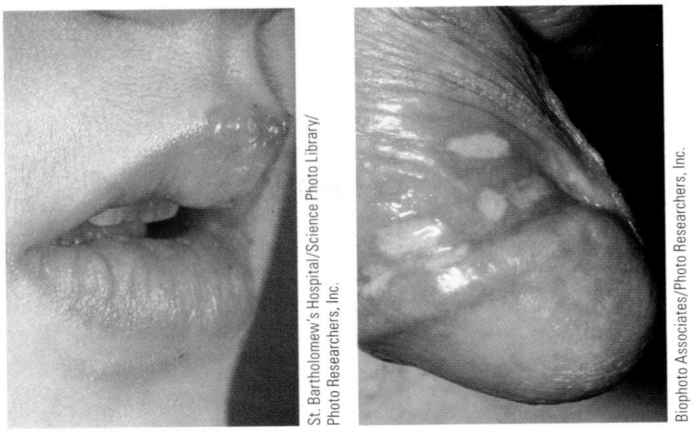

(a) herpes simplex virus (HSV-1) as a mouth sore; (b) herpes simplex virus (HSV-2) as a genital sore.

new cases of genital herpes occur in young people aged 15 to 24. An estimated 4.2 million young adults in this age range—11 percent of the population—have been infected.

Research has shown that individuals without any obvious symptoms shed the virus subclinically, whether or not they have lesions. Most people with herpes contract it from partners who were not aware of any symptoms or of their own contagiousness. Standard methods of diagnosing genital herpes in women, which rely primarily on physical examination and viral cultures, may miss as many as two-thirds of all cases. Newly developed blood tests are more effective in detecting unrecognized and subclinical infections with HSV-2.

The herpes virus is present in genital secretions even when patients do not notice any signs of the disease, and people infected with genital herpes can spread it even between flare-ups when they have no symptoms. There is growing evidence that genital herpes promotes the spread of HIV.

HSV transmission occurs through close contact with mucous membranes or abraded skin. Condoms help prevent infection but aren't foolproof. When herpes sores are present, the infected person is highly contagious and should avoid bringing the lesions into contact with someone else's body through touching, sexual interaction, or kissing.

A newborn can be infected with genital herpes while passing through the birth canal, and the frequency of mother-to-infant transmission seems to be increasing. Most infected infants develop typical skin sores, which can be cultured to confirm a herpes diagnosis. Some physicians recommend treatment with acyclovir. Because of the risk of severe damage and possible death, caesarean delivery may be advised for a woman with active herpes lesions.

The virus that causes herpes never entirely goes away; it retreats to nerves near the lower spinal cord, where it remains for the life of the host. Herpes sores can return without warning weeks, months, or even years after their first occurrence, often during menstruation or times of stress, or with sudden changes in body temperature. Of those who experience HSV recurrence, 10 to 35 percent do so frequently—that is, about six or more times a year. In most people, attacks diminish in frequency and severity over time. Herpes, like other STIs, can trigger feelings of shame, guilt, and depression.

Antiviral drugs, such as acyclovir (Zovirax), have proved effective in treating and controlling herpes. Available as an ointment, in capsules, and in injection form, acyclovir relieves the symptoms but doesn't kill the virus. Whereas the ointment works only for the initial bout with herpes, acyclovir in injectable and pill form dramatically reduces the length and severity of herpes outbreaks. Continuing daily oral acyclovir can reduce recurrences by about 80 percent. However, its safety in pregnant women has not been established. Infection with herpes viruses resistant to acyclovir is a growing problem, especially in individuals with immune-suppressing disorders.

Various treatments—compresses made with cold water, skim milk, or warm salt water; ice packs; or a mild anesthetic cream—can relieve discomfort. Herpes sufferers should avoid heat, hot baths, or nylon underwear. Some physicians have used laser therapy to vaporize the lesions. Clinical trials of an experimental vaccine to protect people from herpes infections are underway.

♀ Pelvic Inflammatory Disease (PID)

Infection of a woman's fallopian tubes or uterus, called **pelvic inflammatory disease (PID),** is not actually an STI, but rather a complication of STIs. About one in every seven women of reproductive age has PID; half of all adult women may have had it. Each year, about 1 million new cases are reported.

Ten to 20 percent of initial episodes of PID lead to scarring and obstruction of the fallopian tubes severe enough to cause infertility. Other long-term complications are ectopic pregnancy and chronic pelvic pain. The risk of these complications rises with subsequent PID episodes, bacterial vaginosis (discussed earlier in this chapter), and use of an IUD. Smoking also may increase the likelihood of PID. Two bacteria—*Gonococcus* (the culprit in gonorrhea) and *Chlamydia*—are

herpes simplex A condition caused by one of the herpes viruses and characterized by lesions of the skin or mucous membranes; herpes virus type 2 is sexually transmitted and causes genital blisters or sores.

pelvic inflammatory disease (PID) An inflammation of the internal female genital tract, characterized by abdominal pain, fever, and tenderness of the cervix.

responsible for one-half to one-third of all cases of PID. Other organisms are responsible for the remaining cases.

Most cases of PID occur among women under age 25 who are sexually active. Gonococcus-caused cases tend to affect poor women; those caused by chlamydia range across all income levels. One-half to one-third of all cases are transmitted sexually, and others have been traced to some IUDs that are no longer on the market. Several studies have shown that women with PID are more likely to have used douches than those without the disease. Consistent condom use may decrease PID risk.

PID is a silent disease that in half of all cases produces no noticeable symptoms as it progresses and causes scarring of the fallopian tubes. Experts are encouraging women with mild symptoms, such as abdominal pain or tenderness, to seek medical evaluation and are encouraging physicians to test these patients for infections. Urine testing is a cost-effective method of detecting gonorrhea and chlamydia in young women and can prevent development of PID. For women with symptoms, magnetic resonance imaging (MRI) is highly accurate in establishing a diagnosis of PID and detecting other diseases that may be responsible for the symptoms. Treatment may require hospitalization and intensive antibiotics therapy. PID causes an estimated 15 to 30 percent of all cases of infertility every year and about half of all cases of ectopic pregnancy.

Gonorrhea

Gonorrhea (sometimes called "the clap" in street language) is one of the most common STIs in the United States. After steady declines from the 1970s to the late 1990s, gonorrhea infections have increased, with about 60 percent of new cases occurring in young adults. The incidence is highest among teenagers and young adults. Sexual contact, including oral-genital sex, is the primary means of transmission.

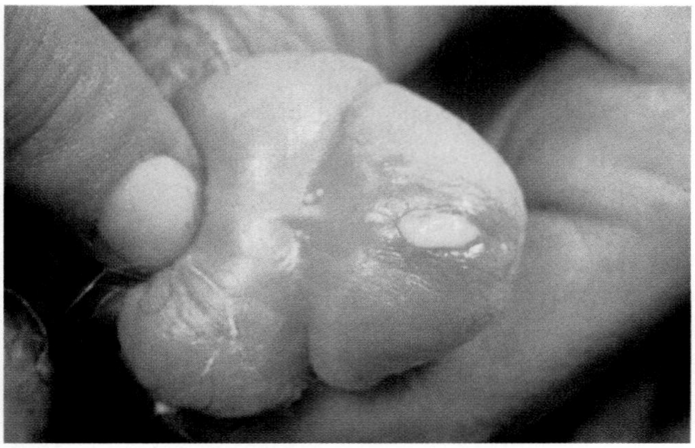

A cloudy discharge is symptomatic of gonorrhea.

Most men who have gonorrhea know it. Thick, yellow-white pus oozes from the penis and urination causes a burning sensation. These symptoms usually develop two to nine days after the sexual contact that infected them. Men have a good reason to seek help: It hurts too much not to. Women also may experience discharge and burning on urination. However, as many as eight out of ten infected women have no symptoms.

Gonococcus, the bacterium that causes gonorrhea, can live in the vagina, cervix, and fallopian tubes for months, even years, and continue to infect the woman's sexual partners. Approximately 5 percent of sexually active American women have positive gonorrhea cultures but are unaware that they are silent carriers.

If left untreated in men or women, gonorrhea spreads through the urinary-genital tract. In women, the inflammation travels from the vagina and cervix, through the uterus, to the fallopian tubes and ovaries. The pain and fever are similar to those caused by stomach upset, so a woman may dismiss the symptoms. Eventually these symptoms diminish, even though the disease spreads to the entire pelvis. Pus may ooze from the fallopian tubes or ovaries into the peritoneum (the lining of the abdominal cavity), sometimes causing serious inflammation. However, this, too, can subside in a few weeks. Gonorrhea, the leading cause of sterility in women, can cause PID. In pregnant women, gonorrhea becomes a threat to the newborn. It can infect the infant's external genitals and can cause a serious form of conjunctivitis, an inflammation of the eye that may lead to blindness. As a preventive step, newborns may have penicillin dropped into their eyes at birth.

In men, untreated gonorrhea can spread to the prostate gland, testicles, bladder, and kidneys. Among the serious complications are urinary obstruction and sterility caused by blockage of the vas deferens (the excretory duct of the testis). In both sexes, gonorrhea can develop into a serious, even fatal, blood-borne infection that can cause arthritis in the joints, attack the heart muscle and lining, cause meningitis, and attack the skin and other organs.

Although a blood test has been developed for detecting gonorrhea, the tried-and-true method of diagnosis is still a microscopic analysis of cultures from the male's urethra, the female's cervix, and the throat and anus of both sexes.

Because gonorrhea often occurs along with chlamydia, practitioners often prescribe an agent effective against both, such as ofloxacin. In some parts of the United States, gonorrhea has become so resistant to certain antibiotics such as fluoroguinolone that they are no longer advised for use in its treatment. Antibiotics taken for other reasons may not affect or cure gonorrhea, because of their dosage or type. And you can't develop immunity to gonorrhea; within days of recovering from one case, you can catch another.

Nongonococcal Urethritis (NGU)

The term **nongonococcal urethritis (NGU)** refers to any inflammation of the urethra that is not caused by gonorrhea. NGU is the most common STI in men, accounting for 4 to 6 million visits to a physician every year. Three microorganisms—*Chlamydia trachomatis, Ureaplasma urealyticum,* and *Mycoplasma genitalium*—are the primary causes; the usual means of transmission is sexual intercourse. Other infectious agents, such as fungi or bacteria, allergic reactions to vaginal secretions, or irritation by soaps or contraceptive foams or gels also may lead to NGU.

In the United States, NGU is more common in men than gonococcal urethritis. The symptoms in men are similar to those of gonorrhea, including discharge from the penis (usually less than with gonorrhea) and mild burning during urination. Women frequently develop no symptoms or very mild itching, burning during urination, or discharge. Symptoms usually disappear after two or three weeks, but the infection may persist and cause cervicitis or PID in women and, in men, may spread to the prostate, epididymis, or both. Treatment usually consists of doxycycline or azithromycin and should be given to both sexual partners after testing.

Syphilis

A corkscrew-shaped, spiral bacterium called *Treponema pallidum* causes **syphilis.** This frail microbe dies in seconds if dried or chilled but grows quickly in the warm, moist tissues of the body, particularly in the mucous membranes of the genital tract. Entering the body through any tiny break in the skin, the germ burrows its way into the bloodstream. Sexual contact, including oral sex or intercourse, is a primary means of transmission. Genital ulcers caused by syphilis may increase the risk of HIV infection, while individuals with HIV may be more likely to develop syphilis.

Public education programs, expanded screening and surveillance, increased tracing of contacts, and condom promotion have helped control the spread of syphilis in some areas. Syphilis rates have fallen to the lowest ever reported in the United States. The decline has been particularly significant in African Americans and people living in the South.

Syphilis has clearly identifiable stages:

- **Primary syphilis.** The first sign of syphilis is a lesion, or *chancre* (pronounced "shanker"), an open lump or crater the size of a dime or smaller, teeming with bacteria. The incubation period before its appearance ranges from 10 to 90 days; three to four weeks is average. The chancre appears exactly where the bacteria entered the body: in the mouth, throat, vagina, rectum, or penis. Any contact with the chancre is likely to result in infection.
- **Secondary syphilis.** Anywhere from one to twelve months after the chancre's appearance, secondary-stage symptoms may appear. Some people have no symptoms. Others develop a skin rash or a small, flat rash in moist regions on the skin; whitish patches on the mucous membranes of the mouth or throat; temporary baldness; low-grade fever; headache; swollen glands; or large, moist sores around the mouth and genitals. These are loaded with bacteria; contact with them, through kissing or intercourse, may transmit the infection. Symptoms may last for several days or several months. Even without treatment, symptoms eventually disappear as the syphilis microbes go into hiding.
- **Latent syphilis.** Although there are no signs or symptoms, no sores or rashes at this stage, the bacteria are invading various organs inside the body, including the heart and brain. For two to four years, there may be recurring infectious and highly contagious lesions of the skin or mucous membranes. However, syphilis loses its infectiousness as it progresses: After the first two years, a person rarely transmits syphilis through intercourse.

  After four years, even congenital syphilis is rarely transmitted. Until this stage of the disease, however, a pregnant woman can pass syphilis to her unborn child. If the fetus is infected in its fourth month or earlier, it may be disfigured or even die. If infected late in pregnancy, the child may show no signs of infection for months or years after birth, but may then become disabled with the symptoms of tertiary syphilis.
- **Tertiary syphilis.** Ten to 20 years after the beginning of the latent stage, the most serious symptoms of syphilis emerge, generally in the organs in which the bacteria settled during latency. Syphilis that has progressed to this stage has become increasingly rare. Victims of tertiary syphilis may die of a ruptured aorta or of other heart damage, or may have progressive brain or spinal cord damage, eventually leading to blindness, insanity, or paralysis. About a third of those who are not treated during the first three stages of syphilis enter the tertiary stage later in life.

Health experts are urging screening for syphilis for everyone who seeks treatment for an STI, especially adolescents; for everyone using illegal drugs; and for the partners

gonorrhea A sexually transmitted disease caused by the bacterium *Neisseria gonorrhoeae;* symptoms include discharge from the penis; women are generally asymptomatic.

nongonococcal urethritis (NGU) Inflammation of the urethra caused by organisms other than the gonococcus bacterium.

syphilis A sexually transmitted disease caused by the bacterium *Treponema pallidum* and characterized by early sores, a latent period, and a final period of life-threatening symptoms, including brain damage and heart failure.

of these two groups. They also recommend that anyone diagnosed with syphilis be screened for other STIs and be counseled about voluntary testing for HIV.

Penicillin is the drug of choice for treating primary, secondary, and latent syphilis. The earlier treatment begins, the more effective it is. Those allergic to penicillin may be treated with doxycycline, ceftriaxone, or erythromycin. An added danger of not getting treatment for syphilis is an increased risk of HIV transmission.

Chancroid

A **chancroid** is a soft, painful sore or localized infection caused by the bacterium *Haemophilus ducrevi* and usually acquired through sexual contact. Half of the cases heal by themselves. In other cases, the infection may spread to the lymph glands near the chancroid, where large amounts of pus can accumulate and destroy much of the local tissue. The incidence of this STI, widely prevalent in Africa and tropical and semitropical regions, is rapidly increasing in the United States, with outbreaks in several states, including Louisiana, Texas, and New York. Chancroids, which may increase susceptibility to HIV infection, are believed to be a major factor in the heterosexual spread of HIV. This infection is treated with antibiotics (ceftriaxone, azithromycin, or erythromycin) and can be prevented by keeping the genitals clean and washing them with soap and water in case of possible exposure.

Pubic Lice and Scabies

These infections are sometimes, but not always, transmitted sexually. *Pubic lice* (or "crabs") are usually found in the pubic hair, although they can migrate to any hairy areas of the body. Lice lay eggs called nits that attach to the base of the hair shaft. Irritation from the lice may produce intense itching. Scratching to relieve the itching can produce sores. *Scabies* is caused by a mite that burrows under the skin, where they lay eggs that hatch and undergo many changes in the course of their life cycle, producing great discomfort, including intense itching.

Lice and scabies are treated with applications of permethrin cream and lindane shampoo to all the areas of the body where there are concentrations of body hair (genitals, armpits, scalp). You must repeat treatment in seven days to kill any newly developed adults. Wash or dry-clean clothing and bedding.

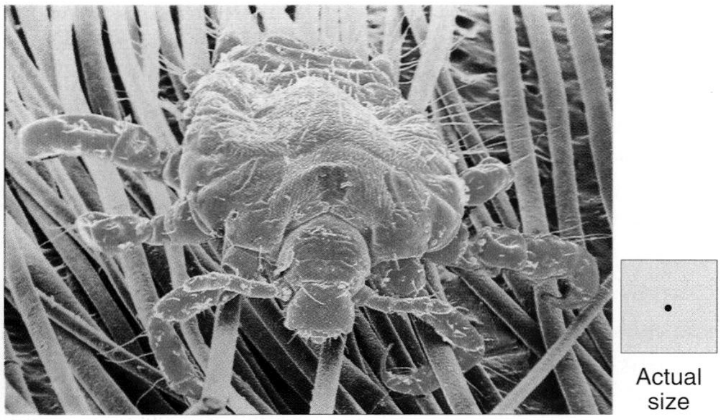

A pubic louse, or "crab."

HIV and AIDS

Thirty years ago, no one knew about **human immunodeficiency virus (HIV).** No one had ever heard of **acquired immune deficiency syndrome (AIDS).** Once seen as an epidemic affecting primarily gay men and injection drug users, AIDS has taken on a very different form. Today, heterosexuals in developing countries have the highest rates of infection and mortality. And HIV infection continues to spread, doubling at an estimated rate of every ten years.

About 39.4 million people worldwide are infected with HIV; 15,000 more individuals are infected every day. AIDS now claims about 3 million lives—more than half children—around the world a year. According to the CDC, 1,039,000 to 1,185,000 people are living with HIV or AIDS in the United States, with about 43,000 new infections every year.

Federal health officials fear that a new generation may not be using adequate safer sex precautions, because they have grown complacent about the dangers of HIV/AIDS. Efforts to prevent sexual transmission of HIV have taken a new focus: counseling those who already have HIV in an attempt to get them to stop spreading it.

Breakthrough drugs are indeed allowing HIV-infected people to live longer. However, new dangers have emerged. Up to 15 percent of new HIV cases in the country may stem from drug-resistant strains of the virus. "Superinfection" with more than one strain of HIV seems more common than previously thought. As a result, HIV-infected people who initially were doing well without drugs may become ill after contracting a second strain of the AIDS virus.

Efforts to prevent nonsexual forms of HIV transmission have been very effective. Screening the blood supply has reduced the rate of transfusion-associated HIV transmission by 99.9 percent. Treatment with antiretroviral drugs during pregnancy and birth has reduced transmission by about 90 percent in optimal conditions.

Among drug users in some settings, programs that combine addiction treatment and needle exchange reduced the incidence of HIV infection by 30 percent.

Men who have sex with men account for 65 percent of AIDS diagnoses among men. Homosexual and bisexual men, particularly those who are young or of color and living in metropolitan areas, are at particularly high risk. The percentage of individuals who acquired HIV through heterosexual contact has increased to 31 percent. Many heterosexuals are not aware of their partners' HIV status and may not see themselves as being at risk of HIV infection. According to the CDC, about a third of the HIV-infected individuals in the United States have not been diagnosed.

African Americans and Latinos account for a disproportionate share of new AIDS diagnoses (Figure 9-7). Almost half of all those living with HIV/AIDS in the United States are African American. The AIDS case rate per 100,000 people is 9.5 times that of whites. African Americans are less likely to survive after a diagnosis of AIDS than other ethnic or racial groups. HIV/AIDS is the third-leading cause of death among African Americans between ages 25 and 34 and the sixth leading cause of death for whites and Latinos in this age group.[25]

HIV/AIDS is seen as a threat to men, but 27 percent of new HIV infections in the United States occur among women. About a quarter of Americans living with HIV/AIDS are women. Women of color, particularly African Americans, have been hardest hit. While African-American women make up just 13 percent of the female population of the United States, they account for 67 percent of newly diagnosed cases. HIV/AIDS is most prevalent among women in their childbearing years (Figure 9.8).[26]

Reducing the Risk of HIV Transmission

HIV/AIDS can be so frightening that some people have exaggerated its dangers, whereas others understate them. The fact is that although no one is immune to HIV, you can reduce the risk if you abstain from sexual activity, remain in a monogamous relationship with an uninfected partner, and do not inject drugs.

If you're not in a long-term monogamous relationship with a partner you're sure is safe, and you're not willing to abstain from sex, there are things you can do to lower your risk of HIV infection. Remember that the risk of HIV transmission depends on sexual behavior, not sexual orientation. Among

chanchroid A soft, painful sore or localized infection usually acquired through sexual contact.

human immunodeficiency virus (HIV) A type of virus that causes a spectrum of health problems, ranging from a symptomless infection to changes in the immune system, to the development of life-threatening diseases because of impaired immunity.

acquired immune deficiency syndrome (AIDS) The final stages of HIV infection, characterized by a variety of severe illnesses and decreased levels of certain immune cells.

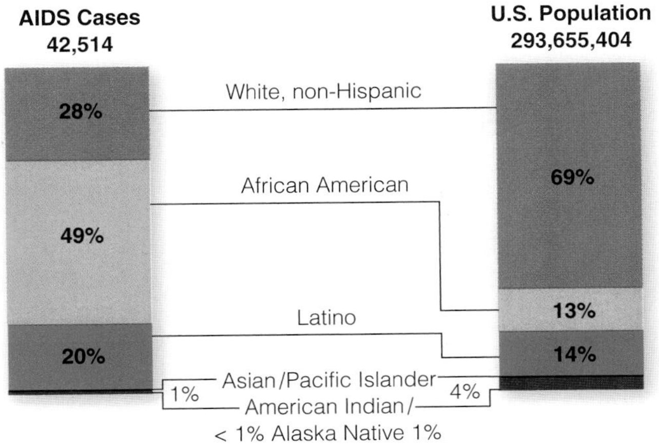

FIGURE 9-7 The Impact of AIDS by Race

Minority Americans represent the majority of new AIDS cases and of those living with AIDS.

Source: "African Americans and HIV/AIDS." *Kaiser Family Foundation HIV/AIDS Fact Sheet,* February 2006. This information is reprinted with permission from the Henry J. Kaiser Family Foundation. The Kaiser Family Foundation, based in Menlo Park, California, is a nonprofit, independent health-care philanthropy and is not associated with Kaiser Permanente or Kaiser Industries.

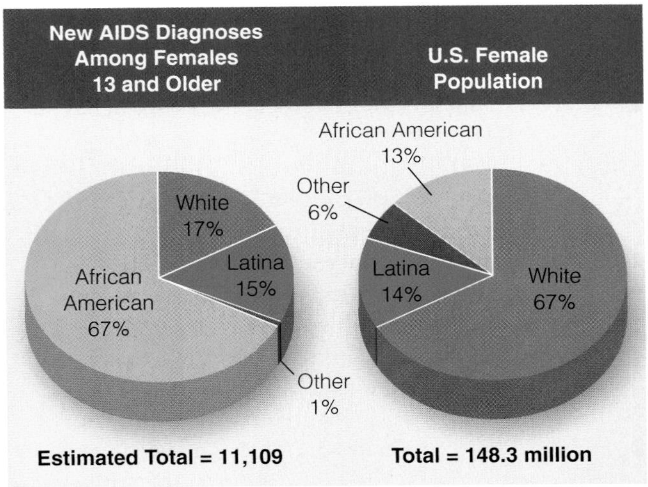

FIGURE 9-8 Women and HIV/AIDS

Women of color, particularly African-American women, have been especially hard hit by the HIV/AIDS epidemic.

Source: "Women and HIV/AIDS in the United States." *Kaiser Family Foundation HIV/AIDS Fact Sheet,* February 2006. This information is reprinted with permission from the Henry J. Kaiser Family Foundation. The Kaiser Family Foundation, based in Menlo Park, California, is a nonprofit, independent health care philanthropy and is not associated with Kaiser Permanente or Kaiser Industries.

young men, the prevalence and frequency of sexual risk behaviors are similar regardless of sexual orientation, ethnicity, or age. Homosexual, heterosexual, and bisexual individuals all need to know about the kinds of sexual activity that increase their risk.

Here's what you should know about HIV transmission:

- Casual contact does *not* spread HIV infection. You cannot get HIV infection from drinking from a water fountain, contact with a toilet seat, or touching an infected person.
- Compared to other viruses, HIV is extremely difficult to get.
- HIV can live in blood, semen, vaginal fluids, and breast milk.
- Many chemicals, including household bleach, alcohol, and hydrogen peroxide, can inactivate HIV.
- In studies of family members sharing dishes, food, clothing, and frequent hugs with people with HIV infection or AIDS, those who have contracted the virus have shared razor blades, toothbrushes, or had other means of blood contact.
- You cannot tell visually whether a potential sexual partner has HIV. A blood test is needed to detect the antibodies that the body produces to fight HIV, thus indicating infection.
- HIV can be spread in semen and vaginal fluids during a single instance of anal, vaginal, or oral sexual contact between heterosexuals, bisexuals, or homosexuals. The risk increases with the number of sexual encounters with an infected partner.
- Teenage girls may be particularly vulnerable to HIV infection because the immature cervix is easily infected.
- Anal intercourse is an extremely high-risk behavior because HIV can enter the bloodstream through tiny breaks in the lining of the rectum. HIV transmission is much more likely to occur during unprotected anal intercourse than vaginal intercourse.
- Other behaviors that increase the risk of HIV infection include having multiple sexual partners, engaging in sex without condoms or virus-killing spermicides, sexual contact with persons known to be at high risk (for example, prostitutes or injection drug users), and sharing injection equipment for drugs.
- Individuals are at greater risk if they have an active sexual infection. Sexually transmitted infections, such as herpes, gonorrhea, and syphilis, facilitate transmission of HIV during vaginal or rectal intercourse.
- No cases of HIV transmission by deep kissing have been reported, but it could happen. Studies have found blood in the saliva of healthy people after kissing; other lab studies have found HIV in saliva. Social (dry) kissing is safe.
- Oral sex can lead to HIV transmission. The virus in any semen that enters the mouth could make its way into the bloodstream through tiny nicks or sores in the mouth. A man's risk in performing oral sex on a woman is smaller because an infected woman's genital fluids have much lower concentrations of HIV than does semen.
- HIV infection is not widespread among lesbians, although there have been documented cases of possible female-to-female HIV transmission. In each instance, one partner had had sex with a bisexual man or male injection drug user or had injected drugs herself.

HIV Infection

HIV infection refers to a spectrum of health problems that results from immunologic abnormalities caused by the virus when it enters the bloodstream. In theory, the body may be able to resist infection by HIV. In reality, in almost all cases, HIV destroys the cell-mediated immune system, particularly the CD4+ T-lymphocytes (also called *T4 helper cells*). The result is greatly increased susceptibility to various cancers and opportunistic infections (infections that take hold because of the reduced effectiveness of the immune system).

Researchers now know that HIV triggers a state of all-out war within the immune system. Almost immediately following infection with HIV, the immune system responds aggressively by manufacturing enormous numbers of CD4 + cells. It eventually is overwhelmed, however, as the viral particles continue to replicate, or multiply. The intense war between HIV and the im-

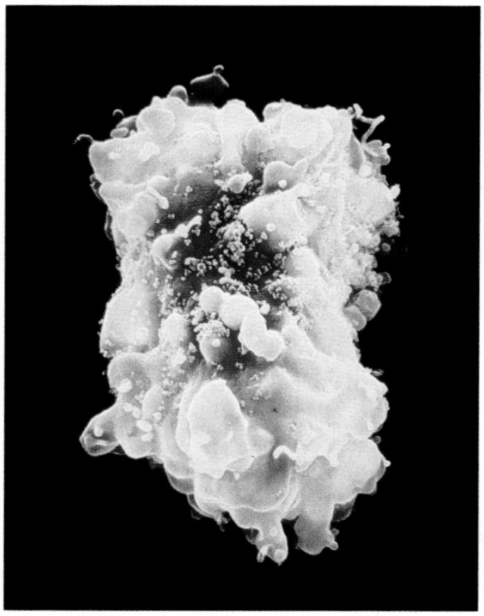

Electron micrograph of a white blood cell being attacked by HIV (*light blue particles*), the virus that causes AIDS.

mune system indicates that the virus itself, not a breakdown in the immune system, is responsible for disease progression.

Shortly after becoming infected with HIV, individuals may experience a few days of flulike symptoms, which most ignore or attribute to other viruses. Some people develop a more severe mononucleosis-type syndrome. After this stage, individuals may not develop any signs or symptoms of disease for a period ranging from weeks to more than 12 years.

HIV symptoms, which tend to increase in severity and number the longer the virus is in the body, may include any of the following:

- Swollen lymph nodes.
- Fever, chills, and night sweats.
- Diarrhea.
- Weight loss.
- Coughing and shortness of breath.
- Persistent tiredness.
- Skin sores.
- Blurred vision and headaches.
- Development of other infections, such as certain kinds of pneumonia.

HIV infection is associated with a variety of HIV-related diseases, including different cancers and dangerous infections including tuberculosis. HIV-infected individuals may develop persistent generalized lymphadenopathy, enlargement of the lymph nodes at two or more different sites in the body. This condition typically persists for more than three months without any other illness to explain its occurrence. Diminished mental function may appear before other symptoms. Tests conducted on infected but apparently healthy men have revealed impaired coordination, problems in thinking, or abnormal brain scans.

HIV Testing

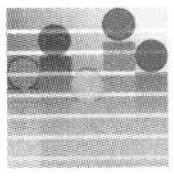

Nearly half of American adults over age 18 have been tested for HIV. In general, minorities are more likely to have sought testing than whites.

All HIV tests measure antibodies, cells produced by the body to fight HIV infection. A negative test indicates no exposure to HIV. It can take three to six months for the body to produce the telltale antibodies, however, so a negative result may not be accurate, depending on the timing of the test.

HIV testing can be either confidential or anonymous. In confidential testing, a person's name is recorded along with the test results, which are made available to medical personnel and in 32 states, the state health department. In anonymous testing, no name is associated with the test results. Anonymous testing is available in 39 states.

The only home HIV test approved by the FDA, Home Access, is available in drug stores or online for \$40 to \$50. An individual draws a blood sample by pricking a finger and sends it to a laboratory along with a personal identification number. Results are given over the phone by a trained counselor, usually within several days.

Newly developed blood tests can determine how recently a person was infected with HIV and distinguish between long-standing infections and those contracted within the previous four to six months.

Diagnosing AIDS

A diagnosis of AIDS applies to anyone with HIV whose immune system is severely impaired, as indicated by a CD4 count of less than 200 cells per cubic millimeter of blood, compared to normal CD4 cell counts in healthy people not infected with HIV of 800 to 1,200 per cubic millimeter of blood. In addition, AIDS is diagnosed in persons with HIV infection who experience recurrent pneumonia, invasive cervical cancer, or pulmonary tuberculosis.

People with AIDS also may experience persistent fever, diarrhea that persists for more than one month, or involuntary weight loss of more than 10 percent of normal body weight. Neurological disease—including dementia (confusion and impaired thinking) and other problems with thinking, speaking, movement, or sensation—may occur. Secondary infectious diseases that may develop in people with AIDS include *Pneumocystis carinii* pneumonia, tuberculosis, or oral candidiasis (thrush). Secondary cancers associated with HIV infection include Kaposi's sarcoma and cancer of the cervix.

Treating HIV/AIDS

New forms of therapy have been remarkably effective in boosting levels of protective T cells and reducing *viral load*—the amount of HIV in the bloodstream. People with high viral loads are more likely to progress rapidly to AIDS than people with low levels of the virus.

The current "gold-standard" approach to combating HIV is known as HAART (highly active antiretroviral therapies), which dramatically reduces viral load even though it does not eradicate the virus. This complex regimen uses one of 250 different combinations of three or more antiretroviral drugs. Since the development of HAART, the number of deaths among persons with AIDS in the United States has declined by 70 percent, and the number of those living with AIDS has risen.

Because HAART can drastically lower viral load, there is some evidence that it also may reduce the risk of

Strategies for Prevention — Should I Be Tested for HIV?

Health officials recommend HIV testing for the following individuals:

- Men who have had sex with other men, regardless of whether they consider themselves homosexual.
- Anyone who uses injection drugs or has shared needles.
- Anyone who has had sex with someone who uses injection drugs or has shared needles.
- Women who have had sex with bisexual men.
- Anyone who has had sex with someone from an area with a high incidence of HIV infection.
- Individuals who have had sex with people they do not know well.
- Individuals diagnosed with an STI such as chlamydia or gonorrhea.
- Anyone who received blood transfusions or blood products between 1978 and 1985, their sexual partners, and, if they are new mothers, their infants.

infectiousness of HIV-positive individuals. Fearing that this could lead to unsafe sex, researchers did a meta-analysis of HAART recipients and found no increased sexual risk behavior. Even when HIV levels are undetectable, they note, this does not mean the infected person is "cured," nor does it eliminate the possibility of transmitting HIV.

In the last few years, several new drugs have become available, and many of these antiretroviral agents can be taken just once or twice a day, rather than more. New antiretroviral agents and new types of drugs are currently in clinical trials. Work is also continuing toward an AIDS vaccine. As more effective therapies have emerged, there has been a major shift in attitude: Physicians are more optimistic about long-term treatments, and hope is replacing despair as more individuals are living productive lives with HIV.

LEARN IT / LIVE IT

The Best Defense

Some day medical science may develop vaccines or other means of providing total protection against infectious diseases. Until then your best defense is to take commonsense steps to promote well-being and reduce the risks of infection. Here are some basic principles of self-defense:

- **Eat a balanced diet** to be sure you get essential vitamins and minerals. Severe deficiencies in vitamins B_6, B_{12}, and folic acid impair immunity. Keep up your iron and zinc intake. Iron influences the number and vigor of certain immune cells, whereas zinc is crucial for cell repair. Too little vitamin C also may increase susceptibility to infectious diseases.
- **Avoid fatty foods.** A low-fat diet can increase the activity of immune cells that hunt down and knock out cells infected with viruses.
- **Get enough sleep.** Without adequate rest, your immune system cannot maintain and renew itself.
- **Exercise regularly.** Aerobic exercise stimulates the production of an immune-system booster called interleukin-2.
- **Don't smoke.** Smoking decreases the levels of some immune cells and increases susceptibility to respiratory infections.
- **Control your alcohol intake.** Heavy drinking interferes with normal immune responses and lowers the number of defender cells.
- **Wash your hands frequently** with hot water and soap. In a public restroom, use a paper towel to turn off the faucet after you wash your hands, and avoid touching the doorknob. Wash objects used by someone with a cold.
- **Don't share food, drinks, silverware, glasses,** and other objects that may carry infectious microbes.
- **Spend as little time as possible in crowds** during cold and flu season, especially closed places, such as elevators and airplanes. When out, keep your distance from sneezers and coughers.
- **Don't touch your eyes, mouth, and nose** after being with someone who has cold symptoms.
- **Use tissues** rather than cloth handkerchiefs, which may harbor viruses for hours or days.

- **Avoid irritating air pollutants** whenever possible.
- **Always use safer sex practices.**
- **Get tested immediately** if you have any reason to suspect that you may have been exposed to an STI.

9 Making This Chapter Work for You

Review Questions

1. Which of the following statements about disease-causing microbes is *false?*
   a. Helminths cause malaria, one of the major worldwide diseases.
   b. AIDS is caused by a virus.
   c. In the United States, the most common protozoan disease is giardiasis.
   d. Salmonella is a foodborne illness caused by bacteria.
2. Which of the following statements about the immune system is *false?*
   a. The immune system has two types of white blood cells: B cells, which produce antibodies that fight bacteria and viruses, and T cells, which protect against other invaders.
   b. Immune system structures include the spleen, tonsils, thymus gland, and lymph nodes located throughout the body.
   c. Inoculation with a vaccine confers active immunity.
   d. The effect of stress on the human immune system depends on whether you can control the stressor and on the mental effort required to cope.
3. College students should have all of the following immunizations *except*
   a. influenza.
   b. pertussis.
   c. measles.
   d. tetanus.
4. Which of the following statements about the common cold and influenza is true?
   a. Influenza is just a more severe form of the common cold.
   b. Aspirin should be avoided by children and young adults who have a cold or influenza.
   c. The flu vaccine is also effective against most of the viruses that cause the common cold.
   d. Antibiotics are appropriate treatments for colds but not for influenza.
5. Which of the following statements about specific infectious diseases is *false?*
   a. Yeast infections can be treated with nonprescription drugs.
   b. Symptoms of UTIs include burning urination, chills, fever, and blood in the urine.
   c. Hepatitis A is usually transmitted through contaminated needles, transfusions, and sexual contact.
   d. College freshmen are at higher risk for contracting meningitis than the general population of young people between the ages of 18 and 23.
6. Sexually transmitted infections
   a. are the major cause of preventable sterility in the United States.
   b. can result in a severe kidney disease called pylonephritis.
   c. have declined in incidence in developing nations due to improving health standards.
   d. do not increase the risk of being infected with HIV.
7. Viral agents cause all of the following STIs *except*
   a. herpes.
   b. genital warts.
   c. hepatitis B.
   d. candidiasis.
8. Jake is sexually active but doesn't want to use a condom. His other choices to protect himself against STIs include all of these *except*
   a. abstinence.
   b. a sexual relationship with a longtime friend.
   c. a sexual relationship with one STI-free partner.
   d. masturbation only.
9. Which of the following statements about HIV transmission is true?
   a. Individuals are not at risk for HIV if they are being treated for chlamydia or gonorrhea.
   b. HIV can be transmitted between lesbians.
   c. Heterosexual men who do not practice safe sex are at less risk for contracting HIV than homosexual men who do practice safe sex.
   d. HIV cannot be spread in a single instance of sexual intercourse.
10. A person with AIDS
    a. has a low viral load and a high number of T4 helper cells.
    b. can no longer pass HIV to a sexual partner.
    c. may suffer from secondary infectious diseases and cancers.
    d. will not respond to treatment.

Answers to these questions can be found on page 422.

Critical Thinking

1. Prior to reading this chapter, describe what you did to avoid contracting infectious disease. Now that you have read the chapter, will you be making any changes in your practices? Briefly explain the convenience,

advantages, and disadvantages of each practice that you have and/or will be using to prevent infection.

2. The U.S. military and some employers routinely screen personnel for HIV. Some hospitals test patients and note their HIV status on their charts. Some insurance companies test for HIV before selling a policy. Do you believe that an individual has the right to refuse to be tested for HIV? Should a physician be able to order an HIV test without a patient's consent? Can a surgeon refuse to operate on an HIV-infected patient or one who refuses HIV testing? Do patients have the right to know if their doctors, dentists, or nurses are HIV-positive?
3. A man who developed herpes sued his former girlfriend. A woman who became sterile as a result of pelvic inflammatory disease (PID) took her ex-husband to court. A woman who contracted HIV infection from her dentist, who had died of AIDS, filed suit against his estate. Do you think that anyone who knowingly transmits a sexually transmitted infection should be held legally responsible? Do you think such an act should be a criminal offense?

Media Menu

ThomsonNOW™ Go to the ThomsonNOW website at **http://www.thomsonedu.com** that will:

- Help you evaluate your knowledge of the material.
- Allow you to take an exam-prep quiz.
- Provide a Personalized Learning Plan targeting resources that address areas you should study.
- Coach you through identifying target goals for behavioral change and creating and monitoring your personal change plan throughout the semester.

INTERNET CONNECTIONS

Immunization Action Coalition
www.immunize.org

This site features comprehensive vaccination information for children, adolescents, and adults.

National Institute of Allergy and Infectious Diseases
www3.niaid.nih.gov

This institute is part of the National Institutes for Health. Its website provides information about current research and includes fact sheets about all manner of topics related to allergies and infectious diseases.

National Center for HIV, STD, and TB Prevention
www.cdc.gov/hiv/dhap.htm

This site, sponsored by the Centers for Disease Control and Prevention (CDC), features current information, fact sheets, conferences, media campaigns, publications, the 20-year history of HIV/AIDS, information on prevention and treatment, a FAQ section, as well as the most current HIV/AIDS statistics.

HIV InSite: Gateway to AIDS Knowledge
http://hivinsite.ucsf.edu

This site, sponsored by the University of California San Francisco School of Medicine, provides statistics, education, prevention, and new developments related to HIV/AIDS.

InfoTrac College Edition Activities Log on, insert **infectious diseases** into the Keyword search box, and limit your search to the past year. When you get the results, Mark articles to review, then Select one to read. Summarize three or four key points from the article.

You can find additional readings related to personal health with InfoTrac College Edition, an online library of more than 900 journals and publications. Follow the instructions for accessing InfoTrac College Edition that were packaged with your textbook; then search for articles using a keyword search.

For additional links, resources, and suggested readings on the InfoTrac College Edition, visit our Health and Wellness Resource Center at **http://health.wadsworth.com.**

Key Terms

The terms listed are used on the page indicated. Definitions of the terms are in the Glossary at the end of this book.

abscess 234
acquired immune deficiency syndrome (AIDS) 254
allergy 234
antibiotics 230
antiviral drug 230
bacteria 230
bacterial vaginosis 244
candidiasis 244
chanchroid 254
chlamydia 249
chronic fatigue syndrome (CFS) 241
cystitis 244
fungi 230
gamma globulin 233
gonorrhea 252
helminth 230
hepatitis 239
herpes simplex 250
host 230
human immunodeficiency virus (HIV) 254
human papilloma virus (HPV) 249
immune deficiency 234
immunity 232
immunotherapy 234
incubation period 231
inflammation 234
influenza 237
Lyme disease 242
lymph nodes 232
meningitis 238
mononucleosis 241

LACC Extra Credit Assignment

9. You have found that you have symptoms of STD. List the steps you would take.

nongonococcal urethritis (NGU) 253
pathogen 230
pelvic inflammatory disease (PID) 251
protozoa 230
sexually transmitted infections (STIs) 245
syphilis 253
systemic disease 234
trichomoniasis 244
tuberculosis (TB) 241
urethritis 244
vector 230
virus 230

10 Lowering Your Risk of Major Diseases

REAL HEALTH

Jamal never forgot the terror he felt when his Dad had his first heart attack. Only ten, he couldn't understand why this towering giant of a man had fallen to the ground. His father seemed different when he came home from the hospital, but he would still flash an impish grin, especially when he'd sneak a cigarette and wink at Jamal so he wouldn't tell his mother. The second heart attack came four years later. This time Jamal's Dad didn't come home.

Jamal promised his mother that he'd take better care of his heart. He wouldn't smoke; he'd watch his blood pressure and weight; he'd keep tabs on his diet; he'd exercise regularly. Jamal didn't forget these promises as time passed. But like many college students, he felt invincible. He was shocked when a sports physical revealed that his blood pressure was high and his levels of the most dangerous type of cholesterol were elevated. But he also felt lucky.

"I got my wake-up call," he says . "And I'm not going to ignore it." His doctor explained that the effort and attention that Jamal invests in lowering his risks now will pay dividends for decades to come. As he now realizes, it's never too soon, or too late, to start being heart smart.

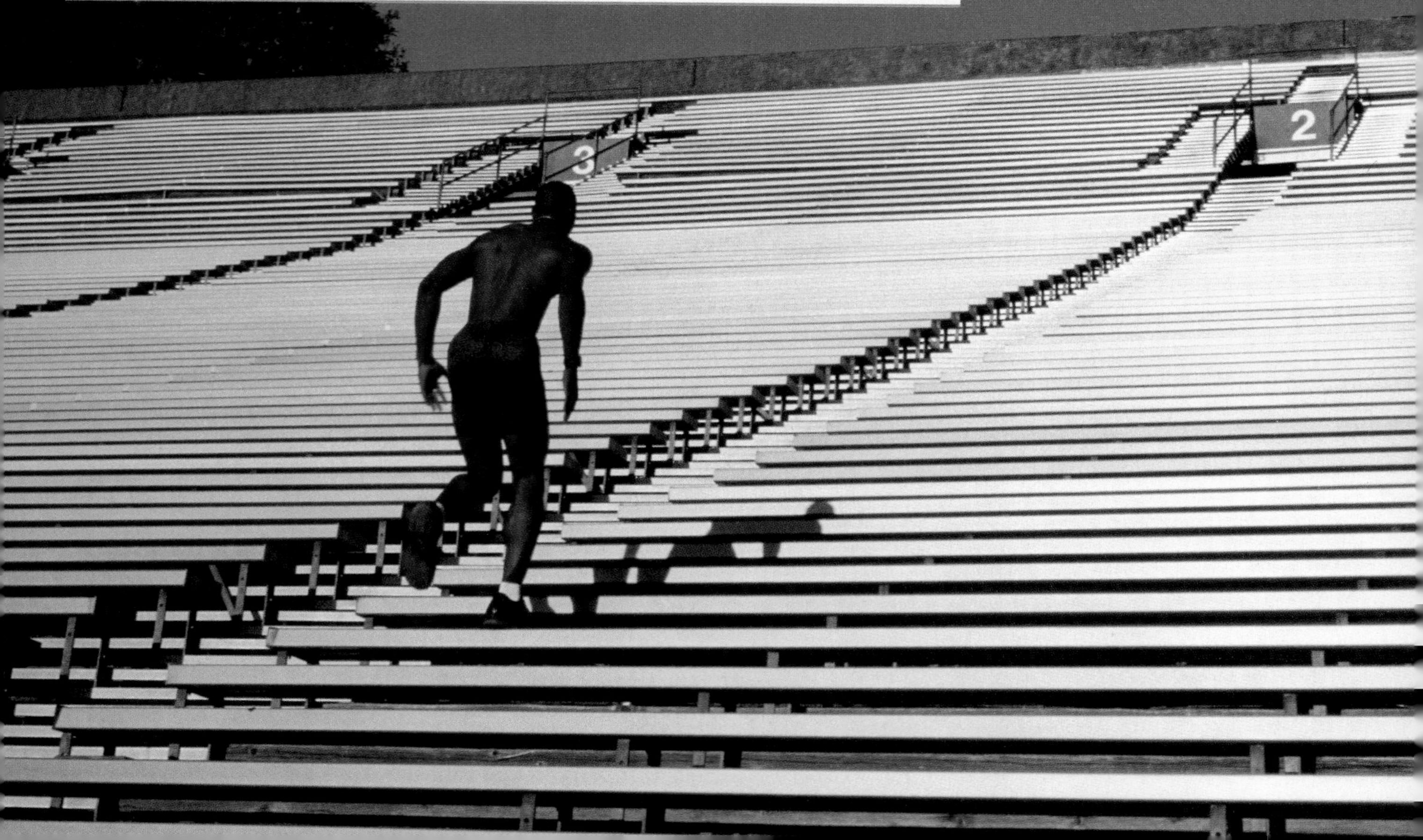

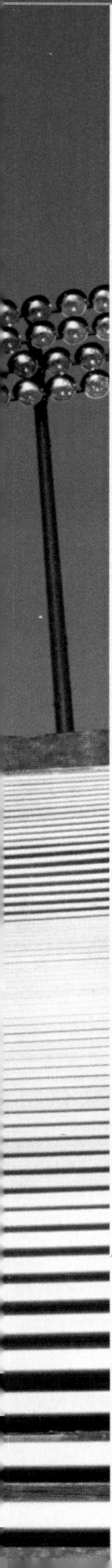

© bread & butter/Photographer's Choice/Getty

Whether or not you will get a serious disease at some time in your life may seem to be a matter of odds. Genetic tendencies, environmental factors, and luck affect your chances of having to face many health threats. However, you do have some control over such risks and often can prevent or delay major illnesses, such as heart disease, for years, even decades.

Despite gains in developed countries, researchers warn that cardiovascular disease will become the leading cause of death and disability worldwide by 2020. A primary reason is that the populations of developing countries have adopted the same harmful habits as industrialized nations, including smoking, overeating, and exercising less. These lifestyle factors also contribute to more than a third of cancer deaths in the United States.

The time to start protecting your health is now. People mistakenly think of heart disease, cancer, and other disorders as illnesses of middle and old age. But the events leading up to these diseases often begin in childhood, progress in adolescence, and become a health threat to men in their thirties and forties and to women in their forties and fifties. This chapter provides the information about the risk factors, silent dangers, and medical advances that can improve your chances of a healthier, longer life.

? FAQ Frequently Asked Questions

- Why should I worry about heart disease? *p. 265*
- What is a healthy blood pressure? *p. 274*
- What is a healthy cholesterol reading? *p. 275*
- How do I know it's a heart attack? *p. 277*
- What causes a stroke? *p. 278*
- Who is at risk for developing cancer? *p. 280*
- Who is at risk for developing diabetes? *p. 290*

After studying the material in this chapter, you should be able to:

- **Explain** how the heart functions.
- **Identify** the risk factors for cardiovascular disease that you can control and those that you cannot control.
- **Define** hypertension, and **discuss** why it is dangerous and ways to prevent it.
- **Describe** the types of cholesterol that compose your lipoprotein profile and the effects of each on heart health.
- **List** the risk factors for cancer, and **describe** ways you can reduce your risk of cancer.
- **Discuss** the most common types of cancer, and **describe** the treatments for each.
- **Describe** the early symptoms and treatment for diabetes mellitus.

ThomsonNOW Log on to ThomsonNOW at **www.thomsonedu.com/thomsonnow** to find your Behavior Change Planner and to explore self-assessments, interactive tutorials, and practice quizzes.

How the Heart Works

The heart is a hollow, muscular organ with four chambers that serve as two pumps (see Figure 10-1). It is about the size of a clenched fist. Each pump consists of a pair of chambers formed of muscles. The upper two—each called an **atrium**—receive blood, which then flows through valves into the lower two chambers, the **ventricles,** which contract to pump blood out into the arteries through a second set of valves. A thick wall divides the right side of the heart from the left side; even though the two sides are separated, they contract at almost the same time. Contraction of the ventricles is called **systole;** the period of relaxation between contractions is called **diastole.** The heart valves, located at the entrance and exit of the ventricular chambers, have flaps that open and close to allow blood to flow through the chambers of the heart.

The *myocardium* (heart muscle) consists of branching fibers that enable the heart to contract, or beat, between 60 and 80 times per minute, or about 100,000 times a day. With each beat, the heart pumps about 2 ounces of blood. This may not sound like much, but it adds up to nearly 5 quarts of blood pumped by the heart in one minute, or about 75 gallons per hour.

The heart is surrounded by the *pericardium,* which consists of two layers of a tough membrane. The space between the two contains a lubricating fluid that allows the heart muscle to move freely. The *endocardium* is a smooth membrane lining the inside of the heart and its valves.

Blood circulates through the body by means of the pumping action of the heart, as shown in Figure 10-2. The right ventricle (on your own right side) pumps blood, via the *pulmonary arteries,* to the lungs, where it picks up oxygen (a gas essential to the body's cells) and gives off carbon dioxide (a waste product of metabolism). The blood returns from the lungs via the *pulmonary veins* to the left side of the heart, which pumps it, via the **aorta,** to the arteries in the rest of the body.

The arteries divide into smaller and smaller branches and finally into **capillaries,** the smallest blood vessels of all (only slightly larger in diameter than a single red blood cell). The blood within the capillaries supplies oxygen and nutrients to the cells of the tissues and takes up various waste products. Blood returns to the heart via the veins: The blood from the upper body (except the lungs) drains into the heart through the *superior vena cava,* while blood from the lower body returns via the *inferior vena cava.*

The workings of this remarkable pump affect your entire body. If the flow of blood to or through the heart or to the rest of the body is reduced, or if a distur-

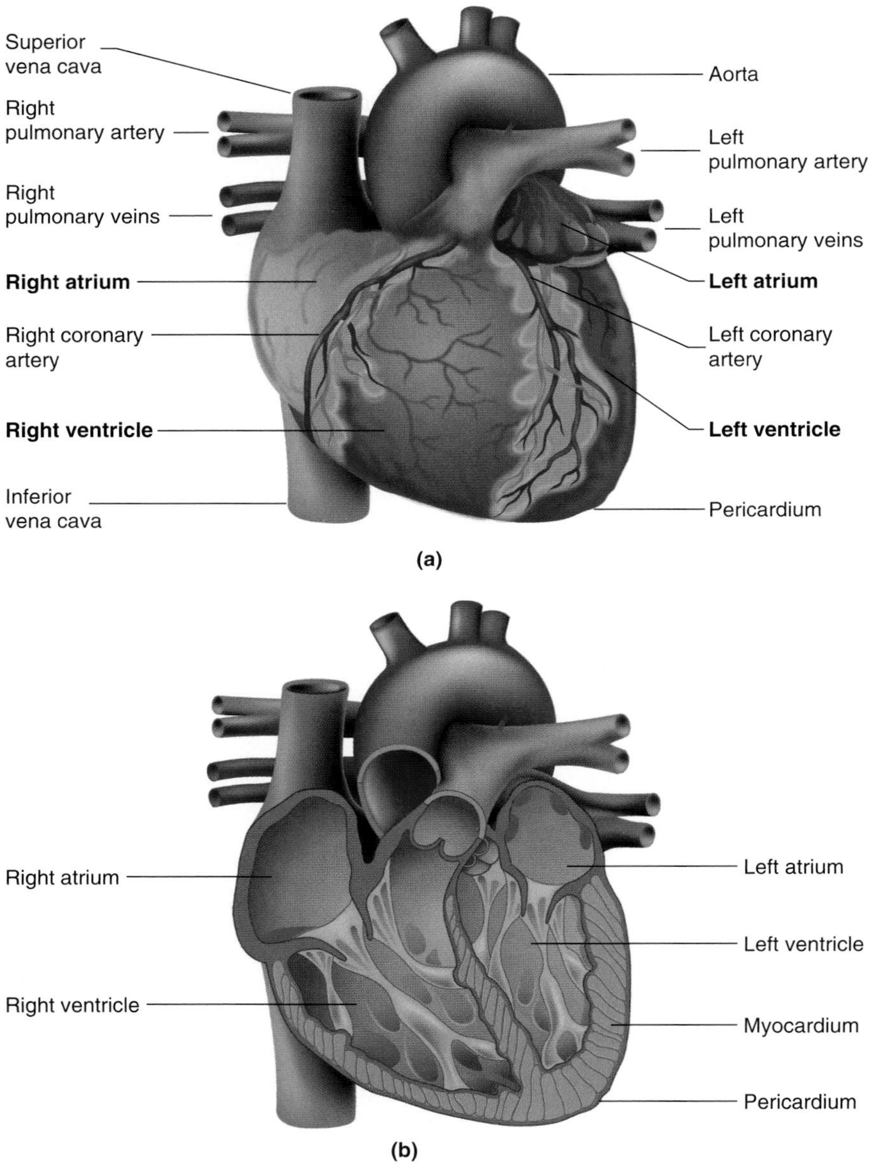

FIGURE 10-1 The Healthy Heart

(a) The heart muscle is nourished by blood from the coronary arteries, which arise from the aorta. (b) The cross section shows the four chambers and the myocardium, the muscle that does the heart's work. The pericardium is the outer covering of the heart.

bance occurs in the small bundle of highly specialized cells in the heart that generate electrical impulses to control heartbeats, the result may at first be too subtle to notice. However, without diagnosis and treatment, these changes could develop into a life-threatening problem.

Perhaps the biggest breakthrough in the field of cardiology has been not a test or a treatment but a realization: Heart disease is not inevitable. We can keep our hearts healthy for as long as we live, but the process of doing so must start early and continue throughout life.

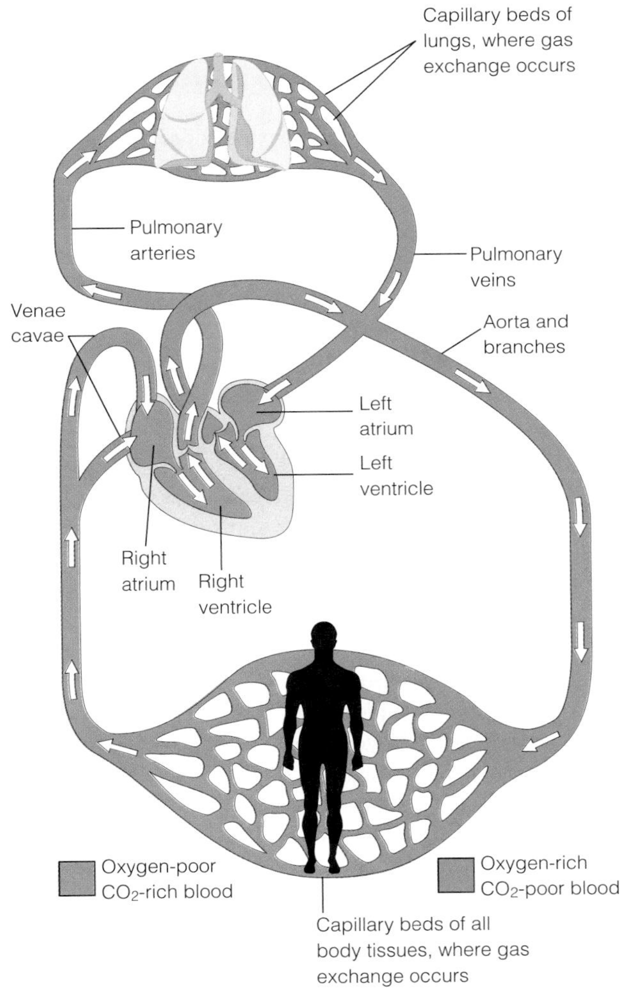

FIGURE 10-2 The Path of Blood Flow
Blood is pumped from the right ventricle into the pulmonary arteries, which lead to the lungs, where gas exchange (oxygen for carbon dioxide) occurs. Oxygenated blood returning from the lungs drains into the left atrium and is then pumped into the left ventricle, which sends the blood into the aorta and its branches. The oxygenated blood flows through the arteries, which extend to all parts of the body. Again, gas exchange occurs in the body tissues; this time oxygen is "dropped off" and carbon dioxide "picked up."

Preventing Heart Problems

For the first time ever, the number of deaths from heart disease for Americans under age 85 has dropped lower than those caused by cancer. This decline reflects the success of new treatments that can save damaged hearts, but it is also testimony to the power of prevention.

? FAQ Why Should I Worry About Heart Disease?

Many people, including college students and other young adults, are unaware of habits and conditions that put their hearts at risk. Many undergraduates view heart disease as mainly a problem for white men and underestimate the risks for women and ethnic groups. Students rate their own knowledge of heart disease as lower than that of sexually transmitted infections and psychological disorders. Yet heart disease is the third-leading cause of death among adults aged 25 to 44. Diabetes, family history, and other risk factors increase their likelihood of heart disease.

Young athletes face special risks. Each year seemingly healthy teens or young adults die suddenly on playing fields and courts. The culprit in one of every three cases of sudden cardiac death in young athletes is a silent condition called hypertrophic cardiomyopathy (HCM), an excessive thickness of the heart muscle. Because of HCM, the heart is more prone to dangerous heart irregularities (see "You Decide").

Because apparently healthy young athletes have died suddenly on playing fields or courts, some health officials argue that colleges should screen competitive athletes before allowing them to join a team. Others argue that screening should be an individual choice. Should college athletes be required to undergo testing for potentially lethal health risks? Or should they have the right to choose whether or not to be tested and whether to take the risks of playing their sport?

You Decide

atrium (plural **atria**) Either of the two upper chambers of the heart, which receive blood from the veins.

ventricle Either of the two lower chambers of the heart, which pump blood out of the heart and into the arteries.

systole The contraction phase of the cardiac cycle.

diastole The period between contractions in the cardiac cycle, during which the heart relaxes and dilates as it fills with blood.

aorta The main artery of the body, arising from the left ventricle of the heart.

capillary A minute blood vessel that connects an artery to a vein.

YOUR LIFE COACH

Making Heart Healthy Changes

Chances are that you don't have any noticeable symptoms of heart disease: no pain, no swelling, no breathlessness when you walk or climb stairs. But that doesn't mean that you're home safe. Depending on your age, family history, blood pressure, cholesterol levels, and other risk factors, your heart's health may be in jeopardy.

Yes, advances in treatment can help if you eventually develop heart disease. But changes in lifestyle can do even more: They can prevent or reverse heart-related symptoms. A 12-week program of therapeutic life changes, sometimes called TLC, helps lower blood pressure, cholesterol, blood sugar, and weight without medications.

If you don't feel any need to make changes, you are in the precontemplation stage of behavioral change (see Chapter 1 for a complete discussion). Read the entire chapter with an open mind, and think of family members or friends who have heart disease or who are clearly at risk because they smoke or are overweight. What effect have their habits had on their health? Make a list of the benefits heart-healthy habits might have for you.

If you do want to make some heart-healthy changes, select some of the behavioral modifications that follow:

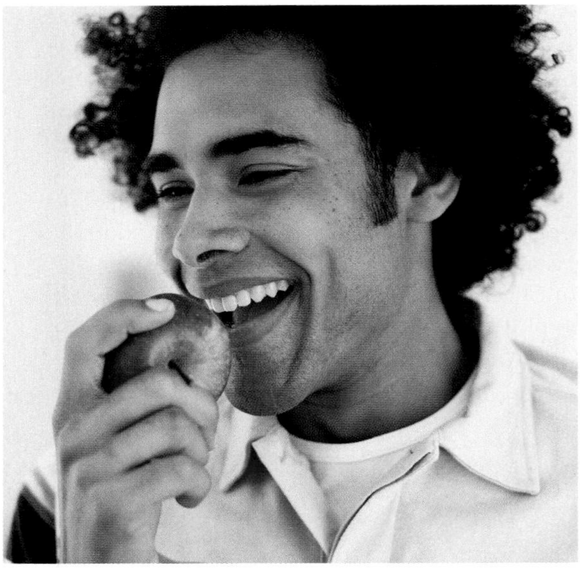

© Stockdisc/Jupiter Images

You can do something today to prevent heart disease in your future: Eat some fruit.

Changes You Can Make Today

- Eat a good breakfast: whole-grain cereal, juice, yogurt, and so forth.
- Take a walk after lunch.
- Skip dessert at dinner.
- Eat one more serving of vegetables.
- Eat one more piece of fruit.
- Drink one more glass of water.
- Take the stairs for one or two flights rather than riding the elevator in your dorm or classroom building.
- Get seven to eight hours of sleep tonight.

Changes You Can Make This Week

- **Block out time for exercise on your calendar.** Try for at least 30 minutes of physical activity most days.
- **If you haven't had your lipoproteins checked** within the last year, schedule a test.
- **If you don't know your blood pressure,** find out what it is. If you know it, compare your reading with those in Table 10-1 (page 274) to determine if it is too high.
- **Make a list of stress-reducing activities,** such as meditation or listening to music. Select two or three to do this week.
- **Get in touch with an old friend,** and enjoy catching up on each other's lives.

Changes You Can Make This Term

- **Look for new ways to meet your goals.** For example, try new and different healthy foods each week, or join a volleyball team.
- **Be patient.** Don't get discouraged if change seems harder and slower than you thought it would be.
- **If you slip up and smoke again or blow your diet, don't give up.** Analyze what triggered your relapse. Was it the smell of smoke at the party Saturday night? Did you try to console yourself for a poor grade with a carton of chocolate ice cream? Think of how you might handle similar situations differently in the future, such as staying away from smokers at parties or taking a walk to lift your mood rather than turning to food.
- **Develop and use a support system of friends and family members.** Identify individuals you can talk to, work out with, or call.

Getting Physical

Physical activity prevents or reduces many of the risk factors for heart disease discussed later in this chapter by:

- **Reducing body weight.**
- **Reducing blood pressure.**

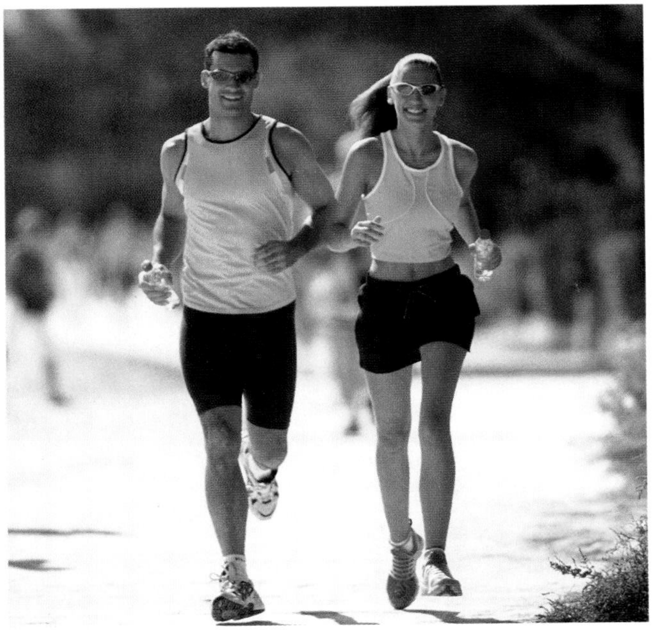

Regular physical activity can lower your risk of heart disease.

- **Reducing harmful low-density lipoprotein** (LDL) and total cholesterol.
- **Increasing beneficial high-density lipoprotein** (HDL) cholesterol.
- **Increasing insulin sensitivity** (and lowering the risk of diabetes).
- **Lowering C-reactive protein,** a marker of inflammation.

Sometimes exercise alone can lower an individual's risk of heart problems; in other cases exercise enhances the benefits of other treatments, such as cholesterol-lowering medications.

To maintain cardiovascular fitness, many medical groups, including the American Heart Association, American College of Sports Medicine, and the CDC, recommend 30 to 60 minutes or more of moderate-intensity physical activity such as brisk walking on most, if not all, days of the week. Simply meeting this recommendation for activity would reduce heart disease by 30 to 40 percent. The greatest cardiovascular gains occur in people who go from being sedentary to engaging in low-intensity to moderate activities, such as gardening, walking, and housecleaning. Their blood pressure falls; they lose weight; their hearts function more efficiently.

The greater the exercise "dose," the more benefits it yields. In studies that compared individuals of different fitness levels, the least fit were at much greater risk of dying. In men, more rigorous exercise, such as jogging, produces greater protection against heart disease and boosts longevity. (See Chapter 4 on fitness.)

In women, exercise capacity, adjusted for a woman's age, is a key predictor of cardiac health. Women who score less than 85 percent of the usual exercise capacity for women their age are more than twice as likely to die of heart disease or any other cause.[1]

Choosing Heart-Healthy Foods

A balanced, low-fat diet is the best recipe for a healthy heart. Fruits and vegetables, in particular, are associated with a reduced risk of cardiovascular disease, including lower blood pressure.

The American Heart Association (AHA) also recommends including cholesterol-lowering foods, such as oats, barley, soy protein, and nuts, in your daily diet. A diet rich in bran, one of the major components of whole grains, lowers the risk of heart disease.

It isn't certain whether you should also eat more fish. Long touted as "good" fats with numerous health benefits, omega-3 fatty acids in oily fish may not live up to expectations. An extensive analysis of 89 studies on omega-3 fatty acids and their impact on cardiovascular disease, cancer, and stroke concluded that they do not improve health outcomes for the general population, although they do not cause harm or increase health risks.[2] Yet another large study resulted in different findings, however, concluding that people who had higher intake of these fatty acids had lower death rates, primarily because of decreased heart attacks and strokes.[3]

Clinical trials generally have found no cardiovascular benefits from antioxidant supplements, such as vitamins C and E, and some evidence suggests that they may have harmful effects, such as interfering with cholesterol-lowering drugs.

Risk Factors for Cardiovascular Disease

Heart disease, contrary to a common misperception, generally does not strike "out of the blue." According to research, 80 to 90 percent of those who develop heart disease and 95 percent of those who suffer a fatal heart attack have at least one major risk factor. Recognition of the risk factors for heart disease has helped prevent many heart-related problems and saved countless lives.

Approximately 25 percent of adults have multiple risk factors, some form of heart disease, or type 2 diabetes. These high-risk men and women should work with their physicians on specific strategies to protect their hearts. Roughly 40 percent of adults with one or more elevated risk factors are at intermediate risk. They should undergo regular testing by a physician.

Risk Factors You Can Control

The choices you make and the habits you follow can have a significant impact on whether or not your heart remains healthy. You can choose to avoid the following potential risks for the sake of your heart's health.

Physical Inactivity

As discussed in Chapter 4, about one-quarter of U.S. adults are sedentary and another third are not active enough to reach a healthy level of fitness. The risk for heart disease is higher for people who are inactive compared with those who engage in regular physical activity.

♀ Women who report higher levels of physical fitness have less risk of cardiovascular disease, regardless of their body mass index (BMI), waist circumference, or waist-hip ratio (see Chapter 4). This suggests that fitness may be more important than overweight or obesity per se for women's cardiovascular risk. A minimum of 30 minutes a day of moderate activity at least five days a week, can lift a woman from the "low-fitness category" and lessen her risk of heart disease.

♂ In men, more rigorous exercise produces greater protection against heart disease. Those who run for an hour or more per week reduce their risk of heart disease by 42 percent, compared with an 18 percent reduction for those who walk briskly for a half-hour per day or more. With walking, pace, not duration, is linked with lower danger of heart disease.

Tobacco

Smoking may be the single most significant risk factor for cardiovascular disease—and quitting may do more to reduce the risk of mortality among heart disease patients who smoke than any other intervention or treatment. Each year smoking causes more than 250,000 deaths from cardiovascular disease—far more than it causes from cancer and lung disease. Smokers who have heart attacks are more likely to die from them than are nonsmokers. Smoking is the major risk factor for *peripheral vascular disease,* in which the vessels that carry blood to the leg and arm muscles become hardened and clogged.

Cigar smoking causes a moderate but significant increase in an individual's risk for coronary artery disease, as well as for cancers of the upper digestive tract and chronic obstructive pulmonary disease.

Both active and passive smoking accelerate the process by which arteries become clogged and increase the risk of heart attacks and strokes. Overall, nonsmokers exposed to environmental tobacco smoke are at a 25 percent higher relative risk of developing coronary heart disease than nonsmokers not exposed to environmental tobacco smoke.

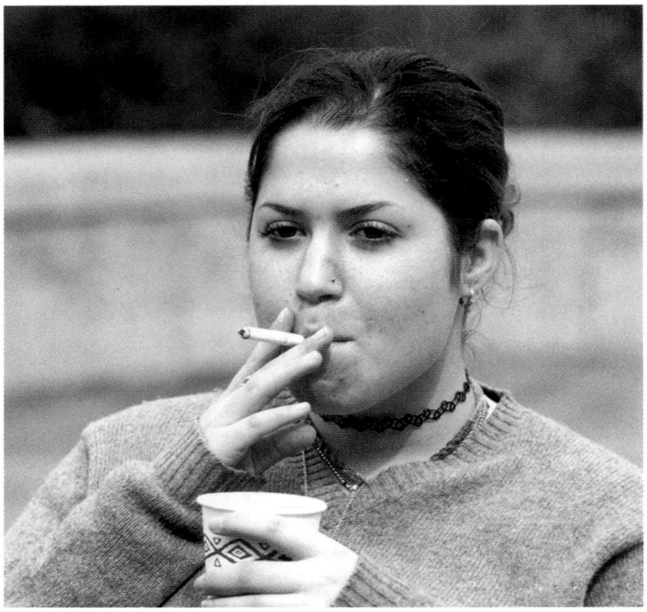

Quitting smoking is the best thing you can do for your heart, regardless of your age.

In various studies, quitting has reduced the risk of heart disease and subsequent death among patients with heart disease by as much as 50 percent. After 18 years without cigarettes, the risk of dying of heart disease among exsmokers is no greater than that of never-smokers.

Obesity

Obesity has emerged as an increasingly common and dangerous risk factor for cardiovascular disease, increasing the risk for hypertension, diabetes, coronary artery disease, and congestive heart failure in both men and women. BMI and measurement of waist circumference, discussed in Chapter 4, are good indicators of increased risk.

According to the National Heart, Lung and Blood Institute (NHLBI), losing weight at any age can help reduce the risk of heart problems. For women, obesity is as great a cause of death and disability from heart disease as smoking and heavy drinking. Even mild-to-moderately obese women are more likely to suffer chest pain or a heart attack than thinner women. Weight loss significantly reduces high blood pressure, another risk factor for heart disease. (See Chapter 6 for a discussion of obesity.)

High Blood Pressure (Hypertension)

Blood pressure is a result of the contractions of the heart muscle, which pumps blood through your body, and the resistance of the walls of the vessels through which the blood flows. Each time your heart beats, your blood pressure goes up and down within a certain range. It's highest when the heart contracts; this is called **systolic blood pressure.** It's lowest between contractions; this is called **diastolic blood pressure.** A blood pressure reading consists of the systolic measurement "over" the diastolic measurement, recorded in millimeters of mercury (mm Hg).

High blood pressure, or **hypertension,** occurs when the artery walls become constricted so that the force exerted as the blood flows through them is greater than it should be. Physicians see blood pressure as a continuum: The higher the reading, the greater the risk of stroke and heart disease.

As a result of the increased work in pumping blood, the heart muscle of a person with hypertension can become stronger and also stiffer. This stiffness increases resistance to filling up with blood between beats, which can cause shortness of breath with exertion. Hypertension can also act on the kidney arteries, which can lead to kidney failure in some cases. In addition, hypertension accelerates the development of plaque buildup within the arteries. Especially when combined with obesity, smoking, high cholesterol levels, or diabetes, hypertension increases the risks of cardiovascular problems several times. However, you can control high blood pressure through diet, exercise, and if necessary, medication.

Blood Fats (Lipids)

Cholesterol is a fatty substance found in certain foods and also manufactured by the body. The measurement of cholesterol in the blood is one of the most reliable indicators of the formation of plaque, the sludgelike substance that builds up on the inner walls of arteries. You can lower blood cholesterol levels by cutting back on high-fat foods and exercising more, thereby reducing the risk of a heart attack. According to the NHLBI, for every 1 percent drop in blood cholesterol, studies show a 2 percent decrease in the likelihood of a heart attack.

Lipoproteins are compounds in the blood that are made up of proteins and fat. The different types are classified by their size or density. The heaviest are *high-density lipoproteins,* or HDLs, which have the highest proportion of protein. These "good guys," as some cardiologists refer to them, pick up excess cholesterol in the blood and carry it back to the liver for removal from the body. An HDL level of 40 mg/dL or lower substantially increases the risk of heart disease. (Cholesterol levels are measured in milligrams of cholesterol per deciliter of blood—mg/dL.) The average HDL for men is about 45 mg/dL; for women, it is about 55 mg/dL.

Low-density lipoproteins, or (LDLs), and very low-density lipoproteins (VLDLs) carry more cholesterol than HDLs and deposit it on the walls of arteries—they're the "bad guys." The higher your LDL cholesterol, the greater your risk for heart disease. If you are at high risk of heart disease, any level of LDL higher than 100 mg/dL may increase your danger. (See "Your Lipoprotein Profile" later in this chapter.)

Triglycerides are fats that flow through the blood after meals and have been linked to increased risk of coronary artery disease, especially in women. Triglyceride levels tend to be highest in those whose diets are high in calories, sugar, alcohol, and refined starches. High levels of these fats may increase the risk of obesity, and cutting back on these foods can reduce high triglyceride levels.

Metabolic Syndrome

Metabolic syndrome, once called Syndrome X or insulin-resistant syndrome, is emerging as a major risk factor for heart disease. This condition is not a disease but a cluster of disorders of the body's metabolism—including high blood pressure, high insulin levels, abdominal obesity, and abnormal cholesterol levels—that make a person more likely to develop diabetes, heart disease, or stroke. Each of these conditions is by itself a risk factor for other diseases. In combination, they dramatically boost the chances of potentially life-threatening illnesses.

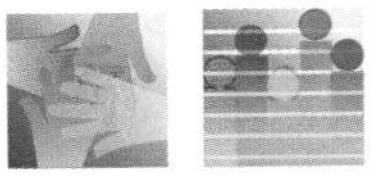

This dangerous syndrome has become so widespread that health officials describe it as an epidemic that affects one in three Americans, especially Hispanic men and women. College-age men and women who maintain their weight as they get older are much less likely to develop metabolic syndrome. However, about one in four undergraduates already has one risk factor for metabolic syndrome. Young adults with metabolic syndrome are more likely than others their age to have thicker neck arteries, an indicator of atherosclerosis, the buildup of fatty plaques in arteries.

systolic blood pressure Highest blood pressure when the heart contracts.

diastolic blood pressure Lowest blood pressure between contractions of the heart.

hypertension High blood pressure occurring when the blood exerts excessive pressure against the arterial walls.

cholesterol An organic substance found in animal fats; linked to cardiovascular disease, particularly atherosclerosis.

lipoprotein A compound in blood that is made up of proteins and fat; a high-density lipoprotein (HDL) picks up excess cholesterol in the blood; a low-density lipoprotein (LDL) carries more cholesterol and deposits it on the walls of arteries.

triglyceride A blood fat that flows through the blood after meals and is linked to increased risk of coronary artery disease.

metabolic syndrome A cluster of disorders of the body's metabolism that make diabetes, heart disease, or stroke more likely.

Strategies for Prevention: Overcoming Metabolic Syndrome

The following steps have proved effective in reversing metabolic syndrome and reducing the risks associated with it:

- Eat a low-fat, low-calorie diet.
- Engage in regular moderate exercise, such as walking, almost everyday.
- Reduce your body weight by 5 to 7 percent.
- If these strategies don't work for you, talk to your doctor about taking a glucose-lowering medication.

Three or more of the following characteristics indicate metabolic syndrome:[4]

- **Waist measurement of 40 inches or more** in men and 35 inches or more in women (for Asians and individuals with a genetic predisposition to diabetes, 37 to 39 inches in men and 31 to 35 inches in women).
- **Triglyceride level of 150 mg/dL** or more.
- **High-density lipoprotein (HDL)**—"good" cholesterol—level of less than 40 mg/dL in men or 50 mg/dL in women.
- **Blood pressure of 130 mmHg** systole over 85 mmHg diastole (130/85), or higher.
- **Fasting blood sugar of 110 mg/dL** or higher.

Men with three factors of metabolic syndrome are nearly twice as likely to have a heart attack or stroke and more than three times more likely to develop heart disease than those with none. Men with four or five characteristics of the syndrome have nearly four times the risk of heart attack or stroke and more than 24 times the risk of diabetes.

Diabetes Mellitus

Diabetes mellitus, a disorder of the endocrine system discussed later in this chapter, increases the likelihood of hypertension and atherosclerosis, thereby increasing the risk of heart attack and stroke. A physician can detect diabetes and prescribe a diet, exercise program, and if necessary, medication to keep it in check. Even before developing diabetes, individuals at high risk for this disease—those who are overweight, have a family history of the disease, have mildly elevated blood pressure and blood sugar levels, and above-ideal levels of harmful blood fats—may already be at increased risk of heart disease. Up to one-half of diabetics also have hypertension, another risk factor.

Diabetics who develop heart disease are more likely to die if they suffer a heart attack or develop heart failure. Two-thirds of people with diabetes die from cardiovascular disease.

Type 2 diabetes, a strong risk factor for coronary heart disease in all women, is especially common in black women. If combined with other risk factors, it puts them at very high risk of cardiovascular disease.

Psychosocial Factors

How you respond to everyday sources of stress can affect your heart as well as your overall health. While you may not be able to control the sources of stress, you can change how you habitually respond to it.

Researchers classify psychological risk factors for heart disease into three categories: chronic, episodic, and acute. Chronic factors, such as job strain or lack of social support, play an important role in the buildup of artery-clogging plaque. Episodic factors, such as depression, can last from several weeks to two years and may lead to the creation of "unstable" plaque, which is more likely to break off and block a blood vessel within the heart. Short-term or acute psychological risk factors, such as an angry outburst, can directly trigger a heart attack in people with underlying heart disease.

These factors may act alone or combine and exert different effects at different ages and stages of life. They may influence behaviors such as smoking, diet, alcohol consumption, and physical activity, as well as directly cause changes in physiology.

Depression and heart disease often occur together. People with heart disease are more likely to be depressed, and some seemingly healthy people with depression are at greater risk of heart problems. Depressed women younger than age 60 are more likely to suffer a heart attack than those who do not suffer from depression. After a heart attack, depression is common in both men and women, but physicians are less likely to recognize and treat depression in women.

Patients who suffer heart attacks and develop clinical depression have higher rates of complications and an increased risk of dying from another heart attack or other heart problems. People who are physically healthy with no risk factors for heart disease but who are prone to anger, hostility, and mild depression have higher levels of C-reactive protein, a substance linked to increased risk of heart disease.

In addition to stress and depression, other psychological traits can increase the risk of heart disease. Based on more than a decade of research, Dutch scientists have identified a "Type D" (for distressed) personality type. Type D people tend to be anxious, self-conscious, irritable, insecure, negative, and go to great lengths not to say or do anything that others might not like.[5] In the Dutch study, almost four times as many Type D individuals as others in cardiac rehabilitation programs died within an eight-year period. Other studies have linked Type D personality to other heart-related problems, such as chronic heart failure.[6]

In the past, other personality types have been linked to disease, for example, hard-charging, hostile Type As to heart disease and conflict-avoiding, emotion-suppressing Type Cs to cancer. However, these traits have not proved to be significant risk factors for these illnesses. Much more research is needed to evaluate the importance of Type D traits. Until we know more, regular aerobic exercise and relaxation techniques such as meditation may ease distress as well as keep the heart healthy.[7]

Risk Factors You Can't Control

Heredity

Anyone whose parents, siblings, or other close relatives suffered heart attacks before age 50 is at increased risk of developing heart disease. Certain risk factors, such as abnormally high blood levels of lipids, can be passed down from generation to generation. Although you can't rewrite your family history, individuals with an inherited vulnerability to cardiovascular disease can lower the danger by changing the risk factors within their control. Your heart's health depends to a great extent on your behavior, including the decisions you make about the foods you eat or the decision not to smoke. As an added preventive step, cardiologists may prescribe a small daily dose of aspirin to individuals with a history of coronary artery disease who are at risk of forming clots that could block blood supplies to the heart, brain, and other organs. (Note: Daily aspirin is not advised for individuals who are not at risk because of their age or health history.)

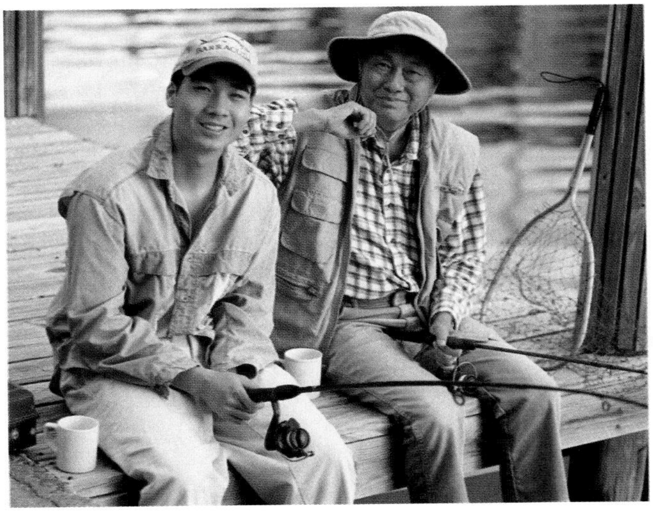

Know your family history. If a close relative had a heart attack before age 50, your risk of heart disease is higher.

Race and Ethnicity

Heart disease and its risk factors occur at higher rates among ethnic minority populations such as African Americans, Hispanic Americans, and Native Americans. Nearly four in every ten black adults have cardiovascular disease. Among Hispanic Americans, nearly three in ten have cardiovascular disease.

African Americans are twice as likely to develop high blood pressure as whites. African Americans also suffer strokes at an earlier age and of greater severity. Poverty may be an unrecognized risk factor for members of this minority group, who are less likely to receive medical treatments or undergo corrective surgery. Family history, lifestyle, diet, and stress may also play a role, starting early in life. However, researchers have found no single explanation for why African-American youngsters, like their parents, tend to have higher blood pressure than white children.

Black women are twice as likely as white women to suffer heart attacks and to die from heart disease. Common risk factors—high blood pressure, diabetes, and high cholesterol—account for this increased jeopardy. In addition, black women are less likely to receive common medications, such as cholesterol-lowering drugs, to lower their risk.

Age

Almost four out of five people who die of a heart attack are over age 65. Heart disease accounts for more than 40 percent of deaths among people between 65 and 74 and almost 60 percent at age 85 and above. However, the risk factors that are likely to cause heart disease later in life, including high blood pressure and high levels of "bad" cholesterol, may begin to develop in childhood. Nevertheless,

diabetes mellitus A disease in which the inadequate production of insulin leads to failure of the body tissues to break down carbohydrates at a normal rate.

although cardiovascular function declines with age, heart disease is not an inevitable consequence of aging. Many 80- and 90-year-olds have strong, healthy hearts.

Gender

Many people still think of heart disease as a "guy problem." Men have a higher incidence of cardiovascular problems than women before age 45. The onset of heart disease in women lags behind that in men by 10 to 15 years. However, for the U.S. population as a whole, as many women as men eventually die of heart disease. Although the same risk factors jeopardize the hearts of men and women, each gender also faces some unique heart-related issues, including male pattern baldness and menopause. A daily low-dose aspirin lowers the risk of heart attack in men, but not women.[8]

Male pattern baldness (the loss of hair at the vertex, or top, of the head) is associated with increased risk of heart attack in men under age 55. The speed at which men lose their hair also may be an indicator of risk. Men with male pattern baldness who lose their hair quickly may metabolize male sex hormones differently than others, thereby increasing the likelihood of heart disease. Although it's premature to say that baldness is definitely bad news for the heart, health experts advise bald men to follow basic guidelines, such as not smoking and controlling their cholesterol levels, to lower any possible risk.

Heart disease is the fourth-leading cause of death among women aged 30 to 34, third among women aged 35 to 39, second among women aged 40 to 64, and first among women over age 65. A woman's risk increases sharply after menopause.

Researchers long believed that postmenopausal hormone therapy protected women from heart disease. However, this has been proved wrong. Based on large-scale studies that showed little, if any, benefit and some potential harm to the hearts of postmenopausal women, neither combined hormone therapy nor estrogen alone is recommended for the prevention of heart disease and stroke.[9]

High Blood Pressure (Hypertension)

Blood pressure refers to the force of blood against the walls of arteries. When blood pressure remains elevated over time—a condition called hypertension—it forces the heart to pump harder than is healthy. Because the heart must force blood into arteries that are offering increased resistance to blood flow, the left side of the heart becomes enlarged. If untreated, high blood pressure can cause a variety of cardiovascular complications, including heart attack and stroke—two of the three leading causes of death among U.S. adults—as well as kidney failure and blindness (Figure 10-3).

The World Health Organization estimates that hypertension causes one in every eight deaths globally, making it the third leading killer in the world. In the United States, high blood pressure is responsible for about a third of cardiovascular problems like heart attack or stroke and a quarter of all premature deaths.

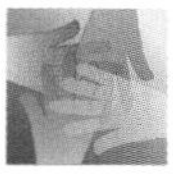

About a third of adults age 18 and older in the United States—some 65 million men and women—have high blood pressure. In the last decade, hypertension grew by about 8 percent, with a 30 percent jump in the total number of adults with high blood pressure. Blood pressure has also increased among children and adolescents over the last decade, with the highest rates among black and Mexican-American children. The primary culprit is the increase in obesity in the young. No one knows why African Americans are more vulnerable, although some speculate that overweight or dietary factors may contribute.

Different races also suffer different consequences of high blood pressure. An African American with the same elevated blood pressure reading as a Caucasian faces a greater risk of stroke, heart disease, and kidney problems.

Family history also plays a role. "If you study healthy college students with normal blood pressures, those who have one parent with hypertension will have blood pressure that's a little higher than average," notes Rose Marie Robertson, M.D., of the American Heart Association. "If two parents have high blood pressure, their levels will be a little higher, and they're destined to go higher still. If your parents have high blood pressure, have yours checked regularly."[10]

Men and women are equally likely to develop hypertension, but in women blood pressure tends to rise around the time of menopause. Half of all women over age 45 have hypertension. For individuals who smoke, are overweight, don't exercise, or have high cholesterol levels, hypertension multiplies the risk of heart disease and stroke. Overweight people with high blood pressure have twice the risk of dying of a heart attack or stroke as those with normal blood pressure. At ultrahigh risk are people with diabetes or kidney disease.

In a young person even mild hypertension can cause organs such as the heart, brain, and kidneys to start to deteriorate. By age 50 or 60, the damage may be irreversible.

Preventing Hypertension

Prevention pays off when it comes to high blood pressure. The most effective preventive measures involve lifestyle changes. Losing weight is the best approach for

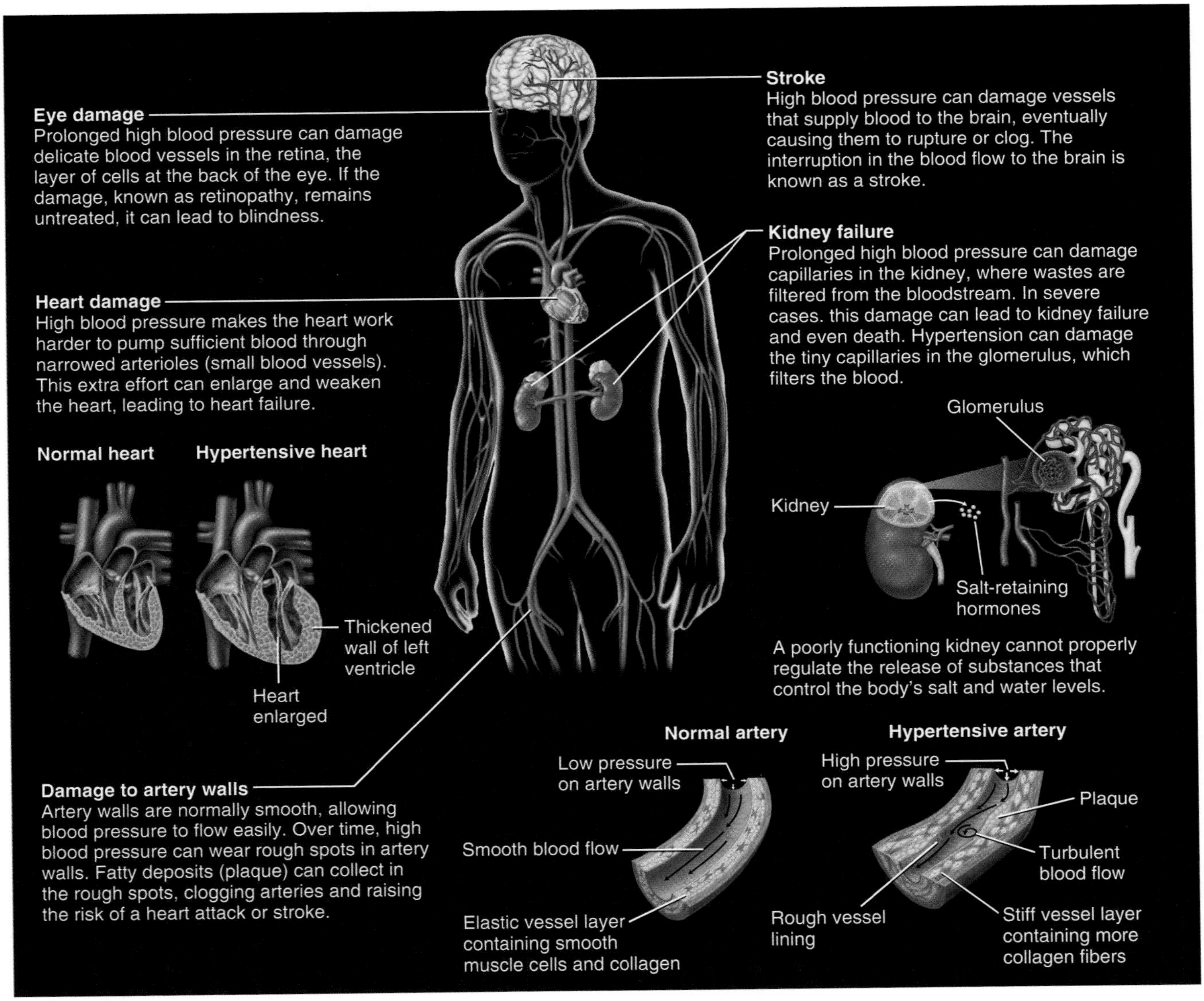

Stroke
High blood pressure can damage vessels that supply blood to the brain, eventually causing them to rupture or clog. The interruption in the blood flow to the brain is known as a stroke.
Eye damage
Prolonged high blood pressure can damage delicate blood vessels in the retina, the layer of cells at the back of the eye. If the damage, known as retinopathy, remains untreated, it can lead to blindness.
Kidney failure
Prolonged high blood pressure can damage capillaries in the kidney, where wastes are filtered from the bloodstream. In severe cases. this damage can lead to kidney failure and even death. Hypertension can damage the tiny capillaries in the glomerulus, which filters the blood.
Heart damage
High blood pressure makes the heart work harder to pump sufficient blood through narrowed arterioles (small blood vessels). This extra effort can enlarge and weaken the heart, leading to heart failure.
Glomerulus
Normal heart
Hypertensive heart
Kidney
Salt-retaining hormones
Thickened wall of left ventricle
Heart enlarged
A poorly functioning kidney cannot properly regulate the release of substances that control the body's salt and water levels.
Normal artery
Hypertensive artery
Low pressure on artery walls
High pressure on artery walls
Damage to artery walls
Artery walls are normally smooth, allowing blood pressure to flow easily. Over time, high blood pressure can wear rough spots in artery walls. Fatty deposits (plaque) can collect in the rough spots, clogging arteries and raising the risk of a heart attack or stroke.
Plaque
Smooth blood flow
Turbulent blood flow
Elastic vessel layer containing smooth muscle cells and collagen
Rough vessel lining
Stiff vessel layer containing more collagen fibers

FIGURE 10-3 Consequences of High Blood Pressure
If left untreated, elevated blood pressure can damage blood vessels in several areas of the body and lead to serious health problems.

individuals with high normal values. Exercise may be effective in lowering mildly elevated blood pressure. High intake of folate, a B vitamin, can significantly reduce the risk of hypertension. In a study of women under age 35, those who consumed the most folate had one-third the risk of developing high blood pressure as those consuming very little. Among the approaches that have not proved effective are dietary supplements, such as calcium, magnesium, potassium, and fish oil.

The National Heart, Lung and Blood Institute has developed what is known as the DASH diet. Following DASH, which stands for Dietary Approaches to Stop Hypertension, has proved as effective as drug therapy in lowering blood pressure. An additional benefit: The DASH diet also lowers harmful blood fats, including cholesterol and low-density lipoprotein, and the amino acid homocysteine (one of the new suspects in heart disease risk).

Restriction of sodium intake also helps. Most Americans consume more salt than they need. The *Dietary Guidelines for Americans* recommend limiting sodium to 2,300 milligrams a day—about a teaspoonful—including salt used at the table and in cooking. Diets of less than 1,500 milligrams of sodium produce greater benefits and help blood pressure medicines work better.

The lower the amount of sodium in the diet, the lower the blood pressure for both those with and those without hypertension and for both genders and all racial and ethnic groups. However, reducing dietary sodium has an even greater

male pattern baldness The loss of hair at the vertex, or top, of the head.

effect on blood pressure in blacks than whites, in women than men, and in individuals with hypertension.

? FAQ What Is a Healthy Blood Pressure?

Current guidelines (Table 10-1) categorize a reading of 120/80 as **prehypertension,** a condition that is likely to worsen in time. A healthy reading is 115/75 mmHg. Once blood pressure rises above this threshold, the risk of cardiovascular disease may increase.

In healthy adults, blood pressure screening should begin at age 21, with repeat evaluations at least every two years, or more often depending on your current health, medical history, and risk factors for cardiovascular disease. According to the National College Health Assessment survey, about nine in ten students have done so. (See Student Snapshot "Healthy Habits on Campus.")

To get an accurate blood pressure reading, you should visit the doctor's office at least twice and have your blood pressure taken two or more times while you're seated. The average of those measurements determines how your blood pressure is classified.

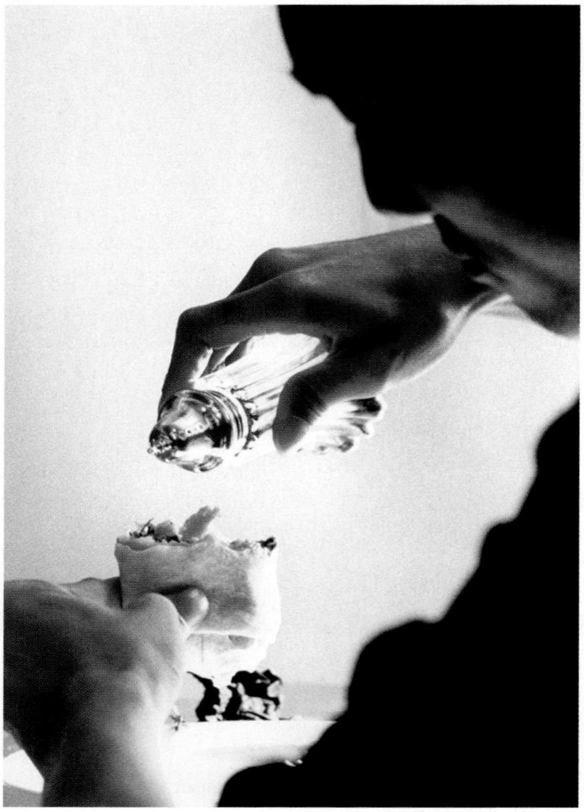

© J. Miles/Photex/zefa/CORBIS

Reducing salt intake can help lower blood pressure.

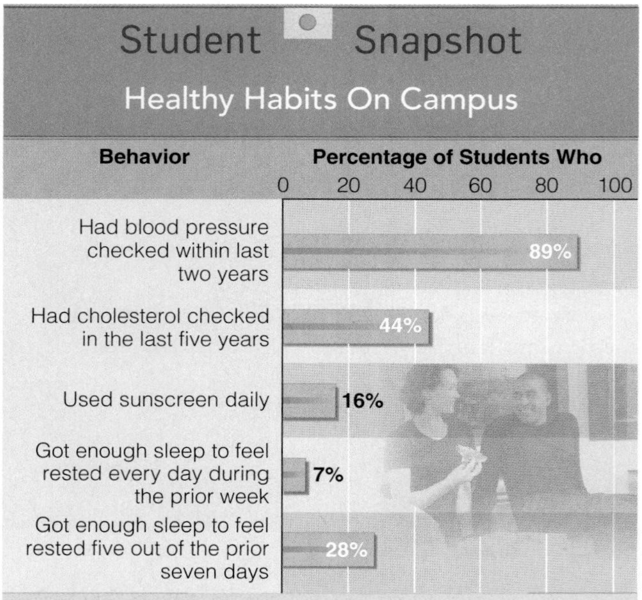

© Jupiter Images

Sources: American College Health Association. "American College Health Association-National College Health Assessment (ACHA-NCHA) Spring 2004 Reference Group Data Report (abridged)." *Journal of American College Health,* Vol. 54, No. 4, January–February 2006, p. 201.

TABLE 10-1 What Your Blood Pressure Means

Top Number (systolic)		Bottom Number (diastolic)	Your Group	What to Do
Below 120	and	Below 80	Normal blood pressure	Maintain a healthy lifestyle
120–139	or	80–89	Prehypertension	Adopt a healthy lifestyle
140–159	or	90–99	Stage 1 hypertension	Adopt a healthy lifestyle; take medication
160 or more	or	100 or more	Stage 2 hypertension	Adopt a healthy lifestyle; take more than one medication

Numbers are expressed in millimeters of mercury (mm Hg).

The new guidelines classify hypertension into two categories:

- **Stage 1.** This consists of a systolic pressure ranging from 140 to 159 or a diastolic pressure ranging from 90 to 99.
- **Stage 2.** The most severe form of hypertension occurs with a systolic pressure of 160 or higher or a diastolic reading of 100 or higher.

Only one of the numbers—the top or bottom—needs to be high to meet these criteria. In people over age 50, systolic pressure is more important than diastolic. If it rises to 140 mmHg or higher, doctors advise treatment regardless of the diastolic pressure.

Controlling High Blood Pressure

Lifestyle changes are a first-line weapon in the fight against high blood pressure. Rather than making a single change, a combination of behavioral changes, including losing weight, eating heart-healthy foods, reducing sodium, and exercising more, yields the best results. For uncomplicated hypertension, the recommended treatment is a thiazide diuretic, either alone or combined with other antihypertensive medications.

Making healthy lifestyle modifications can help reduce Stage 1 hypertension, but most people also require a medication. Those with Stage 2 hypertension typically need at least two types of high blood pressure medications (antihypertensives) to reduce blood pressure to a safer level. The goal for most people with hypertension is to reduce blood pressure to below 140/90 mmHg.

Only about one-third of people with hypertension have it effectively controlled—below 140/90 mmHg. Reducing systolic blood pressure 12 mmHg for 10 years can prevent one death in every 11 people treated for hypertension. In those with existing cardiovascular disease or organ damage, such as kidney disease, that reduction has an even bigger benefit, preventing one death in every nine people treated.

Your Lipoprotein Profile

Medical science has changed the way it views and targets the blood fats that endanger the healthy heart. In the past, the focus was primarily on total cholesterol in the blood. The higher this number was, the greater the risk of heart disease. The NHLBI's National Cholesterol Education Program has recommended more comprehensive testing, called a *lipoprotein profile,* for all individuals age 20 or older (see Savvy Consumer: "What You Need to Know About Your Lipoprotein Profile").

This blood test, which should be performed after a 9- to 12-hour fast and repeated at least once every five years, provides readings of:

- **Total cholesterol.**
- **LDL (bad) cholesterol,** the main culprit in the buildup of plaque within the arteries.
- **HDL (good or *Healthy*)** cholesterol, which helps prevent cholesterol buildup.
- **Triglycerides,** the blood fats released into the bloodstream after a meal.

? FAQ What Is a Healthy Cholesterol Reading?

Total cholesterol is the sum of all the cholesterol in your blood. Less than 200mg/dL total cholesterol is ideal, and 200–239 mg/dL is borderline-high. Total cholesterol above 240 mg/dL is high and doubles your risk of heart disease. However, total cholesterol is not the only crucial number you should know. Because LDL increases your risk for heart disease, you always should find out your LDL level. Even if your total cholesterol is higher than 200, you may not be at high risk for a heart attack. Some people—such as women before menopause and young, active men who have no other risk factors—may have high HDL cholesterol and desirable LDL levels. Ask your doctor to interpret your results so you both know your numbers and understand what they mean.

The updated guidelines of the National Cholesterol Education Program (NCEP) set lower target goals for LDL cholesterol, particularly for those at greatest risk of a heart attack or death from cardiovascular disease (Table 10-2).

prehypertension A condition of slightly elevated blood pressure, which is likely to worsen in time.

TABLE 10-2 New Targets for Lowering LDL

Risk Category	LDL Goal
Low Risk (1 or 0 risk factors for heart disease)	Less than 160 mg/dL
Moderate Risk (2 or more risk factors that create a 10 percent or lower risk of a heart attack in the next 10 years)	Less than 130 mg/dL
Moderately High Risk (2 or more risk factors that create a 10 to 20 percent chance of a heart attack in next 10 years)	Less than 130 mg/dL
High Risk (heart disease or diabetes, diseased blood vessels, 2 or more risk factors)	Less than 100 mg/dL
Very High Risk (heart disease and multiple, severe, or poorly controlled risk factors, especially smoking, or a history of heart attack or angina)	Less than 70 mg/dL

Source: Based on the National Cholesterol Education Program Adult Treatment Panel III Guidelines, www.circulationaha.org.

SAVVY CONSUMER

What You Need to Know About Your Lipoprotein Profile

- Go to your primary health-care provider to get a lipoprotein profile. Although cholesterol tests at shopping malls or health fairs can help identify people at risk, the analyzers are often not certified technicians, and the readings may be inaccurate. In addition, without a health expert to counsel them, some people may be unnecessarily frightened by a high reading—or falsely reassured by a low one.
- Ask about accuracy. Even at first-rate laboratories, cholesterol readings are often inaccurate. Find out if the lab is using the National Institutes of Health standards, and ask about the lab's margin for error (which should be less than 5 percent).
- Fast beforehand. Cholesterol tests are most accurate after a 9- to 14-hour fast. Schedule the test before breakfast if you can. Women may not want to get tested at the end of their menstrual cycles, when minor elevations in cholesterol levels occur because of lower estrogen levels. Cholesterol levels can also rise 5 to 10 percent during periods of stress. Reschedule the test if you come down with an intestinal flu because the viral infection could interfere with the absorption of food and thus with cholesterol levels. Let your doctor know if you're taking any drugs. Common medications, including birth control pills and hypertension drugs, can affect cholesterol levels.
- Sit down before allowing blood to be drawn or your finger to be pricked; fluids pool differently in the body when you're standing than when you're sitting. Don't let a technician squeeze blood from your finger, which forces fluid from cells, diluting the blood sample and possibly leading to a falsely low reading.
- Get real numbers. Don't settle for "normal" or "high," because laboratories can inaccurately label results. Find out exactly what your reading is: your LDL, HDL, and triglyceride levels.

HDL, good cholesterol, also is important, particularly in women. Federal guidelines define an HDL reading of less than 40 mg/dL as a major risk factor for developing heart disease. HDL levels of 60 mg/dL or more are protective and lower the risk of heart disease.

Triglycerides, the free-floating molecules that transport fats in the bloodstream, ideally should be below 150 mg/dL. Individuals with readings of 150 to 199 mg/dL, considered borderline, as well as those with higher readings, may benefit from weight control, physical activity, and if necessary, medication.

Lowering Cholesterol

According to federal guidelines, about one in five Americans may require treatment to lower their cholesterol level. However, nearly half of people who need cholesterol treatment, which can reduce the risk of heart disease by 30 percent over five years, don't get it.[11] The National Cholesterol Education Program (NCEP) estimates that some 36 million Americans should be watching their diet and exercising more. Another 65 million should be taking cholesterol-lowering drugs. Depending on your lipoprotein profile and an assessment of other risk factors, your physician may recommend that you take steps to lower your LDL cholesterol.

Lifestyle Changes

Some individuals with elevated cholesterol can improve their lipoprotein profile with lifestyle changes:

- **Dietary changes.** In the past, dietary changes reduced cholesterol by only 4 to 13 percent, relatively modest improvements compared to the effects of medications, which can cut cholesterol by as much as 35 percent. However, a diet consisting of cholesterol-lowering foods, including nuts, soy, oats, and plant sterols (in margarine and green leafy vegetables), reduced LDL cholesterol by about 30 percent. An added benefit: a reduction in C-reactive protein, discussed below. Researchers are recommending this diet as an effective first treatment for individuals with high cholesterol levels, particularly when coupled with exercise and weight loss.

- **Weight management.** For individuals who are overweight, losing weight can help lower LDL. This is especially true for those with high triglyceride levels and/or low HDL levels and those who have a large waist measurement (more than 40 inches for a man and more than 35 inches for a woman).
- **Physical activity.** The recommended amount is 30 minutes on most, if not all, days. Regular activity can help lower LDL, lower blood pressure, reduce triglycerides, and particularly important, raise HDL. Again, these benefits are especially important for those with high triglyceride levels or large waist measurements.

Lifestyle changes can lower harmful LDL levels by 5 to 10 percent. However, a greater reduction of 30 to 40 percent requires either the kind of intensive lifestyle changes promoted by Dr. Dean Ornish, including an extremely low-fat diet, or the addition of cholesterol-lowering medication.

Medications

The last decade has seen a revolution in treatment for high cholesterol, thanks to a new class of drugs called statins—better known by brand names such as Lipitor, Mevacor, Pravachol, and Zocor. These medications can cut the risk of dying of a heart attack by as much as 40 percent. Initially tested in men, statins have proved equally beneficial for women, including those whose cholesterol levels rise after menopause.

Statins work in the liver to block production of cholesterol. When the liver can't make cholesterol, it draws LDL cholesterol from the blood to use as raw material. This means that less LDL is available to trigger or promote the artery-clogging process known as atherosclerosis. Statins also appear to stabilize cholesterol-filled deposits in artery walls and to cool down inflammation. Long-term therapy with statins reduces the risk for death, heart attack, and stroke among people with heart disease, even when LDL levels are not elevated. The lower the LDL, the lower the risk.

C-Reactive Protein

C-reactive protein (CRP), produced in the liver, rises whenever the body responds to inflammation. As scientists recognized the role of inflammation in heart disease, they developed the high-sensitivity CRP test (hsCRP), which detects coronary artery inflammation by measuring small changes in CRP. Several investi gations have shown that CRP can predict heart disease before any other risk factors become evident, particularly in women. Individuals with the highest CRP levels are two to seven times more likely to develop heart disease than those with the lowest levels. High concentrations of CRP also may predict greater risk of sudden death. The test seems most useful in combination with a lipoprotein profile and assessments of other blood components.

Various strategies can reduce CRP. These include lifestyle changes (healthy diet, exercise, weight control, and not smoking) and medications (aspirin and, as needed, drugs to lower cholesterol and blood pressure).

Heart Attack (Myocardial Infarction)

Each year, about 1.5 million Americans suffer a heart attack. About 500,000 die. Half of the deaths occur within an hour of the start of symptoms and before the person reaches the hospital. The medical name for a heart attack, or coronary, is **myocardial infarction (MI).** The *myocardium* is the cardiac muscle layer of the wall of the heart. It receives its blood supply, and thus its oxygen and other nutrients, from the coronary arteries. If an artery is blocked by a clot or plaque, or by a spasm, the myocardial cells do not get sufficient oxygen, and the portion of the myocardium deprived of its blood supply begins to die. Although such an attack may seem sudden, usually it has been building up for years, particularly if the person has ignored risk factors and early warning signs.

? FAQ How Do I Know It's a Heart Attack?

If they experience the following symptoms, individuals should seek immediate medical care and take an aspirin (325 milligrams) to keep the blood clot in a coronary artery from getting any bigger:

- A tight ache, heavy, squeezing pain, or discomfort in the center of the chest, which may last for 30 minutes or more and is not relieved by rest.
- Chest pain that radiates to the shoulder, arm, neck, back, or jaw.
- Anxiety.
- Sweating or cold, clammy skin.
- Nausea and vomiting.
- Shortness of breath.
- Dizziness, fainting, or loss of consciousness.

myocardial infarction (MI) A condition characterized by the dying of tissue areas in the myocardium, caused by interruption of the blood supply to those areas; the medical name for a heart attack.

Women often experience heart attacks differently than men. In the month before an attack, many report unusual fatigue and disturbed sleep. Far fewer women than men experience chest pain. More common symptoms are shortness of breath, weakness and fatigue, a clammy sweat, dizziness, and nausea. As many as 3 million American women may be at high risk for a heart attack because of a frequently undiagnosed condition in which plaque accumulates in the very small arteries of the heart, reducing oxygen flow and causing pain. Standard methods of assessing the heart's health often fail to detect this hidden danger.[12]

If you're with someone who's exhibiting the classic signs of heart attack, and if they last for two minutes or more, act at once. Expect the person to deny the possibility of anything as serious as a heart attack, but insist on taking prompt action.

Time is of the essence when a heart attack occurs. If you develop symptoms or if you're with someone who does, call the emergency system (911 in most places) immediately. The sooner emergency personnel get to a heart attack and administer cardiac life support, the greater the odds of survival. Yet according to the American Heart Association, most patients wait three hours after the initial symptoms begin before seeking help. By that time, half of the affected heart muscle may already be lost.

Saving Hearts

State-of-the-art treatments for heart attacks include clot-dissolving drugs, early administration of medications to thin the blood, intravenous nitroglycerin, and in some cases, a beta-blocker (which blocks many of the effects of adrenaline in the body, particularly its stimulating impact on the heart).

Emergency balloon **angioplasty** has shown greater effectiveness than clot-dissolving medication in restoring blood flow in arteries immediately after an attack. With this approach, arteries are less likely to close down again and patients have shorter hospital stays and fewer hospital readmissions. Angioplasty patients also are less likely to die of the heart attack or to experience repeat attacks.

Women who have heart attacks are less likely than men to survive over both the short and the long term. A woman's risk of dying within a month of a heart attack is up to 75 percent higher than a man's, in part because women typically take an hour longer to get to the hospital than men. Women also have more complications than men during hospitalization and a higher death rate. Men are more likely to receive therapy with aspirin, beta-blockers, or angiotensin-converting enzyme inhibitors and to undergo angioplasty or bypass surgery.

Stroke

When the blood supply to a portion of the brain is blocked, a cerebrovascular accident, or **stroke,** occurs. Someone in the United States suffers a stroke every 53 seconds; more than a quarter are under age 65. About two-thirds of the 700,000 strokes that occur every year in the United States strike women. However, before age 85, men experience more strokes. Nonetheless, women of every age fare worse than men in the prevention, diagnosis, treatment, and outcome of stroke.[13] An estimated 20 percent of stroke victims die within three months; 50 to 60 percent are disabled. About half of those who have a stroke are partially paralyzed on one side of their body; between a quarter and a half are partially or completely dependent on others for daily living; a third become depressed; a fifth cannot walk. Quick treatment with a clot-busting drug at a hospital can reduce the chance of disability after a stroke, but few people recognize the signs of a stroke (see page 279) and seek medical care within three hours of the first symptoms.[14]

Strokes rank third, after heart disease and cancer, as a cause of death in this country. Worldwide, stroke is second only to heart disease as a cause of death. After decades of steady decline, the number of strokes per year has begun to rise. The main reasons seem to be that more people in the United States are living longer, advanced medical care is allowing more people to survive heart disease, and doctors are better able to diagnose and detect strokes. Yet 80 percent of strokes are preventable, and key risk factors can be modified through either lifestyle changes or drugs. The most important steps are treating hypertension, not smoking, managing diabetes, lowering cholesterol, and taking aspirin, which reduces stroke risk in women, but not men.[15]

? FAQ What Causes a Stroke?

There are two types of stroke: *ischemic stroke,* which is the result of a blockage that disrupts blood flow to the brain, and *hemorrhagic stroke,* which occurs when blood vessels rupture. One of the most common causes of ischemic stroke is the blockage of a brain artery by a thrombus, or blood clot—a *cerebral thrombosis.* Clots generally form around deposits sticking out from the arterial wall. Sometimes a wandering blood clot (embolus), carried in the bloodstream, becomes wedged in one of the cerebral arteries. This is called a *cerebral embolism,* and it can completely plug up a cerebral artery.

In hemorrhagic stroke, a diseased artery in the brain floods the surrounding tissue with blood. The cells

Strategies for Prevention — How to Recognize a Stroke

Prompt treatment can stop a stroke in its tracks—but only with prompt treatment. Researchers have found that the following steps can identify facial weakness, arm weakness, and speech problems, all signs of a stroke:

- Ask the individual to smile.
- Ask him or her to raise both arms.
- Ask the person to speak a simple sentence, such as "It is sunny out today."

If he or she has trouble with any of these tasks, call 9-1-1 immediately and describe the symptoms to the dispatcher.

nourished by the artery are deprived of blood and can't function, and the blood from the artery forms a clot that may interfere with brain function. This is most likely to occur if the patient suffers from a combination of hypertension and atherosclerosis. Hemorrhage (bleeding) may also be caused by a head injury or by the bursting of an aneurysm, a blood-filled pouch that balloons out from a weak spot in the wall of an artery.

Brain tissue, like heart muscle, begins to die if deprived of oxygen, which may then cause difficulty speaking and walking, and loss of memory. These effects may be slight or severe, temporary or permanent, depending on how widespread the damage and whether other areas of the brain can take over the function of the damaged area. About 30 percent of stroke survivors develop dementia, a disorder that robs a person of memory and other intellectual abilities.

Risk Factors for Strokes

Other risk factors, like those for heart disease, include some that can't be changed (such as gender and race) and some that can be controlled:

- **Gender.** Men have a greater risk of stroke than women. However, women are at increased risk at times of marked hormonal changes, particularly pregnancy and childbirth. Past studies have shown an association between oral contraceptive use and stroke, particularly in women over age 35 who smoke. The newer low-dose oral contraceptives have not shown an increased stroke risk among women ages 18 to 44.
- 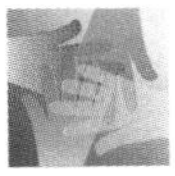 **Race.** The incidence of strokes is two to three times greater in blacks than whites in the same communities. Hispanics also are more likely to develop hemorrhagic strokes than whites.
- **Age.** A person's risk of stroke more than doubles every decade after age 55.
- **Hypertension.** Detection and treatment of high blood pressure are the best means of stroke prevention.
- **High red blood cell count.** A moderate to marked increase in the number of a person's red blood cells increases the risk of stroke.
- **Heart disease.** Heart problems can interfere with the flow of blood to the brain; clots that form in the heart can travel to the brain, where they may clog an artery.
- **Blood fats.** Although the standard advice from cardiologists is to lower harmful LDL levels, what may be more important to lower stroke risk is an increase in the levels of protective HDL.
- **Diabetes mellitus.** Diabetics have a higher incidence of stroke than nondiabetics.
- **Estrogen therapy.** In the Women's Health Initiative—a series of clinical trials of hormone therapy for postmenopausal women—estrogen-only therapy significantly increased the risk of stroke.
- **A diet high in fat and sodium.** Individuals consuming the largest amounts of fatty foods and sodium are at much greater risk then those eating low-fat, low-salt diets.

Understanding Cancer

The uncontrolled growth and spread of abnormal cells causes cancer. Normal cells follow the code of instructions embedded in DNA (the body's genetic material); cancer cells do not. Think of the DNA within the nucleus of a cell as a computer program that controls the cell's functioning, including its ability to grow and reproduce itself. If this program or its operation is altered, the cell goes out of control. The nucleus no longer regulates growth. The abnormal cell divides to create other abnormal cells,

angioplasty Surgical repair of an obstructed artery by passing a balloon catheter through the blood vessel to the area of disease and then inflating the catheter to compress the plaque against the vessel wall.

stroke A cerebrovascular event in which the blood supply to a portion of the brain is blocked.

Strategies for Prevention — **Seven Warning Signs of Cancer**

If you note any of the following seven warning signs, immediately schedule an appointment with your doctor:

- Change in bowel or bladder habits.
- A sore that doesn't heal.
- Unusual bleeding or discharge.
- Thickening or lump in the breast, testis, or elsewhere.
- Indigestion or difficulty swallowing.
- Obvious change in a wart or mole.
- Nagging cough or hoarseness.

which again divide, eventually forming *neoplasms* (new formations), or tumors.

How Cancer Spreads

Tumors can be either *benign* (slightly abnormal, not considered life-threatening) or *malignant* (cancerous). The only way to determine whether a tumor is benign is by microscopic examination of its cells. Cancer cells have larger nuclei than the cells in benign tumors; they vary more in shape and size; and they divide more often.

At one time cancer was thought to be a single disease that attacked different parts of the body. Now scientists believe that cancer comes in countless forms, each with a genetically determined molecular "fingerprint" that indicates how deadly it is. With this understanding, doctors can identify how aggressively a tumor should be treated.

Without treatment, cancer cells continue to grow, crowding out and replacing healthy cells. This process is called **infiltration,** or invasion. Cancer cells may also **metastasize,** or spread to other parts of the body via the bloodstream or lymphatic system (Figure 10-4). For many cancers, as many as 60 percent of patients may have metastases (which may be too small to be felt or seen without a microscope) at the time of diagnosis.

? FAQ Who Is at Risk for Developing Cancer?

For the first time in more than seven decades, annual cancer deaths in the United States are falling. According to the American Cancer Society, 1.4 million individuals are diagnosed with cancer each year; about 565,000 die of it. The five-year survival rate for all cancer is 65 percent, up from 50 percent three decades ago.[16]

Since the occurrence of cancer increases over time, most cases affect adults who are middle-aged or older (Table 10-3). In the United States, men have a one in two lifetime risk of developing cancer; for women, the risk is one in three (Figure 10-5).

The term **relative risk** compares the risk of developing cancer in people with a certain exposure or trait to the risk in those who do not have this exposure or trait. Smokers, for instance, have a ten-times-greater relative risk of developing lung cancer than nonsmokers.

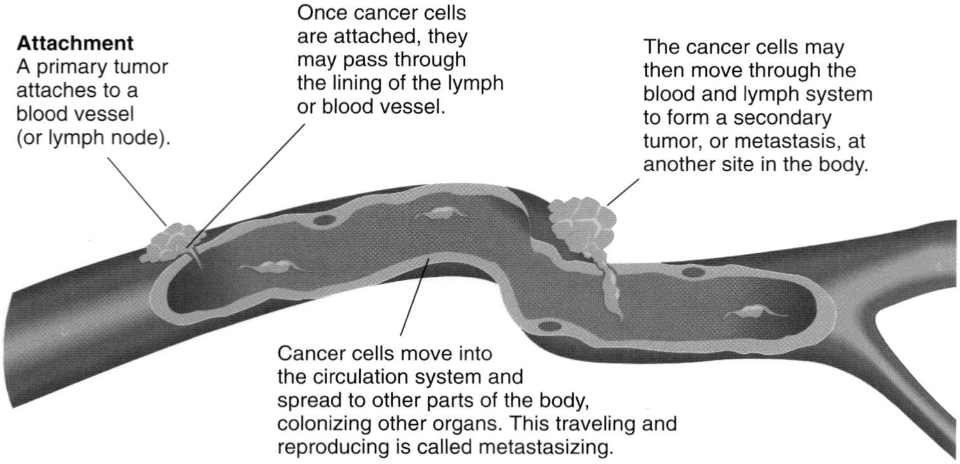

Attachment
A primary tumor attaches to a blood vessel (or lymph node).
Once cancer cells are attached, they may pass through the lining of the lymph or blood vessel.
The cancer cells may then move through the blood and lymph system to form a secondary tumor, or metastasis, at another site in the body.
Cancer cells move into the circulation system and spread to other parts of the body, colonizing other organs. This traveling and reproducing is called metastasizing.

FIGURE 10-4 Metastasis, or Spread of Cancer
Cancer cells can travel through the blood vessels to spread to other organs or through the lymphatic system to form secondary tumors.

Most relative risks are smaller. For example, women who have a first-degree (mother, sister, or daughter) family history of breast cancer have about a twofold increased risk of developing breast cancer compared with women who do not have a family history of the disease. This means that they are about twice as likely to develop breast cancer.

TABLE 10-3 Age and the Risk of Cancer (All Sites)

	Men	Women
Birth to age 39	1 in 64	1 in 51
Ages 40 to 59	1 in 12	1 in 11
Ages 60 to 79	1 in 3	1 in 4
Birth to death	1 in 2	1 in 3

Source: Cancer Facts & Figures 2006. Atlanta, GA: American Cancer Society, 2006.

Heredity

An estimated 13 to 14 million Americans may be at risk of a hereditary cancer. In hereditary cancers, such as retinoblastoma (an eye cancer that strikes young children) or certain colon cancers, a specific cancer-causing gene is passed down from generation to generation. The odds of any child with one affected parent inheriting this gene and developing the cancer are fifty/fifty.

Other people are born with genes that make them susceptible to having certain cells grow and divide uncontrollably, which may contribute to cancer development. The most well-known are mutations of the BRCA gene, linked with increased risk of breast, colon, and ovarian cancer.

infiltration A gradual penetration or invasion.

metastasize To spread to other parts of the body via the bloodstream or lymphatic system.

relative risk The risk of developing cancer in persons with a certain exposure or trait compared to the risk in persons who do not have the same exposure or trait.

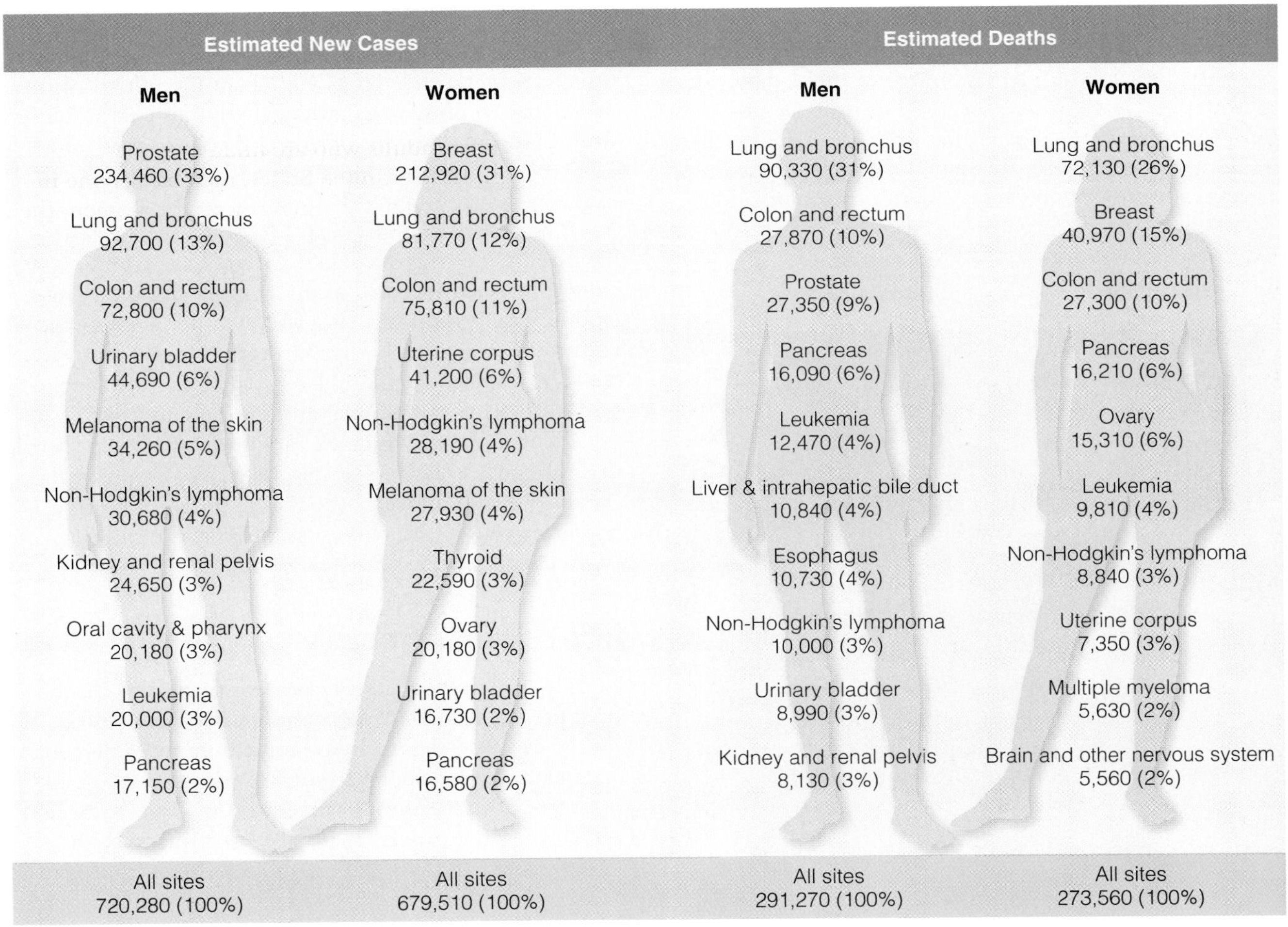
Estimated New Cases
Estimated Deaths
Men
Women
Men
Women
Prostate 234,460 (33%)
Lung and bronchus 92,700 (13%)
Colon and rectum 72,800 (10%)
Urinary bladder 44,690 (6%)
Melanoma of the skin 34,260 (5%)
Non-Hodgkin's lymphoma 30,680 (4%)
Kidney and renal pelvis 24,650 (3%)
Oral cavity & pharynx 20,180 (3%)
Leukemia 20,000 (3%)
Pancreas 17,150 (2%)
All sites 720,280 (100%)
Breast 212,920 (31%)
Lung and bronchus 81,770 (12%)
Colon and rectum 75,810 (11%)
Uterine corpus 41,200 (6%)
Non-Hodgkin's lymphoma 28,190 (4%)
Melanoma of the skin 27,930 (4%)
Thyroid 22,590 (3%)
Ovary 20,180 (3%)
Urinary bladder 16,730 (2%)
Pancreas 16,580 (2%)
All sites 679,510 (100%)
Lung and bronchus 90,330 (31%)
Colon and rectum 27,870 (10%)
Prostate 27,350 (9%)
Pancreas 16,090 (6%)
Leukemia 12,470 (4%)
Liver & intrahepatic bile duct 10,840 (4%)
Esophagus 10,730 (4%)
Non-Hodgkin's lymphoma 10,000 (3%)
Urinary bladder 8,990 (3%)
Kidney and renal pelvis 8,130 (3%)
All sites 291,270 (100%)
Lung and bronchus 72,130 (26%)
Breast 40,970 (15%)
Colon and rectum 27,300 (10%)
Pancreas 16,210 (6%)
Ovary 15,310 (6%)
Leukemia 9,810 (4%)
Non-Hodgkin's lymphoma 8,840 (3%)
Uterine corpus 7,350 (3%)
Multiple myeloma 5,630 (2%)
Brain and other nervous system 5,560 (2%)
All sites 273,560 (100%)

FIGURE 10-5 Sex Differences in Cancer Rates and Deaths

Source: ©2006, American Cancer Society, Inc., Surveillance Research.

Genetic tests can identify some individuals who are born with an increased susceptibility to cancer. By spotting a mutated gene in an individual, doctors can sometimes detect cancer years earlier through increased cancer screening. The most likely sites for inherited cancers to develop are the breast, brain, blood, muscles, bones, and adrenal glands. The telltale signs of inherited cancers include:

- **Early development.** Genetic forms of certain diseases strike earlier than noninherited cancers. For example, the average age of women diagnosed with breast cancer is 62. But if breast cancer is inherited, the average age at diagnosis is 44, an 18-year difference.
- **Family history.** Anyone with a close relative (mother, father, sibling, child) with cancer has about three times the usual chance of getting the same type of cancer.
- **Multiple targets.** The same type of hereditary cancer often strikes more than once—in both breasts or both kidneys, for instance, or in two separate parts of the same organ.
- **Unusual gender pattern.** Genes may be responsible for cancers that generally don't strike a certain gender—for example, breast cancer in a man.
- **Cancer family syndrome.** Some families, with unusually large numbers of relatives affected by cancer, seem clearly cancer-prone. For instance, in Lynch syndrome (a form of colon cancer), more than 20 percent of the family members in at least two generations develop cancer of both the colon and the endometrium.

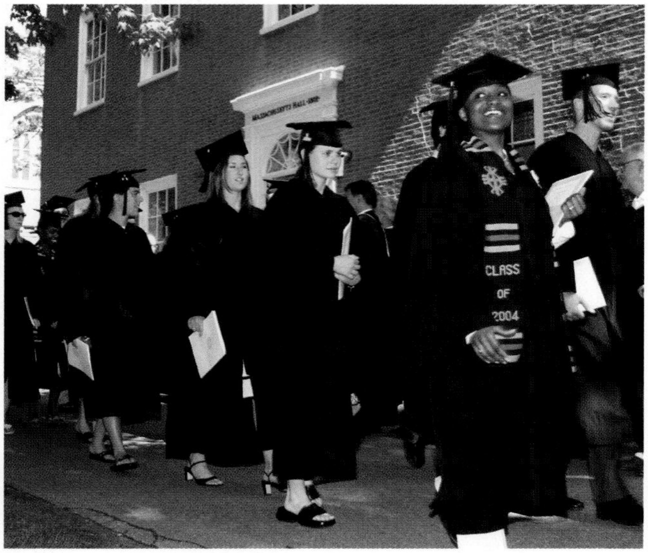

© James Marshall/The Image Works

By age 39, 1 in 64 men and 1 in 51 women will develop cancer. As you look ahead to your future, consider your risk factors and lifestyle: What do you think are your odds of getting cancer?

Racial and Ethnic Groups

More cases of cancer occur in black Americans than in any other racial or ethnic group.[17] Blacks are 30 percent more likely to die of cancer than whites. African-American women have the highest incidence of colorectal and lung cancers of any ethnic group, while black men have the highest rates of prostate, colorectal, and lung cancer. African Americans also have higher rates of incidence and deaths from other cancers, including those of the mouth, throat, esophagus, stomach, pancreas, and larynx.

Cancer rates also vary in other racial and ethnic groups. Hispanics have a six times lower risk of developing melanoma than Caucasians, yet tend to have a worse prognosis than Caucasians when they do develop this skin cancer. The incidence of female breast cancer is highest among white women and lowest among Native American women. Cervical cancer is most common in Hispanic women.

Obesity

Long recognized as threats to cardiovascular health, overweight and obesity may play a role in an estimated 90,000 cancer deaths each year. According to American Cancer Society researchers who examined the relationship between body mass index (BMI) and risk of dying from cancer, 14 percent of cancer deaths in men and 20 percent of cancer deaths in women may stem from excess weight.

The higher an individual's BMI, the greater the likelihood of dying of cancer. An unhealthy body weight increases the risk of many types of cancer, including breast (in postmenopausal women), colon and rectum, kidney, cervix, ovary, uterus, esophagus, gallbladder, stomach (in men), liver, pancreas, prostate, non-Hodgkin's lymphoma, and multiple myeloma.

The degree to which extra pounds affect cancer risk varies by site. Obesity elevates the risk of esophageal cancer fivefold; increases the risk of breast or uterine cancer by two to four times; and boosts the risk for colon cancer by 35 percent to twofold.

Infectious Agents

Worldwide, an estimated 17 percent of cancers can be attributed to infection. In economically developing countries, infections cause or contribute to 26 percent of cancers. In developed countries, they play a role in 7 percent of new cases of cancer.

Among the cancers that have been linked with infectious agents are human papilloma virus (HPV) with cervical cancer and *Helicobacter pylori* with stomach cancer. Viruses have been implicated in certain leukemias (cancers of the blood system) and lymphomas (cancers of the lymphatic system), cancers of the nose and pharynx, liver cancer, and cervical cancer. Human immune deficiency virus (HIV) can lead to certain lymphomas and leukemias and to a type of cancer called Kaposi's sarcoma.

Generally, the presence of a bacterium or a virus per se is not enough to cause cancer. A predisposing environment and other cofactors—most still unknown—are needed for cancer development and growth.

Lowering Your Cancer Risk

Environmental factors may cause between 80 and 90 percent of cancers. At least in theory, these cancers can be prevented by avoiding cancer-causing substances (such as tobacco and sunlight) or using substances that protect against cancer-causing factors (such as antioxidants and vitamin D). How do you start protecting yourself? Simple changes in lifestyle—smart eating, losing excess weight, not smoking, protecting yourself from the sun, exercising regularly—are essential. Despite their initial promise, neither aspirin nor vitamin E has proved effective in preventing specific cancers or cancer in general.

Stay Smoke-Free

Cigarette smoking is the single most devastating and preventable cause of cancer deaths in the United States. If you don't smoke, don't start and limit the time you spend around smokers. If you smoke, read Chapter 12 for advice on quitting. Your life could depend on it.

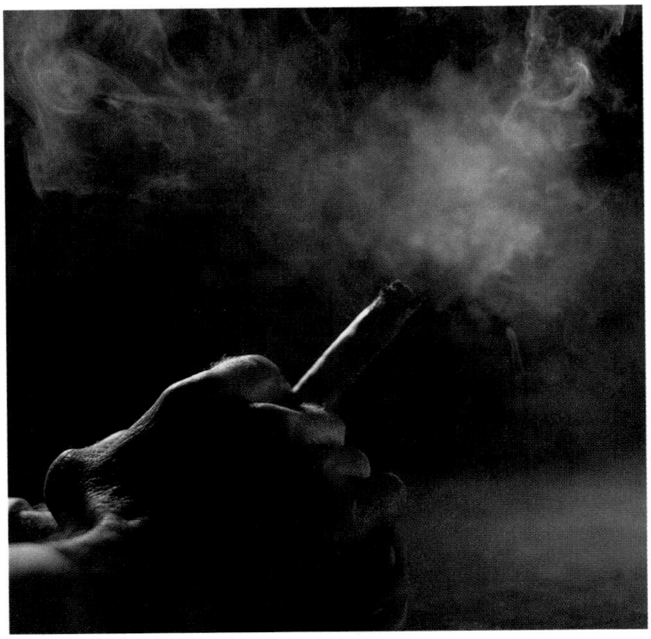

© Eva Mueller/Nonstook/Jupiter Images

Even if you don't smoke, exposure to secondhand smoke can increase your risk of lung cancer and other health problems.

People who smoke two or more packs of cigarettes a day are 15 to 25 times more likely to die of cancer than nonsmokers. Cigarettes cause most cases of lung cancer and increase the risk of cancer of the mouth, pharynx, larynx, esophagus, pancreas, and bladder. Pipes, cigars, and smokeless tobacco also increase the danger of cancers of the mouth and throat.

Environmental tobacco smoke can increase the risk of cancer even among those who've never smoked. For example, exposure to others' tobacco smoke for as little as three hours a day can increase the risk of developing cancer. (See the discussion of environmental tobacco smoke in Chapter 12.)

Eat a Cancer-Smart Diet

The links between diet and cancer are complex, and medical advice is constantly evolving. According to recent studies, cutting down on high-fat foods, particularly after age 50, does little to reduce the risk of breast and colon cancer.[18,19] In large epidemiological studies, increasing fruits and vegetables did not significantly lower rates of breast cancer. However, there is evidence linking red meat consumption and colon cancer.

The best approach is to follow the guidelines designed for overall well-being. The same foods that keep your heart healthy, your blood pressure low, your bones strong, and your weight under control are most likely to help you reduce your risk of cancer and other major illnesses.

Pay attention to food processing and preparation. Whenever possible, select foods close to their natural state, grown locally and without pesticides. Avoid cured, pickled, or smoked meats. When cooking, try not to fry or barbecue often; these cooking methods can produce mutagens that have induced cancer in animal testing. The process of smoking or charcoal-grilling releases carcinogenic tar that may increase the risk of cancer of the stomach and esophagus.

Maintain a Healthy Weight

Obesity, as discussed earlier, causes one in six cancer deaths. Excess weight may account for 14 to 20 percent of all cancers.

♀ Women who gain more than 20 pounds from age 18 to midlife double their risk of breast cancer compared to those whose weight remains stable. Too much body fat increases cancer risk in several ways: It raises the amount of estrogen in a woman's blood, which may contribute to cancers of the female reproductive system. It also raises levels of insulin, which prompts the body to create a hormone that causes cells to multiply. Obesity also makes various types of cancer harder to diagnose and treat.

Limit Exposure to Environmental Risks

Although it may not be feasible to avoid all possible **carcinogens** (cancer-causing chemicals), you can take steps to minimize your danger. Many chemicals used in industry, including nickel, chromate, asbestos, and vinyl chloride, are carcinogens; employees as well as people living near a factory that creates smoke, dust, or gases are at risk. If your job involves their use, follow safety precautions at work. If you are concerned about possible hazards in your community, check with local environmental protection officials.

Very dark shades of permanent coloring have been linked with several types of cancer, but more recent research did not find strong evidence of a marked increase in cancer risk among personal hair dye users. A ban on potential carcinogens in hair dyes may be the reason for the decline.

Chapter 14 discusses pesticides and other environmental threats.

Be Vigilant

Proven methods of cancer prevention and early detection could save more than 60,000 lives a year. Screening examinations, conducted regularly by a health-care professional, can lead to early diagnosis of cancers of the breast, colon, rectum, cervix, prostate, testicles, and oral cavity and can improve the odds of successful treatment. Self-examinations for cancers of the breast, testicles, and skin may also result in detection of tumors at earlier stages. The five-year relative survival rate for all these cancers is about 81 percent. If all Americans participated in regular cancer screenings, this rate could increase to more than 95 percent. (See Your Action Plan in The Self-Assessment Booklet for the latest guidelines on cancer screenings.)

Common Types of Cancer

Cancer refers to a group of more than a hundred diseases characterized by abnormal cell growth. Although all cancers have similar characteristics, each is distinct. Some cancers are relatively simple to cure, whereas others are more threatening and mysterious. The earlier any cancer is found, the easier it is to treat and the better the patient's chances of survival.

Cancers are classified according to the type of cell and the organ in which they originate, such as the following:

- **Carcinoma,** the most common kind, which starts in the epithelium, the layers of cells that cover the body's surface or line internal organs and glands.
- **Sarcoma,** which forms in the supporting, or connective, tissues of the body: bones, muscles, blood vessels.
- **Leukemia,** which begins in the blood-forming tissues: bone marrow, lymph nodes, and the spleen.
- **Lymphoma,** which arises in the cells of the lymph system, the network that filters out impurities.

Skin Cancer

One of every five Americans can expect to develop skin cancer in their lifetimes. Once scientists thought exposure to the B range of ultraviolet light (UVB), the wavelength of light responsible for sunburn, posed the greatest danger. However, longer-wavelength UVA, which penetrates deeper into the skin, also plays a major role in skin cancers. An estimated 80 percent of total lifetime sun exposure occurs during childhood, so sun protection is especially important in youngsters. Tanning salons and sunlamps also increase the risk of skin cancer because they produce ultraviolet radiation. A half-hour dose of radiation from a sunlamp can be equivalent to the amount you'd get from an entire day in the sun.

Young adults spend the most time in the sun and also frequent tanning salons. Even when they perceive the seriousness of skin cancer, college students—particularly women—describe suntanned skin as attractive, healthy, and athletic-looking and view the benefits of getting a suntan as outweighing the risks of skin cancer or premature aging. However, a CDC report concluded that indoor tanning is "simply not safe" and causes sunburn, infection, eye damage, and increased risk of skin cancer.[20]

The most common skin cancers are *basal cell* (involving the base of the epidermis, the top level of the skin) and *squamous cell* (involving cells in the epidermis). Their incidence is increasing among men and women under the age of 40. Long-term exposure to the sun is the biggest risk factor for these cancers.

Every year more than 5 million Americans develop skin lesions known as actinic keratoses (AKs), rough red or brown scaly patches that develop in the upper layer of the skin, usually on the face, lower lip, bald scalp, neck, and back of the hands and forearms. Forty percent of squamous cell carcinomas, the second leading cause of skin cancer deaths, begin as AKs. Treatments include surgical removal, cryosurgery (freezing the skin), electrodesiccation (heat generated by an electric current), topical chemotherapy, and removal with lasers, chemical peels, or dermabrasion.

Smoking and exposure to certain hydrocarbons in asphalt, coal tar, and pitch may increase the risk of squamous cell skin cancer. Other risk factors include occupational exposure to carcinogens and inherited skin

Strategies for Prevention — Scanning and Saving Your Skin

- Once a month, stand in front of a full-length mirror to examine your front and back, and your left and right sides with your arms raised. Check the backs of your legs, the tops and soles of your feet, and the surfaces between your toes. Use a hand mirror to check the back of your neck, behind your ears, and your scalp.
- Watch for changes in the size, color, number, and thickness of moles. Suspicious moles are likely to be asymmetrical (one half doesn't match the other), with ragged, notched, or blurred edges. Also look for any signs of darkly pigmented growth, oozing, scaliness, bleeding, or a change in sensation, itchiness, tenderness, or pain.
- Don't put too much faith in sunscreens. Wearing sunscreen (with a sun protection factor, or SPF, of at least 15) is good, but protective clothing is better—and staying in the shade is best. Check your shadow. One simple guideline for reducing the risk of skin cancer is avoiding the sun anytime your shadow is shorter than you are. According to the National Cancer Institute (NCI), this shadow method—based on the principle that the closer the sun comes to being directly overhead, the stronger its ultraviolet rays—works for any location and at any time of year.
- Check for photosensitivity. If you are taking any drugs, ask your doctor or pharmacist to see if the medication could make you more sensitive to sun damage. Be especially cautious about sun exposure if you have been using a synthetic preparation derived from vitamin A (Retin A) as an acne or anti-wrinkle treatment; it can increase your susceptibility.
- Use extra caution near water, snow, and sand since they reflect the damaging rays of the sun and increase the risk of sunburn. Wear protective clothing, such as a wide-brimmed cap or hat, whenever possible.

disorders, such as xeroderma pigmentosum and familial atypical multiple-mole melanoma.

Malignant *melanoma,* the deadliest type of skin cancer, causes 1 to 2 percent of all cancer deaths. During the 1930s, the lifetime risk of melanoma was about 1 in 1,500. Today it is 1 in 75. This increase in risk is due mostly to overexposure to UV radiation. The use of a tanning bed ten times or more a year doubles the risk for individuals over age 30.

Both the amount and the intensity of lifetime sun exposure play key roles in determining risk for melanoma. People living in areas where the sun's ultraviolet rays reach the earth with extra intensity, such as tropical or high-altitude regions, are at increased risk. Although melanoma occurs more often among people over 40, it is increasing in younger people, particularly those who had severe sunburns in childhood. The rate of increase in melanoma also has risen more in men (4.6 percent a year) than in women (3.2 percent). Men are more likely than women to be diagnosed with melanoma after age 40.

Individuals with any of the following characteristics are at increased risk:

- **Fair skin,** light eyes, or fair hair.
- **A tendency to develop freckles** and to burn instead of tan.
- **A history of childhood sunburn** or intermittent, intense sun exposure.
- **A personal or family history** of melanoma.
- **A large number of nevi,** or moles (200 or more, or 50 or more if under age 20), or dysplastic (atypical) moles.

Detection

The most common predictor for melanoma is a change in an existing mole or development of a new and changing pigmented mole. The most important early indicators are change in color, an increase in diameter, and changes in the borders of a mole (Figure 10-6). An increase in height signals a corresponding growth in depth under the skin. Itching in a new or long-standing mole also should not be ignored.

Treatment

If caught early, melanoma is highly curable, usually with surgery alone. Once it has spread, chemotherapy with a single drug or a combination can temporar-

carcinogen A substance that produces cancerous cells or enhances their development and growth.

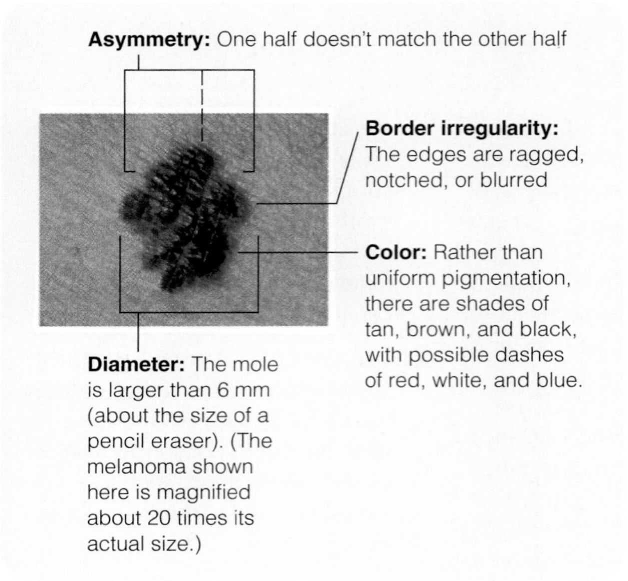

Asymmetry: One half doesn't match the other half
Border irregularity: The edges are ragged, notched, or blurred
Color: Rather than uniform pigmentation, there are shades of tan, brown, and black, with possible dashes of red, white, and blue.
Diameter: The mole is larger than 6 mm (about the size of a pencil eraser). (The melanoma shown here is magnified about 20 times its actual size.)

FIGURE 10-6 ABCD: The Warning Signs of Melanoma
An estimated 95 percent of cases of melanoma arise from an existing mole. A normal mole is usually round or oval, less than 6 millimeters (about 1/4 inch) in diameter, and evenly colored (black, brown, or tan). Seek prompt evaluation of any moles that change in ways shown in the photo.
Source: American Academy of Dermatology. All rights reserved.

By age 25	1 in 19,608
By age 30	1 in 2,525
By age 35	1 in 622
By age 40	1 in 217
By age 45	1 in 93
By age 50	1 in 50
By age 55	1 in 33
By age 60	1 in 24
By age 65	1 in 17
By age 70	1 in 14
By age 75	1 in 11
By age 80	1 in 10
By age 85	1 in 9
Ever	1 in 8

FIGURE 10-7 A Woman's Risk of Developing Breast Cancer
Source: Surveillance Program, National Cancer Institute.

ily shrink tumors in some people. However, the five-year survival rate for metastatic melanoma is 14 percent.

Breast Cancer

Every 3 minutes, a woman in the United States learns that she has breast cancer. Every 12 minutes, a woman dies of breast cancer. Many women misjudge their own likelihood of developing breast cancer, either overestimating or underestimating their susceptibility. In a national poll, one in every ten surveyed considered herself at no risk at all. This is never the case. Every woman is at risk for breast cancer simply because she's female.

However, not all women's risks are equal. The National Cancer Institute (NCI) has developed a computerized Breast Cancer Risk Assessment Tool, based on data from more than 280,000 women, that allows a woman to sit down with her doctor and discuss her own odds of developing breast cancer within the next five years and over her entire lifetime.

The most common risk factors include the following:

- **Age.** As shown in Figure 10-7, at 25, a woman's chance of developing breast cancer is 1 in 19,608; by age 45, it has increased to 1 in 93; by 65, it is 1 in 17. The mean age at which women are diagnosed is 63.
- **Family history.** The overwhelming majority of breast cancers—90 to 95 percent—are not due to

Strategies for Change: Are You Addicted to Tanning?

You know that exposure to ultraviolet rays increases your risk of developing skin cancer, but maybe you still can't stay out of the sun or a tanning booth. Why? Researchers theorize that repetitive tanning behavior may be the result of a kind of addiction.[21]

Texas beachgoers, asked questions about their tanning habits, gave replies similar to those who gamble or drink compulsively. About a quarter of those interviewed were classified as "ultraviolet light (UVL) dependent" because of their answers to the CAGE screening test, which asks the following questions:

- **C**ut: Ever felt you ought to cut down on your behavior?
- **A**nnoyed: Have people annoyed you by criticizing your behavior?
- **G**uilt: Ever felt bad or guilty about your behavior?
- **E**ye Opener: Ever engaged in your behavior to steady your nerves in the morning?

Answering yes to two of the CAGE questions is a strong indication for an addictive behavior; answering yes to three confirms it.

strong genetic factors. However, having a first-degree relative—mother, sister, or daughter—with breast cancer does increase risk, and if the relative developed breast cancer before menopause, the cancer is more likely to be hereditary.

- **Long menstrual history.** Women who had their first period before age 12 are at greater risk than women who began menstruating later. The reason is that the more menstrual cycles a woman has, the longer her exposure to estrogen, a hormone known to increase breast cancer danger. For similar reasons, childless women, who menstruate continuously for several decades, are also at greater risk.
- **Age at birth of first child.** An early pregnancy—in a woman's teens or twenties—changes the actual maturation of breast cells and decreases risk. But if a woman has her first child in her forties, precancerous cells may actually flourish with the high hormone levels of the pregnancy.
- **Breast biopsies.** Even if laboratory analysis finds no precancerous abnormalities, women who require such tests are more likely to develop breast cancer. Fibrocystic breast disease, a term often used for "lumpy" breasts, is not a risk factor.
- 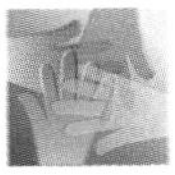 **Race.** Breast cancer rates are lower in Hispanic and Asian populations than in whites and in African-American women. Caucasian women over 40 have the highest incidence rate for breast cancer in this country, but African-American women at every age have a greater likelihood of dying from breast cancer.
- **Occupation.** Based on two decades of following more than a million women, Swedish researchers have developed a list of jobs linked with a high risk of breast cancer. These include pharmacists, certain types of teachers, schoolmasters, systems analysts and programmers, telephone operators, telegraph and radio operators, metal platers and coaters, and beauticians.
- **Alcohol.** Women's risk of breast cancer increases with the amount of alcohol they drink. Those who take two or more drinks per day are 40 percent more likely to develop breast cancer than women who don't drink at all. For a nondrinking woman, the lifetime risk of breast cancer by age 80 is 1 in 11. For heavy drinkers it's about 1 in 7, regardless of race, education, family history, use of hormone therapy, or other risk factors.
- **Hormone therapy (HT).** Several studies confirm an increased risk with a combination of estrogen and progestin, particularly in women who use combination HT for five years or longer. Women taking combination HT are more likely to have abnormal mammograms requiring further testing and to be diagnosed at a more advanced stage of breast cancer. Women taking only estrogen for shorter periods did not have an elevated rate of breast cancer, but their risk increased significantly after 15 years of use.[22] In African-American women, estrogen use has been linked to higher breast cancer risk, particularly in leaner women.[23]
- **Obesity.** Excess weight, particularly after menopause, increases the risk of getting breast cancer. Overweight women, both pre- and postmenopausal, with breast cancer are more likely to die of their disease.
- **Sedentary lifestyle.** According to the World Health Organization, regular physical activity may cut the risk of developing breast cancer by 20 to 40 percent, regardless of a woman's menopausal status or the type or intensity of the activity. The reason may be that exercise lowers levels of circulating ovarian hormones.

Detection

Doctors have long advised women to perform monthly breast self-exams (BSE) after their periods (Figure 10-8). In its newest guidelines, the American Cancer Society now describes BSE as "an option" for women starting in their twenties and urges all women to report any breast changes promptly. It recommends a breast exam by a trained practitioner every three years for women in their twenties and thirties and every year for women 40 and over and a yearly mammogram for all women, starting at age 40.

The best tool for early detection is the diagnostic X-ray exam called **mammography.** Women whose breast cancer is detected by screening mammography have a significantly better prognosis than those whose cancer is found another way—even if the cancer has already spread to their lymph nodes. A likely reason is that mammography can detect tumors that are both slower growing and less biologically lethal than others. Digital mammography, which allows doctors to break down images of breast cancer into slices and magnetic resonance imaging (MRI) can reveal cancerous tissue even sooner.

Treatment

Breast cancer can be treated with surgery, radiation, and drugs (chemotherapy and hormonal therapy). Doctors may use one of these options or a combination, depending on the type and location of the cancer and whether the disease has spread.

Most women undergo some type of surgery. **Lumpectomy,** or breast-conserving surgery, removes only the cancerous tissue and a surrounding margin of normal tissue. A

mammography A diagnostic X-ray exam used to detect breast cancer.

lumpectomy The surgical removal of a breast tumor and its surrounding tissue.

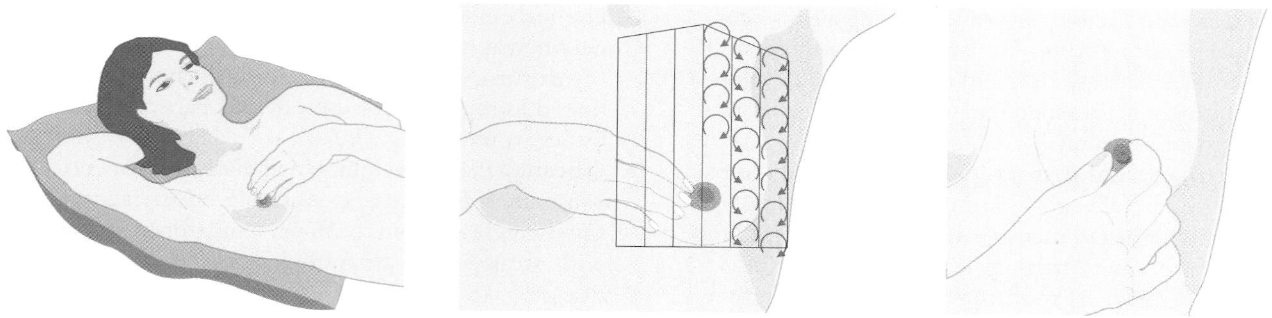

1. Lie flat on your back. Place a pillow or towel under one shoulder, and raise that arm over your head. With the opposite hand, you'll feel with the pads, not the fingertips, of the three middle fingers, for lumps or any change in the texture of the breast or skin.

2. The area you'll examine is from your collarbone to your bra line and from your breastbone to the center of your armpit. Imagine the area divided into vertical strips. Using small circular motions (the size of a dime), move your fingers up and down the strips. Apply light, medium, and deep pressure to examine each spot. Repeat this same process for your other breast.

3. Gently squeeze the nipple of each breast between your thumb and index finger. Any discharge, clear or bloody, should be reported to your doctor immediately.

FIGURE 10-8 Breast Self-Exam
The best time to examine your breasts is after your menstrual period every month.

modified radical **mastectomy** includes the entire breast and some of the underarm lymph nodes. Removing underarm lymph nodes is important to determine if the cancer has spread, but a technique called sentinel node biopsy allows physicians to pinpoint the first lymph node into which a tumor drains (the sentinel node) and remove only the nodes most likely to contain cancer cells.

Radiation therapy is treatment with high-energy rays or particles to destroy cancer. In almost all cases, lumpectomy is followed by six to seven weeks of radiation. Chemotherapy is used to reach cancer cells that may have spread beyond the breast—in many cases even if no cancer is detected in the lymph nodes after surgery.

The use of drugs such as tamoxifen and aromatase inhibitors, in addition to standard chemotherapy, can significantly lower the risk of recurrence.

Cervical Cancer

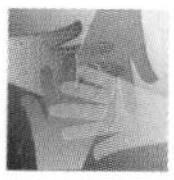

An estimated 9,710 cases of invasive cervical cancer are diagnosed in the United States every year. The highest incidence rate occurs among Vietnamese women; Alaskan Native, Korean, and Hispanic women also have higher rates than the national average. The mortality rate for African-American women is more than twice that of whites, largely because of a high number of deaths among older black women.

The primary risk factor for cervical cancer is infection with certain types of the human papilloma virus (HPV), discussed in Chapter 9. HPV occurs in more than 99.7 percent of cervical cancer cases. However, not every HPV infection becomes cervical cancer, and while HPV infection is very common, cervical cancer is not. Other risk factors for cervical cancer include early age of first intercourse, multiple sex partners, genital herpes, and smoking or significant exposure to passive smoke.

The standard screening test for cervical cancer is the Pap smear. New, more precise forms of Pap testing and new screening tests for HPV may help detect cases of cervical cancer at earlier stages. Warning signs for cervical cancer include irregular bleeding or unusual vaginal discharge. In precancerous stages, cervical cells can be destroyed by laser surgery or freezing during a visit to a doctor's office.

The National Cancer Institute (NCI) recommends a combination of chemotherapy and radiation rather than the standard use of radiation alone for invasive tumors. For women whose cervical cancer is detected early, cryotherapy (use of extreme cold), electrocoagulation (intense heat), or surgery are standard treatments.

Ovarian Cancer

Ovarian cancer is the leading cause of death from gynecological cancers. Risk factors include a family history of ovarian cancer; personal history of breast cancer; obesity; infertility (because the abnormality that interferes with conception may also play a role in cancer development); and low levels of transferase, an enzyme involved in the metabolism of dairy foods. Often women develop no obvious symptoms until the advanced stages, although they may experience painless swelling of the abdomen, irregular bleeding, lower abdominal pain, digestive and urinary

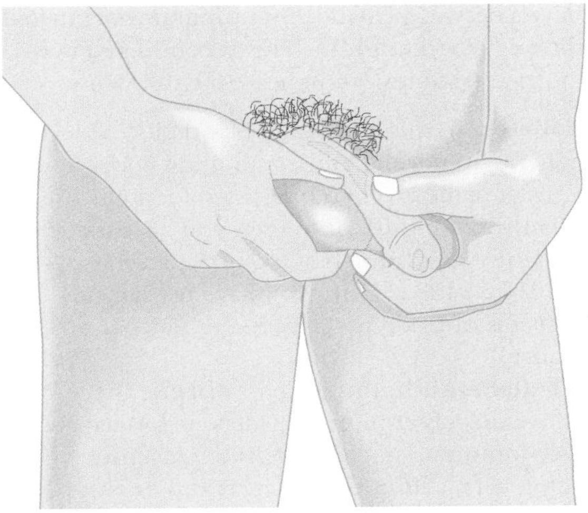

FIGURE 10-9 Testicular Self-Exam
The best time to examine your testicles is after a hot bath or shower, when the scrotum is most relaxed. Place your index and middle fingers under each testicle and the thumb on top, and roll the testicle between the thumb and fingers. If you feel a small, hard, usually painless lump or swelling, or anything unusual, consult a urologist.

abnormalities, fatigue, backache, bloating, and weight gain. Ovarian cancer may be diagnosed by pelvic examination, ultrasound, MRI, computed tomography, or PET (positron emission tomography) scan.[24]

Testicular Cancer

In the last 20 years the incidence of testicular cancer has risen 51 percent in the United States—from 3.61 to 5.44 per 100,000. It is not clear why testicular cancer is on the rise, although researchers speculate that changing environmental or socioeconomic risk factors could have a role. Testicular cancer occurs mostly among young men between the ages of 18 and 35, who are not normally at risk of cancer. At highest risk are men with an undescended testicle (a condition that is almost always corrected in childhood to prevent this danger). To detect possibly cancerous growths, men should perform monthly testicular self-exams, as shown in Figure 10-9.

Although college-age men are among those at highest risk of testicular cancer, three in four do not know how to perform a testicular self-examination.

Often the first sign of this cancer is a slight enlargement of one testicle. There also may be a change in the way it feels when touched. Sometimes men with testicular cancer report a dull ache in the lower abdomen or groin, along with a sense of heaviness or sluggishness. Lumps on the testicles also may indicate cancer.

A man who notices any abnormality should consult a physician. If a lump is indeed present, a surgical biopsy is necessary to find out if it is cancerous. If the biopsy is positive, a series of tests generally is needed to determine whether the disease has spread.

Treatment for testicular cancer generally involves surgical removal of the diseased testis, sometimes along with radiation therapy, chemotherapy, and the removal of nearby lymph nodes. The remaining testicle is capable of maintaining a man's sexual potency and fertility. Only in rare cases is removal of both testicles necessary. Testosterone injections following such surgery can maintain potency. The chance for a cure is very high if testicular cancer is spotted early.

Colon and Rectal Cancer

Colon and rectal, or colorectal, cancer is the third most common cancer and accounts for 10 percent of cancer deaths. Most cases occur after age 50. Both age and gender influence the risk of colon cancer. Older individuals and men are more likely to develop polyps (nonmalignant growths that may turn cancerous at some point) and tumors in the colon than young people and women.

Risk factors include age (over 50), personal or family history of colon and rectal cancer, polyps in the colon or rectum, ulcerative colitis, smoking, alcohol consumption, prolonged high consumption of red and processed meat, high-fat or low-fiber diet, and inadequate intake of fruits and vegetables. In the landmark Women's Health Initative trials, a low-fat diet did not reduce the risk of colon and rectal cancer in postmenopausal women.[25] Nonsteroidal anti-inflammatory drugs, such as aspirin and ibuprofen, and regular exercise may reduce the risk. Vitamin B_6, whether from food or supplements, may help prevent colorectal cancer in women.

New guidelines recommend screening for colon cancer beginning at age 50, earlier for those at higher risk based on personal, family, or medical history. The initial screening is crucial because it detects the largest, most dangerous polyps, which can then be removed.[26]

Early signs of colorectal cancer are bleeding from the rectum, blood in the stool, or a change in bowel habits. Treatment may involve surgery, radiation therapy, and/or chemotherapy.

Prostate Cancer

After skin cancer, prostate cancer is the most common form of cancer in American men. The risk of prostate cancer is 1 in 6; the risk of death due to metastatic prostate cancer is 1 in 30. More than a quarter of men diagnosed with cancer have prostate cancer. The disease strikes African-American men more often than white; Asian and American Indian men are affected less often.

The risk of prostate cancer increases with age,

mastectomy The surgical removal of an entire breast.

family history, exposure to the heavy metal cadmium, high number of sexual partners, and history of frequent sexually transmitted diseases. An inherited predisposition may account for 5 to 10 percent of cases. A purported link between vasectomy and prostate cancer has been disproved.

The development of a simple annual screening test that measures levels of a protein called prostate-specific antigen (PSA) in the blood has revolutionized the diagnosis of prostate cancer. PSA testing is recommended for men at high risk (African Americans and men with close relatives with prostate cancer) starting at age 45 and for all men at age 50. It remains controversial, however. Some claim that PSA testing saves lives; others, that it leads to unnecessary and potentially harmful treatments.

Treatment may include hormones, chemotherapy, and radiation. About 60,000 men undergo radical prostate surgery in the United States every year. The five-year survival rate has increased from 67 percent to 99 percent over the past 20 years.[27]

Diabetes Mellitus

About 100 million people around the world, including more than 18 million in the United States, have diabetes mellitus, a disease in which the body doesn't produce or respond properly to insulin, a hormone essential for daily life. In those with diabetes, the pancreas, which produces insulin (the hormone that regulates carbohydrate and fat metabolism) doesn't function as it should. When the pancreas either stops producing insulin or doesn't produce sufficient insulin to meet the body's needs, almost every body system can be damaged.

The prevalence of diabetes has nearly doubled since 1990, and health experts describe it as a global epidemic. About 6.3 percent of Americans have diabetes; a third are not aware that they have it because certain types develop insidiously with no visible symptoms.

The risk of premature death among people with diabetes is about twice that of people without the disease. According to the American Diabetes Association, the total economic cost of diabetes totals more than $132 billion a year. Diabetes accounts for $1 of every $10 spent on health care in the United States.[28]

Types of Diabetes

Diabetes includes several conditions in which the body has difficulty controlling levels of glucose in the bloodstream. After an overnight fast, most people have blood glucose levels between 70 and 100 milligrams of glucose per deciliter of blood (mg/dL). This is considered normal. Abnormal readings can indicate the following:

- **Prediabetes.** In this condition, blood glucose levels are higher than normal but are not high enough for a diagnosis of diabetes. If your fasting blood glucose is consistently 126 mg/dL or higher, you have diabetes. However, if your fasting blood glucose level is between 101 and 125 mg/dL, you have prediabetes, which also is called hyperglycemia or glucose intolerance.
- **Type 1 diabetes.** In this form of diabetes (once called juvenile-onset or insulin-dependent diabetes), the body's immune system attacks the insulin-producing beta cells in the pancreas and destroys them. The pancreas then produces little or no insulin and therefore blood glucose cannot enter the cells to be used for energy. Type 1 diabetes develops most often in young people but can appear in adults. Individuals with type 1 diabetes require insulin therapy because their own bodies no longer supply this vital hormone.
- **Type 2 diabetes.** In type 2 diabetes (once called adult-onset or non-insulin-dependent diabetes), either the pancreas does not make enough insulin or the body is unable to use insulin correctly.

Type 2 diabetes, which accounts for 90 percent of cases of diabetes, develops most often in middle-aged and older adults, but increasingly is appearing in young people, including adolescents and children.

? FAQ Who Is at Risk for Developing Diabetes?

Although type 1 and type 2 diabetes have different causes, two factors are important in both: an inherited predisposition to the disease and something in the environment that triggers diabetes. Genes alone are not enough. In most cases of type 1 diabetes, people need to inherit risk factors from both parents and to experience some environmental trigger, which might involve prenatal nutrition, a virus, or an unknown agent.

In type 2 diabetes, family history is one of the strongest risk factors for getting the disease, but only in Westernized countries. African Americans, Mexican Americans, and Native Americans have the highest rates, but people who live in less developed nations tend not to get type 2 diabetes, no matter how high their genetic risk.

Other risk factors for type 2 diabetes include:

- **Weight.** Excess weight is most risky for young people and for people who have been obese for a long time. However, you can improve your glucose levels simply by losing weight. Even a small loss can be beneficial.[29]

- **Waist circumference.** As discussed in Chapter 4, apple-shaped people who carry most of their excess weight around their waists are at greater risk of diabetes than are pear-shaped individuals who carry most of their excess weight below their waist. The more visceral fat that you have, the more resistant your body's cells become to the effects of your own insulin. A measurement of more than 40 inches in men and more than 35 inches in women indicates increased health risks.
- **Metabolic syndrome.** As discussed earlier, this condition is a cluster of disorders of your body's metabolism—including high blood pressure, high insulin levels, excess body weight, and abnormal cholesterol levels—that make you more likely to develop diabetes as well as heart disease or stroke.
- **Inactivity.** The less active you are, the greater your risk of diabetes. Physical activity helps you control your weight, uses up glucose, makes your cells more sensitive to insulin, increases blood flow, and improves circulation in even the smallest blood vessels. Exercise also helps build muscle mass, which is important because most of the glucose in your blood is absorbed into your muscles. When you have less muscle tissue, more glucose stays in your blood.
- **Age.** Your risk of type 2 diabetes increases as you get older, especially past the age of 45.
- 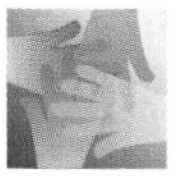 **Race.** For reasons that aren't entirely clear, people of some races are more likely to develop diabetes. Blacks and Hispanics have double the rate for whites. The incidence is even higher among Native Americans. Among the Pima Indians of Arizona, half of all adults have type 2 diabetes.
- **Depression.** If you're a younger adult who has received a diagnosis of depression, you may be at higher risk of developing type 2 diabetes than someone without depression. Researchers speculate that this is because people with depression often gain weight and are inactive.

Diabetes Signs and Symptoms

About a third of individuals with type 2 diabetes do not realize they have the illness. If you have risk factors for the disease, watch for the following warning signs:

- **Increased thirst and frequent urination.** Excess glucose circulating in your body draws water from your tissues, making you feel dehydrated. Drinking water and other beverages to quench thirst leads to more frequent urination.
- **Flu-like symptoms.** Type 2 diabetes can sometimes feel like a viral illness, with such symptoms as extreme fatigue and weakness. When glucose, your body's main fuel, doesn't reach cells, you may feel tired and weak.
- **Weight loss or weight gain.** Because your body is trying to compensate for lost fluids and glucose, you may eat more than usual and gain weight, or the opposite may occur. Although eating more than normal, you may lose weight because your muscle tissues don't get enough glucose to generate growth and energy.
- **Blurred vision.** High levels of blood glucose pull fluid from body tissues, including the lenses of the eyes, which affects ability to focus. Vision should improve with treatment of diabetes.
- **Slow-healing sores or frequent infections.** Diabetes affects the body's ability to heal and fight infection. Bladder and vaginal infections can be a particular problem for women.
- **Nerve damage (neuropathy).** Excess blood glucose can damage the small blood vessels to your

Strategies for Prevention — How to Lower Your Risk of Prediabetes and Type 2 Diabetes

The Diabetes Prevention Program (DPP), a landmark study sponsored by the National Institutes of Health, found that people at increased risk for type 2 diabetes can prevent or delay the onset of the disease by taking the following steps:

- Exercise 30 minutes on at least five days of the week.
- If you're overweight or obese, lose weight. Aim for 5 to 7 percent of your initial weight.
- Eat a diet rich in complex carbohydrates (bread and other starches) and high-fiber foods, and low in sodium and fat.
- Eat fruits and vegetables that are rich in antioxidants, substances that prevent oxygen damage to cells.
- If your doctor advises, take medications, such as metformin (Glucophage), to help lower your blood sugar.

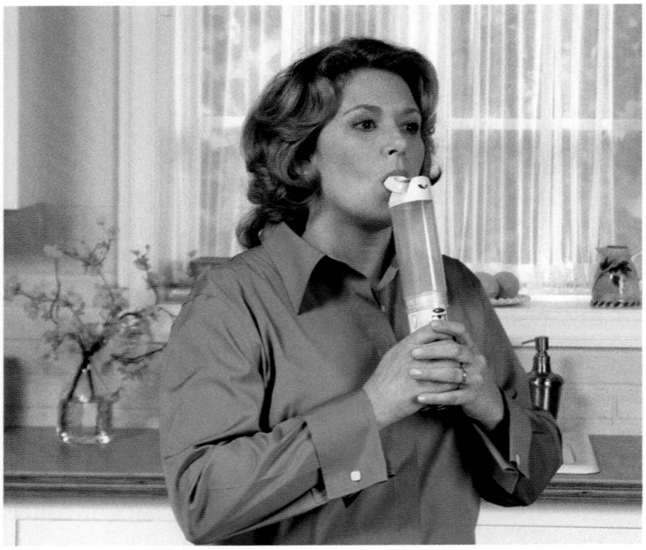

Courtesy of Pfizer Inc.

Some diabetics can control their blood sugar by using a new insulin-delivery device: an insulin powder inhaler.

nerves, leading to symptoms such as tingling and loss of sensation in hands and feet.

- **Red, swollen, tender gums.** Diabetes increases the risk of infection in your gums and in the bones that hold your teeth in place.

Treatment

The goal for diabetics is to keep blood sugar levels as stable as possible to prevent complications, such as kidney damage. Home glucose monitoring including new continuous glucose monitors, allow diabetics to check their blood sugar levels as many times a day as necessary and to adjust their diet or insulin doses as appropriate.

Types of insulin differ in how long it takes to start working after injection (onset), when it works hardest (peak), and how long it lasts in the body (duration). Individuals with diabetes may use different types in various combinations, depending on time of day and timing of meals. New insulin inhalers offer an alternative to injections for those with type 2 diabetes.

Those with type 1 diabetes require daily doses of insulin via injections, an insulin infusion pump, or oral medication. Those with type 2 diabetes can control their disease through a well-balanced diet, exercise, and weight management. However, insulin therapy may be needed to keep blood glucose levels near normal or normal, thereby reducing the risk of damage to the eyes, nerves, and kidneys. New medications help control weight and lower blood pressure and cholesterol.

Medical advances hold out bright hopes for diabetics. Laser surgery, for instance, is saving eyesight. Bypass operations are helping restore blood flow to the heart and feet. Dialysis machines and kidney and pancreas transplants save many lives. Researchers are exploring various approaches to prevention, including antibody therapies that delay the onset of type 1 diabetes. Transplanting insulin-producing cells from healthy pancreases has helped a small number of patients, but many problems remain.

LEARN IT / LIVE IT

Preventing Serious Illness

You may not be able to control every risk factor in your life or environment, but you can protect yourself from the obvious ones.

- **Don't smoke.** There's no bigger favor you can do for your heart and lungs.
- **Cut down on saturated fats and cholesterol.** This can help prevent high blood cholesterol levels, obesity, and heart disease.
- **Watch your weight.** Even relatively modest gains can have a big effect on your risk of heart disease. Overweight and obesity are associated with increased risk for cancers at several sites: breast (among postmenopausal women), colon, endometrium, esophagus (adenocarcinoma), and kidney.
- **Get moving.** Regular exercise can help lower your blood pressure, lower LDLs, and reduce triglycerides.
- **Know your family history.** Inheriting a predisposition to high blood pressure, heart disease, or cancer means that you need extra preventive care.
- **Lower your stress levels.** If too much stress is a problem in your life, try the relaxation techniques described in Chapter 3.
- **Get your blood pressure checked regularly.** Knowing your numbers can alert you to a potential problem long before you develop any symptoms.
- **Avoid excessive exposure to ultraviolet light.** If you spend a lot of time outside, protect your skin by using sunscreen and wearing long-sleeve shirts and a hat. Also, wear sunglasses to protect your eyes. Don't purposely

put yourself at risk by binge-sunbathing or by using sunlamps.

- **Control your alcohol intake.** The risk of cancers of the mouth, pharynx, larynx, esophagus, liver, and breast increases substantially with intake of more than two drinks per day for men or one drink for women.
- **Be alert to changes in your body.** You know your body's rhythms and appearance better than anyone else, and only you will know if certain things aren't right. Changes in bowel habits, skin changes, unusual lumps or discharges—anything out of the ordinary—may be clues that require further medical investigation.

10 Making This Chapter Work for You

Review Questions

1. The heart
   a. has four chambers, which are responsible for pumping blood into the veins for circulation through the body.
   b. pumps blood first to the lungs where it picks up oxygen and discards carbon dioxide.
   c. beats about 10,000 times and pumps about 75 gallons of blood per day.
   d. has specialized cells that generate electrical signals to control the amount of blood that circulates through the body.
2. You can control all of these risk factors for heart disease *except*
   a. male pattern baldness.
   b. diabetes mellitus.
   c. sedentary lifestyle.
   d. blood fat cells.
3. Hypertension
   a. is diagnosed when blood pressure is consistently lower than 130/85 mmHg.
   b. may be treated with dietary changes, which include eating low-fat foods and avoiding sodium.
   c. can cause fatty deposits to collect on the artery walls.
   d. usually does not respond to medication, especially in severe cases.
4. In your lipoprotein profile, having a high level of this blood element is a good thing:
   a. LDL cholesterol
   b. HDL cholesterol
   c. C-reactive protein
   d. triglyceride
5. A heart attack
   a. occurs when the myocardium receives an excessive amount of blood from the coronary arteries.
   b. is typically suffered by individuals who have irregular episodes of atherosclerosis.
   c. can be treated successfully up to four hours after the event.
   d. occurs when the myocardial cells are deprived of oxygen-carrying blood, causing them to die.
6. You can protect yourself from certain types of cancer by
   a. not smoking.
   b. avoiding people who have had cancer.
   c. wearing sunscreen with an SPF of less than 15.
   d. using condoms during sexual intercourse.
7. Which of the following statements about skin cancer is true?
   a. Individuals with a large number of moles are at decreased risk for melanoma.
   b. The most serious type of skin cancer is squamous cell carcinoma.
   c. The safest way to get a tan and avoid skin cancer is to use tanning salons and sunlamps instead of sunbathing in direct sunlight.
   d. Individuals with a history of childhood sunburn are at increased risk for melanoma.
8. A woman's risk of developing breast cancer increases if
   a. she is Caucasian over the age of 40.
   b. she had her first child when in her teens or twenties.
   c. her husband's mother had breast cancer.
   d. she began menstruating when she was 15 or 16.
9. Prostate cancer
   a. occurs mostly among men between the ages of 18 and 35.
   b. is usually more aggressive in white men.
   c. has a low survival rate.
   d. can be detected through a screening test that measures the levels of prostate-specific antigen in the blood.
10. Which of the following statements about diabetes mellitus is *false?*
    a. Individuals with type 2 diabetes can often control the disease without taking insulin.
    b. The incidence of diabetes has decreased in the last decade, especially among African Americans, Native Americans, and Latinos.
    c. Individuals with diabetes must measure the levels of glucose in their blood to ensure that it does not rise to unsafe levels.

d. Untreated or uncontrolled diabetes can lead to coma and eventual death.

Answers to these questions can be found on page 422.

Critical Thinking

1. Have you had your blood pressure checked lately? If your reading was high, what steps are you now taking to help reduce your blood pressure?
2. Have you had a lipoprotein profile lately? Do you think it's necessary for you to obtain one? If your reading was/is borderline or high, what lifestyle changes can you make to help control your cholesterol level?
3. Do you have family members who have had cancer? Were these individuals at risk for cancer because of specific environmental factors, such as long-term exposure to tobacco smoke? If no particular cause was identified, what other factors could have triggered their diseases? Are you concerned that you might have inherited a genetic predisposition to any particular type of cancer because of your family history?
4. A friend of yours, Karen, discovered a small lump in her breast during a routine self-examination. When she mentions it, you ask if she has seen a doctor. She tells you that she hasn't had time to schedule an appointment; besides, she says, she's not sure it's really the kind of lump one has to worry about. It's clear to you that Karen is in denial and procrastinating about seeing a doctor. What advice would you give her?

Media Menu

ThomsonNOW™ Go to the ThomsonNOW website at **http://www.thomsonedu.com** that will:

- Help you evaluate your knowledge of the material
- Allow you to take an exam-prep quiz
- Provide a Personalized Learning Plan targeting resources that address areas you should study
- Coach you through identifying target goals for behavioral change and creating and monitoring your personal change plan throughout the semester.

INTERNET CONNECTIONS

American Heart Association
www.americanheart.org

This comprehensive site features a searchable database of all major cardiovascular diseases, plus information on healthy lifestyles, current research, CPR, cardiac warning signs, risk awareness, low-cholesterol diets, and family health. The interactive Heart Profilers® provides personalized information about treatment options for common cardiovascular conditions such as hypertension, heart failure, and cholesterol.

The Heart: An Online Exploration
www.fi.edu/biosci/heart.html

This interesting site, developed by the Franklin Institute of Science, provides an interactive multimedia tour of the heart, as well as statistics, resources, links, and information on how to monitor your heart's health by becoming aware of your vital signs.

Cancer Prevention and Control
www.cdc.gov/cancer/

This site, sponsored by the Centers for Disease Control and Prevention (CDC), features current information on cancer of the breast, cervix, prostate, skin, and colon. The site also provides monthly spotlights on specific cancers, as well as links to the National Comprehensive Cancer Control Program and the National Program of Cancer Registries.

American Diabetes Association
www.diabetes.org

Here you will find the latest information on both type 1 and type 2 diabetes mellitus, including suggestions regarding diet and exercise. The online bookstore features meal planning guides, cookbooks, and self-care guides. Type in your zip code to find community resources.

• **InfoTrac College Edition Activities** Log on, insert **cardiovascular disease** or **skin cancer** into the Keyword search box, and limit your search to the past year. When you get the results, Mark articles to review, then Select one to read. Summarize three or four key points from the article.

You can find additional readings related to personal health with InfoTrac College Edition, an online library of more than 900 journals and publications. Follow the instructions for accessing InfoTrac College Edition that were packaged with your textbook; then search for articles using a keyword search.

For additional links, resources, and suggested readings on the InfoTrac College Edition, visit our Health and Wellness Resource Center at **http://health.wadsworth.com.**

Key Terms

The terms listed are used on the page indicated. Definitions of the terms are in the Glossary at the end of this book.

angioplasty 278
aorta 264
atrium 264
capillary 264
carcinogen 284
cholesterol 269
diabetes mellitus 270
diastole 264
diastolic blood pressure 269
hypertension 269
infiltration 280
lipoprotein 269

LACC Extra Credit Assignment

10. Discuss preventive measures for the top three chronic diseases.

lumpectomy 287
male pattern baldness 272
mammography 287
mastectomy 288
metabolic syndrome 269
metastasize 280
myocardial infarction (MI) 277
prehypertension 274
relative risk 280
stroke 278
systole 264
systolic blood pressure 269
triglyceride 269
ventricle 264

11 Drug Use, Misuse, and Abuse

REAL HEALTH

Amanda thought of drug users as losers who end up as desperate addicts craving a fix. She wasn't like that.

One term when Amanda had too many papers to write and too little time to finish them, one of the girls in her sorority suggested some Ritalin that a friend took for an attention deficit disorder (discussed in Chapter 2). "Doctors prescribe it all the time," she said. "It's perfectly safe."

During midterms Amanda bought Ritalin from a classmate. As finals approached, she started hoarding stimulants from several people. When she still had several pills left, Amanda popped a few at the last-bash parties of the school year.

As Amanda started preparing for her sophomore year, she considered faking symptoms of an attention disorder to get a prescription from her family doctor. She was rehearsing what she would say when she suddenly realized that a drug had become so important to her that she was ready to lie and steal to get it. Although she wasn't physically addicted, she'd become psychologically dependent on stimulants. When she thought about it, she realized that the drugs hadn't improved her grades or helped her have a better time at parties. All they had done is turn her into what she'd never wanted to be or to become.

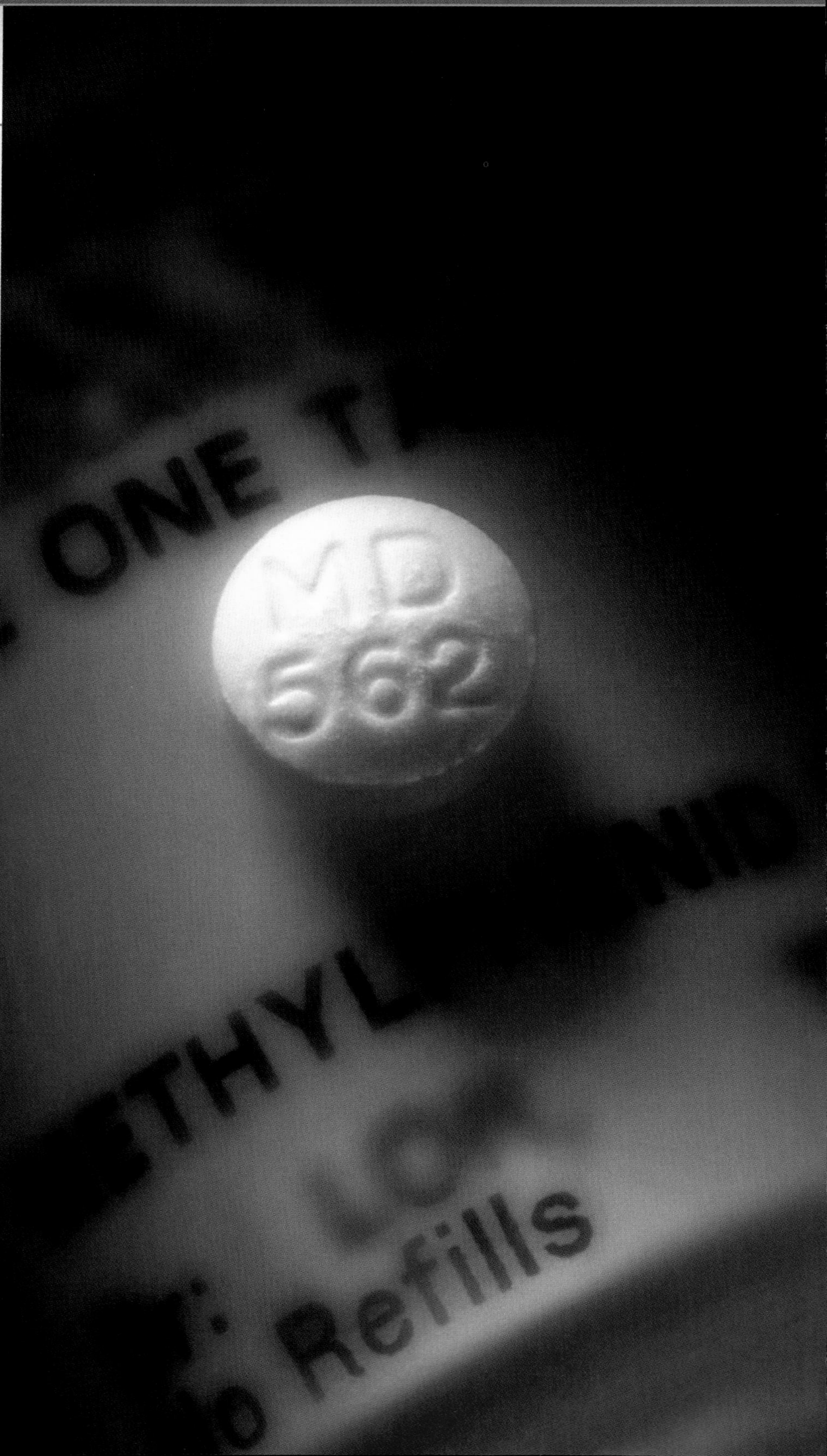

People who try illegal drugs don't think they'll ever lose control. Even regular drug users are convinced that they are smart enough, strong enough, lucky enough not to get caught and not to get hooked. But with continued use, drugs produce changes in an individual's body, mind, and behavior. In time, a person's need for a drug can outweigh everything else, including the values, people, and relationships he or she once held dearest.

Drug use among older teens has declined steadily in recent years.[1] Among college students, rates of illicit drug abuse are lower than they were several decades ago. About two-thirds of undergraduates in the National College Health Assessment say they have never smoked marijuana. Nine in ten have never used amphetamines, cocaine, club drugs, or ecstasy (See Student Snapshot: "Drugs on Campus.")[2] However, a significant percentage of students abuse or misuse prescription drugs, including painkillers and stimulants.[3]

The impact of drug-taking in college ranges from short-term consequences, such as academic difficulties, to long-term physical and psychological problems. This chapter provides information on addictive behaviors, the nature and effects of drugs, and the drugs Americans most commonly use, misuse, and abuse. It also offers practical strategies for preventing, recognizing the signs of, and seeking help for drug-related problems.

? FAQ Frequently Asked Questions

- What should I know about over-the-counter drugs? *p. 301*
- Do many college students abuse prescription drugs? *p. 303*
- Is it possible to overdose on caffeine? *p. 305*
- What causes drug dependence and abuse? *p. 306*

After studying the material in this chapter, you should be able to:

- **Describe** the factors affecting individuals' response to drugs.
- **Give examples** of appropriate and inappropriate use of over-the-counter and prescription medications.
- **Identify** the types of drug dependence, and discuss the factors affecting drug dependence.
- **Describe** the effects and health risks of common drugs of abuse.
- **Describe** the treatment methods available for individuals seeking help for drug dependence.

ThomsonNOW™ Log on to ThomsonNOW at **www.thomsonedu.com/thomsonnow** to find your Behavior Change Planner and to explore self-assessments, interactive tutorials, and practice quizzes.

Drug Use on Campus

Although the majority of college students have never used illicit drugs, drugs are available on most campuses. White men have the highest rates of drug use, although drug use has increased among minority students, including African-Americans and Pacific Islanders.[4] Students who engage in other risky behaviors, such as binge drinking and smoking, are more likely to use illicit drugs.

Students tend to overestimate how many of their peers take drugs. Even though the majority of undergraduates report never having used marijuana, for instance, students believe that most of their peers smoke pot at least once a month. While nine in ten do not use cocaine or amphetamines, students believe that more than half of undergraduates are taking these drugs.[5] Students' perceptions of their friends' drug use can affect their own use.[6]

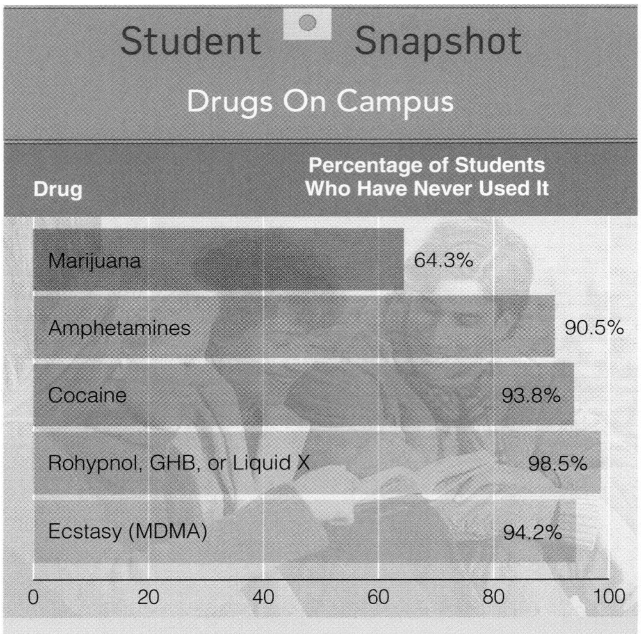

© 2006 Jupiter Images

Source: American College Health Association. "American College Health Association-National College Health Assessment (ACHA-NCHA) Spring 2004 Reference Group Data Report (abridged)." *Journal of American College Health,* Vol. 54, No. 4, January–February 2006, p. 201.

Why Students Use Drugs

Various factors influence which students use drugs, including the following:

- **Perception of risk.** Students seem most likely to try substances they perceive as being "safe," or low risk. Of these, the top three are caffeine, alcohol, and tobacco; marijuana is listed fourth in terms of perceived safety. Other agents—barbiturates, heroin, cocaine, PCP, speed, LSD, crack, and inhalants—are viewed as more risky and are used much less often.
- **Alcohol use.** Often individuals engage in more than one "risk behavior," and researchers have documented correlations among smoking, drinking, and drug use. Among college students, researchers have found that those who report binge drinking are much more likely than other students to report current or past use of marijuana, cocaine, or other illegal drugs.
- **Environment.** As with alcohol use, students are influenced by their friends, their residence, the general public's attitude toward drug use, and even the Internet. College health officials are realizing that rather than simply trying to change students' substance abuse, they also must change the environment to promote healthier lifestyle choices. Rather than simply educating students about the dangers of drugs, more colleges are offering substance-free dormitories and providing treatment for students who violate college substance abuse policies.[7]
- 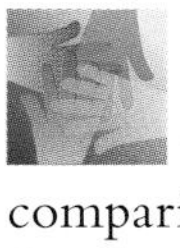 **Race/ethnicity.** In general, white students have higher levels of alcohol and drug use than do African-American students. In a comparison of African-American students at predominantly white and predominantly black colleges, those at historically black colleges had lower rates of alcohol and drug use than did either white or African-American students at white schools. The reason, according to the researchers, may be that these colleges provide a greater sense of self-esteem, which helps prevent alcohol and drug use.
- **Sexual identity.** Gay, lesbian, and bisexual teens may rely on alcohol and marijuana to lessen social anxiety and boost self-confidence when they first come out. However, once they become more involved in the gay community, many are less likely to do so. Nonetheless, self-identified lesbian women are significantly more likely than heterosexual women to use marijuana, ecstasy, and other drugs. Gay and bisexual men are significantly less likely than heterosexual men to drink heavily but more likely to use some drugs.
- **Gambling.** In a study at four Connecticut universities, one in nine students had a gambling problem significantly connected to a substance-related issue. Problem/pathological gamblers report a higher number of drug and alcohol problems than nongamblers or social gamblers.
- **Disability.** About 6 percent of college students—at least 720,000 individuals—have some form of disability. In the general population, the risk for substance abuse problems is five times that of other adults. Although there has not been much research, this also may be true of undergraduates.[8]

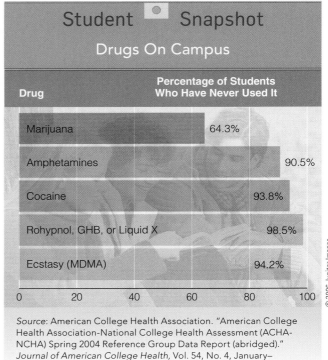

Strategies for Change — Do You Have a Gambling Problem?

- Have you ever felt that your gambling or betting was out of control?
- Have you ever gotten into a fight with your family or friends because of gambling or betting?
- Have you ever felt that you lost too much money in gambling or betting?
- Have you ever felt the need to bet more and more money?
- Have you ever had to lie to people important to you about how much you gamble?

Even a single yes answer may indicate a problem. Go online or check with a counselor on campus to find resources, such as a local chapter of Gamblers Anonymous.

Gambling

Although gambling is illegal for anyone under 18 to 21 years of age, depending on individual state law, underage gambling is a significant and growing problem across the country. In a survey of almost 1,000 university students, a majority had gambled—60 percent of the 18-year-olds, 73 percent of the 19-year-olds, 86 percent of the 20-year-olds, and 93 percent of those over 21 years of age—had gambled at least once in a casino.[9] College students who gamble do so for fun or excitement, to socialize, to win money, or to "just have something to do"—reasons similar to those for adults who gamble. Simply having access to casino machines, ongoing card games, or Internet gambling sites increases the likelihood that students will gamble.

Although most people who gamble limit the time and money they spend, some cross the line and lose control of their gambling "habit." The term *problem gambling* refers to all individuals with gambling-related problems, including mild or occasional ones. Pathological or compulsive gambling is defined as "persistent and recurrent maladaptive behavior." Researchers now view problem or pathological gambling as an addiction that runs in families.[10] Individuals predisposed to gambling because of their family history are more likely to develop a problem if they are regularly exposed to gambling. Alcoholism and drug abuse often occur along with gambling, leading to chaotic lives and dysfunctional relationships.[11]

YOUR LIFE COACH

Developing Positive Addictions

When you're anxious, bored, restless, or confused, when drugs seem all too appealing as a "quick fix," there are real solutions, "positive addictions" that can help you solve your problems without creating new and bigger ones. A positive addiction—whether it is exercising, mountain-climbing, or listening to music—can produce very real "highs." But there's a crucial difference between this sort of stimulation and drug dependency: one is real, the other is chemical. With one, you're in control; with the other, drugs are.

Here are some examples:

- **If you feel a need for physical relaxation,** if you want more energy or distraction from physical discomforts, you can turn to athletics, exercise (including walking and hiking), dance, or outdoor hobbies.
- **If you want to stimulate your senses,** enhance sexual stimulation, or magnify the sensations of sight, sound, and touch, train yourself to be more sensitive to nature and beauty. Take time to appreciate the sensations you experience when you're walking in the woods or embracing a person you love. Through activities like sailing or sky-diving, you can literally fill up your senses without relying on chemicals.
- **If you have psychological troubles,** if you're anxious or depressed, if you feel inhibited or uptight, if you don't know how to solve complex personal problems and want relief from emotional pain, turn to people who can offer lasting help: in some cases, friends; in others, professional counselors or support groups.
- **If you want peer acceptance,** if you'd like to overcome your shyness, if you want to communicate and relate more effectively, you can join expertly managed sensitivity or encounter groups, enroll in confidence-building seminars, seek counseling, or volunteer in programs in which you can assist others and not focus only on your self-consciousness.
- **If you want to escape mental boredom,** gain new understanding of the world around you, study better, experiment with your levels of awareness, or indulge your intellectual curiosity, challenge

your mind through reading, classes, creative games, discussion groups, memory training, or travel.

- **If you want to enhance your creativity** or your appreciation of the arts, pursue training in music, art, singing, gardening, or writing. Sign up for a nongraded course in art history or music appreciation. Attend more concerts, ballets, museum shows.
- **If you want to promote political or social change,** defy the establishment, change drug legislation, or gain power, you can volunteer in political campaigns, work on nonpartisan projects, or join lobbying and political action groups.
- **If you want to find meaning in life,** understand the nature of the universe, or expand your personal awareness, explore various philosophical theories through classes, seminars, and discussion groups. Study different religious orientations, including mysticism, or try yoga and meditation.
- **If you're looking for kicks,** adventure, danger, and excitement, sign up for a wilderness survival course. Take up an adventurous sport, like hang gliding or rock climbing. Set a challenging professional or personal goal and direct your energies to meeting it.

Understanding Drugs and Their Effects

A **drug** is a chemical substance that affects the way you feel and function. In some circumstances, taking a drug can help the body heal or relieve physical and mental distress. In other circumstances, taking a drug can distort reality, undermine well-being, and threaten survival. No drug is completely safe; all drugs have multiple effects that vary greatly in different people at different times. Knowing how drugs affect the brain, body, and behavior is crucial to understanding their impact and making responsible decisions about their use.

Drug misuse is the taking of a drug for a purpose or by a person other than that for which/whom it was medically intended. Borrowing a friend's prescription for penicillin when your throat feels scratchy is an example of drug misuse. The World Health Organization defines **drug abuse** as excessive drug use that's inconsistent with accepted medical practice. Taking prescription painkillers to get high is an example of drug abuse.

Risks are involved with all forms of drug use. Even medications that help cure illnesses or soothe symptoms have side effects and can be misused. Some substances that millions of people use every day, such as caffeine, pose some health risks. Others—like the most commonly used drugs in our society, alcohol and tobacco—can lead to potentially life-threatening problems. With some illicit drugs, any form of use can be dangerous.

Many factors determine the effects a drug has on an individual. These include how the drug enters the body, the dosage, the drug action, and the presence of other drugs in the body—as well as the physical and psychological makeup of the person taking the drug and the setting in which the drug is used.

Routes of Administration

Drugs can enter the body in a number of ways (Figure 11-1). The most common way of taking a drug is by swallowing a tablet, capsule, or liquid. However, drugs taken orally don't reach the bloodstream as quickly as drugs introduced into the body by other means. A drug taken orally may not have any effect for 30 minutes or more.

Drugs can enter the body through the lungs either by inhaling smoke, for example, from marijuana, or by inhaling gases, aerosol sprays, or fumes from solvents or other compounds that evaporate quickly. Young users of such inhalants, discussed later in this chapter, often soak a rag with fluid and press it over their nose. Or they may place inhalants in a plastic bag, put the bag over their nose and mouth, and take deep breaths—a practice called *huffing* and one that can produce serious, even fatal consequences.

Drugs can also be injected with a syringe subcutaneously (beneath the skin), intramuscularly (into muscle tissue, which is richly supplied with blood vessels), or intravenously (directly into a vein). **Intravenous** (IV) injection gets the drug into the bloodstream immediately (within seconds in most cases); **intramuscular** injection, moderately fast (within a few minutes); and **subcutaneous** injection, more slowly (within ten minutes).

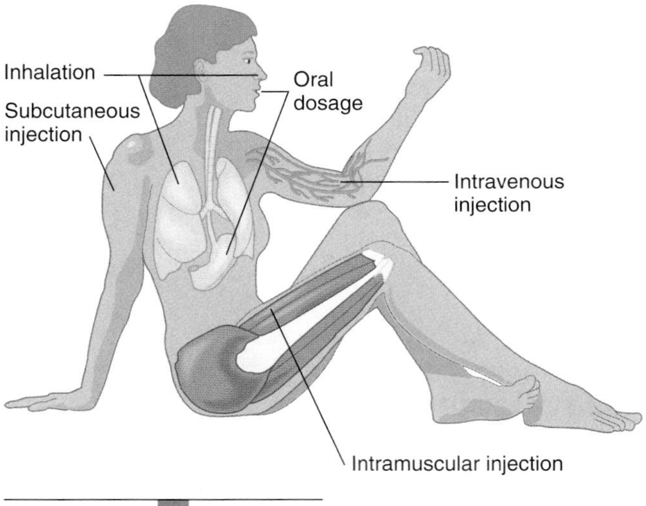

FIGURE 11-1 Routes of Administration of Drugs

Injecting drugs is extremely dangerous because many diseases, including hepatitis and infection with human immune deficiency virus (HIV), can be transmitted by sharing contaminated needles. Injection-drug users who are HIV-positive are a major source of transmission of HIV among heterosexuals (see Chapter 9).

Dosage and Toxicity

The effects of any drug depend on the amount an individual takes. Increasing the dose usually intensifies the effects produced by smaller doses. Also, the kind of effect may change at different dose levels. For example, low doses of barbiturates may relieve anxiety, while higher doses can induce sleep, loss of sensation, even coma and death.

The dosage level at which a drug becomes poisonous to the body, causing either temporary or permanent damage, is called its **toxicity.** In most cases, drugs are eventually broken down in the liver by special body chemicals called *detoxification enzymes.*

Individual Differences

Each person responds differently to different drugs, depending on circumstances or setting. The enzymes in the body reduce the levels of drugs in the bloodstream; because there can be 80 variants of each enzyme, every person's body may react differently.

Often drugs intensify the emotional state a person is in. If you're feeling depressed, a drug may make you feel more depressed. A generalized physical problem, such as having the flu, may make your body more vulnerable to the effects of a drug. Genetic differences among individuals also may account for varying reactions.

Personality and psychological attitude also play a role in drug effects. Each user's *mind-set*—his or her expectations or preconceptions about using the drug—affects the experience. Someone who takes a "club drug" (discussed further later in this chapter) to feel more "connected" may feel more sociable simply because that's what he or she expects.

Medications

As many as half of all patients take the wrong medications, in the wrong doses, at the wrong times, or in the wrong ways. Every year these inadvertent errors lead to an estimated 125,000 deaths and more than $8.5 billion in hospital costs.[12] Mistakes occur among people of all ages, both genders, and every race, occupation, level of education, and personality type. Their number-one cause: not understanding directions (see Savvy Consumer: "Avoiding Medication Mistakes").

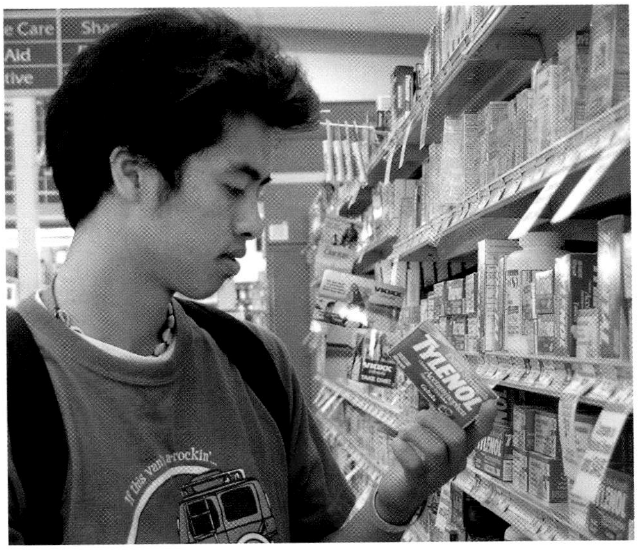

Geri Engberg Photography

Practically all of these packages carry warnings to consumers. Read them before using an over-the-counter drug.

According to a survey of office-based physicians, about one-fifth of medications are prescribed "off-label" to treat conditions for which they are not approved by the FDA. Psychiatric and allergy medications are especially likely to be prescribed off-label with limited or no scientific support.[13]

? FAQ What Should I Know About Over-The-Counter Drugs?

More than half a million health products—remedies for everything from bad breath to bunions—are readily available without a doctor's prescription. This doesn't mean that they're necessarily safe or effective. Indeed, many widely used **over-the-counter (OTC) drugs** pose unsuspected hazards.

Federal regulators have issued warnings for many popular painkillers, including over-the-counter pills

drug Any substance, other than food, that affects bodily functions and structures when taken into the body.

drug misuse The use of a drug for a purpose (or person) other than that for which it was medically intended.

drug abuse The excessive use of a drug in a manner inconsistent with accepted medical practice.

intravenous Into a vein.

intramuscular Into or within a muscle.

subcutaneous Under the skin.

toxicity Poisonousness; the dosage level at which a drug becomes poisonous to the body, causing either temporary or permanent damage.

over-the-counter (OTC) drugs Medications that can be obtained legally without a prescription from a medical professional.

SAVVY CONSUMER

Avoiding Medication Mistakes

- Whenever you get a prescription, be sure to find out from your doctor and pharmacist the name of the drug, what it's supposed to do, and how and when to take it and for how long. Are there foods, drinks, other medications, or activities you should avoid while taking the medication?
- Ask if the drug causes any side effects and what you should do if any occur.
- Keep a record of all your medicines, listing both their brand and generic (chemical) names and the reason you are taking them, and update it regularly. Give a copy of this list to every physician and every pharmacy providing health-care services.
- Inform your doctors of any over-the-counter drugs, vitamins, and herbal products you use regularly. Popular herbal supplements like gingko bilboa and common over-the-counter drugs like aspirin can interact with many prescription drugs to cause serious problems, such as excessive bleeding.
- Always turn on the lights when you take your medication. Familiarize yourself with the imprint on each tablet or capsule so you can recognize each pill. If a refill looks different, check with your pharmacist or doctor before taking it.
- Don't crush or chew a medicine without checking with your doctor or pharmacist first. Some medications are designed for gradual release rather than all at once and could be harmful if absorbed too quickly.
- Don't use a kitchen spoon to dispense liquid medications. Household teaspoons can hold between 3 and 7 milliliters; a prescription "teaspoon" means 5 milliliters. Either measure the dose in the cup or dropper that came with the medicine or ask the pharmacist for a measuring device.
- Never take someone else's medications. They could interact with your medications or the dose may be different.
- Always check labels for warnings on interactions with alcohol and instructions on whether or not to take before, with, or after meals.
- Don't take medicine with grapefruit juice, which can interact with more than 200 medications, including cholesterol-lowering statins, sleeping pills, and anti-anxiety agents.
- Plan ahead to make sure you have adequate amounts of the medications you need.
- Don't leave medicines in a car for prolonged periods. Temperature extremes, along with moisture, light, and oxygen, can affect the potency of many medications.
- Use cues, such as the alarm on your cell phone or Palm Pilot or Post-it notes, to remind you to take your medication on schedule.

like Advil and Aleve. Their labels cite risks to the heart, stomach, and skin. Tylenol (acetaminophen) and aspirin are generally considered safe for people with temporary pain like headaches and muscle aches. However, aspirin can cause stomach irritation and bleeding. Tylenol and other products containing acetaminophen account for 40 to 50 percent of all acute cases of liver failure, many the result of unintentional overdose. Doctors caution against taking more than eight Tylenol Extra Strength pills (which contain 500 mg per tablet) in a 24-hour period.[14]

Like other drugs, OTC medications can be used improperly, often simply because of a lack of education about proper use. Among those most often misused are the following:

- **Nasal sprays.** Nasal sprays relieve congestion by shrinking blood vessels in the nose. If they are used too often or for too many days in a row, the blood vessels widen instead of contracting, and the surrounding tissues become swollen, causing more congestion. To make the vessels shrink again, many people use more spray more often. The result can be permanent damage to nasal membranes, bleeding, infection, and partial or complete loss of smell.
- **Laxatives.** Believing that they must have one bowel movement a day (a common misconception), many people rely on laxatives. Brands that contain phenolphthalein irritate the lining of the intestines and cause muscles to contract or tighten, often making constipation worse rather than better. Bulk laxatives are less dangerous, but regular use is not advised. A high-fiber diet and more exercise are safer and more effective remedies for constipation.

- **Eye drops.** Eye drops make the blood vessels of the eye contract. However, as in the case of nasal sprays, with overuse (several times a day for several weeks), the blood vessels expand, making the eye look redder than before.
- **Sleep aids.** Although OTC sleeping pills are widely used, there has been little research on their use and possible risks. A national consensus panel on insomnia concluded that they are not effective and cause side effects such as morning-after grogginess.[15] Medications like Tylenol PM and Excedrin PM combine a pain reliever with a sleep-inducing antihistamine, the same ingredient that people take for hay fever or cold symptoms. Although they make people drowsy, they can leave you feeling groggy the next day, and they dry out the nose and mouth.
- **Cough syrup.** As discussed in Chapter 9, many of the "active" ingredients in over-the-counter cough preparations may be ineffective. Chugging cough syrup (also called *roboing,* after the OTC medication Robitussin) is a growing problem, in part because young people think of dextromethorphan (DXM), a common ingredient in cough medicine, as a "poor man's version" of the popular drug ecstasy.

Prescription Drugs

In a recent study of about 9,000 undergraduates at a large midwestern university, 57 percent reported that they had used prescription drugs for medical reasons at some point in their lives. The most widely used ones were pain medications, sedative or anxiety medications, sleeping medications, and stimulant medications. College women used more pain, anxiety, and sleeping pills; college men used more medically prescribed stimulants.[16]

Both doctors and patients make errors when it comes to prescription drugs. The most frequent mistakes doctors make are over- or under-dosing, omitting information from prescriptions, ordering the wrong dosage form (a pill instead of a liquid, for example), and not recognizing a patient's allergy to a drug.

National attention focused on widely used prescription painkillers after Vioxx and Bextra, two popular medications for pain, were taken off the market. Evidence suggested that these drugs, called COX-2 inhibitors (which block a hormone that promotes inflammation), may double the risk of heart attacks and strokes. Bextra was also linked to serious but rare skin conditions. Celebrex remains on the market but with a black box on the label that warns of possible cardiovascular and gastrointestinal problems. High doses of the rheumatoid arthritis drugs Humira or Remicade significantly increase the risks of several kinds of cancer, including skin, breast, and lung tumors, and serious infections such as tuberculosis and pneumonia.[17]

FAQ: Do Many College Students Abuse Prescription Drugs?

The abuse or prescription medications on college campuses has increased in the last 15 years. As many as one in five college students misuses or abuses a prescription medication every year. The rates of illicit use of prescribed drugs are higher than for the use of cocaine, ecstasy, inhalants, LSD, other psychedelics, crystal methamphetamine, heroin, GHB, or Ketamine. Only marijuana use is more widespread on campus.[18]

College students are more likely to abuse stimulant medications, such as Ritalin (discussed on page 314), than their same-age peers who are not attending college. College men have higher rates of prescription drug abuse than women. White and Hispanic undergraduates are significantly more likely to abuse medications than African-American and Asian students. Many students taking prescription drugs for medical purposes report being approached by classmates seeking drugs. Undergraduates who misuse or abuse prescription medications are much more likely to report heavy binge drinking and use of illicit drugs.[19]

Nonadherence

Many prescribed medications aren't taken the way they should be; millions simply aren't taken at all. As many as 70 percent of adults have trouble understanding dosage information and 30 percent can't read standard labels, according to the FDA, which has called for larger, clearer drug labeling. The dangers of nonadherence (not properly taking prescription drugs) include recurrent infections, serious medical complications, and emergency hospital treatment. The drugs most likely to be taken incorrectly are those that treat problems with no obvious symptoms (such as high blood pressure), require complex dosage schedules, treat psychiatric disorders, or have unpleasant side effects.

The most common reason that college students fail to take medicines as directed is forgetting. Others are concerned about cost, or they stop when they feel better. Students' underlying health beliefs, such as a conviction that taking medicine reflects weakness, can affect their compliance.[20]

Physical Side Effects

Most medications, taken correctly, cause only minor complications. However, no drug is entirely without side effects for all individuals taking it. Serious complications that may occur include heart failure, heart attack, seizures, kidney and liver failure, severe blood disorders, birth defects, blindness, memory problems, and allergic reactions.

Allergic reactions to drugs are common. The drugs that most often provoke allergic responses are penicillin and other antibiotics (drugs used to treat infection). Aspirin, sulfa drugs, barbiturates, anticonvulsants, insulin, and local anesthetics can also provoke allergic responses.

Psychological Side Effects

Dozens of drugs—both over-the-counter and prescription—can cause changes in the way people think, feel, and behave. Unfortunately, neither patients nor their physicians usually connect such symptoms with medications. Doctors may not even mention potential mental and emotional problems because they don't want to scare patients away from what otherwise may be a very effective treatment. What you don't know about a drug's effects on your mind *can* hurt you.

Among the medications most likely to cause psychiatric side effects are drugs for high blood pressure, heart disease, asthma, epilepsy, arthritis, Parkinson's disease, anxiety, insomnia, and depression. Some drugs—such as the powerful hormones called *corticosteroids,* used for asthma, autoimmune diseases, and cancer—can cause different psychiatric symptoms, depending on dosage and other factors. The older you are, the sicker you are, and the more medications you're taking, the greater your risk of developing some psychiatric side effects.

Drug Interactions

OTC and prescription drugs can interact in a variety of ways. For example, mixing some cold medications with tranquilizers can cause drowsiness and coordination problems, thus making driving dangerous. Moreover, what you eat or drink can impair or completely wipe out the effectiveness of drugs or lead to unexpected effects on the body. For instance, aspirin takes five to ten times as long to be absorbed when taken with food or shortly after a meal than when taken on an empty stomach. If tetracyclines encounter calcium in the stomach, they bind together and cancel each other out.

To avoid potentially dangerous interactions, check the label(s) for any instructions on how or when to take a medication, such as "with a meal." If the directions say that you should take a drug on an empty stomach, take it at least one hour before eating or two or three hours after eating. Don't drink a hot beverage with a medication; the temperature may interfere with the effectiveness of the drug.

Whenever you take a drug, be especially careful of your intake of alcohol, which can change the rate of metabolism and the effects of many different drugs. Because it dilates the blood vessels, alcohol can add to the dizziness sometimes caused by drugs for high blood pressure, angina, or depression. Also, its irritating effects on the stomach can worsen stomach upset from aspirin, ibuprofen, and other anti-inflammatory drugs.

Caffeine and Its Effects

Caffeine, which has been drunk, chewed, and swallowed since the Stone Age, is the most widely used **psychoactive** (mind-affecting) drug in the world. Eighty percent of Americans drink coffee, our principal caffeine source—an average of 3.5 cups a day. Coffee contains 100 to 150 milligrams of caffeine per cup; tea, 40 to 100 milligrams; cola, about 45 milligrams. Most medications that contain caffeine are one-third to one-half the strength of a cup of coffee. However, some, such as Excedrin, are very high in caffeine (Table 11-1).

Despite 20 years of reassuring research, many people still avoid caffeinated coffee because they worry about its health effects. In moderation—a few cups a day—coffee is a safe beverage that may offer some health benefits, including lowering the risk for type 2 diabetes. Coffee also may reduce the likelihood of gallstones, Parkinson's disease, and colon cancer.

As a stimulant, caffeine relieves drowsiness, helps in the performance of repetitive tasks, and improves the capacity for work. Caffeine improves performance and endurance during prolonged, exhaustive exercise and to a lesser degree, enhances short-term, high-intensity athletic performance. Additional benefits include improved concentration, reduced fatigue, and sharpened alertness.

Various studies have linked increased coffee intake with an increased risk of heart attacks, but only individuals whose bodies metabolize caffeine slowly may be at risk.[21]

Caffeinated energy drinks such as Red Bull, which typically contain sugar, caffeine, and an amino acid called taurine, are popular on campus. Health experts caution that they should not be mixed with alcohol. Also, do not drink them before

TABLE 11-1 Caffeine Counts

Substance (typical serving)	Caffeine (milligrams)
No Doz, one pill	200
Coffee (drip), one 5-ounce cup	130
Excedrin, two pills	130
Espresso, one 2-ounce cup	100
Energy drink, one can	80
Instant coffee, one 5-ounce cup	74
Coca-Cola, 12 ounces	46
Tea, one 5-ounce cup	40
Dark chocolate, 1 ounce	20
Milk chocolate, 1 ounce	6
Cocoa, 5 ounces	4
Decaffeinated coffee, one 5-ounce cup	3

intense exercise because of the increased risk of dehydration. In a study of college men and women who normally consumed fewer than three caffeinated beverages per day, caffeine boosted anxiety but did not significantly affect performance on various low-intensity tasks, except for hand-eye coordination, which improved.

You'll stay more alert, particularly if you are fighting sleep deprivation, if you spread your coffee consumption over the course of the day. For instance, rather than drinking two 8-ounce cups in the morning, try consuming smaller servings of an ounce or two during the course of the day.

? FAQ Is It Possible to Overdose on Caffeine?

Yes, you can overdose on caffeine. The characteristic symptoms of caffeine intoxication are restlessness, nervousness, excitement, insomnia, flushed face, increased urination, digestive complaints, muscle twitching, rambling thoughts and speech, rapid heart rate or arrhythmias, periods of inexhaustibility, and physical restlessness. Some people develop these symptoms after as little as 250 milligrams of caffeine a day; others, only with much larger doses. Higher doses may produce ringing in the ears or flashes of light, grand mal seizures, and potentially fatal respiratory failure.

Caffeine withdrawal for those dependent on this substance can cause headaches and other neurological symptoms. Those who must cut back should taper off gradually. One approach is to mix regular and decaffeinated coffee, gradually decreasing the quantity of the former.

Men, Women, and Drugs

Beginning at a very early age, males and females show different patterns in drug use. Men generally encounter more opportunities to use drugs than women, but given an opportunity to use drugs for the first time, both genders are equally likely to do so and to progress from initial use to dependence. Vulnerability to some drugs varies with gender. Both are equally likely to become addicted to or dependent on cocaine, heroin, hallucinogens, tobacco, and inhalants. Women are more likely than men to become addicted to or dependent on sedatives and drugs designed to treat anxiety or sleeplessness and less likely than men to abuse alcohol and marijuana.

Males and females may differ in their biological responses to drugs. In studies of animals given the opportunity to self-administer intravenous doses of cocaine or heroin, females began self-administration sooner than males and administered larger amounts of the drugs. Male and female long-term cocaine users showed similar impairment in tests of concentration, memory, and academic achievement following sustained abstinence, even though women in the study had substantially greater exposure to cocaine. Women cocaine users also were less likely than men to exhibit abnormalities of blood flow in the brain's frontal lobes. These findings suggest a gender-related mechanism that may protect women from some of the damage cocaine inflicts on the brain. However, women are more vulnerable to poor nutrition and below-average weight, depression, physical abuse, and if pregnant, preterm labor or early delivery.

Substance abuse compounds the risk of AIDS for women, who may become infected with HIV by sharing needles with other injection-drug users and by engaging in unprotected sex. In all, drug abuse is nearly twice as likely to be directly or indirectly associated with AIDS in women as in men.

Substance Use Disorders

People have been using psychoactive chemicals for centuries. Citizens of ancient Mesopotamia and Egypt used opium. More than 3,000 years ago, Hindus included cannabis products in religious ceremonies. For centuries the Inca in South America have chewed the leaves of the coca bush. Yet while drugs existed in most societies, their use was usually limited to small groups. Today millions of people regularly turn to drugs to pick them up, bring them down, alter perceptions, or ease psychological pain.

The word **addiction,** as used by the general population, refers to the compulsive use of a substance, loss of control, negative consequences, and denial. Mental health professionals describe drug-related problems in terms of *dependence* and *abuse.*

Dependence

Individuals may develop **psychological dependence** and feel a strong craving for a drug because it produces pleasurable feelings or relieves stress and anxiety. **Physical dependence** occurs when a person develops *tolerance* to the effects of a drug and needs larger and larger doses to achieve intoxication or another desired effect.

psychoactive Mind-affecting.

addiction A behavioral pattern characterized by compulsion, loss of control, and continued repetition of a behavior or activity in spite of adverse consequences.

psychological dependence The emotional or mental attachment to the use of a drug.

physical dependence The physiological attachment to, and need for, a drug.

Individuals who are physically dependent and have a high tolerance to a drug may take amounts many times those that would produce intoxication or an overdose in someone who was not a regular user.

Men and women with a substance dependence disorder may use a drug to avoid or relieve withdrawal symptoms, or they may consume larger amounts of a drug or use it over a longer period than they'd originally intended. They may repeatedly try to cut down or control drug use without success; spend a great deal of time obtaining or using drugs or recovering from their effects; give up or reduce important social, occupational, or recreational activities because of their drug use; or continue to use a drug despite knowledge that the drug is likely to cause or worsen a persistent or recurring physical or psychological problem.

Specific symptoms of dependence vary with particular drugs. Some drugs, such as marijuana, hallucinogens, and phencyclidine, do not cause withdrawal symptoms. The degree of dependence also varies. In mild cases, a person may function normally most of the time. In severe cases, the person's entire life may revolve around obtaining, using, and recuperating from the effects of a drug.

Individuals with drug dependence become intoxicated or high on a regular basis—whether every day, every weekend, or several binges a year. They may try repeatedly to stop using a drug and yet fail, even though they realize their drug use is interfering with their health, family life, relationships, and work.

Abuse

Some drug users do not develop the symptoms of tolerance and withdrawal that characterize dependence, yet they use drugs in ways that clearly have a harmful effect on them. These individuals are diagnosed as having a *psychoactive substance abuse disorder.* They continue to use drugs despite their awareness of persistent or repeated social, occupational, psychological, or physical problems related to drug use, or they use drugs in dangerous ways or situations (before driving, for instance).

Intoxication and Withdrawal

Intoxication refers to maladaptive behavioral, psychological, and physiologic changes that occur as a result of substance use. **Withdrawal** is the development of symptoms that cause significant psychological and physical distress when an individual reduces or stops drug use. (Intoxication and withdrawal from specific drugs are discussed later in this chapter.)

Polyabuse

Most users prefer a certain type of drug but also use several others; this behavior is called **polyabuse.** The average user who enters treatment is on five different drugs. The more drugs anyone uses, the greater the chance of side effects, complications, and possibly life-threatening interactions.

Coexisting Conditions

Mental disorders and substance abuse disorders have a great deal of overlap. Many individuals with substance abuse disorders also have another psychiatric disorder, such as depression. Individuals with such *dual diagnoses* require careful evaluation and appropriate treatment for the complete range of complex and chronic difficulties they face. However, they can benefit from participation in 12-step groups, like Double Trouble in Recovery, that provide treatment for both.

? FAQ What Causes Drug Dependence and Abuse?

No one fully understands why some people develop drug dependence or abuse disorders, whereas others, who may experiment briefly with drugs, do not. Inherited body chemistry, genetic factors, and sensitivity to drugs may make some individuals more susceptible. These disorders may stem from many complex causes.

The Biology of Dependence

Scientists now view drug dependence as a brain disease triggered by frequent use of drugs that change the biochemistry and anatomy of neurons and alter the way they work. A major breakthrough in understanding dependence has been the discovery that certain mood-altering substances and experiences—a puff of marijuana, a slug of whiskey, a snort of cocaine, a big win at blackjack—trigger a rise in a brain chemical called *dopamine,* which is associated with feelings of satisfaction and euphoria. This brain chemical or neurotransmitter is one of the crucial messengers that links nerve cells in the brain and its level rises during any pleasurable experience, whether it be a loving hug or a taste of chocolate.

Addictive drugs have such a powerful impact on dopamine and its receptors that they change the pathways within the brain's pleasure centers. Various psychoactive chemicals create a craving for more of the same. According to this hypothesis, addicts do not specifically yearn for heroin, cocaine, or nicotine but for the rush of dopamine that these drugs produce. Other brain chemicals, including glutamate, GABA (gamma-aminobutyric acid), and possibly norepinephrine, may also be involved. Some individuals, born with low levels of dopamine, may be particularly susceptible to addiction.

The Psychology of Vulnerability

Although scientists do not believe there is an addictive personality, certain individuals are at greater risk of drug dependence because of psychological factors, in-

Strategies for Prevention — Saying No to Drugs

If people offer you a drug, here are some ways to say no.

- Let them know you're not interested. Change the subject. If the pressure seems threatening, just walk away.
- Have something else to do: "No, I'm going for a walk now."
- Be prepared for different types of pressure. If your friends tease you, tease them back.
- Keep it simple. "No, thanks," "No," or "No way" all get the point across.
- Hang out with people who won't offer you drugs.

cluding difficulty controlling impulses, a lack of values that might constrain drug use (whether based in religion, family, or society), low self-esteem, feelings of powerlessness, and depression. The one psychological trait most often linked with drug use is denial. Young people in particular are absolutely convinced that they will never lose control or suffer in any way as a result of drug use.

Many diagnosed drug users have at least one mental disorder, particularly depression or anxiety. Disorders that emerge in adolescence, such as bipolar disorder, may increase the risk of substance abuse. Many people with psychiatric disorders abuse drugs. Individuals may self-administer drugs to treat psychiatric symptoms; for example, they may take sedating drugs to suppress a panic attack.

Early Influences

Teen drug abuse has declined in the last decade, but some teens remain more vulnerable. Young people from lower socioeconomic backgrounds are more likely to use drugs than their more affluent peers, possibly because of economic disadvantage; family instability; a lack of realistic, rewarding alternatives and role models; and increased hopelessness.

Those whose companions are substance abusers are far more likely to use drugs. Peer pressure to use drugs can be a powerful factor for adolescents, although having a drug-using roommate does not increase the odds that a college student will use drugs.[22] The likelihood of drug abuse is also related to family instability, parental rejection, and divorce.

Parents' own attitudes and drug-use history affect their children's likelihood of using marijuana, according to the Substance Abuse and Mental Health Services Administration. Parents who perceive little risk associated with marijuana use have children with similar attitudes, and the children of parents who used marijuana are more likely to try the drug than children whose parents never used the drug.

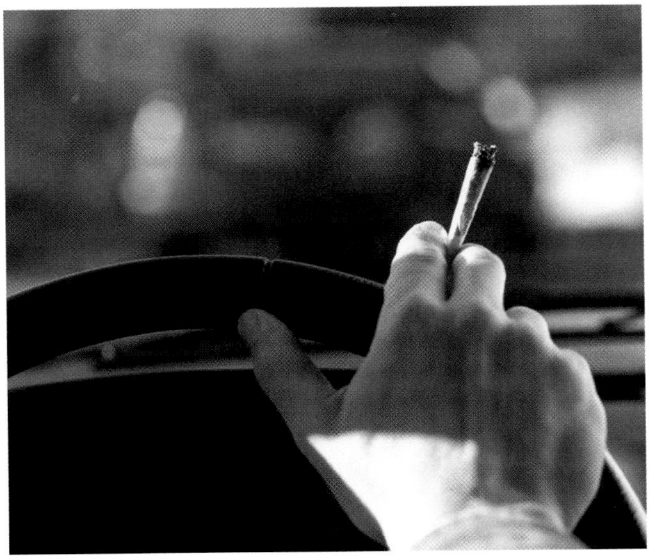

Oliver DIGOIT/Alamy

All psychoactive drugs affect driving ability. For instance, marijuana decreases the ability to stay in the lane through curves and to brake quickly, and it slows thinking and reflexes.

Common Drugs of Abuse

Table 11-2 describes the common drugs of abuse within these categories: cannabis, "club drugs," stimulants, depressants, hallucinogens, and inhalants.

Cannabis

Marijuana (pot) and **hashish** (hash)—the most widely used illegal drugs—are derived from the cannabis plant. The major psychoactive ingredient in both is *THC*

intoxication Maladaptive behavioral, psychological, and physiologic changes that occur as a result of substance abuse.

withdrawal Development of symptoms that cause significant psychological and physical distress when an individual reduces or stops drug use.

polyabuse The misuse or abuse of more than one drug.

marijuana The drug derived from the cannabis plant, containing the psychoactive ingredient THC, which causes a mild sense of euphoria when inhaled or eaten.

hashish A concentrated form of a drug, derived from the cannabis plant, containing the psychoactive ingredient TCH, which causes a sense of euphoria when inhaled or eaten.

TABLE 11-2 Commonly Abused Drugs

Drug	Street Names	How It's Used	Intoxication Effects / Potential Health Consequences
Cannabis			
Marijuana	Pot, grass, reefer, weed, blunt, dope, ganja, grass, herb, joints, Mary Jane, sinsemilla, skunk	Smoked, swallowed	Euphoria, slowed thinking and reaction time, confusion, impaired balance and coordination / Cough, frequent respiratory infections; impaired memory and learning; increased heart rate, anxiety; panic attacks; tolerance, addiction
Club Drugs			
MDMA	Ecstasy, E, Eve, X, XTC, clarity, lover's speed, peace, STP	Swallowed	Mild hallucinogenic effects, increased tactile sensitivity, empathic feelings / Impaired memory and learning, hyperthermia, cardiac toxicity, renal failure, liver toxicity
GHB	G, Georgia home boy, grievous bodily harm, liquid ecstasy	Swallowed	Reduced anxiety, feeling of well-being, lowered inhibitions, slowed pulse and breathing, lowered blood pressure, poor concentration / Fatigue; confusion; impaired coordination, memory, judgment; addiction, drowsiness, nausea/vomiting, headache, loss of consciousness, loss of reflexes, seizures, coma, death
Ketamine	Cat, Valiums, K, Special-K, vitamin K	Injected, snorted, smoked	Increased heart rate and blood pressure, impaired motor function / Memory loss; numbness; nausea/vomiting; at high doses, delirium, depression, respiratory depression, and arrest
Nitrites	Poppers	Inhaled	Stimulation, loss of inhibition; headache; nausea/vomiting; slurred speech; loss of motor coordination; wheezing / Unconsciousness, cramps, weight loss, muscle weakness, depression, memory impairment, damage to cardiovascular and nervous systems, sudden death
Stimulants			Increased heart rate, blood pressure, metabolism; feelings of exhilaration, energy, increased mental alertness / Rapid or irregular heart beat; reduced appetite, weight loss, heart failure, nervousness, insomnia
Amphetamine	Bennies, black beauties, crosses, hearts, LA turnaround, speed, truck drivers, uppers	Injected, swallowed, smoked, snorted	In addition to preceding: Rapid breathing / Tremor, loss of coordination; irritability, anxiousness, restlessness, delirium, panic, paranoia, impulsive behavior, aggressiveness, tolerance, addiction, psychosis
Methamphetamine	Chalk, crank, crystal, fire, glass, go fast, ice, meth, speed	Injected, swallowed, smoked, snorted	In addition to preceding: Aggression, violence, psychotic behavior / Memory loss, cardiac and neurological damage; impaired memory and learning, tolerance, addiction
Cocaine	Blow, bump, C, candy, Charlie, coke, crack, flake, rock, snow, toot	Injected, smoked, snorted	In addition to preceding: Increased temperature / Chest pain, respiratory failure, nausea, abdominal pain, strokes, seizures, headaches, malnutrition, panic attacks
Depressants			Reduced anxiety; feeling of well-being; lowered inhibitions; slowed pulse and breathing; lowered blood pressure; poor concentration / Fatigue; confusion; impaired coordination, memory, judgment; addiction; respiratory depression and arrest, death
Benzodiazepines	Candy, downers, sleeping pills, tranks	Swallowed, injected	In addition to preceding: Sedation, drowsiness / Dizziness

TABLE 11-2 (*continued*)

Drug	Street Names	How It's Used	Intoxication Effects / Potential Health Consequences
Rohypnol	Forget-me pill, Mexican Valium, R2, Roche, roofies, roofinol, rope, rophies	Swallowed, snorted	Visual and gastrointestinal disturbances, urinary retention, memory loss for the time under the drug's effects
Barbiturates	Barbs, reds, red birds, phennies, tooies, yellows, yellow jackets	Injected, swallowed	In addition to preceding: Sedation, drowsiness / Depression, unusual excitement, fever, irritability, poor judgment, slurred speech, dizziness, life-threatening withdrawal
Opioids			Pain relief, euphoria, drowsiness / Nausea, constipation, confusion, sedation, respiratory depression and arrest, tolerance, addiction, unconsciousness, coma, death
Heroin	Brown sugar, dope, H, horse, junk, skag, skunk, smack, white horse	Injected, smoked, snorted	
Morphine	Miss Emma, monkey, white stuff	Injected, swallowed, smoked	
Codeine	Captain Cody, Cody, schoolboy	Injected, swallowed	
OxyContin	Oxy, OC, Killer	Swallowed, snorted, injected	
Vicodin	Vike, Watson-387	Swallowed	
Hallucinogens			Altered states of perception and feeling / Nausea; persisting perception disorder (flashbacks)
LSD	Acid, blotter, boomers, cubes, microdot, yellow sunshines	Swallowed, absorbed through mouth tissues	In addition to preceding: Increased body temperature, heart rate, blood pressure; loss of appetite, sleeplessness, numbness, weakness, tremors, persistent mental disorders
PCP	Angel dust, boat, hog, love boat, peace pill	Injected, swallowed, smoked	Impaired motor function, possible decrease in blood pressure and heart rate, panic, aggression, violence / Memory loss; numbness, nausea/vomiting, loss of appetite, depression
Inhalants			
Solvents (paint thinners, gasoline, glues) Gases (butane, propane, aerosol propellants, nitrous oxide)		Inhaled through nose or mouth	Stimulation, loss of inhibition; headache; nausea/vomiting; slurred speech, loss of motor coordination; wheezing / Unconsciousness, cramps, weight loss, muscle weakness, depression, memory impairment, damage to cardiovascular and nervous systems, sudden death

Source: National Institute on Drug Abuse, www.nida.nih.gov/DrugPages/DrugsofAbuse.html

(delta-9-tetrahydrocannabinol). Marijuana is the most widely abused substance, with more than 150 million people reporting they've used it at least once in the last year. Some 12 million Americans use cannabis; more than 1 million cannot control this use.

Teens and young adults who use marijuana are more likely to develop serious mental health problems. According to the National Survey on Drug Use and Health, among individuals age 18 years or older, those who first used marijuana before age 12 were twice as likely to have a serious mental illness as those who first used marijuana at age 18 or older.[23]

Marijuana use is generally less pervasive than binge drinking (see Chapter 12) on most campuses, although at some schools as many as a third of students report smoking pot. Students who used marijuana in high school are more likely to do so in college. Roommates have very little impact on drug use. Men who have not used marijuana before college seem, if anything, turned off rather than turned on by roommates who have smoked pot. Peers have no clear impact on women's marijuana use.

Different types of marijuana have different percentages of THC. Because of careful cultivation, the strength of today's marijuana is much greater than that used in the 1970s. Today a marijuana joint contains 150 mg of THC, compared to 10 mg in the 1960s. Usually, marijuana is smoked in a joint (hand-rolled cigarette) or pipe; it may also be eaten as an ingredient in other foods (as when baked in brownies), though with a less predictable effect.

Marijuana has shown some medical benefits, including boosting appetite in patients who are HIV-positive or undergoing chemotherapy, alleviating cancer and neck pain, reducing pressure on the eyeball in glaucoma patients, and helping people with spasticity (extreme muscle tension) due to multiple sclerosis or injuries.

A growing number of states have passed voter referenda (or legislative actions) making marijuana to smoke available for a variety of medical conditions upon a doctor's recommendation. However, the FDA, after a comprehensive investigation, concluded that "no sound scientific studies supported medical use of marijuana for treatment in the United States, and no animal or human data supported the safety or efficacy of marijuana for general medical use." FDA-approved medications are available as treatment alternatives for many of the proposed uses of smoked marijuana, such as relief of nausea and vomiting induced by chemotherapy. Synthetic versions of the active ingredient in marijuana, developed for medical use, act on the brain like the THC in smoked marijuana but eliminate the need to inhale harmful smoke.[24]

Advocates for the legalization of marijuana contend that making pot legal would reduce the black market and violence associated with its sale and ensure its availability for medicinal purposes. Opponents argue that legalization would increase the number of people who use marijuana and suffer harmful effects such as slowed brain function and lung damage. Should marijuana possession remain a criminal offense? Or should individuals have the right to choose to use this drug?

You decide.

How Users Feel

The circumstances in which marijuana is smoked, the communal aspects of its use, and the user's experience all can affect the way a marijuana-induced high feels.

In low to moderate doses, marijuana typically creates a mild sense of euphoria, a sense of slowed time (five minutes may feel like an hour), a dreamy sort of self-absorption, and some impairment in thinking and communicating. Users report heightened sensations of color, sound, and other stimuli, relaxation, and increased confidence. The sense of being stoned peaks within half an hour and usually lasts about three hours. Even when alterations in perception seem slight, it is not safe to drive a car for as long as four to six hours after smoking a single joint.

Some users—particularly those smoking marijuana for the first time or taking a high dose in an unpleasant or unfamiliar setting—experience acute anxiety, which may be accompanied by a panicky fear of losing control. They may believe that their companions are ridiculing or threatening them and experience a panic attack, a state of intense terror.

The immediate physical effects of marijuana include increased pulse rate, bloodshot eyes, dry mouth and throat, slowed reaction times, impaired motor skills, increased appetite, and diminished short-term memory (Figure 11-2). High doses reduce the ability to perceive and to react; all the reactions experienced with low doses are intensified, leading to sensory distortion and, in the case of hashish, vivid hallucinations and LSD-like, psychedelic reactions. The drug remains in the body's fat cells 50 hours or more after use, so people may experience psychoactive effects for several days after use. Drug tests may produce positive results for days or weeks after last use.

Risks

Marijuana produces a range of effects in different bodily systems, such as depression, diminished immune responses, and impaired fertility in men. Other risks include damage to the brain, lungs, and heart and to babies born to mothers who use marijuana during pregnancy or while nursing (see Figure 11-2).

Brain THC produces changes in the brain that affect learning, memory, and the way the brain integrates sensory experiences with emotions and motivations. Short-term effects include problems with memory and learning; distorted perceptions; difficulty thinking and problem solving; loss of coordination; increased anxiety; and panic attacks. Long-term use produces changes in the brain similar to those seen with other major drugs of abuse. Long-term heavy users of marijuana perform significantly worse on tests of verbal fluency, memory, and coordination than short-term users or non-users, even after abstaining from pot for more than 24 hours.[25]

Over time, continued heavy marijuana use can interfere with students' ability to learn and perform well in school and in challenging careers. Marijuana contributes significantly to accidental death and injury among adolescents, especially through motor vehicle crashes.

Lungs Smoking cannabis may cause similar effects to smoking tobacco, with many of them appearing at a younger age. They include chronic bronchitis, emphysema, and other lung disorders and increased risk of heart attacks and sudden death. The amount of tar inhaled by marijuana smokers and the level of carbon monoxide absorbed are three to five times greater than among tobacco smokers. The reasons may be that marijuana users inhale more deeply, hold the smoke in the lungs longer, and do not use filters. Smoking a single joint can be as damaging to the lungs as smoking five tobacco cigarettes. Someone who smokes five joints a week may take in as many cancer-causing chemicals as a person who smokes a pack of cigarettes a day.

Heart Otherwise healthy people have suffered heart attacks shortly after smoking marijuana. Experiments

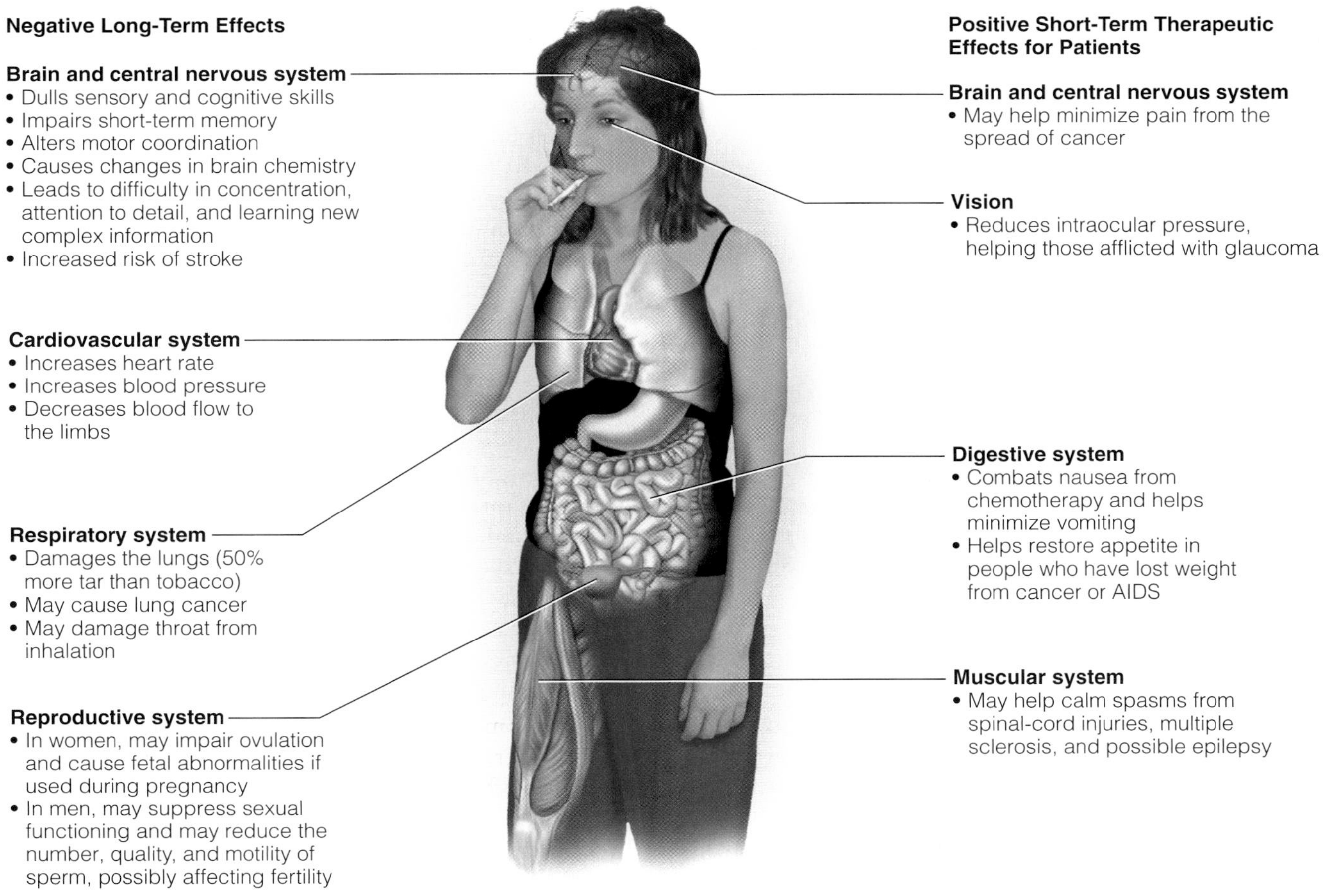
Negative Long-Term Effects
Brain and central nervous system
• Dulls sensory and cognitive skills
• Impairs short-term memory
• Alters motor coordination
• Causes changes in brain chemistry
• Leads to difficulty in concentration, attention to detail, and learning new complex information
• Increased risk of stroke
Cardiovascular system
• Increases heart rate
• Increases blood pressure
• Decreases blood flow to the limbs
Respiratory system
• Damages the lungs (50% more tar than tobacco)
• May cause lung cancer
• May damage throat from inhalation
Reproductive system
• In women, may impair ovulation and cause fetal abnormalities if used during pregnancy
• In men, may suppress sexual functioning and may reduce the number, quality, and motility of sperm, possibly affecting fertility
Positive Short-Term Therapeutic Effects for Patients
Brain and central nervous system
• May help minimize pain from the spread of cancer
Vision
• Reduces intraocular pressure, helping those afflicted with glaucoma
Digestive system
• Combats nausea from chemotherapy and helps minimize vomiting
• Helps restore appetite in people who have lost weight from cancer or AIDS
Muscular system
• May help calm spasms from spinal-cord injuries, multiple sclerosis, and possible epilepsy

FIGURE 11-2 Impact of Marijuana
Marijuana may have positive short-term therapeutic effects for people with cancer, glaucoma, or AIDS, but the long-term effects for healthy users are all negative.

have also linked marijuana use to elevated blood pressure and decreased oxygen supply to the heart muscle. The risk of heart attack triples within an hour of smoking pot. Smoking marijuana while shooting cocaine can potentially cause deadly increases in heart rate and blood pressure.

Pregnancy Babies born to mothers who use marijuana during pregnancy are smaller than those born to mothers who did not use the drug, and the babies are more likely to develop health problems. A nursing mother who uses marijuana passes some of the THC to the baby in her breast milk. This may impair the infant's motor development (control of muscle movement).

Withdrawal

Marijuana users can develop a compulsive, often uncontrollable craving for the drug. More than 120,000 people enter treatment every year for marijuana addiction. In addition, animal studies suggest that marijuana causes physical dependence. Stopping after long-term marijuana use can produce *marijuana withdrawal syndrome,* which is characterized by insomnia, restlessness, loss of appetite, and irritability. People who smoke marijuana daily for many years may become aggressive after they stop using it and may relapse to prevent aggression and other symptoms.

Club Drugs (Designer Drugs)

The National Institute on Drug Abuse identifies a variety of drugs—alcohol, LSD (acid), MDMA (ecstasy), GHB, GBL, ketamine (Special-K), fentanyl, Rohypnol, and nitrites—as **"club drugs."** They first became popular among teens and young adults at nightclubs, bars, or raves and trances—night-long dances often held in warehouses or other unusual settings. Their use by teenagers has been dropping in recent years.

Young people may take club drugs to relax, energize, and enhance their social interactions, but a large number also experience negative consequences. As many as three

club drugs Illegally manufactured psychoactive drugs that have dangerous physical and psychological effects.

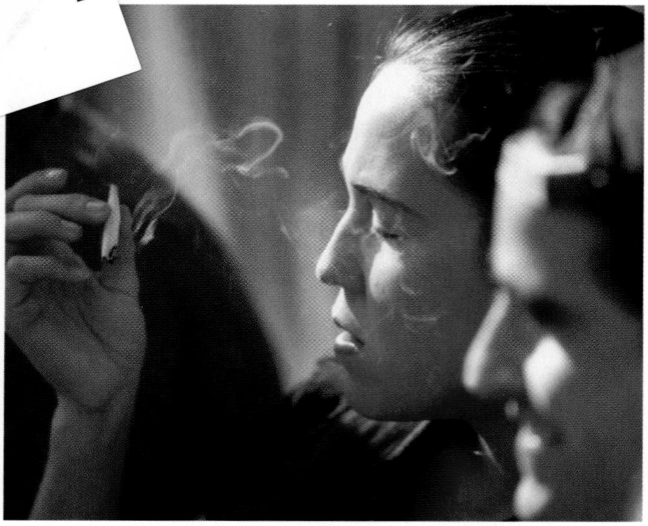

© Tom & Dee Ann McCarthy/CORBIS

Marijuana and other drugs of abuse can produce physical and psychological effects.

in four report side effects such as profuse sweating, hot and cold flashes, tingling or numbness, blurred vision, trouble sleeping, hallucinations, depression, confusion, anxiety, irritability, paranoia, and loss of libido (sex drive). Some also experience difficulty with their usual daily activities and financial and work troubles.

Ecstasy

Ecstasy (E, XTC, X, hug, beans, love drug) is the most common street name for methylenedioxymethamphetamine (MDMA), a synthetic compound with both stimulant and mildly hallucinogenic properties.

According to various studies, students who take ecstasy were more likely to use marijuana, binge-drink, smoke cigarettes, have multiple sexual partners, spend more time socializing with friends and less time studying, and consider parties important and religion as less important. However, researchers who compared students who used ecstasy and other illicit drugs with those who used only marijuana have concluded that undergraduates who use ecstasy may be a subgroup of marijuana users who tend to engage in many risk-taking behaviors. Ecstasy users also think that their peers smoke more marijuana and use more ecstasy than they actually do.

How It Feels Although it can be smoked, inhaled (snorted), or injected, ecstasy is almost always taken as a pill or tablet. Its effects begin in 45 minutes and last for two to four hours.

MDMA belongs to a family of drugs called *enactogens,* which literally means "touching within." As a mood elevator, it produces a relaxed, euphoric state but does not produce hallucinations. Users of ecstasy often say they feel at peace with themselves and a sense of connectedness with others. In some settings, they reveal intimate details of their lives (which they may later regret); in other settings, they join in collective rejoicing. Like hallucinogenic drugs, MDMA can enhance sensory experience, but it rarely causes visual distortions, sudden mood changes, or psychotic reactions. Regular users may experience depression and anxiety the week after taking MDMA.

Risks Ecstasy poses risks similar to those of cocaine and amphetamines. These include psychological difficulties (confusion, depression, sleep problems, drug craving, severe anxiety, and paranoia) and physical symptoms (muscle tension, involuntary teeth clenching, nausea, blurred vision, rapid eye movement, faintness, chills, sweating, and increases in heart rate and blood pressure that pose a special risk for people with circulatory or heart disease).

Ecstasy can produce nausea, vomiting, and dizziness. When combined with extended physical exertion like dancing, club drugs can lead to hyperthermia (severe overheating), severe dehydration, serious increases in blood pressure, stroke, and heart attack. Without sufficient water, dancers at raves may suffer dehydration and heat stroke, which can be fatal. Individuals with high blood pressure, heart trouble, or liver or kidney disease are in the greatest danger. Several deaths have occurred in teens who suffered brain damage by drinking large amounts of water to counteract the raised body temperature induced by the drug.

MDMA has been implicated in some cases of acute hepatitis, which can lead to liver failure. Even after liver transplantation, the mortality rate for individuals with this condition is 50 percent. Another danger comes from the practice of taking SSRIs (see Chapter 2), which modulate the mood-altering brain chemical serotonin, before ecstasy. This can cause jaw clenching, nausea, tremors, and in extreme cases, potentially fatal elevations in body temperature.

Although not a sexual stimulant (if anything, MDMA has the opposite effect), ecstasy fosters strong feelings of intimacy that may lead to risky sexual behavior. The psychological effects of ecstasy become less intriguing with repeated use, and the physical side effects become more uncomfortable. Ecstasy poses risks to a developing fetus, including a greater likelihood of heart and skeletal abnormalities and long-term learning and memory impairments in children born to women who used MDMA during pregnancy.

Because ecstasy is *neurotoxic* (damaging to brain cells), it depletes the brain of serotonin, a messenger chemical involved with mood, sleep, and appetite, and can lead to depression, anxiety, and impaired thinking and memory. Even short-term use of ecstasy can have long-term neurological consequences that may affect memory and the brain's ability to perform complex thought processes.[26]

According to brain-imaging studies, users, although as mentally alert as nonusers, fared far worse on measures of memory, learning, and general intelligence. The more frequently they took ecstasy, the worse they did, probably because ecstasy alters neuronal function in a brain structure called the hippocampus, which helps create short-term memory. The effect on memory persists for years after discontinuing use.

GHB and GBL

Once sold in health food stores for its muscle-building and alleged fat-burning properties, **gammahydroxybutyrate** (**GHB,** G, Georgia home boy) was banned because of its effects on the brain and nervous system. The main ingredient is **GBL (gamma butyrolactone),** an industrial solvent often used to strip floors. Once ingested, GBL converts into GHB, an odorless, colorless sedative that can be slipped into a beverage to knock an individual out. Once taken, GHB acts as a sedative while producing feelings of euphoria and heightened sexuality. Because of its amnesic properties, GHB has been used as a "date rape" drug, similar to Rohypnol. Alcohol intensifies its effects.

Larger doses can cause someone to pass out in 15 minutes and fall into a coma within half an hour. Other side effects include nausea, amnesia, hallucinations, decreased heart rate, convulsions, and sometimes blackouts. Long-term use at high doses can lead to a withdrawal reaction: rapid heartbeat, tremor, insomnia, anxiety, and occasionally hallucinations that last a few days to a week.

GHB is addictive. Users who attempt to quit may experience significant withdrawal symptoms, including anxiety, tremors, and insomnia. Most symptoms decrease within one to two weeks of cessation, but severe psychological effects can last for weeks to months.

Ketamine

Ketamine—called K, Special-K, and Vitamin K—is an anesthetic used by veterinarians. When cooked, dried, and ground into a powder for snorting, K blocks chemical messengers in the brain that carry sensory input. As a result, the brain fills the void with hallucinations. Users may report an "out-of-body" experience with distorted perceptions of time and space. The effects typically begin within 30 minutes and last for approximately two hours.

Ketamine has become common in club and rave scenes and has been used as a date rape drug. It can cause anxiety, agitation, paranoia, and vomiting. Higher doses can cause lethal breathing impairments, stroke, and heart attack. Repeated ketamine use can be addictive and even a single use can occasionally produce audiovisual "flashbacks," similar to those described by phencyclidine (PCP) users, and long-term memory loss.

Nitrites

Nitrites (amyl, butyl, and isobutyl nitrite) are clear, amber-colored liquids that have had a history of abuse for more than three decades, especially in gay and bisexual men. Popular in dance clubs, they are used recreationally for a high feeling, a slowed sense of time, a carefree sense of well-being, and intensified sexual experiences.

Sold in small glass ampules containing individual doses, nitrites are usually inhaled and rapidly absorbed into the bloodstream. Users feel their physiological and psychological impact in seconds. Acute adverse effects include headache, dizziness, a drop in blood pressure, changes in heart rate, increased pressure within the eye, and skin flushing. Some individuals develop respiratory irritation and cough, sneezing, or difficulty breathing. Chronic use can lead to crusty skin lesions and chemical burns around the nose, mouth, and lips.

Herbal Ecstasy

Herbal ecstasy, also known as herbal bliss, cloud 9, and herbal X, is a mixture of stimulants such as ephedrine, pseudoephedrine, and caffeine. Sold in tablet or capsule form as a "natural" and safe alternative to ecstasy, its ingredients vary greatly. Herbal ecstasy can have dangerous and unpleasant side effects, including stroke, heart attack, and a disfiguring skin condition.

Stimulants

Central nervous system **stimulants** are drugs that increase activity in some portion of the brain or spinal cord. Some stimulants increase motor activity and enhance mental alertness, and some combat mental fatigue. Amphetamine, methamphetamine, caffeine,

ecstasy (MDMA) A synthetic compound, also known as methylenedioxymethamphetamine, that is similar in structure to methamphetamine and has both stimulant and hallucinogenic effects.

GHB gamma hydroxybutyrate A brain messenger chemical that stimulates the release of human growth hormone; commonly abused for its high and its alleged ability to trim fat and build muscles. Also known as "blue nitro" or the "date rape drug."

GBL gamma butyrolactone The main ingredient in gamma hydroxybutyrate (GHB), also known as the "date rape drug"; once ingested, GBL converts to GHB and can cause the ingestor to lose consciousness.

stimulant An agent, such as a drug, that temporarily relieves drowsiness, helps in the performance of repetitive tasks, and improves capacity for work.

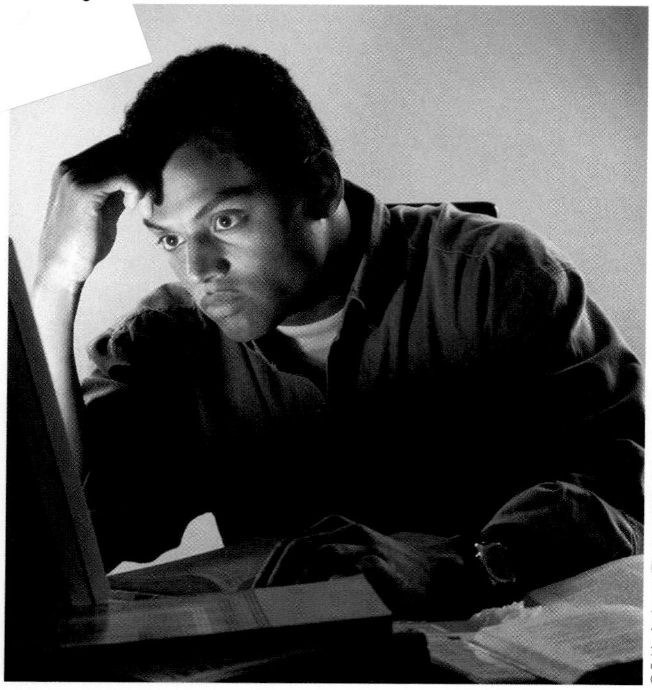

Some college students try stimulants to stay alert while cramming for exams, but these medications do not improve academic performance and cause harmful side effects.

cocaine, and khat are stimulants. Stimulant medications are used to treat conditions such as ADHD.

Abuse of Prescription Stimulants on Campus

The most widely abused prescription drugs are stimulant medications, such as Ritalin, which are prescribed for attention deficit disorders (discussed in Chapter 2). Although medical use of this agent appears safe, misuse or abuse of any stimulant medication can be dangerous, even deadly. When taken in high doses, either orally or nasally, the risk of addiction increases. Physical side effects include cardiovascular complications, increased blood pressure, and headache. High doses can trigger panic attacks, aggressive behavior, and suicidal or homicidal impulses. Overdoses can kill.[27]

In a recent survey at a northeastern university, 16 percent of students—about equal numbers of men and women—reported misuse or abuse of stimulants. About half used the drugs two or three times a year; a third took them two or three times a month. About 69 percent of the students said they took stimulants to improve attention, usually when staying up to write a paper or prepare for exams. Almost as many—65 percent—did so for the sake of partying. Most swallowed pills, but a high percentage reported snorting the drug. The majority expressed little concern about the potential negative effects of stimulants.[28]

Amphetamine

Amphetamines trigger the release of epinephrine (adrenaline), which stimulates the central nervous system. They were once widely prescribed for weight control because they suppress appetite, but they have emerged as a global danger. Amphetamines are sold under a variety of names: amphetamine (brand name Benzedrine, street-name bennies), dextroamphetamine (Dexedrine, dex), methamphetamine (Methedrine, meth, speed, crank), and Desoxyn (copilots). Related *uppers* include the prescription drugs methylphenidate (Ritalin), pemoline (Cylert), and phenmetrazine (Preludin). Amphetamines are available in tablet or capsule form.

How Users Feel Amphetamines produce a state of hyper-alertness and energy. Users feel confident in their ability to think clearly and to perform any task exceptionally well—although amphetamines do not, in fact, significantly boost performance or thinking. Higher doses make users feel *wired:* talkative, excited, restless, irritable, anxious, moody.

If taken intravenously, amphetamines produce a characteristic rush of elation and confidence, as well as adverse effects, including confusion, rambling or incoherent speech, anxiety, headache, and palpitations. Individuals may become paranoid; be convinced they are having profound thoughts; feel increased sexual interest; and experience unusual perceptions, such as ringing in the ears, a sensation of insects crawling on their skin, or hearing their name called. Methamphetamine users may feel high and sleepy or may hallucinate and lose contact with reality.

Risks Dependence on amphetamines can develop with episodic or daily use. Bingeing—taking high doses over a period of several days—can lead to an extremely intense and unpleasant *crash,* characterized by a craving for the drug, shakiness, irritability, anxiety, and depression. Two or more days are required for recuperation.

Amphetamine intoxication may cause the following symptoms:

- **Feelings of grandiosity,** anxiety, tension, hypervigilance, anger, social hypersensitivity, fighting, jitteriness or agitation, paranoia, and impaired judgment in social or occupational functioning.
- **Increased heart rate,** dilated pupils, elevated blood pressure, perspiration or chills, and nausea or vomiting.
- **Less frequent effects such as speeding up** or slowing down of physical movement; muscular weakness; impaired breathing, chest pain, heart arrhythmia; confusion, seizures, impaired movements or muscle tone; or even coma.
- **In high doses, a rapid or irregular heartbeat,** tremors, loss of coordination, and collapse.

The long-term effects of amphetamine abuse include malnutrition, skin disorders, ulcers, insomnia, depression, vitamin deficiencies, and in some cases, brain damage that results in speech and thought disturbances. Sexual dysfunction and impaired concentration or memory also may occur.

Withdrawal When the immediate effects of amphetamines wear off, users experience a *crash* and become shaky, irritable, anxious, and depressed. Amphetamine withdrawal usually persists for more than 24 hours after cessation of prolonged, heavy use. Its characteristic features include fatigue, disturbing dreams, much more or less than usual sleep, increased appetite, and speeding up or slowing down of physical movements. Those who are unable to sleep despite their exhaustion often take sedative-hypnotics (discussed later in this chapter) to help them rest and may then become dependent on them in addition to amphetamines. Symptoms usually reach a peak in two to four days, although depression and irritability may persist for months. Suicide is a major risk.

Methamphetamine

Methamphetamine, an addictive stimulant that is less expensive and possibly more addictive than cocaine or heroin, has become America's leading drug problem. More than 12 million Americans have tried methamphetamine, and 1.5 million are regular users, according to federal estimates.[29]

Methamphetamine is chemically related to amphetamine, but its effects on the central nervous system are greater. Made in illegal laboratories, street methamphetamine is referred to by many names, such as speed, meth, and chalk. Methamphetamine hydrochloride, clear chunky crystals resembling ice that can be inhaled by smoking, is called ice, crystal, glass, and tina. Methamphetamine can be snorted, smoked, or injected.

How Users Feel Methamphetamine causes the release of large amounts of dopamine, which creates a sensation of euphoria, increased self-esteem, and alertness. Users also report a marked increase in sexual appetite, which often leads to risky sexual behaviors while under the drug's influence.

Smoking or intravenous injection leads to an intense, pleasurable sensation, called a rush or flash, that lasts only a few minutes. Oral or intranasal use produces a high but not a rush. Users may become addicted quickly, using more methamphetamine more and more frequently. Despair and suicidal thinking can develop when the stimulant effect wears off.

Risks Even small amounts of methamphetamine can increase wakefulness and physical activity, depress appetite, and raise body temperature. Other effects on the central nervous system include irritability, insomnia,

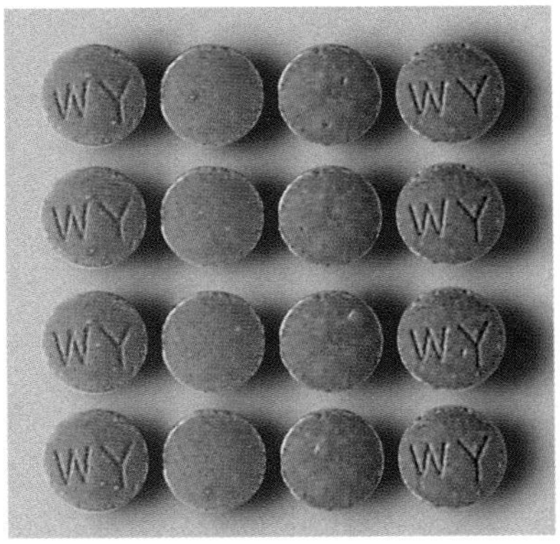

DEA/Office of Forensic Sciences

Ya-ba/Thai Tabs are a powerful form of methamphetamine that tastes sweet like candy.

confusion, tremors, convulsions, anxiety, paranoia, and aggressiveness.

Methamphetamine increases heart rate and blood pressure and can cause irreversible damage to blood vessels in the brain, producing strokes. Other effects of methamphetamine include respiratory problems, irregular heartbeat, and extreme loss of appetite and weight. During intoxication, the body (and probably brain) temperature rises, sometimes resulting in convulsions. High fevers or collapse of the circulatory system can cause death.

Common psychiatric symptoms are insomnia, irritability, and aggressive behavior. The drug causes intellectual impairment, anxiety, and depression. Chronic users become disorganized and unable to cope with everyday problems. The risk of developing psychotic symptoms—hallucinations and delusions—is very high. They may persist for months or years after use stops.[30]

Another side effect is called meth mouth. In short periods of time, sometimes just months, teeth can turn a grayish-brown, twist, begin to fall out, and take on a peculiar texture. This may be the result of methamphetamine's effects on the metabolic system, plus the huge quantities of sugary soft drinks that users consume for the dry mouth caused by the drug.[31]

Meth users engage in more sex, more carelessly. Meth has become popular among gay and bisexual men, and it has been linked to an increase in unsafe sex practices. Methamphetamine use and needle sharing has been linked to a spike in HIV and hepatitis C infections in gay communities.

Methamphetamine causes abnormalities in brain regions associated with selective attention and in those associated with memory. The brain may recover somewhat after months of abstinence, but

amphetamine Any of a class of stimulants that trigger the release of epinephrine, which stimulates the central nervous system; users experience a state of hyperalertness and energy, followed by a crash as the drug wears off.

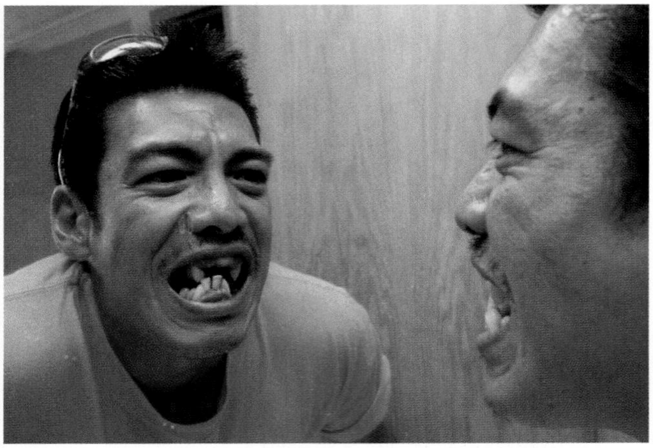

In addition to respiratory damage, brain damage, and mental impairment, methamphetamine turns users' teeth from white to grayish-brown. This is how "meth mouth" looks.

problems often remain. Former methamphetamine addicts may suffer from chronic apathy and anhedonia (inability to experience pleasure) for years.

The Toll on Society Law enforcement officials consider methamphetamine their biggest drug problem. Meth-related arrests have soared. Meth addicts are pouring into prisons and recovery centers at an ever-increasing rate. "Meth babies" are crowding the foster-care system. Meth-making operations have been uncovered in all 50 states, with the greatest number in Missouri. Production releases poisonous gases and results in toxic waste that is often dumped down household drains, in a backyard, or at a roadside. The cost of cleaning up the environment is a growing problem for many communities.

Over-the-counter cold medicines (ephedrine and pseudoephedrine) are commonly used in meth production, which is one reason for federal and state restrictions on their sale. As drug stores and retailers have placed nonprescription cold pills behind the pharmacy counter, meth manufacturing has moved into Mexico, where labs produce hundreds of pounds of meth a year and smuggle it into the United States.

Withdrawal Methamphetamine addiction is difficult to treat. As with cocaine, coming off methamphetamine causes intense distress, so users often seek out the drug to relieve their pain. Treatment usually requires the intervention of the patient's family as well as a substance abuse specialist team experienced in treating methamphetamine addiction. Standard substance abuse treatment methods such as education, behavior therapy, individual and family counseling, and support groups may be effective for some. Methamphetamine abusers often use other illicit drugs as well, a problem that can be addressed as part of a comprehensive program.

Cocaine

Cocaine (coke, snow, lady) is a white crystalline powder extracted from the leaves of the South American coca plant. Usually mixed with various sugars and local anesthetics like lidocaine and procaine, cocaine powder is generally inhaled. When sniffed or snorted, cocaine anesthetizes the nerve endings in the nose and relaxes the lung's bronchial muscles.

Cocaine can be dissolved in water and injected intravenously. The drug is rapidly metabolized by the liver, so the high is relatively brief, typically lasting only about 20 minutes. This means that users will commonly inject the drug repeatedly, increasing the risk of infection and damage to their veins.

Cocaine alkaloid, or *freebase,* is obtained by removing the hydrochloride salt from cocaine powder. *Freebasing* is smoking the fumes of the alkaloid form of cocaine. *Crack,* pharmacologically identical to freebase, is a cheap, easy-to-use, widely available, smokeable, and potent form of cocaine named for the popping sound it makes when burned. Because it is absorbed rapidly into the bloodstream and large doses reach the brain very quickly, it is particularly dangerous. However, its low price and easy availability have made it a common drug of abuse in poor urban areas.

How Users Feel A powerful stimulant to the central nervous system, cocaine targets several chemical sites in the brain, producing feelings of soaring well-being and boundless energy. Users feel they have enormous physical and mental ability, yet are also restless and anxious. After a brief period of euphoria, users slump into a depression. They often go on cocaine binges, lasting from a few hours to several days, and consume large quantities of cocaine.

With crack, dependence develops quickly. As soon as crack users come down from one high, they want more crack. Whereas heroin addicts may shoot up several times a day, crack addicts need another hit within minutes. Thus, a crack habit can quickly become more expensive than heroin addiction.

Risks Cocaine dependence is an easy habit to acquire. With repeated use, the brain becomes tolerant of the drug's stimulant effects, and users must take more of it to get high. Those who smoke or inject cocaine can develop dependence within weeks. Those who sniff cocaine may not become dependent on the drug for months or years. It is thought that 5 to 20 percent of all coke users—a group as large as the estimated total number of heroin addicts—are dependent on the drug.

The physical effects of acute cocaine intoxication include dilated pupils, elevated or lowered blood pressure, perspiration or chills, nausea or vomiting, speeding up or slowing down of physical activity, muscular weakness, impaired breathing, chest pain, and impaired movements or muscle tone. Prolonged cocaine snorting can result in ulceration of the mucous membrane of the nose and damage to the nasal septum (the membrane between the nostrils) severe enough to cause it to collapse.

Although some users initially try cocaine as a sexual stimulant, it does not enhance sexual performance. At low doses, it may delay orgasm and cause heightened sensory awareness, but men who use cocaine regularly have problems maintaining erections and ejaculating. They also tend to have low sperm counts, less active sperm, and more abnormal sperm than nonusers. Both male and female chronic cocaine users tend to lose interest in sex and have difficulty reaching orgasm.

Cocaine use can cause blood vessels in the brain to clamp shut and can trigger a stroke, bleeding in the brain, and potentially fatal brain seizures. Cocaine users can also develop psychiatric or neurological complications (Figure 11-3). Repeated or high doses of cocaine can lead to impaired judgment, hyperactivity, nonstop babbling, feelings of suspicion and paranoia, and violent behavior. The brain never learns to tolerate cocaine's negative effects; users may become incoherent and paranoid and may experience unusual sensations, such as ringing in their ears, feeling insects crawling on the skin, or hearing their name called.

Cocaine can damage the liver and cause lung damage in freebasers. Smoking crack causes bronchitis as well as lung damage and may promote the transmission of HIV through burned and bleeding lips. Some smokers have died of respiratory complications, such as pulmonary edema (the buildup of fluid in the lungs).

Cocaine causes the heart rate to speed up and blood pressure to rise suddenly. Its use is associated with many cardiac complications, including arrhythmia (disruption of heart rhythm), angina (chest pain), and acute myocardial infarction (heart attack).

The combination of alcohol and cocaine is particularly lethal. The liver combines the two agents and manufactures cocaethylene, which intensifies cocaine's euphoric effects, while possibly increasing the risk of sudden death. Cocaine users who inject the drug and share needles put themselves at risk for another potentially lethal problem: HIV infection.

Cocaine is dangerous for pregnant women and their babies, causing miscarriages, developmental disorders, and life-threatening complications during birth. Cocaine can reduce the fetal oxygen supply, possibly interfering with the development of the fetus's nervous system.

Withdrawal When addicted individuals stop using cocaine, they often become depressed. This may lead to further cocaine use to alleviate depression. Other symptoms of cocaine withdrawal include fatigue, vivid and disturbing dreams, excessive or too little sleep, irritability, increased appetite, and physical slowing down or speeding up. This initial crash may last one to three days after cutting down or stopping the heavy use of cocaine. Some individuals become violent, paranoid, and suicidal.

Symptoms usually reach a peak in two to four days, although depression, anxiety, irritability, lack of pleasure in usual activities, and low-level cravings may continue for weeks. As memories of the crash fade, the desire for cocaine intensifies. For many weeks after stopping, individuals may feel an intense craving for the drug.

Despite years of research, there is no drug approved in the United States for treating cocaine dependence. Some cocaine abusers fare better with cognitive-behavioral therapy (discussed in Chapter 2); others, with 12-step programs.

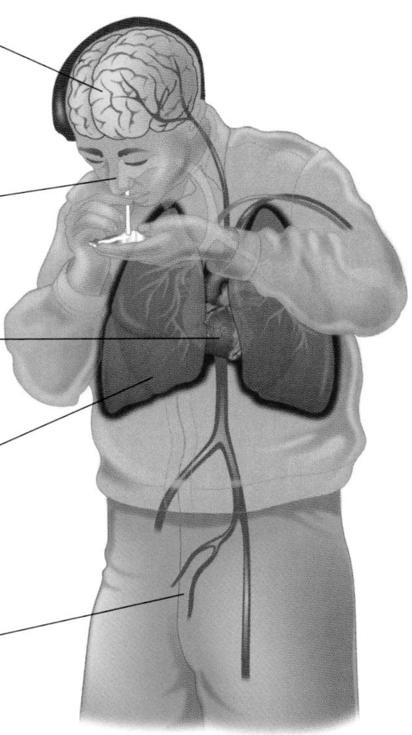
Central nervous system
• Repeated use or high dosages may cause severe psychological problems
• Suppresses desire for food, sex, and sleep
• Can cause strokes, seizures, and neurological damage
Nose
• Damages mucous membrane
Cardiovascular system
• Increases blood pressure by constricting blood vessels
• Causes irregular heartbeat
• Damages heart tissue
Respiratory system
• Freebasing causes lung damage
• Overdose can lead to respiratory arrest
Reproductive system
• In men, affects ability to maintain erections and ejaculate; also causes sperm abnormalities
• In women, may affect ability to carry pregnancy to term

FIGURE 11-3 Some Effects of Cocaine on the Body

Khat (Kat, Catha, Chat, Abyssinian Tea)

For centuries people in East Africa and the Arabian peninsula consumed the fresh young leaves of the *Catha edulis* shrub in ways similar to our drinking

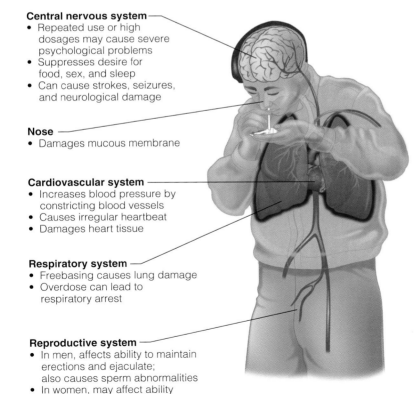

cocaine A white crystalline powder extracted from the leaves of the coca plant that stimulates the central nervous system and produces a brief period of euphoria followed by a depression.

coffee. Its active ingredients are two controlled substances, cathinone and cathine. Chewing alleviates fatigue and reduces appetite. Compulsive use may result in manic behavior, grandiose illusions, paranoia, and hallucinations.

Depressants

Depressants depress the central nervous system, reduce activity, and induce relaxation, drowsiness, or sleep. They include the benzodiazepines and the barbiturates, the opioids, and alcohol.

Benzodiazepines and Barbiturates

These depressants are the sedative-hypnotics, also known as anxiolytic or antianxiety drugs. The **benzodiazepines**—the most widely used drugs in this category—are commonly prescribed for tension, muscular strain, sleep problems, anxiety, panic attacks, anesthesia, and in the treatment of alcohol withdrawal. They include such drugs as *chlordiazepoxide* (Librium), *diazepam* (Valium), *oxazepam* (Serax), *lorazepam* (Ativan), *flurazepam* (Dalmane), and *alprazolam* (Xanax). They differ widely in their mechanism of action, absorption rate, and metabolism, but all produce similar intoxication and withdrawal symptoms.

Rohypnol, a trade name for flunitrazepam, is one of the benzodiazepines, and it has been of particular concern for the last few years because of its abuse in date rape. When mixed with alcohol, Rohypnol can incapacitate victims and prevent them from resisting sexual assault. It produces "anterograde amnesia," which means individuals may not remember events they experienced while under the effects of the drug. Rohypnol may be lethal when mixed with alcohol or other depressants.

Benzodiazepine sleeping pills have largely replaced the **barbiturates,** which were used medically in the past for inducing relaxation and sleep, relieving tension, and treating epileptic seizures. These drugs are usually taken by mouth in tablet, capsule, or liquid form. When used as a general anesthetic, they are administered intravenously.

How Users Feel Low doses of these drugs may reduce or relieve tension, but increasing doses can cause a loosening of sexual or aggressive inhibitions. Individuals using this class of drugs may experience rapid mood changes, impaired judgment, and impaired social or occupational functioning.

Risks All sedative-hypnotic drugs can produce physical and psychological dependence within two to four weeks. A complication specific to sedatives is *cross-tolerance* (cross-addiction), which occurs when users develop tolerance for one sedative or become dependent on it and develop tolerance for other sedatives as well.

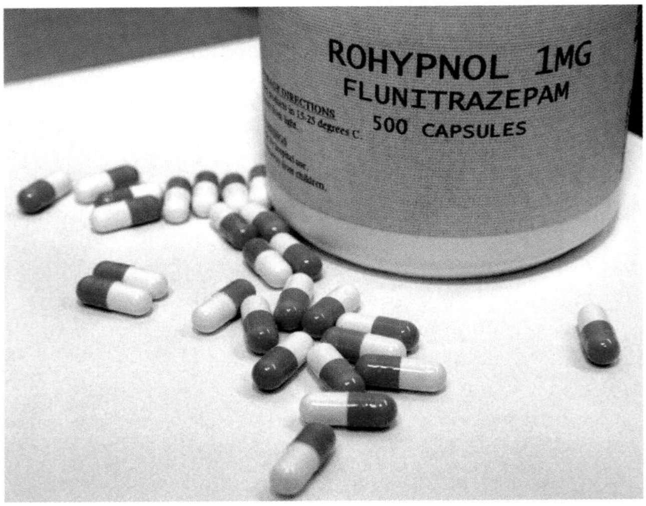

Merja OJala/AFP/Getty Images

Because Rohypnol is colorless, tasteless, and odorless, it can be added to beverages without your knowledge. Never let your drink out of your sight!

Intoxication with these drugs can produce changes in mood or behavior, such as inappropriate sexual or aggressive acts, mood swings, and impaired judgment. Physical signs include slurred speech, poor coordination, unsteady gait, involuntary eye movements, impaired attention or memory, and stupor or coma.

Taken in combination with alcohol, these drugs have a synergistic effect that can be dangerous or even lethal. For example, an individual's driving ability, already impaired by alcohol, will be made even worse, increasing the risk of an accident. Alcohol in combination with sedative-hypnotics leads to respiratory depression and may result in respiratory arrest and death. Regular users of any of these drugs who become physically dependent should not try to cut down or quit on their own. If they try to quit suddenly, they run the risk of seizures, coma, and death.

Withdrawal Withdrawal from sedative-hypnotic drugs may range from relatively mild discomfort to a severe syndrome with grand mal seizures, depending on the degree of dependence. Withdrawal symptoms include malaise or weakness, sweating, rapid pulse, coarse tremors (of the hands, tongue, or eyelids), insomnia, nausea or vomiting, temporary hallucinations or illusions, physical restlessness, anxiety or irritability, and grand mal seizures. Withdrawal may begin within two to three days after stopping drug use, and symptoms may persist for many weeks.

Opioids

The **opioids** include *opium* and its derivatives (*morphine, codeine,* and *heroin*) and synthetic drugs that have similar sleep-inducing and pain-relieving properties. The opioids come from a resin taken from the seedpod of the

Asian poppy. Synthetic opioids, such as *meperidine* (Demerol), *methadone,* and *propoxyphene* (Darvon), are synthesized in a chemical laboratory. Whether natural or synthetic, these drugs are powerful *narcotics,* or painkillers.

Heroin (also known as horse, junk, smack, or downtown), the most widely abused opioid, is illegal in this country. In other nations it is used as a potent painkiller for conditions such as terminal cancer. There are an estimated 600,000 heroin addicts in the United States, with men outnumbering women addicts by three to one. Among people aged 18 to 25, the percentage of heroin users who inject the drug has doubled in the last decade. While the number of young heroin users in major cities has dropped by 50 percent, their numbers almost tripled in suburban and rural areas.

Heroin users typically inject the drug into their veins. However, individuals who experiment with recreational drugs often prefer *skin-popping* (subcutaneous injection) rather than *mainlining* (intravenous injection); they also may snort heroin as a powder or dissolve it and inhale the vapors. To try to avoid addiction, some users begin by *chipping,* taking small or intermittent doses. Regardless of the method of administration, tolerance can develop rapidly.

Morphine, used as a painkiller and anesthetic, acts primarily on the central nervous system, eyes, and digestive tract. By producing mental clouding, drowsiness, and euphoria, it does not decrease the physical sensation of pain as much as it alters a person's awareness of the pain; in effect, he or she no longer cares about it.

Prescription Opioids

Two semisynthetic derivatives of morphine are *hydromorphone* (trade name Dilaudid, street name little D), with two to eight times the painkilling effect of morphine, and *oxycodone* (OxyContin, Percocet, Percodan, perkies), similar to codeine but more potent. The synthetic narcotic *meperidine* (Demerol, demies) is now probably second only to morphine for use in relieving pain. It is also used by addicts as a substitute for morphine or heroin.

Abuse of prescription painkillers, such as OxyContin and Vicodin, is widespread on campuses. In a survey of more than 10,000 students attending 119 colleges, 12 percent of undergraduates reported lifetime use of a prescription painkiller for nonmedical reasons; 7 percent did so in the previous year. Students who are members of fraternities and sororities, enrolled at more competitive schools, earning lower grade point averages, and engaging in substance use and other risky behaviors are more likely to abuse these drugs.[32]

Codeine, a weaker painkiller than morphine, is an ingredient in liquid products prescribed for relieving coughs and in tablet and injectable form for relieving pain. The synthetic narcotic *propoxyphene* (Darvon), a somewhat less potent painkiller than codeine, is no more effective than aspirin in usual doses. It has been one of the most widely prescribed drugs for headaches, dental pain, and menstrual cramps. At higher doses, Darvon produces a euphoric high, which may lead to misuse.

Like other addictions, a prescription drug "habit" is a treatable brain disease. Recovery usually requires carefully supervised detoxification, appropriate medications (similar to those used for opioid dependence), behavioral therapy, and ongoing support.

How Users Feel All opioids relax the user. When injected, they can produce an immediate *rush* (high) that lasts 10 to 30 minutes. For two to six hours thereafter, users may feel indifferent, lethargic, and drowsy; they may slur their words and have problems paying attention, remembering, and going about their normal routine. The primary attractions of heroin are the euphoria and pain relief it produces. However, some people experience very unpleasant feelings, such as anxiety and fear. Other effects include a sensation of warmth or heaviness, dry mouth, facial flushing, and nausea and vomiting (particularly in first-time users).

Risks Addiction is common. Almost all regular users of opioids rapidly develop drug dependence, which can lead to lethargy, weight loss, loss of sex drive, and the continual effort to avoid withdrawal symptoms through repeated drug administration. In addition, they experience anxiety, insomnia, restlessness, and craving for the drug. Users continue taking opioids as much to avoid the discomfort of withdrawal, a classic sign of opioid addiction, as to experience pleasure.

Physical symptoms include constricted pupils (although pupils may dilate from a severe overdose), drowsiness, slurred speech, and impaired attention or memory. Morphine affects blood pressure, heart rate, and blood circulation in the brain. Both morphine and heroin slow down the respiratory system; overdoses can cause fatal respiratory arrest.

Over time, users who inject opioids may develop infections of the heart lining and valves, skin abscesses, and lung congestion. Infections from unsterile solutions, syringes, and shared needles can lead to hepatitis, teta-

benzodiazepines Antianxiety drugs that depress the central nervous system, reduce activity, and induce relaxation, drowsiness, or sleep; often prescribed to relieve tension, muscular strain, sleep problems, anxiety, and panic attacks; also used as an anesthetic and in the treatment of alcohol withdrawal.

barbiturates Antianxiety drugs that depress the central nervous system, reduce activity, and induce relaxation, drowsiness, or sleep; often prescribed to relieve tension and treat epileptic seizures or as a general anesthetic.

opioids Drugs that have sleep-inducing and pain-relieving properties, including opium and its derivatives and nonopioid, synthetic drugs.

nus, liver disease, and HIV transmission. Depression is common and may be both an antecedent and a risk factor for needle-sharing.

Opioid abuse during pregnancy can cause miscarriage, stillbirth, or low birth weight. Babies born to addicted mothers experience withdrawal symptoms after birth.

Withdrawal If a regular user stops taking an opioid, withdrawal begins within 6 to 12 hours. The intensity of the symptoms depends on the degree of the addiction; they may grow stronger for 24 to 72 hours and gradually subside over a period of 7 to 14 days, though some symptoms, such as insomnia, may persist for several months. Individuals may develop craving for an opioid, irritability, nausea or vomiting, muscle aches, runny nose or eyes, dilated pupils, sweating, diarrhea, yawning, fever, and insomnia. Opioid withdrawal usually is not life-threatening.

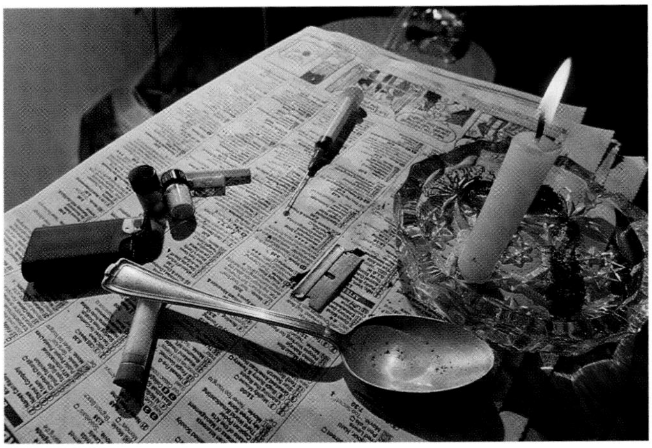

Opioid drugs, made from the Asian poppy, come in both legal and illegal forms. All are highly addictive.

Hallucinogens

The drugs known as **hallucinogens** produce vivid and unusual changes in thought, feeling, and perception. Hallucinogens do not produce dependence in the same way as cocaine or heroin. Individuals who have an unpleasant experience after trying a hallucinogen may stop using the drug completely without suffering withdrawal symptoms. Others continue regular or occasional use because they enjoy the effects.

LSD and Mescaline

LSD (*lysergic acid diethylamide,* acid) was initially developed as a tool to explore mental illness. It became popular in the 1960s and resurfaced among teenagers in the 1990s. LSD is taken orally, either blotted onto pieces of paper that are held in the mouth or chewed along with another substance, such as a sugar cube. Peyote (whose active ingredient is *mescaline*) is another hallucinogen, but it is much less commonly used in this country.

Phencyclidine (PCP)

PCP (**phencyclidine,** brand name Sernyl; street names angel dust, peace pill, lovely, and green) is an illicit drug manufactured as a tablet, capsule, liquid, flake, spray, or crystal-like white powder that can be swallowed, smoked, sniffed, or injected. Sometimes it is sprinkled on crack, marijuana, tobacco, or parsley, and smoked. A fine-powdered form of PCP can be snorted or injected.

PCP use peaked in the 1970s, but it remains a popular drug of abuse in both inner-city ghettos and suburban high schools. Users often think that the PCP they take together with another illegal psychoactive substance, such as amphetamines, coke, or hallucinogens, is responsible for the highs they feel, so they seek it out specifically.

How Users Feel The effects of PCP are utterly unpredictable. It may trigger violent behavior or irreversible psychosis the first time it is used, or the twentieth time, or never. In low doses, PCP produces changes—from hallucinations or euphoria to feelings of emptiness or numbness—similar to those produced by other psychoactive drugs. Higher doses may produce a stupor that lasts several days, increased heart rate and blood pressure, skin flushing, sweating, dizziness, and numbness.

Risks Some people experience repetitive motor movements (such as facial grimacing), hallucinations, and paranoia. Suicide is a definite risk. Intoxication typically lasts four to six hours, but some effects can linger for several days. Delirium may occur within 24 hours of taking PCP or after recovery from an overdose and can last as much as a week.

Inhalants

Inhalants or *deleriants* are chemicals that produce vapors with psychoactive effects. The most commonly abused inhalants are solvents, aerosols, model-airplane glue, cleaning fluids, and petroleum products like kerosene and butane. Some anesthetics and nitrous oxide (laughing gas) are also abused.

Young people who have been treated for mental health problems, have a history of foster care, or already abuse other drugs have an increased risk of abusing or becoming dependent on inhalants. In addition, adolescents who first begin using inhalants at an early age are more likely to become dependent on them. Approximately 9 percent of adolescents nationwide report having used inhalants in their lifetime. Teens with inhalant use disorders report coexisting multiple drug abuse and dependence, mental health treatment, and delinquent behaviors.

How Users Feel Inhalants very rapidly reach the lungs, bloodstream, and other parts of the body. At low doses, users may feel slightly stimulated; at higher doses, they may feel less inhibited. Intoxication often occurs within five minutes and can last more than an hour. Inhalant users do not report the intense rush associated with other drugs; nor do they experience the perceptual changes associated with LSD. However, inhalants interfere with thinking and impulse control, so users may act in dangerous or destructive ways.

Often there are visible external signs of use: a rash around the nose and mouth; breath odors; residue on face, hands, and clothing; redness, swelling, and tearing of the eyes; and irritation of throat, lungs, and nose that leads to coughing and gagging. Nausea and headache also may occur.

Risks Regular use of inhalants leads to tolerance, so the sniffer needs more and more to attain the desired effects. Younger children who use inhalants several times a week may develop dependence. Older users who become dependent may use the drugs many times a day.

Although some young people believe inhalants are safe, this is far from true. Inhalation of butane from cigarette lighters displaces oxygen in the lungs, causing suffocation. Users also can suffocate while covering their heads with a plastic bag to inhale the substance or from inhaling vomit into their lungs while high. The effects of inhalants are unpredictable, and even a single episode can trigger asphyxiation or cardiac arrhythmia, leading to disability or death. Abusers also can develop difficulties with memory and abstract reasoning, problems with coordination, and uncontrollable movements of the extremities.

Treating Substance Dependence and Abuse

An estimated 6.1 million Americans are in need of drug treatment, but the vast majority—some 5 million—never get treatment.[33] The most difficult step for a drug user is to admit that he or she *is* in fact an addict. If drug abusers are not forced to deal with their problem through some unexpected trauma, such as being fired or going bankrupt, those who care—family, friends, coworkers, doctors—may have to confront them and insist that they do something about their addiction. Often this *intervention* can be the turning point for addicts and their families. Treatment has proved equally successful for young people and for older adults.

Some universities offer interventions for students who violate college substance abuse policies. *Motivational interviewing,* a brief intervention in which counselors express empathy to support personal change, has proved effective in reducing alcohol and drug consumption.[34]

Treatment may take place in an outpatient setting, a residential facility, or a hospital. Increasingly, treatment thereafter is tailored to address coexisting or dual diagnoses. A personal treatment plan may consist of individual psychotherapy, marital and family therapy, medication, and behavior therapy. Once an individual has made the decision to seek help for substance abuse, the first step usually is detoxification, which involves clearing the drug from the body.

Controlled and supervised withdrawal within a medical or psychiatric hospital may be recommended if an individual has not been able to stop using drugs as an outpatient or in a residential treatment program. Detoxification is most likely to be complicated in a polysubstance abuser, who may require close monitoring and treatment of potentially fatal withdrawal symptoms. Other reasons for inpatient treatment include lack of psychosocial support for maintaining abstinence and the absence of a drug-free living environment. Restrictions on insurance coverage may limit the number of days of inpatient care. Increasingly, once individuals complete detoxification, they continue treatment in residential programs or as outpatients.

Medications are used in detoxification to alleviate withdrawal symptoms and prevent medical and psychiatric complications. Once withdrawal is complete, these medications are discontinued, so the individual is in a drug-free state. However, individuals with mental disorders may require appropriate psychiatric medication to manage their symptoms and reduce the risk of relapse. For example, a person suffering from major depression or panic disorder may require ongoing treatment with antidepressant medication.

The aim of chemical dependence treatment is to help individuals establish and maintain their recovery from alcohol and drugs of abuse. Recovery is a dynamic process of personal growth and healing in which the drug user makes the transition from a lifestyle of active substance use to a drug-free lifestyle.

Whatever their setting, chemical dependence treatment programs initially involve some period of intensive treatment followed by one or two years of continuing aftercare. Most freestanding programs (those not affiliated with a hospital) follow what is known as the *Minnesota model,* a treatment approach developed at Hazelden Recovery Center in Center City, Minnesota, more than 30 years ago. Its key principles include a focus on drug use as the primary problem, not as a symptom of underlying emotional problems; a multidisciplinary approach that addresses the physical, emotional, spiritual, family,

hallucinogen A drug that causes hallucinations.

PCP (phencyclidine) A synthetic psychoactive substance that produces effects similar to other psychoactive drugs when swallowed, smoked, sniffed, or injected, but also may trigger unpredictable behavioral changes.

inhalants Substances that produce vapors having psychoactive effects when sniffed.

and social aspects of the individual; a supportive community; and a goal of abstinence and health.

12-Step Programs

Since its founding in 1935, Alcoholics Anonymous (AA)—the oldest, largest, and most successful self-help program in the world—has spawned a worldwide movement. As many as 200 different recovery programs are based on the spiritual **12-step program** of AA. Participation in 12-step programs for drug abusers, such as Substance Anonymous, Narcotics Anonymous, and Cocaine Anonymous, is of fundamental importance in promoting and maintaining long-term abstinence.

The basic precept of 12-step programs is that members have been powerless when it comes to controlling their addictive behavior on their own. These programs don't recruit members. The desire to stop must come from the individual, who can call the number of a 12-step program, listed in the telephone book, and find out when and where the next nearby meeting will be held. A representative may offer to send someone to the caller's house to talk about the problem and to escort him or her to the next meeting.

Meetings of various 12-step programs are held daily in almost every city in the country. (Some chapters, whose members often include the disabled or those in remote areas, meet via Internet chat rooms or electronic bulletin boards.) There are no dues or fees for membership. Many individuals belong to several programs because they have several problems, such as alcoholism, substance abuse, and pathological gambling. All have only one requirement for membership: a desire to stop an addictive behavior.

To get the most out of a 12-step program:

- Try out different groups until you find one you like and in which you feel comfortable.
- Once you find a group in which you feel comfortable, go back several times (some recommend a minimum of six meetings) before making a final decision on whether to continue.
- Keep an open mind. Listen to other people's stories and ask yourself if you've had similar feelings or experiences.
- Accept whatever feels right to you and ignore the rest. One common saying in 12-step programs is, "Take what you like and leave the rest."

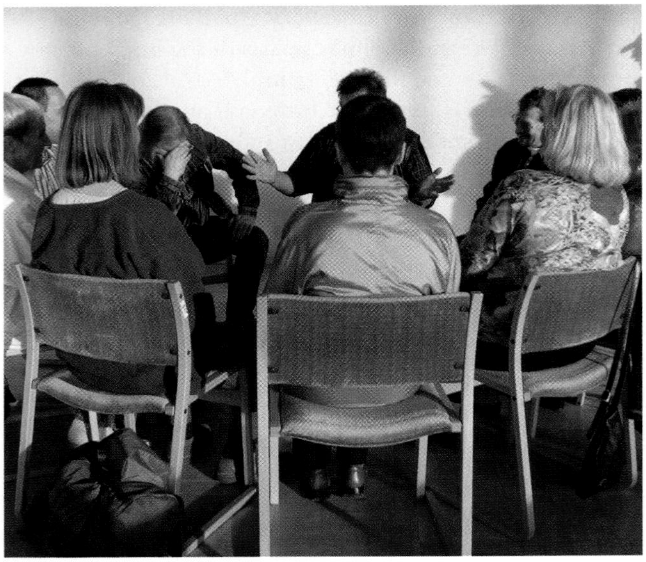

Based on the Alcoholics Anonymous model, 12-step programs have helped many people overcome addictions. The one requirement for membership is a desire to end a pattern of addictive behavior.

Relapse Prevention

The most common clinical course for substance abuse disorders involves a pattern of multiple relapses over the course of a lifespan. It is important for individuals with these problems and their families to recognize this fact. When relapses do occur, they should be viewed as nei-

Strategies for Prevention: Relapse-Prevention Planning

The following steps from Terence Gorski and Merlene Miller's *Staying Sober: A Guide for Relapse Prevention*, can lower the likelihood of relapses:

- **Stabilization and self-assessment**. Get control of yourself. Find out what's going on in your head, heart, and life.
- **Education.** Learn about relapse and what to do to prevent it.
- **Warning-sign identification and management.** Make a list of your personal relapse warning signs. Learn how to interrupt them before you lose control.
- **Inventory training.** Learn how to become consciously aware of warning signs as they develop.
- **Review of the recovery program.** Make sure your recovery program is able to help you manage your warning signs of relapse.
- **Involvement of significant others.** Teach them how to help you avoid relapses.

ther a mark of defeat nor evidence of moral weakness. While painful, they do not erase the progress that has been achieved and ultimately may strengthen self-understanding. They can serve as reminders of potential pitfalls to avoid in the future.

One key to preventing relapse is learning to avoid obvious cues and associations that can set off intense cravings. This means staying away from the people and places linked with past drug use. Some therapists use conditioning techniques to give former users some sense of control over their urge to use the drug. The theory behind this approach, which is called *extinction* of conditioned behavior, is that with repeated exposure—for example, to videotapes of dealers selling crack cocaine—the arousal and craving will diminish. While this technique by itself cannot ward off relapses, it does seem to enhance the overall effectiveness of other therapies.

Another important lesson that therapists emphasize is that every lapse does not have to lead to a full-blown relapse. Users can turn to the skills acquired in treatment—calling people for support or going to meetings—to avoid a major relapse. Ultimately, users must learn much more than how to avoid temptation; they must examine their entire view of the world and learn new ways to live in it without turning to drugs. This is the underlying goal of the recovery process.

LEARN IT / LIVE IT

Choosing an Addiction-Free Lifestyle

People with substance abuse disorders and addictive behaviors lose control of their choices and their lives. Their compulsion to gamble or to use a drug seems irresistible. You, in contrast, have a choice. You can create a life and a lifestyle with no need and no room for reliance on a substance or a self-destructive behavior. Here are some ways to go about it:

- **Set goals for yourself.** Think about who you want to become, what you'd like to do, the future you wish for yourself. Focus on what it will take—years of education, perhaps, or specialized training—to achieve these goals. Understand that drugs can only get in the way and diminish your potential.
- **Participate in drug-free activities.** If you're bored or unfocused, drugs may appeal to you simply as something to do. Take charge of your time. Play a sport. Work out at the gym. Join a club. Volunteer. Start a blog.
- **Educate yourself.** Much of the information that young people hear from friends, particularly drug-using friends, is wrong. Drugs that are used as medicines are not safe for recreational use. The fact that many people at a rave are having fun doesn't mean that some aren't endangering their brains and their lives by taking club drugs. Get the facts for yourself from sites such as those on page 324–325.
- **Choose friends with a future.** The world of drug users shrinks. Nothing matters more than the next hit, the next high, the next fix. Losing all sense of tomorrow, they focus on getting through the day with the help of drugs. Are these the people you want to spend time with? Choose friends who can broaden your world with new ideas, ambitious plans, and great dreams for tomorrow.

11 Making This Chapter Work for You

Review Questions

1. Which of the following statements about drugs is *false?*
   a. Toxicity is the dosage level of a prescription.
   b. Drugs can be injected into the body intravenously, intramuscularly, or subcutaneously.
   c. Drug misuse is the taking of a drug for a purpose other than that for which it was medically intended.
   d. An individual's response to a drug can be affected by the setting in which the drug is used.
2. To help ensure that an over-the-counter or prescription drug is safe and effective:
   a. take smaller dosages than indicated in the instructions.
   b. test your response to the drug by borrowing a similar medication from a friend.
   c. ask your doctor or pharmacist about possible interactions with other medications.
   d. buy all of your medications online.
3. Prescription drug abuse on college campuses
   a. is not a problem.
   b. is higher among college women than college men.
   c. is more widespread than the use of marijuana.
   d. is more widespread than the use of ecstasy, cocaine, and meth.

twelve-step programs Self-help group programs based on the principles of Alcoholics Anonymous.

4. Individuals with substance use disorders
   a. are usually not physically dependent on their drug of choice.
   b. have a compulsion to use one or more addictive substances.
   c. require less and less of the preferred drug to achieve the desired effect.
   d. suffer withdrawal symptoms when they use the drug regularly.
5. Amphetamine is very similar to which of the following in its effects on the central nervous system?
   a. marijuana
   b. heroin
   c. cocaine
   d. alcohol
6. Which of the following statements about marijuana is *false?*
   a. People who have used marijuana may experience psychoactive effects for several days after use.
   b. Marijuana has shown some effectiveness in treating chemotherapy-related nausea.
   c. Unlike long-term use of alcohol, regular use of marijuana does not have any long-lasting health consequences.
   d. Depending on the amount of marijuana used, its effects can range from a mild sense of euphoria to extreme panic.
7. Cocaine dependence can result in all of the following *except*
   a. stroke.
   b. paranoia and violent behavior.
   c. heart failure.
   d. enhanced sexual performance.
8. Which of the following statements about club drugs is true?
   a. Club drugs can produce many unwanted effects, including hallucinations and paranoia.
   b. Most club drugs do not pose the same health dangers as "hard" drugs such as heroin.
   c. MDMA is the street name for ecstasy.
   d. When combined with extended physical exertion, club drugs can lead to hypothermia (lowered body temperature).
9. The opioids
   a. are not addictive if used in a prescription form such as codeine or Demerol.
   b. produce an immediate but short-lasting high and feeling of euphoria.
   c. include morphine, which is typically used for cough suppression.
   d. are illegal in the United States, although they are allowed in other countries to help control severe pain.
10. Which of the following statements about drug dependence treatment is *false?*
    a. Chemical dependence treatment programs usually involve medications to alleviate withdrawal symptoms.
    b. Detoxification is usually the first step in a drug treatment program.
    c. Relapses are not uncommon for a person who has undergone drug treatment.
    d. The 12-step recovery program associated with Alcoholics Anonymous has been shown to be ineffective with individuals with drug dependence disorders.

Answers to these questions can be found on p. 422.

Critical Thinking

1. Some state programs send nonviolent drug offenders into drug treatment rather than jail. In one case, about a quarter of those diverted into rehabilitation from prison, including those addicted to methamphetamine, completed their alternative treatment successfully. Would you support more programs like this? Why or why not?
2. Some Web enthusiasts oppose any kind of government regulations on the Internet. Do you agree or disagree? How would you address the problems associated with distributing drugs online?
3. Suppose that a close friend is using amphetamines to keep her energy levels high so that she can continue to attend school full-time and hold down a job to pay her school expenses. You fear that she is developing a substance abuse disorder. What can you do to help her realize the dangers of her behavior? What resources are available at your school or in your community to help her deal with both her drug problem and her financial needs?

Media Menu

ThomsonNOW™ Go to the ThomsonNOW website at **http://www.thomsonedu.com** that will:

- Help you evaluate your knowledge of the material.
- Allow you to take an exam-prep quiz.
- Provide a Personalized Learning Plan targeting resources that address areas you should study.
- Coach you through identifying target goals for behavioral change and creating and monitoring your personal change plan throughout the semester.

INTERNET CONNECTIONS

National Institute on Drug Abuse
www.nida.nih.gov

This government site—a virtual clearinghouse of information for students, parents, teachers, researchers, and health professionals—features current treatment and research, as well as a comprehensive database on common drugs of abuse. The science of drug abuse and addictions is discussed with a focus on the major illegal drugs in use, with additional resources on drug testing, treatment research, and trends/statistics.

LACC Extra Credit Assignment

11. Discuss both the legal and illegal uses of drugs; their benefits and detriments.

Partnership for a Drug-Free America
www.drugfree.org

This site features current resources and photographs on a wide spectrum of drugs, including performance-enhancing drugs, club drugs, and commonly abused prescription drugs. The drug guide even allows you to search for a drug using its slang name.

Club Drugs
www.clubdrugs.gov

This site is a service of the National Institute of Drug Abuse to provide information on club drugs.

Drug Help
www.drughelp.org

This is a national nonprofit information and referral service providing information on specific drugs and treatment options in addition to referrals to public and private treatment programs, self-help groups, family support groups, and crisis centers.

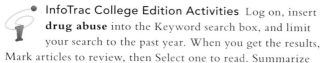

InfoTrac College Edition Activities Log on, insert **drug abuse** into the Keyword search box, and limit your search to the past year. When you get the results, Mark articles to review, then Select one to read. Summarize three or four key points from the article.

You can find additional readings related to personal health with InfoTrac College Edition, an online library of more than 900 journals and publications. Follow the instructions for accessing InfoTrac College Edition that were packaged with your textbook; then search for articles using a keyword search.

For additional links, resources, and suggested readings on the InfoTrac College Edition, visit our Health and Wellness Resource Center at **http://health .wadsworth.com.**

Key Terms

The terms listed are used on the page indicated. Definitions of the terms are in the Glossary at the end of this book.

addiction 305
amphetamines 314
barbiturates 318
benzodiazepines 318
club drugs 311
cocaine 316
drug 300
drug abuse 300
drug misuse 300
ecstasy (MDMA) 312
GBL (gamma butyrolactone) 313
GHB (gamma hydroxybutyrate) 313
hallucinogens 320
hashish 307
inhalants 320
intoxication 306
intramuscular 300
intravenous 300
marijuana 307
opioids 318
over-the-counter (OTC) drugs 301
PCP (phencyclidine) 320
physical dependence 305
polyabuse 306
psychoactive 304
psychological dependence 305
stimulant 313
subcutaneous 300
toxicity 301
12-step program 322
withdrawal 306

12 Alcohol and Tobacco Use, Misuse, and Abuse

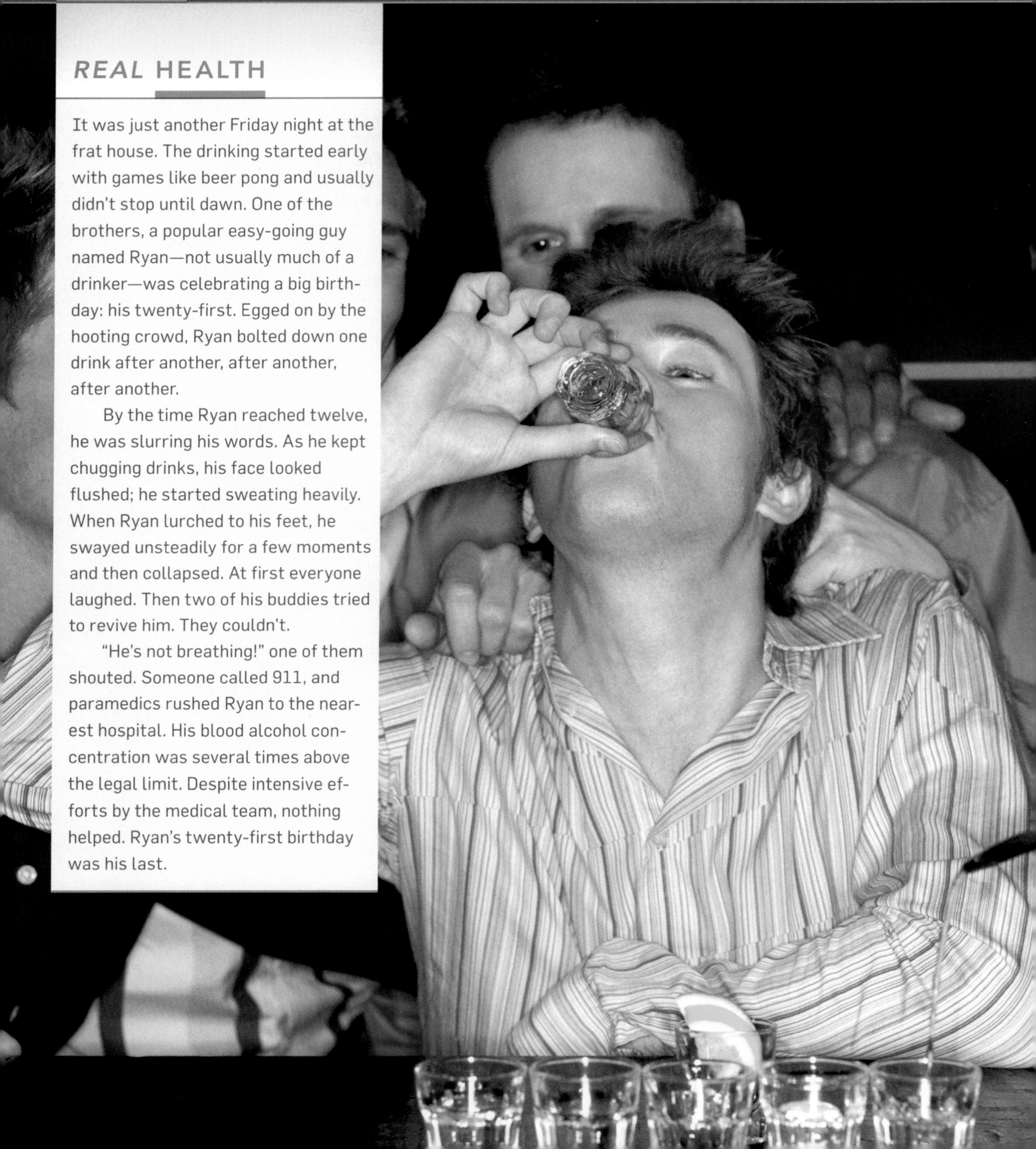

REAL HEALTH

It was just another Friday night at the frat house. The drinking started early with games like beer pong and usually didn't stop until dawn. One of the brothers, a popular easy-going guy named Ryan—not usually much of a drinker—was celebrating a big birthday: his twenty-first. Egged on by the hooting crowd, Ryan bolted down one drink after another, after another, after another.

By the time Ryan reached twelve, he was slurring his words. As he kept chugging drinks, his face looked flushed; he started sweating heavily. When Ryan lurched to his feet, he swayed unsteadily for a few moments and then collapsed. At first everyone laughed. Then two of his buddies tried to revive him. They couldn't.

"He's not breathing!" one of them shouted. Someone called 911, and paramedics rushed Ryan to the nearest hospital. His blood alcohol concentration was several times above the legal limit. Despite intensive efforts by the medical team, nothing helped. Ryan's twenty-first birthday was his last.

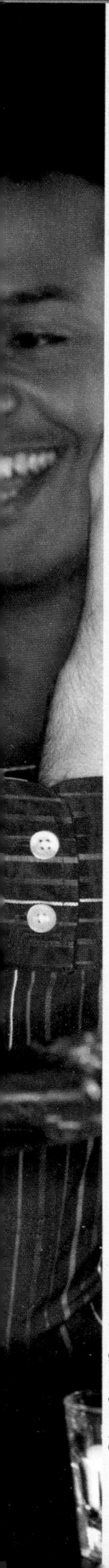

© Image Source/Getty Images

Alcohol and tobacco are the most widely used mind-altering substances in the world. College campuses are no exception. About eight in ten college students drink, at least occasionally. About two in five engage in the dangerous practice of binge drinking and put themselves at physical, legal, academic, and psychological risk.[1]

About one in five college students smoke.[2] The more and the longer they smoke, the greater their risks of heart disease, respiratory problems, several types of cancer, and a shortened lifespan.

Each dangerous in itself, drinking and smoking tend to go together. Heavy drinking is more common among current smokers than former or nonsmokers. The more individuals smoke and drink, the less likely they are to eat a nutritious diet and follow a healthy lifestyle.

Even if you never drink to excess and don't smoke, you live with the consequences of others' drinking and smoking. That's why it's important for everyone to know about these harmful habits. This chapter provides information that can help you understand, avoid, and change behaviors that could destroy your health, happiness, and life.

? FAQ Frequently Asked Questions

- How can I tell if someone has alcohol poisoning? *p. 331*
- What is binge drinking? *p. 332*
- Why do students binge? *p. 336*
- What are colleges doing to prevent alcohol abuse? *p. 339*
- Is social smoking less risky? *p. 349*
- What are bidis? *p. 354*

After studying the material in this chapter, you should be able to:

- **List** the effects of alcohol on the body systems.
- **Define** alcohol abuse, dependence, and alcoholism, and **list** their symptoms.
- **List** the negative consequences to individuals, and to our society, from alcohol abuse.
- **List** the health effects of smoking tobacco or using smokeless tobacco.
- **Describe** some of the tobacco-control policies on college campuses.

Your Body's Response to Alcohol

Pure alcohol is a colorless liquid obtained through the fermentation of a liquid containing sugar. **Ethyl alcohol,** or *ethanol,* is the type of alcohol in alcoholic beverages. Another type—methyl, or wood, alcohol—is a poison that should never be drunk. Any liquid containing 0.5 to 80 percent ethyl alcohol by volume is an alcoholic beverage. However, different drinks contain different amounts of alcohol.

Do you know what a "drink" is? Most students don't. In one experiment undergraduates defined a "drink" as one serving, regardless of how big it was or how much alcohol it contained.[3] In fact, one standard drink can be any of the following:

- **One bottle or can** (12 ounces) of beer, which is 5 percent alcohol.
- **One glass** (4 or 5 ounces) of table wine, such as burgundy, which is 12 percent alcohol.
- **One small glass** (2½ ounces) of fortified wine, which is 20 percent alcohol.
- **One shot** (1 ounce) of distilled spirits (such as whiskey, vodka, or rum), which is 50 percent alcohol.

All of these drinks contain close to the same amount of alcohol—that is, if the number of ounces in each drink is multiplied by the percentage of alcohol, each drink contains the equivalent of approximately ½ ounce of 100 percent ethyl alcohol.

But the words *bottle* and *glass* can be deceiving. Drinking a 16-ounce bottle of malt liquor, which is 6.4 percent alcohol, is not the same as drinking a 12-ounce glass of light beer (3.2 percent alcohol): The malt liquor contains 1 ounce of alcohol and is the equivalent of two drinks. Two bottles of high-alcohol wines (such as Cisco), packaged to resemble much less powerful wine coolers, can lead to alcohol poisoning, especially in those who weigh less than 150 pounds.

With distilled spirits (such as bourbon, scotch, vodka, gin, and rum), alcohol content is expressed in terms of **proof,** a number that is twice the percentage of alcohol: 100-proof bourbon is 50 percent alcohol; 80-proof gin is 40 percent alcohol. Many mixed drinks are equivalent to one and a half or two standard drinks; for instance, see the margarita in Figure 12-1.

Blood-Alcohol Concentration

The amount of alcohol in your blood at any given time is your **blood-alcohol concentration (BAC).** It is expressed in terms of the percentage of alcohol in the blood and is often measured from breath or urine samples.

Law enforcement officers use BAC to determine whether a driver is legally drunk. All the states have followed the recommendation of the federal Department of Transportation to set 0.08 percent—the BAC that a 150-pound man would have after consuming about three mixed drinks within an hour—as the threshold at which a person can be cited for drunk driving (Figure 12-2).

Using a formula for blood-alcohol concentration developed by highway transportation officials, researchers calculate that when college students drink, their typical BAC is 0.079, dangerously close to the legal limit.[4]

A BAC of 0.05 percent indicates approximately 5 parts alcohol to 10,000 parts other blood components. Most people reach this level after consuming one or two drinks and experience all the positive sensations of drinking—relaxation, euphoria, and well-being—without feeling intoxicated. If they continue to drink past the 0.05 percent BAC level, they start feeling worse rather than better, gradually losing control of speech, balance, and emotions. At a BAC of 0.2 percent, they

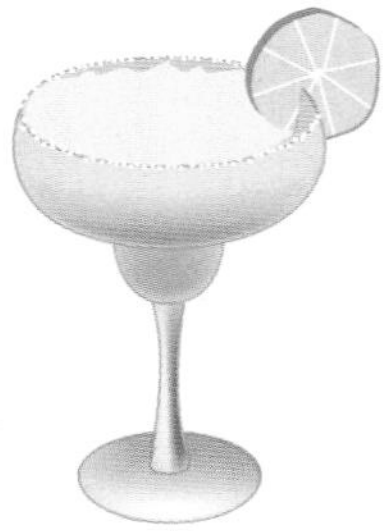

Margarita:

1 1/2 oz. tequila (80 proof) = 1.5 oz. × 40 percent alcohol = 0.6 oz. alcohol

3/4 oz. triple sec (60 proof) = 0.75 oz. × 30 percent alcohol = 0.23 oz. alcohol

Splash of sour mix — 0.83 oz. alcohol = 1 1/2 drinks

Dash of lime juice

Salt for the rim

Malt liquor:

16 oz. × 6.4 percent alcohol = 1 oz. alcohol = 2 drinks

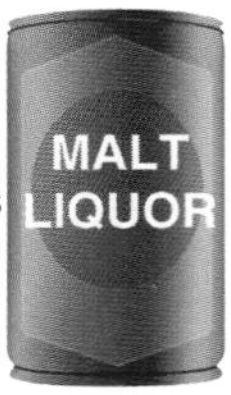

FIGURE 12-1 How many standard drinks are you drinking?

Men	Approximate blood alcohol percentage								
	Body weight in pounds								
Drinks	100	120	140	160	180	200	220	240	
0	.00	.00	.00	.00	.00	.00	.00	.00	Only safe driving limit
1	.04	.03	.03	.02	.02	.02	.02	.02	Impairment begins
2	.08	.06	.05	.05	.04	.04	.03	.03	Driving skills significantly affected Possible criminal penalties
3	.11	.09	.08	.07	.06	.06	.05	.05	
4	.15	.12	.11	.09	.08	.08	.07	.06	
5	.19	.16	.13	.12	.11	.09	.09	.08	
6	.23	.19	.16	.14	.13	.11	.10	.09	
7	.26	.22	.19	.16	.15	.13	.12	.11	Legally intoxicated Criminal penalties
8	.30	.25	.21	.19	.17	.15	.14	.13	
9	.34	.28	.24	.21	.19	.17	.15	.14	
10	.38	.31	.27	.23	.21	.19	.17	.16	

Subtract 0.01 percent for each 40 minutes of drinking.
One drink is 1.25 oz. of 80 proof liquor, 12 oz. of beer, or 5 oz. of table wine.

Women	Approximate blood alcohol percentage									
	Body weight in pounds									
Drinks	90	100	120	140	160	180	200	220	240	
0	.00	.00	.00	.00	.00	.00	.00	.00	.00	Only safe driving limit
1	.05	.05	.04	.03	.03	.03	.02	.02	.02	Impairment begins
2	.10	.09	.08	.07	.06	.05	.05	.04	.04	Driving skills significantly affected Possible criminal penalties
3	.15	.14	.11	.10	.09	.08	.07	.06	.06	
4	.20	.18	.15	.13	.11	.10	.09	.08	.08	
5	.25	.23	.19	.16	.14	.13	.11	.10	.09	
6	.30	.27	.23	.19	.17	.15	.14	.12	.11	Legally intoxicated Criminal penalties
7	.35	.32	.27	.23	.20	.18	.16	.14	.13	
8	.40	.36	.30	.26	.23	.20	.18	.17	.15	
9	.45	.41	.34	.29	.26	.23	.20	.19	.17	
10	.51	.45	.38	.32	.28	.25	.23	.21	.19	

Subtract 0.01 percent for each 40 minutes of drinking.
One drink is 1.25 oz. of 80 proof liquor, 12 oz. of beer, or 5 oz. of table wine.

FIGURE 12-2 Alcohol Impairment Chart

Source: Adapted from data supplied by the Pennsylvania Liquor Control Board.

may pass out. At a BAC of 0.3 percent, they could lapse into a coma; at 0.4 percent, they could die.

Many factors affect an individual's BAC and response to alcohol, including the following:

- **How much and how quickly you drink.** The more alcohol you put into your body, the higher your BAC. If you chug drink after drink, your liver, which metabolizes about ½ ounce of alcohol an hour, won't be able to keep up—and your BAC will soar.
- **What you're drinking.** The stronger the drink, the faster and harder the alcohol hits. Straight shots of liquor and cocktails such as martinis will get alcohol into your bloodstream faster than beer or table wine. Beer and wine not only contain lower

ethyl alcohol The intoxicating agent in alcoholic beverages; also called ethanol.

proof The alcoholic strength of a distilled spirit, expressed as twice the percentage of alcohol present.

blood-alcohol concentration (BAC) The amount of alcohol in the blood, expressed as a percentage.

concentrations of alcohol, but they also contain nonalcoholic substances that slow the rate of **absorption** (passage of the alcohol into your body tissues). If the drink contains water, juice, or milk, the rate of absorption will be slowed. However, carbon dioxide—whether in champagne, ginger ale, or a cola—whisks alcohol into your bloodstream. Also, the alcohol in warm drinks—such as a hot rum toddy or warmed sake—moves into your bloodstream more quickly than the alcohol in chilled wine or scotch on the rocks.

- **Your size.** If you're a large person (whether due to fat or to muscle), you'll get drunk more slowly than someone smaller who's drinking the same amount of alcohol at the same rate. Heavier individuals have a larger water volume, which dilutes the alcohol they drink.
-  **Your gender.** Women have lower quantities of a stomach enzyme that neutralizes alcohol, so one drink for a woman has the impact that two drinks have for a man. Hormone levels also affect the impact of alcohol. Women are more sensitive to alcohol just before menstruation, and birth control pills and other forms of estrogen can intensify alcohol's impact.
- **Your age.** The same amount of alcohol produces higher BACs in older drinkers, who have lower volumes of body water to dilute the alcohol than younger drinkers do.
- 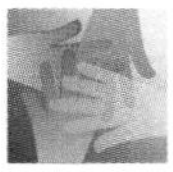 **Your race.** Many members of certain ethnic groups, including Asians and Native Americans, are unable to break down alcohol as quickly as Caucasians. This can result in higher BACs, as well as uncomfortable reactions, such as flushing and nausea, when they drink.
- **Other drugs.** Some common medications—including aspirin, acetaminophen (Tylenol), and ulcer medications—can cause blood-alcohol levels to increase more rapidly. Individuals taking these drugs can be over the legal limit for blood-alcohol concentration after as little as a single drink.
- **Family history of alcoholism.** Some children of alcoholics don't develop any of the usual behavioral symptoms that indicate someone is drinking too much. It's not known whether this behavior is genetically caused or is a result of growing up with an alcoholic.
- **Eating.** Food slows the absorption of alcohol by diluting it, by covering some of the membranes through which alcohol would be absorbed, and by prolonging the time the stomach takes to empty.
- **Expectations.** In various experiments, volunteers who believed they were given alcoholic beverages but were actually given nonalcoholic drinks acted as if they were guzzling the real thing and became more talkative, relaxed, and sexually stimulated.
- **Physical tolerance.** If you drink regularly, your brain becomes accustomed to a certain level of alcohol. You may be able to look and behave in a seemingly normal fashion, even though you drink as much as would normally intoxicate someone your size. However, your driving ability and judgment will still be impaired.

Once you develop tolerance, you may drink more to get the desired effects from alcohol. In some people, this can lead to abuse and alcoholism. On the other hand, after years of drinking, some people become exquisitely sensitive to alcohol. Such reverse tolerance means that they can become intoxicated after drinking only a small amount of alcohol.

Intoxication

If you drink too much, the immediate consequence is that you get drunk—or, more precisely, intoxicated. Alcohol *intoxication,* which can range from mild inebriation to loss of consciousness, is characterized by at least one of the following signs: slurred speech, poor coordination, unsteady gait, abnormal eye movements, impaired attention or memory, stupor, or coma.

Strategies for Prevention — *What To Do When Someone Is Intoxicated*

- Continually monitor the intoxicated person.
- Check breathing, waking the person often to be sure he or she is not unconscious.
- Do not force the person to walk or move around.
- Do not allow the person to drive a car or ride a bicycle.
- Do not give the person food, liquid (including coffee), medicines, or drugs to sober them up.
- Do not give the person a cold shower; the shock of the cold could cause unconsciousness.

Medical risks of intoxication include falls, hypothermia in cold climates, and increased risk of infections because of suppressed immune function. Time and a protective environment are the recommended treatments for alcohol intoxication.

Alcohol Poisoning

Incidents like the one in Real Health (page 326) occur every year on college campuses. Because federal law requires colleges to publish all student deaths, the stories of young lives ended by alcohol poisoning have gained national attention. Yet many students remain unaware that alcohol, in large enough doses, can and does kill.

Alcohol depresses nerves that control involuntary actions, such as breathing and the gag reflex (which prevents choking). A fatal dose of alcohol will eventually suppress these functions. Because alcohol irritates the stomach, people who drink an excessive amount often vomit. If intoxication has led to a loss of consciousness, a drinker is in danger of choking on vomit, which can cause death by asphyxiation. Blood alcohol concentration can rise even after a drinker has passed out because alcohol in the stomach and intestine continues to enter the bloodstream and circulate throughout the body.

? FAQ How Can I Tell If Someone Has Alcohol Poisoning?

- If the person is breathing less than twelve times per minute or stops breathing for periods of ten seconds or more, **call 911.**
- If the person is asleep and you are unable to wake him or her up, **call 911.**
- Look at the person's skin. If it is cold, clammy, pale, bluish in color, **call 911.**
- Stay with a person who is vomiting. Try to keep him or her sitting up. If the person must lie down, keep him on his side with head turned to the side. Watch for choking; if the person begins to choke, **call 911.**

Alcohol poisoning is a medical emergency requiring immediate treatment. Black coffee, a cold shower, or letting a person "sleep it off" does not help. Without medical treatment, breathing slows, becomes irregular, or stops. The heart beats irregularly. Body temperature falls, which can cause cardiac arrest. Blood sugar plummets, which can lead to seizures. Vomiting creates severe dehydration, which can cause seizures, permanent brain damage, or death. Even if the victim lives, an alcohol overdose can result in irreversible brain damage.

Rapid binge drinking is especially dangerous because the victim can ingest a fatal dose before becoming unconscious. If you suspect alcohol poisoning, call 911 for help. Don't try to guess the level of drunkenness. Tell emergency medical technicians the symptoms and, if you know, how much alcohol the victim drank. Prompt action may save a life.

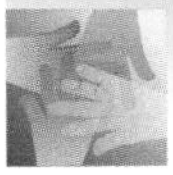

Drinking in America

According to the most recent statistics available from the National Institute on Alcohol Abuse and Alcoholism, about 60 percent of American adults use alcohol, although they vary in how much and how often they drink. Whites are more likely to be daily or near-daily drinkers than nonwhites. Men tend to drink more and more often than women. In general the rates of women who drink have not changed much in the last twenty years. However, the drinking behavior of women in their twenties has changed in two seemingly contradictory ways: More young women don't drink at all, and more of the women who do consume alcohol drink to intoxication.[5]

The median age of first alcohol use is 15. Drinking typically accelerates in the late teens, peaks in the early 20s, and decreases as people age.[6] The median age of onset for alcohol-use disorders is 19 to 20.

Abstinence

Because of concern about alcohol's health effects, increasing numbers of Americans are choosing not to drink.

According to the National College Health Assessment, about one in five students (18 percent) reports never using alcohol.[7] With alcohol consumption in the United States at its lowest level in 30 years, nonalcoholic beverages have grown in popularity. They appeal to drivers, boaters, individuals with health problems that could worsen with alcohol, those who are older and can't tolerate alcohol, anyone taking medicines that interact with alcohol (including antibiotics, antidepressants, and muscle relaxers), and everyone interested in limiting alcohol intake. Under federal law, these drinks can contain some alcohol but a much smaller amount than regular beer or wine. Nonalcoholic beers and wines on the market also are lower in calories than alcoholic varieties.

Some people—such as women who are pregnant or trying to conceive; individuals with problems, such as ulcers, that might be

absorption The passage of substances into or across membranes or tissues.

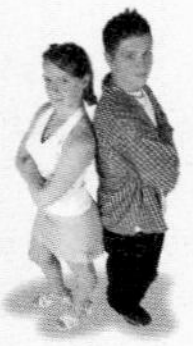

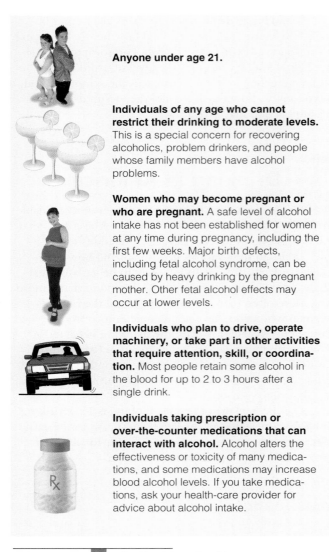

Anyone under age 21.

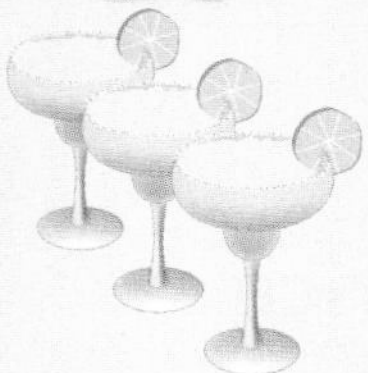

Individuals of any age who cannot restrict their drinking to moderate levels. This is a special concern for recovering alcoholics, problem drinkers, and people whose family members have alcohol problems.

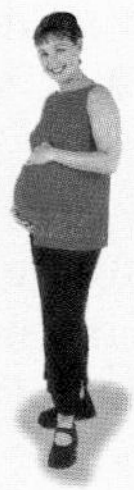

Women who may become pregnant or who are pregnant. A safe level of alcohol intake has not been established for women at any time during pregnancy, including the first few weeks. Major birth defects, including fetal alcohol syndrome, can be caused by heavy drinking by the pregnant mother. Other fetal alcohol effects may occur at lower levels.

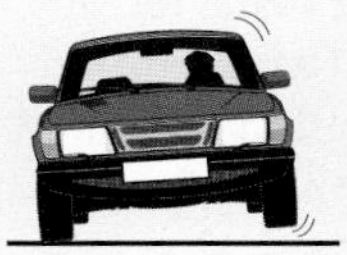

Individuals who plan to drive, operate machinery, or take part in other activities that require attention, skill, or coordination. Most people retain some alcohol in the blood for up to 2 to 3 hours after a single drink.

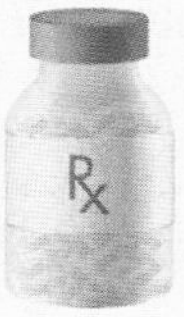

Individuals taking prescription or over-the-counter medications that can interact with alcohol. Alcohol alters the effectiveness or toxicity of many medications, and some medications may increase blood alcohol levels. If you take medications, ask your health-care provider for advice about alcohol intake.

FIGURE 12-3 Who Should Not Drink?

Source: National Council an Alcoholism and Drug Dependence, www.ncadd.org/facts/heath.html.

aggravated by alcohol; those taking medications such as sleeping pills or antidepressants; and those driving or operating any motorized equipment—shouldn't drink at all (Figure 12-3).

Why People Drink

The most common reason people drink alcohol is to relax. Because it depresses the central nervous system, alcohol can make people feel less tense. Some psychologists theorize that men engage in *confirmatory drinking;* that is, they drink to reinforce the image of masculinity associated with alcohol consumption. Both genders may engage in *compensatory drinking,* consuming alcohol to heighten their sense of masculinity or femininity.

Here are some other reasons why men and women, drink:

- **Inherited susceptibility.** In both women and men, genetics accounts for 50 to 60 percent of a person's vulnerability to a serious drinking problem. Female alcoholics are more likely than males to have a parent who abused drugs or alcohol, who had psychiatric problems, or who attempted suicide.
- **Childhood traumas.** Female alcoholics often report that they were physically or sexually abused as children or suffered great distress because of poverty or a parent's death.
- **Depression.** Women are more likely than men to be depressed prior to drinking and to suffer from both depression and a drinking problem at the same time.
- **Relationship issues.** Single, separated, or divorced men and women drink more and more often than married ones.
- **Psychological factors.** Both men and women may drink to compensate for feelings of inadequacy. Women who tend to ruminate or mull over bad feelings may find that alcohol increases this tendency and makes them feel more distressed.
- **Self-medication.** More so than men, some women feel it's permissible to use alcohol as if it were a medicine. As long as they're taking it for a reason, it seems acceptable to them, even if they're drifting into a drinking problem.
- **Social ease.** When people use alcohol, they may seem bolder, wittier, sexier. At the same time, they become more relaxed and seem to enjoy each other's company more. Because alcohol lowers inhibitions, some people see it as a prelude to seduction.
- **Role models.** Athletes, some of the most admired celebrities in our country, have a long history of appearing in commercials for alcohol. Many advertisements feature glamorous women holding or sipping alcoholic beverages.
- **Advertising.** Brewers and beer distributors spend \$15 to \$20 million a year promoting the message: If you want to have fun, have a drink. Young people may be especially responsive to such sales pitches.

? FAQ What is Binge Drinking?

Binge drinking consists of having five or more drinks in a single sitting for a man or four drinks in a single sitting for a woman. Although this definition is widely used, some criticize it for overlooking body weight and the length of time over which drinking occurs—both factors that influence the effects of alcohol consumption.[8] It also does not take into account alcohol tolerance, metabolism, and medications.

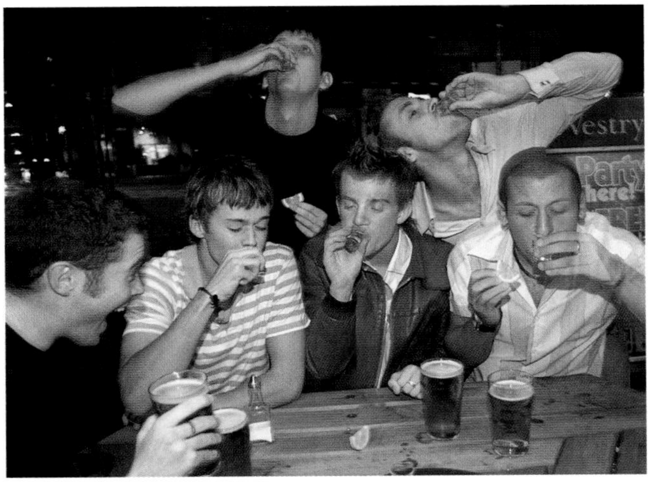

© Topham/The Image Works

Drinking games and binges, which are common on college campuses, are dangerous in themselves and increase the likelihood of other risky behaviors, such as driving while intoxicated.

By any measure, drinking multiple drinks at a single setting is common—and hazardous. About half of the alcohol consumed by adults—and 90 percent of alcohol drunk by underage young people—is in the form of binge drinks.[9] Binge drinking accounts for half of alcohol-related deaths and a wide range of serious health and social problems, including motor vehicle accidents, injuries from falls, drowning, hypothermia, and burns; heart attacks; suicide; unplanned pregnancy; and sexually transmitted infection. It also is strongly linked to violence, including murders, assaults, robberies, and sexual offenses.

Among high school students who drink, 60 percent report binge-drinking, as do about 40 percent of college students (see page 335). Among adults, about 32 percent of current drinkers report having engaged in a binge in the last months.[10]

Binge drinking among women of child-bearing age endangers not only a woman's health but that of her unborn child. Binge drinking during pregnancy, not the total amount of alcohol consumed, doubles the risk of mental retardation and delinquent behavior in children.

Among the solutions public health officials have suggested to halt binge drinking are increased taxes to raise the price of alcohol, enforcing strict restrictions on sales to underage minors, and screening and brief counseling for individuals identified as binge drinkers. But taking personal responsibility also is critical to ending binge drinking and preventing its harmful consequences.

Drinking and Driving

Drunk driving is the most frequently committed crime in the United States. Alcohol impairs driving-related skills regardless of the age of the driver or the time of day it is consumed. However, younger drinkers and drivers are at greatest risk. Underage drinkers are more likely to drive after drinking, to ride with intoxicated drivers, and to be injured after drinking—at least in part because they believe that people can drive safely and legally after drinking.

The number of alcohol-related fatalities on American highways has dropped in recent years, but more than 42,000 people still die on the nation's highways each year. Safety groups attribute the decline in alcohol-related deaths to enforcement tools like sobriety checkpoints and to the states' adoption of a uniform drunken-driving standard of a BAC of 0.08 percent.

However, among college students ages 18 to 24, deaths from alcohol-related accidents and other unintentional injuries have increased to more than 1,700 a year.[11] In one survey, 29 percent of college students drove after drinking some alcohol; 10 percent after five or more drinks; 23 percent rode in a car with a driver who was high or drunk. The rates of drinking and driving are higher at larger schools and schools in the southern and north-central regions.[12]

In the last two decades, families of the victims of drunk drivers have organized to change the way the nation treats its drunk drivers. Because of the efforts of MADD (Mothers

binge drinking For a man, having five or more alcoholic drinks at a single sitting; for a woman, having four drinks or more at a single sitting.

Strategies for Prevention — How to Prevent Drunk Driving

- When going out in a group, always designate one person who won't drink at all to serve as the driver.
- Never get behind the wheel if you've had more than two drinks within two hours, especially if you haven't eaten.
- Never let intoxicated friends drive home. Call a taxi, drive them yourself, or arrange for them to spend the night in a safe place.

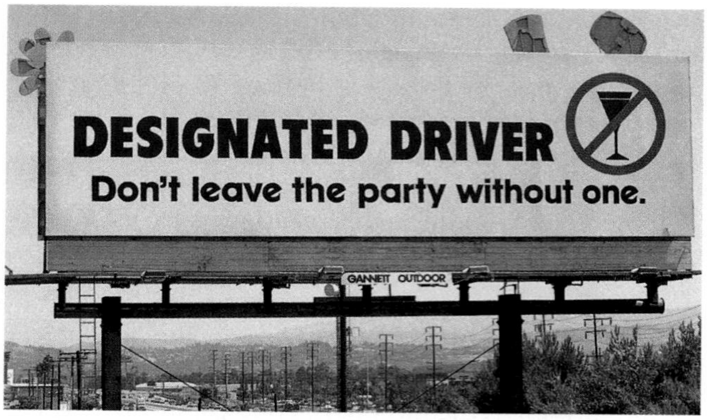

© Tony Freeman/PhotoEdit

Public awareness campaigns like this one for designated drivers can help prevent the high incidence of fatalities caused by drunk drivers.

Against Drunk Driving), SADD (Students Against Destructive Decisions), and other lobbying groups, cities, counties, and states are cracking down on drivers who drink. Since courts have held establishments that serve alcohol liable for the consequences of allowing drunk customers to drive, many bars and restaurants have joined the campaign against drunk driving. Many communities also provide free rides home on holidays and weekends for people who've had too much to drink. Designated drivers can help save lives—if they refrain from drinking.

Student Snapshot

Drinking and Smoking on Campus

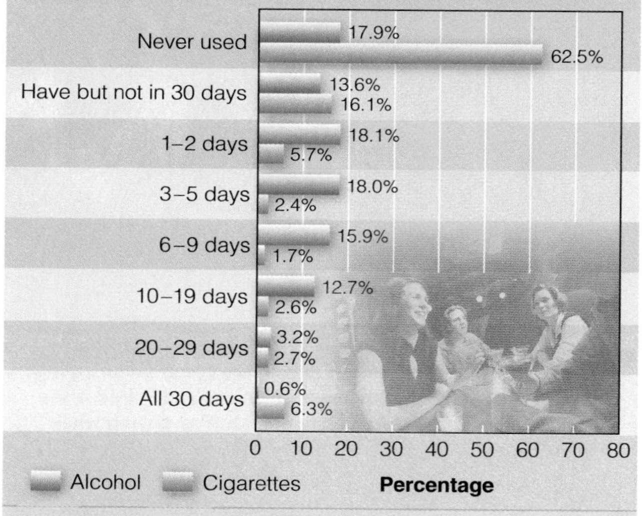

© Jupiter Image

Source: American College Health Association. "American College Health Association-National College Health Assessment (ACHA-NCHA) Spring 2004 Reference Group Data Report (abridged)." *Journal of American College Health*, Vol. 54, No. 4, January–February 2006, p. 201.

Drinking on Campus

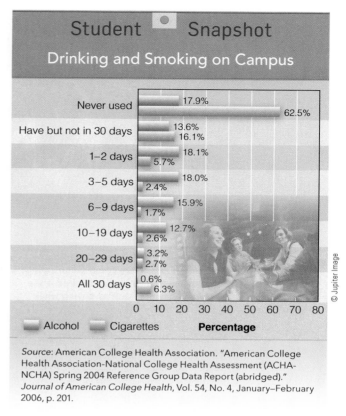

College students drink more, more often, and more dangerously than young people of the same age not attending college.[13] About eight in ten undergraduates drink, at least occasionally, although this figure varies on different campuses. College men drink more, more often, and more intensely than women. Caucasians drink more than African Americans or Asians. Fraternity and sorority members also use more alcohol more often than non-Greeks.[14] (See Student Snapshot: "Drinking and Smoking on Campus.")

For most, alcohol usually does not interfere with their school and work responsibilities. However, an increasing number—about two in five—engage in the dangerous practice of binge drinking. A single binge, combined with poor judgment or bad luck, can lead to life-altering and sometimes life-threatening consequences.

When asked how many drinks they had the last time they partied, 22 percent of students said none, while 44 percent of the women and 28 percent of the men had one to four. About a quarter of men and women had five to eight drinks. About three times as many men as women—25 versus 7 percent—reported more than nine drinks.[15]

According to the National College Health Assessment, 18 percent of students report never using alcohol. Students who don't drink give various reasons for their choice, including not having access to alcohol, parental or peer pressure, being underage, costs, religious reasons, and not liking the taste.[16]

African-American students are more likely than white undergraduates to abstain and to report never having had an alcoholic drink and not having a drink in the past 30 days. They also drink less frequently and consume fewer drinks per occasion than whites. Black undergraduates experience fewer negative consequences of drinking and more regularly use strategies to prevent problem drinking, such as eating before drinking and keeping track of how many drinks they consume.

Social Norms and Student Drinking

More than 50 studies have documented that college students overestimate how much their peers drink. In one recent poll, 23 percent of students at a northeastern university reported drinking no alcohol in the last month. Yet the students believed that only 1 percent of their peers hadn't had a drink during that period. Only 3 percent reported daily drinking, but the students estimated that 43 percent of their peers drank every day for the last month.[17] In one nationwide study, 70 percent of students overestimated the quantity of alcohol consumed by their peers.[18]

This extraordinarily common misperception has a greater influence on how much a student drinks than the actual campus drinking norm.[19] Students who overestimated how much undergraduates drink to celebrate their twenty-first birthdays, for instance, drank heavily on their own twenty-first birthdays.[20] Schools that educate students about actual drinking norms report less high-risk drinking and fewer negative consequences.

Other misperceptions also affect how much students drink. In one recent study, undergraduates significantly overestimated the number of drinks it would take to vomit, feel hungover, have unwanted sexual experiences, or black out. Even after such experiences, heavy-drinking students continued to overestimate how much alcohol they could consume without negative consequences.[21]

Social norms also can affect a student's readiness to change drinking behavior (see Chapter 1). Students in the precontemplation stage see no reason for behavioral change because they believe heavy drinking is the norm in their social group. Once they realize that heavy drinking is not accepted and puts them at risk, they move to the contemplation stage. Students who are encouraged to feel confident in their ability to change—their self-efficacy—proceed to the action stage.[22]

Why College Students Drink

Most college students drink for the same reasons undergraduates have always turned to alcohol: Away from home, often for the first time, many are excited by and apprehensive about their newfound independence. When new pressures seem overwhelming, when they feel awkward or insecure, when they just want to let loose and have a good time, they reach for a drink. In one recent survey, peer pressure was the top-rated reason students gave for drinking. Other motives include to escape, for the effects, to reduce stress, to relax, and for social reasons.[23]

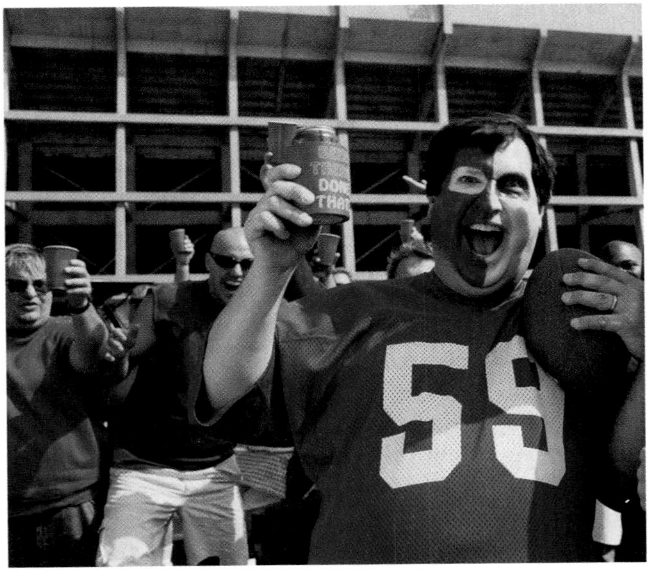

© Sean Murphy/Taxi/Getty Images

Do you drink at sports events? Why?

Freshmen may be especially vulnerable to dangerous drinking as they struggle to adapt to an often bewildering new world. Many who were nondrinkers as high school seniors start to drink in college. They are less likely to do so if friends discourage them from drinking. The heaviest drinking occurs among male freshmen and at the beginning of each academic year. By senior year, drinking moderates.

About half of college men and a third of college women report drinking to excess. Male athletes drink more often, consume more alcohol, and drink to intoxication more than other students, while female athletes consume the lowest quantities of alcohol. Of all students, male athletes are the most likely to drink for social reasons and to drink to get high. College women (athletes or not) and men who are not athletes are more likely to drink as a way of coping, for instance, to feel better.

College sports events intensify heavy drinking. In one study, drinking before and after a men's National College Athletic Association basketball championship increased. Collegiate sporting events appear to be a particularly heavy-drinking context; sports-related alcohol use can occur in many places (for example, at home, at a bar, at the stadium) and celebratory drinking is a frequently endorsed reason for drinking. College students who are sports fans are more likely to drink heavily and experience more alcohol-related negative consequences compared with those who are not sports fans.[24] Heavy drinking is most likely to occur at events where many people become intoxicated, illicit drugs are available, and drinking games are played.

On average, students tend to drink more on days when they are feeling good—possibly because of what researchers call the "celebratory and social" nature of college drinking. Drinking—and positive emotions—also peak on weekends.

Students who believe that their parents approve of drinking are more likely to drink and to report a drinking-related problem. This relationship is even stronger in younger students and those who perceive that their mothers approve of drinking.[25]

Binge Drinking on Campus

Binge drinking—is the leading cause of preventable death among undergraduates and the most serious threat to their intellectual, physical, and psychological development. In spite of great efforts across U.S. college campuses to decrease binge drinking, the national average—two out of five students report bingeing—remained steady for 20 years.

According to the National College Health Assessment, most students—68 percent of women and 54 percent of men—reported no binges in the previous two weeks. However, 46 percent of men and 32 percent of women had five or more drinks at one sitting at least once in the previous two weeks (Figure 12-4).

Frequent binge drinkers account for almost 70 percent of all alcohol consumed by college students. Students in four-year colleges are more likely to binge than those in two-year colleges.[26]

Binge drinkers are most likely to be white, fraternity and sorority members, under 24 years of age, involved in athletics, and frequent socializers. White males binge-drink the most; African-American women, the least. Students who study a great deal or are involved in community service or the arts are less likely to binge-drink.

Binge drinking has jumped from one in four women to almost one in three: Women who report binge-drinking are more likely to have greater weight concerns than those who did not binge. Women who think their peers drink frequently engage in more binge drinking episodes than others.[27]

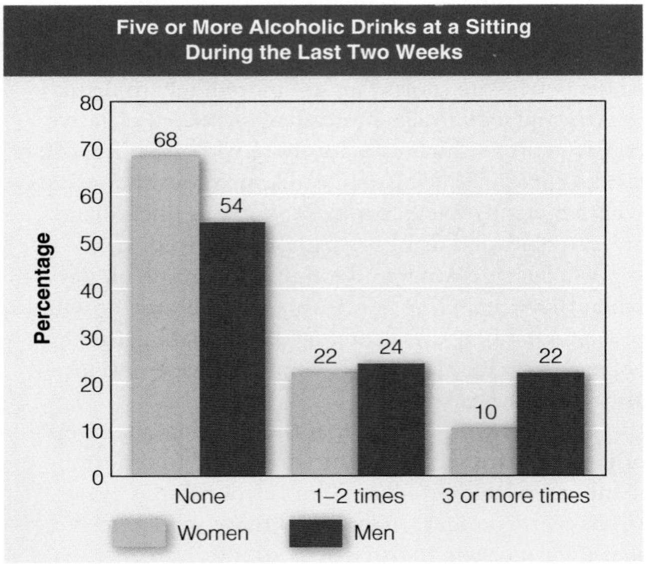

FIGURE 12-4 Binge Drinking on Campus

*Based on surveys of 54,111 students on 71 campuses

Source: American College Health Association. American College Health Association-National College Health Assessment (ACHA-NCHA) Web Summary. Available at www.acha.org/projects_programs/ncha_sampledata.cfm.

Unplanned sexual activities, date rape, and sexual assault are 150 percent more likely among women who drink than among those who do not. Sophomore, junior, and senior women are much less likely to engage in heavy episodic drinking than freshmen women.

Surveys consistently show that students who engage in binge drinking, particularly those who do so more than once a week, experience a far higher rate of problems than other students. Frequent binge drinkers are likely to miss classes, vandalize property, drive after drinking, and abuse other substances, including nicotine, marijuana, cocaine, and LSD.

? FAQ Why Do Students Binge?

Young people who came from, socialized within, or were exposed to "wet" environments—settings in which alcohol is cheap and accessible and drinking is prevalent—are more likely to engage in binge drinking. Students who report drinking at least once a month during their final year of high school are over three times more likely to binge-drink in college than those who drank less frequently in high school.

The factors that most influence students to binge-drink are:

- **Low price** for alcohol.
- **Easy access to alcohol.** In one study, the density of alcohol outlets (such as bars) near campus affected the drinking of students.
- **Attending a school** or living in a residence with many binge drinkers.
- **Belief** that close friends were likely to binge.
- **Drinking games**—such as tongue twisters or drinking whenever a certain phrase is mentioned in a song or on a TV program—are dangerous because they can result in high levels of intoxication in a short period of time.
- **Parents who drank** or did not disapprove of their children drinking.
- **Recreational drinking** before age 16.

Some educators view binging as a product of the college environment. More students binge-drink at the beginning of the school year and then cut back as the semester progresses and academic demands increase. Binge drinking also peaks following exam times, during home football weekends, and during spring break. Many new students engage in binge drinking for the first time very soon after they arrive on campus. Binges become less common in their subsequent years at school and almost always end with education. Real life, one educator notes, is "a strong disincentive" to this type of drinking.

Colleges and health authorities are trying innovative approaches to prevent or stop binge drinking. One school has found that four weekly electronic "newsletters" are as likely to reach students as print ones. The Internet may be a particularly appealing means of communication because of its anonymity, nonjudgmental nature, and 24-7 availability.

Spring breaks, which have become notorious for wild partying, promote the most dangerous forms of drinking. In an American Medical Association poll, 83 percent of college women and recent graduates said that spring breaks involve more or heavier drinking than occurs on college campuses. The majority of the respondents agreed that women use drinking as an excuse for outrageous behavior, including unprotected sex. One in five regretted sexual activity they had engaged in during a spring break.[28] (See You Decide.)

No Mom. No Dad. No rules. Nothing to do but party. Spring break has long been an anything-goes celebration. However medical authorities are leading a campaign against what the American Medical Association calls a "dangerous binge-fest" that leads to risky sexual behavior, sexual assaults and rapes, alcohol poisoning, and alcohol-related injuries and deaths. College women in particular put themselves in danger of sexually transmitted infections, blackouts, and sexual violence. Do you think that spring break is just a way for undergraduates to blow off steam after months of hitting the books? Or have the promoters of spring break trips gone too far and now exploit female students and endanger their health?

You Decide

Underage Drinking on Campus

Students under age 21 drink less often than older students, but tend to drink more heavily and to experience more negative alcohol-related consequences. More underage students report drinking "to get drunk" and drinking at binge levels when they consumed alcohol.

Underage college students are most likely to drink if they can easily obtain cheap alcohol, especially beer. They tend to drink in private settings, such as dorms and fraternity parties, and are more likely than students of legal age to experience a host of negative drinking-related consequences, including doing something they regretted; forgetting where they were or what they did; causing property damage; getting into trouble with police; and being hurt or injured. The drinking behavior of underage students also depends on their living arrangements. Those in controlled settings, such as their parents' home or a substance-free dorm, are less likely to binge-drink. Students living in fraternities or sororities were most likely to binge-drink, regardless of age.

Students under age 21 in states with tough laws against underage drinking are less likely to drink than those in states with fewer restrictions.

The Toll of College Drinking

According to research summarized in a College Task Force report to the National Institute on Alcohol Abuse and Alcoholism (NIAAA), the consequences of excessive drinking by college students are more significant, more destructive, and more costly than many students or parents realize. These consequences affect students whether or not they drink. Drinking by college students aged 18 to 24 contributes to an estimated 1,700 student deaths, 599,000 injuries, and 97,000 cases of sexual assault or date rape each year.[29]

According to the Commission on Substance Abuse at Colleges and Universities, alcohol is involved in two-thirds of college student suicides, nine of ten rapes, and 95 percent of violent crimes on campus. A national survey released by the Higher Education Center for Alcohol and Other Drug Prevention reported that 75 to 90 percent of all violence on college campuses is alcohol-related. About 300,000 of today's college students will eventually die from alcohol-related causes, including drunk-driving accidents, cirrhosis of the liver, various cancers, and heart disease, estimates the Core Institute, an organization that studies college drinking.

In the National College Health Assessment, 38 percent of students who drank did something they later regretted; 31 percent forgot who they were with or what they did. Men were more likely than women to injure themselves, have unprotected sex, get involved in a fight, or physically injure another person. Women were more likely to have someone use force or threat of force to have sex with them.[30] In a recent study of first-year students, about one in seven reported at least one drinking-related problem. More than half reported a headache (hangover) or getting sick and throwing up after drinking. More than a fourth experienced memory loss, missing work or school, or regrettable sexual situations. (Figure 12-5).[31]

"Secondhand" Drinking Problems

Heavy alcohol use can endanger both drinkers and others. Secondhand problems caused by other's alcohol use include loss of sleep, interruption of studies,

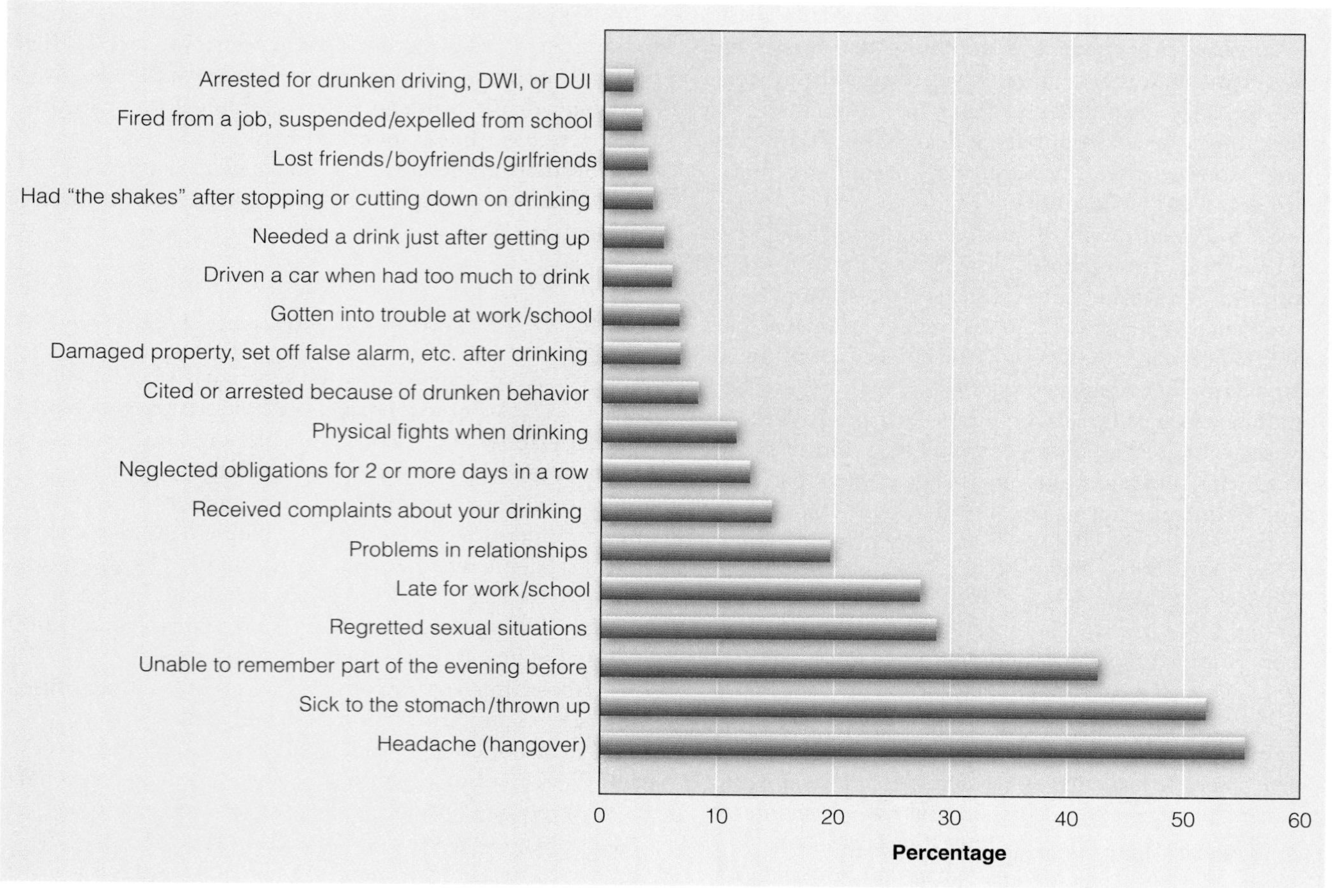

FIGURE 12-5 Occurrence of Drinking Problems Among First-Year Students Since Beginning College

Source: Boyle, Jennifer, et al. "Perceived Parental Approval of Drinking and Its Impact on Problem Drinking Behaviors among First Year College Students." *Journal of American College Health*, Vol. 54, No. 4, January–February 2006, p. 238.

assaults, vandalism, and unwanted sexual advances. Students living on campuses with high rates of binge drinking are two or more times as likely to experience these secondhand effects as those living on campuses with low rates. In one study, nearly three-quarters of campus rapes happened when the victims were so intoxicated that they were unable to consent or refuse.

YOUR LIFE COACH

Taking Charge of Alcohol Use

Drinking, like other behaviors, is a choice. You—and no one else but you—have the right to decide not to drink, and you owe no one an explanation if you say no to alcohol. As with other risk-taking behaviors, never let anyone intimidate you into doing anything that violates your values.

How Students Protect Themselves from Unsafe Drinking

Smart choices can help you avoid many of the negative consequences of drinking. Various "self-protective" behaviors, such as designating a driver, eating before or during drinking, and keeping track of the number of drinks consumed, have proved effective in reducing alcohol-related problems. Women employ these strategies more often when partying or socializing than men; black students use them more often than white men. The students who used these strategies most often had the fewest problem behaviors.[32]

How do you compare with the students surveyed by the National College Health Assessment?

Behavior	Students Who Always or Usually Use the Strategy
Eat before and/or during drinking	77%
Use a designated driver	76%
Keep track of how many drinks they're having	65%
Avoid drinking games	42%
Decide in advance how many drinks to have	34%
Have a friend let you know when you've had enough	28%
Choose not to drink	26%
Pace yourself to no more than one drink an hour	28%
Alternate alcoholic and nonalcoholic beverages	27%

Staying in Control of Your Drinking

If you do drink, take responsibility for how much and how often you drink. Here are some guidelines that can help:

- **Keep a diary.** Writing down how much you drink each day can make you more aware of exactly how much you drink.
- **Pace yourself.** Try having a "spacer," a nonalcoholic drink every second or third drink.
- **Stay busy.** You will drink less if you play pool or dance rather than just sitting and drinking.
- **Try low-alcohol alternatives,** such as light beers and low- or no-alcohol wines
- **Have alcohol-free days.** Don't drink at all at least two days a week.
- **Start with a soft drink.** You will drink much faster if you are thirsty, so have a nonalcoholic drink to quench your thirst before you start drinking alcohol.
- **Use standard drinks.** Monitor how much alcohol you drink. By converting what you drink into standard drinks, it is easier to keep track.
- **Drink slowly.** Take sips and not gulps. Put your glass down between sips.
- **Avoid salty snacks.** Salty food like chips or nuts make you thirsty so you drink more.
- **Have one drink at a time.** Don't let people top up your drinks. It makes it harder to keep track of how much alcohol you're consuming.
- **Be assertive.** Don't be pressured into drinking more than you want or intend to. Say "Thanks, but no thanks."
- **Pay attention.** Watch as your drink is poured. Don't let your drink out of your sight.
- **Never leave a party with someone you don't know.** This is especially true if you've been drinking and are feeling somewhat intoxicated.
- **Abstain for 48 hours** if you do have an episode of heavy drinking to let your body recover.
- **When you throw a party, be a responsible host.** Collect car keys from your guests. Serve high-protein food like pepperoni pizza, shrimp, or spareribs. Serve nonalcoholic beverages. Do not force drinks on your guests or rush to refill their glasses when empty. Stop serving alcohol about two hours before the party is over.

? FAQ What Are Colleges Doing to Prevent Alcohol Abuse?

Because drinking problems are so common and cause so many harmful consequences, colleges have placed a high priority on changing the drinking culture on their campuses. The National Institute on Alcohol Abuse and Alcoholism has studied interventions that effectively deal with college drinking problems. Programs that address alcohol-related attitudes and behaviors, use survey data to counter students' misconceptions about their fellow students' drinking practices, and increase students' motivation to change their drinking habits have proved effective.[33]

The social norm approach, which communicates actual facts about drinking behavior to dispel myths, is simple, cost-efficient, and effective. Its positive message is that most students on virtually every campus believe in and practice safety, responsibility, and moderation, rather than excess drinking.

Motivational interviewing, a nonjudgmental, supportive approach to personal change, also has proved beneficial.[34] In brief interventions, specially trained counselors help build students' self-efficacy (discussed in Chapter 1), in this case, their belief in their ability to change their drinking behavior.[35]

First-year students are at particular risk for alcohol-related problems, and those who begin to drink heavily may continue to do so throughout college. Some schools focus on incoming freshmen with interventions that include self-surveys, group discussions about normal drinking behavior, and practical strategies for high-risk situations.[36] Other approaches include self-monitoring with monthly drinking diaries for high-risk students, such as athletes and Greeks, and those

motivational interviewing A nonjudgmental but directive method for supporting motivation to change.

who violate campus alcohol policies. Researchers report less drinking and fewer drinking-related problems following such interventions.[37]

Other university alcohol policies include campus alcohol bans, no alcohol at university-sponsored events, prohibition of beer kegs, limits on the maximum number of drinks served per student, and dry rushing activities. Studies suggest that student who attend schools that ban alcohol are less likely to engage in heavy binge drinking, more likely to abstain from using alcohol, and less likely to experience the secondhand effects of drinking.[38]

Most colleges and universities offer some type of alcohol education program for students. Some schools post their policies online, but in many cases they are difficult to find among all of the other information on a school's website. Can you find the policy for your school?

The U.S. Department of Education has begun highlighting innovative antidrinking practices on campus. There has been an increase in on-campus chapters of national support groups such as AA, Al-Anon, Adult Children of Alcoholics, and a peer-education program called BACCHUS: Boost Alcohol Consciousness Concerning the Health of University Students.

Alcohol's Effects on the Body

Unlike food or drugs in tablet form, alcohol is directly and quickly absorbed into the bloodstream through the stomach walls and upper intestine. The alcohol in a typical drink reaches the bloodstream in 15 minutes and rises to its peak concentration in about an hour. The bloodstream carries the alcohol to the liver, heart, and brain (Figure 12-6).

Most of the alcohol you drink can leave your body only after metabolism by the liver, which converts about 95 percent of the alcohol to carbon dioxide and water. The other 5 percent is excreted unchanged, mainly through urination, respiration, and perspiration.

Alcohol is a diuretic, a drug that speeds up the elimination of fluid from the body, so drink water when you drink alcohol to maintain your fluid balance. And

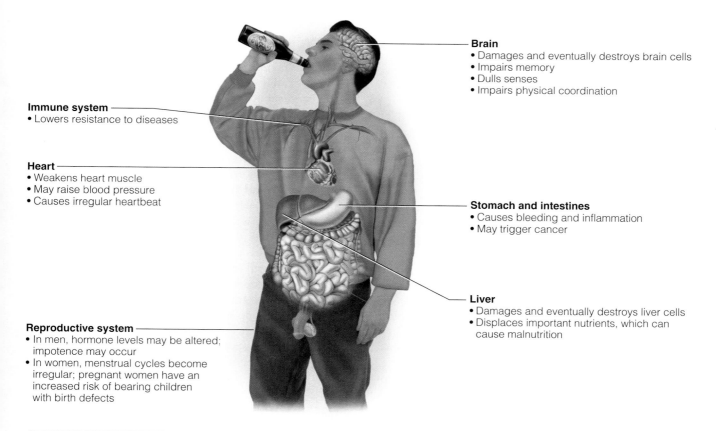

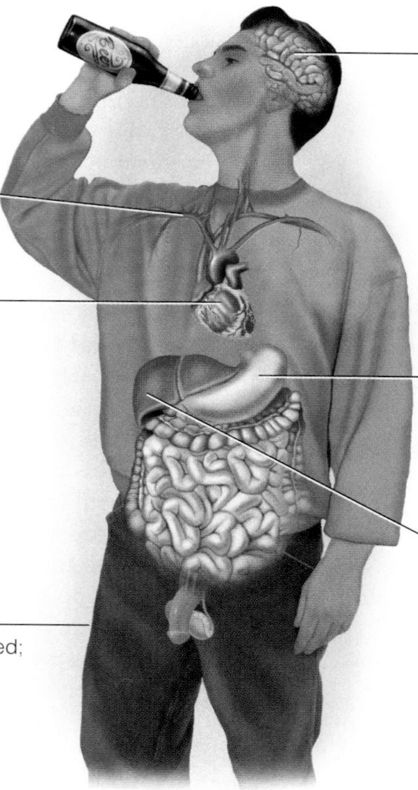
Brain
• Damages and eventually destroys brain cells
• Impairs memory
• Dulls senses
• Impairs physical coordination
Immune system
• Lowers resistance to diseases
Heart
• Weakens heart muscle
• May raise blood pressure
• Causes irregular heartbeat
Stomach and intestines
• Causes bleeding and inflammation
• May trigger cancer
Liver
• Damages and eventually destroys liver cells
• Displaces important nutrients, which can cause malnutrition
Reproductive system
• In men, hormone levels may be altered; impotence may occur
• In women, menstrual cycles become irregular; pregnant women have an increased risk of bearing children with birth defects

FIGURE 12-6 The Effects of Alcohol Abuse on the Body

Alcohol has a major effect on the brain, damaging brain cells, impairing judgment and perceptions, and often leading to accidents and altercations. Alcohol also damages the digestive system, especially the liver.

alcohol lowers body temperature, so you should never drink to get or stay warm.

Digestive System

Alcohol reaches the stomach first, where it is partially broken down. The remaining alcohol is absorbed easily through the stomach tissue into the bloodstream. In the stomach, alcohol triggers the secretion of acids, which irritate the stomach lining. Excessive drinking at one sitting may result in nausea; chronic drinking may result in peptic ulcers (breaks in the stomach lining) and bleeding from the stomach lining.

The alcohol in the bloodstream eventually reaches the liver. The liver, which bears the major responsibility of fat metabolism in the body, converts this excess alcohol to fat. After a few weeks of four or five drinks a day, liver cells start to accumulate fat. Alcohol also stimulates liver cells to attract white blood cells, which normally travel throughout the bloodstream engulfing harmful substances and wastes. If white blood cells begin to invade body tissue, such as the liver, they can cause irreversible damage.

Weight and Waists

At 7 calories per gram, alcohol has nearly as many calories as fat (9 calories per gram) and significantly more than carbohydrates or protein (which have 4 calories per gram). Since a standard drink contains 12–15 grams of alcohol, the alcohol in a single drink adds about 100 calories to your daily intake. A glass of wine contains as many calories as some candy bars; you would have to walk a mile to burn them off. In addition to being a calorie-dense food, alcohol stimulates the appetite so you're likely to eat more.

"Beer bellies" earn their name. In a study of men and women over age 20 in Copenhagen, those who drank the most beer or spirits had wider waists on a ten-year follow-up. Wine did not have a similar impact.

Cardiovascular System

Alcohol gets mixed reviews regarding its effects on the cardiovascular system. As several studies have shown, people who drink moderate amounts of alcohol have lower mortality rates after a heart attack, as well as a lower risk of heart attack compared to abstainers and heavy drinkers.

How does alcohol enhance heart health? Researchers believe that it boosts beneficial high-density lipoproteins (HDL), lowers the risk of blood clots, and also may have an anti-inflammatory effect. According to recent studies, alcohol may lower two blood components, C-reactive protein and fibrinogen, that indicate increased heart disease risk (discussed in Chapter 10).

Some cardiologists contend that the benefits of moderate drinking may be overstated, especially because of alcohol's contribution to the epidemic of obesity around the world. Heavier drinking triggers the release of harmful oxygen molecules called free radicals, which can increase the risk of heart disease, stroke, and cirrhosis of the liver. Alcohol use can weaken the heart muscle directly, causing a disorder called cardiomyopathy. The combined use of alcohol and other drugs, including tobacco and cocaine, greatly increases the likelihood of damage to the heart.

Breast Cancer

According to several large studies, women who have three drinks per day are 18 percent more likely to develop breast cancer than women who don't drink at all. The risk occurs with all forms of alcohol—beer, wine, and spirits—and increases the more women drink.

In the Nurses' Health Study, breast cancer rates rose slightly even in women who took as little as half a drink per day. A single daily drink of 1 ounce of spirits, such as whiskey, gin, or vodka, or 3 ounces of wine increases a woman's breast cancer risk slightly—perhaps 3 or 4 percent. Every additional daily drink increases the risk by 7 percent. By four drinks a day, a woman's risk increases 30 percent.

Brain and Behavior

At first, when you drink, you feel up. In low dosages, alcohol affects the regions of the brain that inhibit or control behavior, so you feel looser and act in ways you might not otherwise. However, you also experience losses of concentration, memory, judgment, and fine motor control; and you have mood swings and emotional outbursts.

Moderate amounts of alcohol can have disturbing effects on perception and judgment, including the following:

- **Impaired perceptions.** You're less able to adjust your eyes to bright lights because glare bothers you more. Although you can still hear sounds, you can't distinguish between them or judge their direction well.
- **Dulled smell and taste.** Alcohol itself may cause some vitamin deficiencies, and the poor eating habits of heavy drinkers result in further nutrition problems.
- **Diminished sensation.** On a freezing winter night, you may walk outside without a coat and not feel the cold.
- **Altered sense of space.** You may not realize, for instance, that you have been in one place for several hours.

- **Impaired motor skills.** Writing, typing, driving, and other abilities involving your muscles are impaired. This is why law enforcement officers sometimes ask suspected drunk drivers to touch their nose with a finger or to walk a straight line. Drinking large amounts of alcohol impairs reaction time, speed, accuracy, and consistency, as well as judgment.
- **Impaired sexual performance.** While drinking may increase your interest in sex, it may also impair sexual response, especially a man's ability to achieve or maintain an erection. As Shakespeare wrote, "It provokes the desire, but it takes away the performance."

Moderate and heavy drinkers show signs of impaired intelligence, slowed-down reflexes, and difficulty remembering. Because alcohol is a central nervous system depressant, it slows down the activity of the neurons in the brain, gradually dulling the responses of the brain and nervous system. One or two drinks act as a tranquilizer or relaxant. Additional drinks result in a progressive reduction in central nervous system activity, leading to sleep, general anesthesia, coma, and even death.

Heavy alcohol use may pose special dangers to the brains of drinkers at both ends of the age spectrum. Adolescents who drink regularly show impairments in their neurological and cognitive functioning. Elderly people who drink heavily appear to have more brain shrinkage, or atrophy, than those who drink lightly or not at all. In general, moderate drinkers have healthier brains and a lower risk of dementia than those who don't drink and those who drink to excess.

Immune System

Chronic alcohol use can inhibit the production of both white blood cells, which fight off infections, and red blood cells, which carry oxygen to all the organs and tissues of the body. Alcohol may increase the risk of infection with human immunodeficiency virus (HIV), by altering the judgment of users so that they more readily engage in activities, such as unsafe sexual practices, that put them in danger. If you drink when you have a cold or the flu, alcohol interferes with the body's ability to recover. It also increases the chance of bacterial pneumonia in flu sufferers.

Increased Risk of Dying

Alcohol kills. Alcohol is responsible for 100,000 deaths each year and is the third-leading cause of death after tobacco and improper diet and lack of exercise. The leading alcohol-related cause of death is injury. Alcohol plays a role in almost half of all traffic fatalities, half of all homicides, and a quarter of all suicides. The second leading cause of alcohol-related deaths is cirrhosis of the liver, a chronic disease that causes extensive scarring and irreversible damage. In addition, as many as half of patients admitted to hospitals and 15 percent of those making office visits seek or need medical care because of the direct or indirect effects of alcohol.

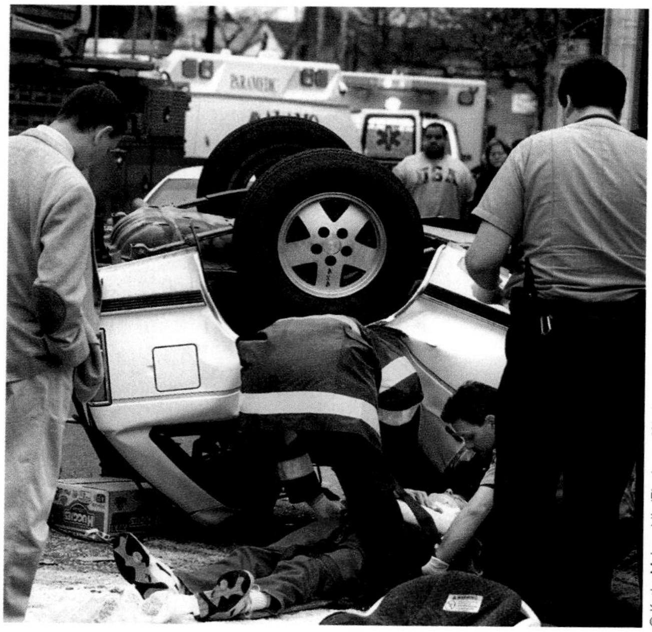

Alcohol plays a role in 40 percent of motor vehicle fatalities.

Young drinkers—teens and those in their early twenties—are at highest risk of dying from injuries, mostly car accidents. Older drinkers over age 50 face the greatest danger of premature death from cirrhosis of the liver, hepatitis, and other alcohol-linked illnesses.

Most studies of the relationship between alcohol consumption and death from all causes show that moderate drinkers—those who consume approximately seven drinks per week—have a lower risk of death than abstainers, while heavy drinkers have a higher risk than either group. In one ten-year study, never-drinkers showed no elevated risk of dying, while consistent heavier drinkers were at higher risk of dying of any cause than other men.

Fetal Alcohol Effects and Syndrome

An estimated 15 percent of women drink alcohol while pregnant, most having one drink or less per day. Even light consumption of alcohol can lead to **Fetal Alcohol Effects (FAE):** low birthweight, irritability as newborns, and permanent mental impairment.

The babies of women who consume three or more ounces of alcohol (the equivalent of six or seven cocktails) are at risk of more severe problems. One of every 750 newborns has a cluster of physical and mental defects called **Fetal Alcohol Syndrome (FAS):** small head, abnormal facial features, jitters, poor muscle tone, sleep disorders, sluggish motor development, failure to thrive, short stature, delayed speech, mental retardation, and hyperactivity.

Interaction with Other Drugs

Alcohol can interact with other drugs—prescription and nonprescription, legal and illegal. Of the 100 most frequently prescribed drugs, more than half contain at least one ingredient that interacts adversely with alcohol. Because alcohol and other psychoactive drugs may work on the same areas of the brain, their combination can produce an effect much greater than that expected of either drug by itself. The consequences of this synergistic interaction can be fatal. Alcohol is particularly dangerous when combined with other depressants and antianxiety medications.

Alcohol, Gender, and Race

Experts in alcohol treatment are increasingly recognizing racial and ethnic differences in risk factors for drinking problems, patterns of drinking, and most effective types of treatment.

Gender

According to conventional gender stereotypes, drinking is a symbol of manliness. In the past, far more men than women drank. In the United States today, both genders are likely to consume alcohol. However, there are well-documented differences in how often and how much men and women drink. In general, men drink more frequently, consume a larger quantity of alcohol per drinking occasion, and report more problems related to drinking. More than half of women drink: Of these, 45 percent are light drinkers; 3 percent, moderate drinkers; 2 percent, heavy drinkers; and 21 percent, binge drinkers.

The bodies of men and women respond to alcohol in different ways. Because they have a far smaller quantity of a protective enzyme in the stomach to break down alcohol before it's absorbed into the bloodstream, women absorb about 30 percent more alcohol into their bloodstream than men. The alcohol travels through the blood to the brain, so women become intoxicated much more quickly. And because there's more alcohol in the bloodstream to break down, the liver may also be adversely affected. In alcoholic women, the stomach seems to completely stop digesting alcohol, which may explain why women alcoholics are more likely to suffer liver damage than men.

Race

African-American Community

Overall, African Americans consume less alcohol per person than whites, yet twice as many blacks die of cirrhosis of the liver each year. In some cities, the rate of cirrhosis is ten times higher among African-American than white men. Alcohol also contributes to high rates of hypertension, esophageal cancer, and homicide among African-American men.

Hispanic Community

The various Hispanic cultures tend to discourage any drinking by women but encourage heavy drinking by men as part of machismo, or feelings of manhood. Hispanic men have higher rates of alcohol use and abuse than the general population and suffer a high rate of cirrhosis. Moreover, American-born Hispanic men drink more than those born in other countries.

Few Hispanics enter treatment, partly because of a lack of information, language barriers, and poor community-based services. Hispanic families generally try to resolve problems themselves, and their cultural values discourage the sharing of intimate personal stories, which characterizes Alcoholics Anonymous and other support groups. Churches often provide the most effective forms of help.

Native American Community

European settlers introduced alcohol to Native Americans. Because of the societal and physical problems resulting from excessive drinking, at the request of tribal leaders, the U.S. Congress in 1832 prohibited the use of alcohol by Native Americans. Many reservations still ban alcohol use, so Native Americans who want to drink may have to travel long distances to obtain alcohol, which may contribute to the high death rate from hypothermia and pedestrian and motor-vehicle accidents among Native Americans. (Injuries are the leading cause of death among this group.)

Certainly, not all Native Americans drink, and not all who drink do so to excess. However, they have three times the general population's rate of alcohol-related injury and illness. Cirrhosis of the liver is the fourth-leading cause of death among this cultural group. While many Native American women don't drink, those who do have

fetal alcohol effects (FAE) Milder forms of FAS, including low birthweight, irritability as newborns, and permanent mental impairment as a result of the mother's alcohol consumption during pregnancy.

fetal alcohol syndrome (FAS) A cluster of physical and mental defects in the newborn, including low birthweight, smaller-than-normal head circumference, intrauterine growth retardation, and permanent mental impairment caused by the mother's alcohol consumption during pregnancy.

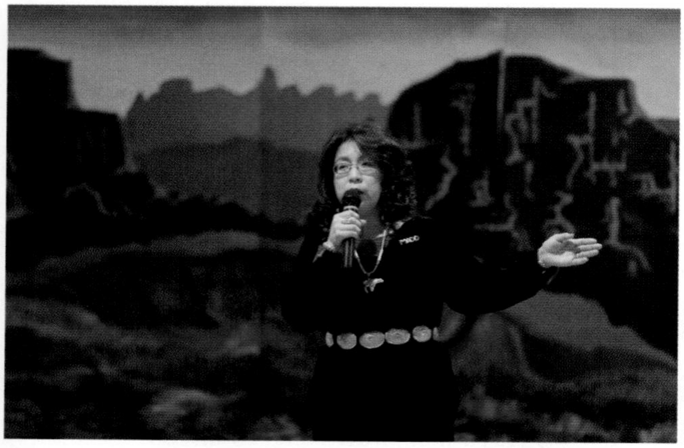

Navajo Vikki Shirley speaks to parents at Rough Rocks Elementary School in Rough Rocks, Arizona. Shirley, who lost her daughter in an alcohol-related crash, travels to remote Navajo Nation villages to speak to parents throughout Arizona, New Mexico, Utah, and Colorado.

high rates of alcohol-related problems, which affect both them and their children. Their rate of cirrhosis of the liver is 36 times that of white women. In some tribes, 10.5 out of every 1,000 newborns have fetal alcohol syndrome, compared with 1 to 3 out of 1,000 in the general population.

Asian-American Community

Asian Americans tend to drink very little or not at all, in part because of an inborn physiological reaction to alcohol that causes facial flushing, rapid heart rate, lowered blood pressure, nausea, vomiting, and other symptoms. A very high percentage of women of all Asian-American nationalities abstain completely. Some sociologists have expressed concern, however, that as Asian Americans become more assimilated into American culture, they'll drink more—and possibly suffer very adverse effects from alcohol.

Alcohol Problems

By the simplest definition, problem drinking is the use of alcohol in any way that creates difficulties, potential difficulties, or health risks for an individual. Like alcoholics, problem drinkers are individuals whose lives are in some way impaired by their drinking. The only difference is one of degree. Alcohol becomes a problem, and a person becomes an alcoholic, when the drinker can't "take it or leave it." He or she spends more and more time anticipating the next drink, planning when and where to get it, buying and hiding alcohol, and covering up secret drinking. As many as one in six adults in the United States may have a problem with drinking.

Alcohol abuse involves continued use of alcohol despite awareness of social, occupational, psychological, or physical problems related to drinking, or drinking in dangerous ways or situations (before driving, for instance). A diagnosis of alcohol abuse is based on one or more of the following occurring at any time during a 12-month period:

- **A failure to fulfill major role obligations** at work, school, or home (such as missing work or school).
- **The use of alcohol in situations in which it is physically hazardous** (such as before driving).
- **Alcohol-related legal problems** (such as drunk-driving arrests).
- **Continued alcohol use despite persistent or recurring social or interpersonal problems** caused or exacerbated by alcohol (such as fighting while drunk).[39]

Alcohol dependence is a separate disorder in which individuals develop a strong craving for alcohol because it produces pleasurable feelings or relieves stress or anxiety. Over time they experience physiological changes that lead to *tolerance* of its effects; this means that they must consume larger and larger amounts to achieve

Strategies for Prevention: How to Recognize the Warning Signs of Alcoholism

- Experiencing the following symptoms after drinking: frequent headaches, nausea, stomach pain, heartburn, gas, fatigue, weakness, muscle cramps, irregular or rapid heartbeats.
- Needing a drink in the morning to start the day.
- Denying any problem with alcohol.
- Doing things while drinking that are regretted afterward.
- Dramatic mood swings, from anger to laughter to anxiety.
- Sleep problems.
- Depression and paranoia.
- Forgetting what happened during a drinking episode.
- Changing brands or going on the wagon to control drinking.
- Having five or more drinks a day.

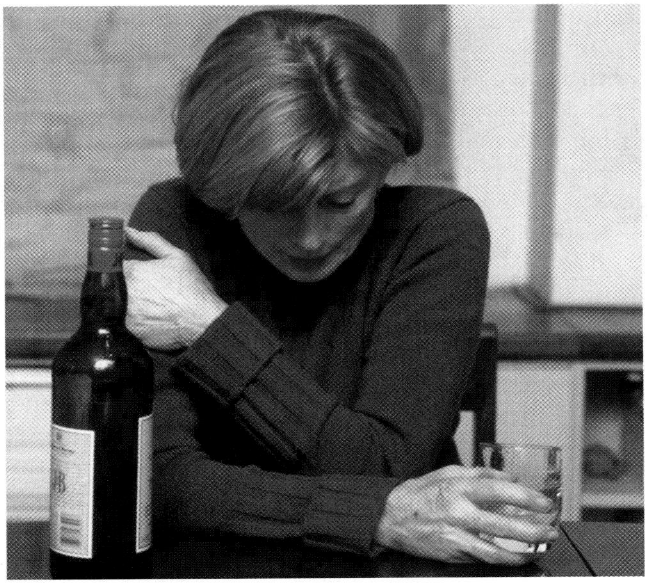

Catherine Ursillo/Photo Researchers, Inc.

Daytime drinking and drinking alone can be signs of a serious problem, even though the drinker may otherwise appear to be in control.

intoxication. If they abruptly stop drinking, they suffer *withdrawal,* a state of acute physical and psychological discomfort. A diagnosis of alcohol dependence is based on three or more of the following symptoms occurring during any 12-month period:

- **Tolerance,** as defined by either a need for markedly increased amounts of alcohol to achieve intoxication or desired effect, or a markedly diminished effect with continued drinking of the same amount of alcohol as in the past.
- **Withdrawal,** including at least two of the following symptoms: sweating, rapid pulse, or other signs of autonomic hyperactivity; increased hand tremor; insomnia; nausea or vomiting; temporary hallucinations or illusions; physical agitation or restlessness; anxiety; or grand mal seizures.
- **Drinking to avoid** or relieve the symptoms of withdrawal.
- **Consuming larger amounts of alcohol,** or drinking over a longer period than was intended.
- **Persistent desire** or unsuccessful efforts to cut down or control drinking.
- **A great deal of time spent** in activities necessary to obtain alcohol, drink it, or recover from its effects.
- **Important social, occupational, or recreational activities given up** or reduced because of alcohol use.
- **Continued alcohol use** despite knowledge that alcohol is likely to cause or exacerbate a persistent or recurring physical or psychological problem.

According to a survey of more than 14,000 undergraduates at four-year colleges, 6 percent of college students met criteria for a diagnosis of alcohol dependence or alcoholism, 31 percent for alcohol abuse. More than two of every five students reported at least one symptom of these conditions and were at increased risk of developing a true alcohol disorder. Few reported seeking treatment since coming to college.

Alcoholism, as defined by the National Council on Alcoholism and Drug Dependence and the American Society of Addiction, is a primary, chronic disease in which genetic, psychosocial, and environmental factors influence its development and manifestations. The disease is often progressive and fatal. Its characteristics include an inability to control drinking, a preoccupation with alcohol, continued use of alcohol despite adverse consequences, and distorted thinking, most notably denial. Like other diseases, alcoholism is not simply a matter of insufficient willpower but a complex problem that causes many symptoms, can have serious consequences, yet can improve with treatment.

A lack of obvious signs of alcoholism can be deceiving. A person who doesn't drink in the morning but feels that he or she must always have a drink at a certain time of the day may have lost control over his or her drinking. A person who never drinks alone but always drinks socially with others may be camouflaging loss of control. A person who is holding a job or taking care of the family may still spend every waking hour thinking about that first drink at the end of the day (preoccupation).

Alcohol Dependence and Abuse

Although the exact cause of alcohol dependence and abuse is not known, certain factors—including biochemical imbalances in the brain, heredity, cultural acceptability, and stress—all seem to play a role. They include the following:

- **Genetics.** Scientists have not yet identified conclusively a specific gene that puts people at risk for alcoholism. However, epidemiological studies have shown evidence of heredity's role. Studies of twins suggest that heredity accounts for two-thirds of the risk of becoming alcoholic in both men and women.

alcohol abuse Continued use of alcohol despite awareness of social, occupational, psychological, or physical problems related to its use, or use of alcohol in dangerous ways or situations, such as before driving.

alcohol dependence Development of a strong craving for alcohol due to the pleasurable feelings or relief of stress or anxiety produced by drinking.

alcoholism A chronic, progressive, potentially fatal disease characterized by impaired control of drinking, a preoccupation with alcohol, continued use of alcohol despite adverse consequences, and distorted thinking, most notably denial.

- **Stress and traumatic experiences.** Many people start drinking heavily as a way of coping with psychological problems.
- **Parental alcoholism.** According to researchers, alcoholism is four to five times more common among the children of alcoholics, who may be influenced by the behavior they see in their parents.
- **Drug abuse.** Alcoholism is also associated with the abuse of other psychoactive drugs, including marijuana, cocaine, heroin, amphetamines, and various antianxiety medications.

Medical Complications of Alcohol Abuse and Dependence

Excessive alcohol use adversely affects virtually every organ system in the body, including the brain, the digestive tract, the heart, muscles, blood, and hormones (look back at Figure 12-6, page 340). In addition, because alcohol interacts with many drugs, it can increase the risk of potentially lethal overdoses and harmful interactions. Among the major risks and complications are:

- **Liver disease.** Chronic heavy drinking can lead to alcoholic hepatitis (inflammation and destruction of liver cells) and in the 15 percent of people who continue drinking beyond this stage, cirrhosis (irreversible scarring and destruction of liver cells). The liver eventually may fail completely, resulting in coma and death.
- **Cardiovascular disease.** Heavy drinking can weaken the heart muscle (causing cardiac myopathy), elevate blood pressure, and increase the risk of stroke.
- **Cancer.** Heavy alcohol use may contribute to cancer of the liver, stomach, and colon, as well as malignant melanoma, a deadly form of skin cancer.
- **Brain damage.** Long-term heavy drinkers may suffer memory loss and be unable to think abstractly, recall names of common objects, and follow simple instructions. Chronic brain damage resulting from alcohol consumption is second only to Alzheimer's disease as a cause of cognitive deterioration in adults.
- **Vitamin deficiencies.** Alcoholism is associated with vitamin deficiencies, especially of thiamin (B_1). Lack of thiamin may result in Wernicke-Korsakoff syndrome, which is characterized by disorientation, memory failure, hallucinations, and jerky eye movements, and can be disabling enough to require lifelong custodial care.
- **Digestive problems.** Alcohol triggers the secretion of acids in the stomach that irritate the mucous lining and cause gastritis. Chronic drinking may result in peptic ulcers (breaks in the stomach lining) and bleeding from the stomach lining.
- **Accidents and injuries.** Alcohol may contribute to almost half of the deaths caused by car accidents, burns, falls, and choking. Nearly half of those convicted and jailed for criminal acts committed these crimes while under the influence of alcohol.
- **Higher mortality.** As discussed earlier, the mortality rate for alcoholics is two to three times higher than that for nonalcoholics of the same age. Injury is the leading alcohol-related cause of death, chiefly in auto accidents involving a drunk driver. Alcohol is a factor in about 30 percent of all suicides.

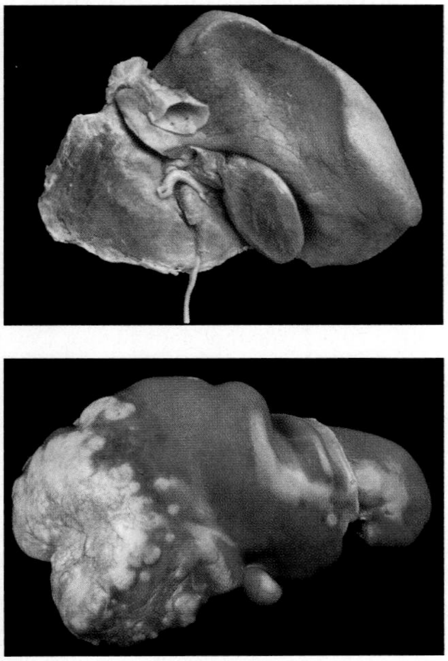

Mark Nielsen (both)

A normal liver (top) compared to one with cirrhosis.

Alcoholism Treatments

An estimated 8 million adults in the United States have alcohol dependence. Only a minority ever undergo treatment for alcohol-related problems. Until recent years, the only options for professional alcohol treatment were, as one expert puts it, "intensive, extensive, and expensive," such as residential programs at hospitals or specialized treatment centers. Today individuals whose drinking could be hazardous to their health may choose from a variety of approaches, including medication, behavioral therapy, or both.[40] Treatment that works well for one person may not work for another. As research into the outcomes of alcohol treatments has grown, more attempts have been made to match individuals to approaches tailored to their needs and more likely to help them overcome their alcohol problems.[41]

Men and women who have seriously remained sober for more than a decade credit a variety of approaches, including Alcoholics Anonymous (AA), individual psychotherapy, and other groups, such as Women for Sobriety. There is no one sure path to sobriety—

Strategies for Change — If Someone Close to You Drinks Too Much

- Try to remain calm, unemotional, and factually honest in speaking about the drinker's behavior. Include the drinker in family life.
- Discuss the situation with someone you trust: a member of the clergy, social worker, friend, or someone who has experienced alcoholism directly.
- Never cover up or make excuses for the drinker or shield him or her from the consequences of drinking. Assuming the drinker's responsibilities undermines his or her dignity and sense of importance.
- Refuse to ride with the drinker if he or she is driving while intoxicated.
- Encourage new interests and participate in leisure-time activities that the drinker enjoys.
- Try to accept setbacks and relapses calmly.

a wide variety of treatments may offer help and hope to those with alcohol-related problems.

Smoking in America

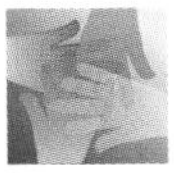

Americans are snuffing out cigarettes. The prevalence of smoking in the United States has declined more than 40 percent in recent decades. According to federal surveys, 20.9 percent of Americans smoke. Of these, about eight in ten smoke every day. As Table 12-1 indicates, more men (23.4 percent) than women (18.5 percent) are current smokers. American Indians have the highest smoking rates, while Asians and Hispanics have the lowest. Individuals with undergraduate and graduate degrees are least likely to smoke.[42]

The drop in smoking in the overall population still falls short of the national health objective of reducing cigarette smoking among adults to 12 percent by 2010. However, some groups have met this goal. They include women with undergraduate or graduate degrees, men with graduate degrees, Hispanic and Asian women, and people over age 65. Smoking among high school sophomores and seniors has fallen to an all-time low.[43]

TABLE 12-1 Who Smokes In America?

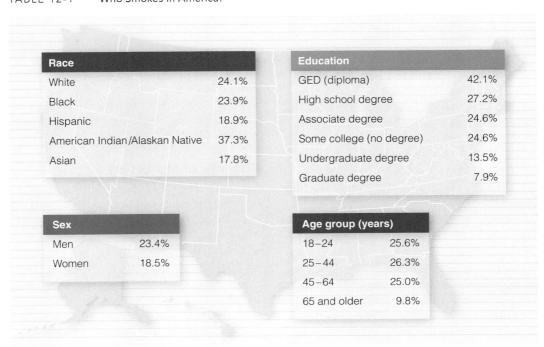

Race	
White	24.1%
Black	23.9%
Hispanic	18.9%
American Indian/Alaskan Native	37.3%
Asian	17.8%

Education	
GED (diploma)	42.1%
High school degree	27.2%
Associate degree	24.6%
Some college (no degree)	24.6%
Undergraduate degree	13.5%
Graduate degree	7.9%

Sex	
Men	23.4%
Women	18.5%

Age group (years)	
18–24	25.6%
25–44	26.3%
45–64	25.0%
65 and older	9.8%

Source: "Cigarette Smoking Among Adults—United States, 2004." *Journal of the American Medical Association*, Vol. 295, No. 7, January 15, 2006, p. 749.

Another big drop has occurred in young adults between ages 18 and 24. This was the only age group in which smoking increased from 1993 to 2002, when 28.5 percent of college-age Americans reported smoking. According to the National College Health Assessment, 21.4 percent of students smoked in the last month; 27.5 percent have never smoked.[44]

Why Do People Start Smoking?

Most people are aware that an enormous health risk is associated with smoking, but many don't know exactly what that risk is or how it might affect them.

The two main factors linked with the onset of a smoking habit are age and education. The vast majority of white men with less than a high school education are current or former daily cigarette smokers. White women with a similar educational background are also very likely to smoke or to have smoked every day. Hispanic men and women without a high school education are less likely to be or become daily smokers. These factors are associated with reasons for smoking.

Limited Education

People who have graduated from college are much less likely to smoke than high school graduates; those with fewer than 12 years of education are more likely to smoke. An individual with 8 years or less of education is 11 times more likely to smoke than someone with postgraduate training.

Adolescent Experimentation and Rebellion

For teenagers, smoking may be a coping mechanism for dealing with boredom and frustration; a marker of the transition into high school or college; a bid for adult status; a way of gaining admission to a peer group; or a way to have fun, reduce stress, or boost energy. The teenagers most likely to begin smoking are those least likely to seek help when their emotional needs are not met. They might smoke as a means of gaining social acceptance or to self-medicate when they feel helpless, lonely, or depressed. Depressed teens are more susceptible to cigarette ads than their counterparts. For example, they are more likely to have a favorite cigarette ad or own clothing with cigarette logos.

Genetics

Researchers speculate that genes may account for about 50 percent of smoking behavior, with environment playing an equally important role. Studies have shown that identical twins, who have the same genes, are more likely to have matching smoking profiles than fraternal twins. If one identical twin is a heavy smoker, the other is also likely to be; if one smokes only occasionally, so does the other.

According to NIDA research, genetic factors play a more significant role for initiation of smoking in women than men, but they play a less significant role in smoking persistence for women.

Parental Role Models

Children who start smoking are 50 percent more likely than youngsters who don't smoke to have at least one smoker in their family. A mother who smokes seems a particularly strong influence on making smoking seem acceptable. The majority of youngsters who smoke say that their parents also smoke and are aware of their own tobacco use.

Adolescents are more likely to smoke, express an intention to smoke, or smoke longer if their parents smoke.

Mental Disorders

The percentage of smokers jumps to more than 90 percent among those with alcoholism and other addictions, 85 percent among schizophrenia patients, and 80 percent among depressed patients. The relationship between depression and smoking is complex. Smokers are more likely to be depressed, while adults who are depressed are 40 to 50 percent more likely to smoke than adults who are not depressed. Research has identified biological connections between smoking and depression, suggesting a biological similarity between substance use and depressive disorders.

Weight Control

Concern about weight is a significant risk factor for smoking among young women. Daily smokers are two to four times more likely to fast, use diet pills, and purge to control their weight than nonsmokers. Although black girls smoke at substantially lower rates than white girls, the common factor in predicting daily smoking among all girls, regardless of race, is concern with weight.

Aggressive Marketing

Cigarette companies spend billions of dollars each year on advertisements and promotional campaigns, with manufacturers targeting ads especially at women, teens, minorities, and the poor. Most controversial are cigarette advertisements in magazines and media aimed at teenagers and even younger children.

Stress

In studies that have analyzed the impact of life stressors, depression, emotional support, marital status, and income, researchers have concluded that an individual with a high stress level is approximately 15 times more likely to be a smoker than a person with low stress.

About half of smokers identify workplace stress as a key factor in their smoking behavior.

Addiction

Nicotine addiction is as strong or stronger than addiction to drugs such as cocaine and heroin. The first symptoms of nicotine addiction can begin within a few days of starting to smoke and after just a few cigarettes, particularly in teenagers. Smoking a single cigarette before age 11 increases the odds of becoming dependent on nicotine. (See Self Survey: "Are You Addicted to Nicotine?" in the Self-Assessment Booklet.)

Tobacco Use on Campus

After increasing for several years, smoking has dropped in college-age adults, but about one in every four to five students currently smoke. (Figure 12-7). College students smoke for many reasons, including defiance of their parents and relaxed smoking standards in their dorms. Many students who had never tried smoking may experiment with cigarettes in college. Students who were occasional smokers in high school are more likely to become more frequent, heavier smokers once in college.

Many college students say they smoke as a way of managing depression or stress. Studies consistently link smoking with depression and low life satisfaction. Smokers are significantly more likely to have higher levels of perceived stress than nonsmokers. In one study, students who had been diagnosed or treated for depression were seven times as likely as other students to use tobacco.

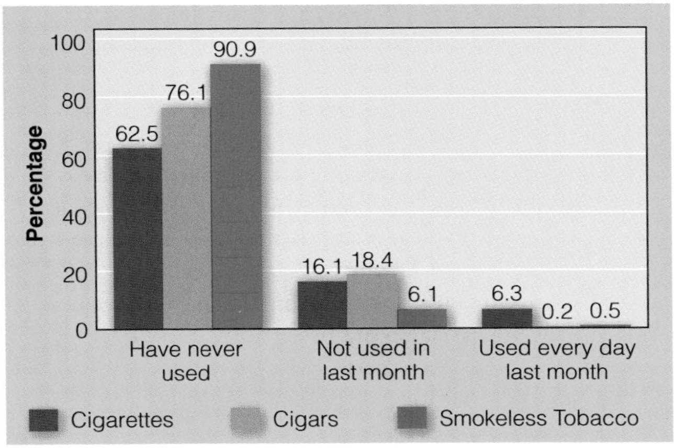

FIGURE 12-7 Tobacco Use on Campus

Source: American College Health Association. "American College Health Association-National College Health Assessment (ACHA-NCHA), Spring 2004 Reference Group Data Report (abridged)." *Journal of American College Health*, Vol. 54, No. 4, January–February 2006, p. 201.

Male students who smoke are more likely to say that smoking makes them feel more masculine and less anxious. More than half of female smokers feel that smoking helps them control their weight. Overweight female students are more likely to smoke to lose weight and to see weight gain as a barrier to quitting.

College students are more likely to have tried smoking if they are female, are Hispanic, participate in intercollegiate sports, have ever tried a tobacco product, and estimate that 20 to 30 percent of their friends smoke.[45]

FAQ Is Social Smoking Less Risky?

About half of college students who smoke say they are "social smokers" who average less than one cigarette a day and smoke mainly in the company of others. On the positive side, social smokers smoke less often and less intensely than other smokers and are less dependent on tobacco. However, they are still jeopardizing their health. The more they smoke, the greater the health risks they face. Even smokers who don't inhale or nonsmokers who breathe in secondhand smoke are at increased risk for negative health effects.

In research studies, smoking less than a pack a week of cigarettes has proved to damage the lining of blood vessels and to increase the risk of heart disease as well as of cancer. In women taking birth control pills, even a few cigarettes a week can increase the likelihood of

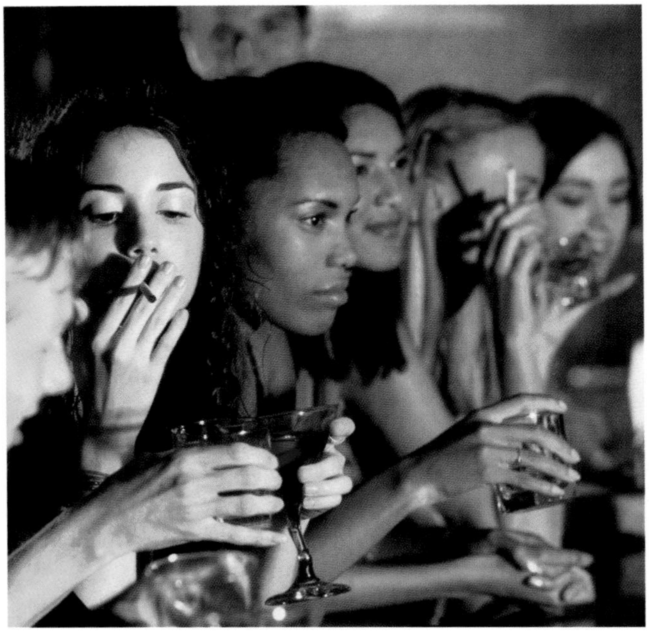

Jim Arbogast6/Photodisc/Getty Images

Social smoking has negative short- and long-term health effects and can lead to dependence.

heart disease, blood clots, stroke, liver cancer, and gallbladder disease. Pregnant women who smoke only occasionally still run a higher risk of giving birth to unhealthy babies. Another risk is addiction. Social smokers are less motivated to quit and make fewer attempts to do so. Many end up smoking more cigarettes for many more years than they intended.

College Tobacco-Control Policies

Other than religious institutions, colleges and universities have traditionally had few smoking restrictions. This has changed. Several national health organizations, including the American College Health Association and National Center on Addiction and Substance Abuse, have recommended that colleges ban smoking in and around all campus buildings, including student housing, and prohibit the sale, advertisement, and promotion of tobacco products on campus. Although some schools, particularly large public universities, have made progress in adopting such policies, most still fall short of the national recommendations.[46]

Although many colleges now provide smoke-free housing, others have not done so because of concern about increased costs, such as the need for outdoor cigarette receptacles. However, universities that have banned smoking from designated residence halls report decreased damage to the buildings, increased retention of students, and improved enforcement of marijuana policies.[47] Two-thirds of schools do not allow tobacco sales on campus; a third of student newspapers do not allow tobacco advertising. None have specifically banned tobacco industry sponsorships and promotions on college property. In general, schools in the West have done the most to implement tobacco policies. Those in the South, particularly in the major tobacco-growing states, have done the least.

Smoking, Gender, and Race

On average, girls who begin smoking during adolescence continue smoking for 20 years, four years longer than boys. Women are at greater risk for developing smoking-related illnesses compared with men who smoke the same amount. Lung cancer now claims more women's lives than breast cancer. In men, cigarette smoking increases the risk of aggressive prostate cancer.

Smoking is a risk factor for developing rheumatoid arthritis for men, but not for women. Women who smoke are more likely to develop osteoporosis, a bone-weakening disease.

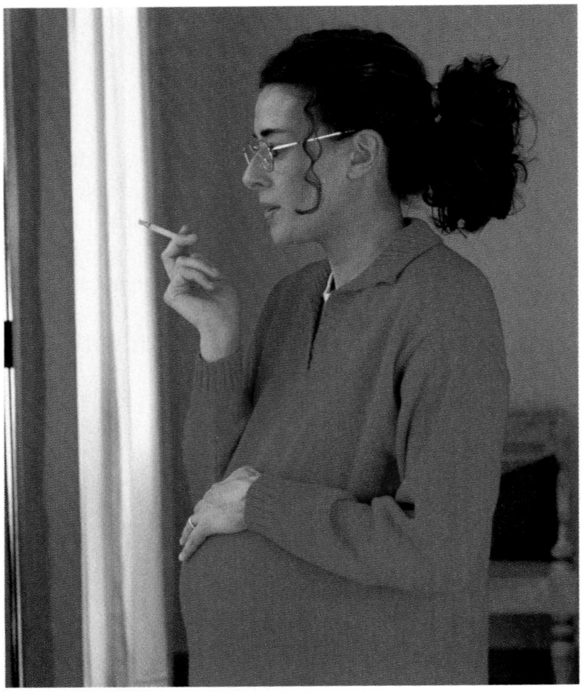

© Pixtal/SuperStock

Smoking late in pregnancy can endanger the physical and intellectual development of the fetus.

According to the U.S. Surgeon General, women account for 39 percent of smoking-related deaths each year, a proportion that has doubled since 1965. Each year, American women lose an estimated 2.1 million years of life due to premature deaths attributable to smoking. If she smokes, a woman's annual risk of dying more than doubles after age 45 compared with a woman who has never smoked.

High nicotine intake may affect male hormones, including testosterone. Smoking also can reduce blood flow to the penis, impairing a man's sexual performance and increasing the likelihood of erectile dysfunction.

Smoking directly affects women's reproductive organs and processes. Women who smoke are less fertile and experience menopause one or two years earlier than women who don't smoke. Smoking also greatly increases the possible risks associated with taking oral contraceptives.

Women who smoke during pregnancy increase their risk of miscarriage and pregnancy complications, including bleeding, premature delivery, and birth defects such as cleft lip or palate. Smoking during the third trimester affects both physical and intellectual development. In one study, the more cigarettes a mother smoked, the lower her son's birth weight and IQ as he matured.

Cigarette smoking is a major cause of disease and death in all population groups. However, tobacco use varies within and among racial and ethnic minority groups. Among adults, Native Americans and Alaska Natives have the highest rates of tobacco use. African-American and Southeast Asian men also have a high smoking rate. Asian-American and Hispanic women have the lowest rates of smoking. Tobacco use is significantly higher among white college students than among Hispanic, African-American, and Asian students.

Tobacco is the substance most abused by Hispanic youth, whose smoking rates have soared in the last ten years. In general, smoking rates among Hispanic adults increase as they adopt the values, beliefs, and norms of American culture. Recent declines in the prevalence of smoking have been greater among Hispanic men with at least a high school education than among those with less education.

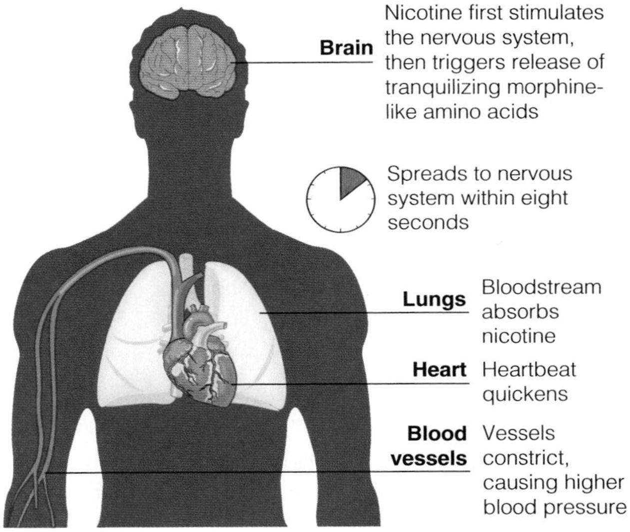

FIGURE 12-8 The Immediate Effects of Nicotine on the Body

The primary active ingredient in tobacco is nicotine, a fast-acting and potent drug.

Source: American Cancer Society, National Cancer Institute.

Tobacco's Immediate Effects

Tobacco, an herb that can be smoked or chewed, directly affects the brain. While its primary active ingredient is nicotine, tobacco smoke contains almost 400 other compounds and chemicals, including gases, liquids, particles, tar, carbon monoxide, cadmium, pyridine, nitrogen dioxide, ammonia, benzene, phenol, acrolein, hydrogen cyanide, formaldehyde, and hydrogen sulfide.

How Nicotine Works

A colorless, oily compound, **nicotine** is poisonous in concentrated amounts. If you inhale while smoking, 90 percent of the nicotine in the smoke is absorbed into your body. Even if you draw smoke only into your mouth and not into your lungs, you still absorb 25 to 30 percent of the nicotine. The FDA has concluded that nicotine is a dangerous, addictive drug that should be regulated.

Faster than an injection, smoking speeds nicotine to the brain in seconds (Figure 12-8). Nicotine affects the brain in much the same way as cocaine, opiates, and amphetamines, triggering the release of dopamine, a neurotransmitter associated with pleasure and addiction, as well as other messenger chemicals. Because nicotine acts on some of the same brain regions stimulated by interactions with loved ones, smokers come to regard cigarettes as a friend that they turn to when they're stressed, sad, or mad.

Nicotine may enhance smokers' performance on some tasks but leaves other mental skills unchanged. Nicotine also acts as a sedative. How often you smoke and how you smoke determine nicotine's effect on you. If you're a regular smoker, nicotine will generally stimulate you at first, then tranquilize you. Shallow puffs tend to increase alertness because low doses of nicotine facilitate the release of the neurotransmitter *acetylcholine,* which makes the smoker feel alert. Deep drags, on the other hand, relax the smoker because high doses of nicotine block the flow of acetylcholine.

Nicotine stimulates the adrenal glands to produce adrenaline, a hormone that increases blood pressure, speeds up the heart rate by 15 to 20 beats a minute, and constricts blood vessels (especially in the skin). Nicotine also inhibits the formation of urine, dampens hunger, irritates the membranes in the mouth and throat, and dulls the taste buds so foods don't taste as good as they would otherwise.

Nicotine withdrawal usually begins within hours. Symptoms include craving, irritability, anxiety, restlessness, and increased appetite.

Tar and Carbon Monoxide

As it burns, tobacco produces **tar,** a thick, sticky dark fluid made up of several hundred different chemicals—many of them poisonous, some of them *carcinogenic* (enhancing the growth of cancerous cells). As you inhale tobacco smoke, tar and other particles settle in the forks of the branchlike bronchial tubes in your lungs, where precancerous changes are apt to occur. In addition, tar and smoke damage the mucus and the cilia in the bronchial tubes,

nicotine The addictive substance in tobacco; one of the most toxic of all poisons.

tar A thick, sticky dark fluid produced by the burning of tobacco, made up of several hundred different chemicals, many of them poisonous, some of them carcinogenic.

which normally remove irritating foreign materials from your lungs.

Smoke from cigarettes, cigars, and pipes also contains **carbon monoxide,** the deadly gas that comes out of the exhaust pipes of cars, in levels 400 times those considered safe in industry. Carbon monoxide interferes with the ability of the hemoglobin in the blood to carry oxygen, impairs normal functioning of the nervous system, and is at least partly responsible for the increased risk of heart attacks and strokes in smokers.

Health Effects of Cigarette Smoking

Figure 12-9 shows a summary of the physiological effects of tobacco and the other chemicals in tobacco smoke. If you're a smoker who inhales deeply and started smoking before the age of 15, you're trading a minute of future life for every minute you now spend smoking. On average, smokers die nearly seven years earlier than nonsmokers. Smoking not only eventually kills, it also ages you: Smokers get more wrinkles than nonsmokers.

But the effects of smoking are far more than skin-deep. A cigarette smoker is 10 times more likely to develop lung cancer than a nonsmoker and 20 times more likely to have a heart attack. Daily smokers also are more likely to have suicidal thoughts or attempt suicide, although the reasons are not clear (see Chapter 2).

Heart Disease and Stroke

The toxic chemicals in tobacco signal the heart to beat faster and harder. Blood vessels constrict, forcing blood to travel through a narrower space. Blood pressure increases—temporarily at first. Over time, smokers develop chronic high blood pressure. Smoking increases harmful cholesterol (LDL) and lowers beneficial cholesterol (HDL). It also leads to the buildup of plaque, or fatty deposits within the arteries; hardening of the arteries; and greater risk of blood clots.

Although a great deal of publicity has been given to the link between cigarettes and lung cancer, heart attack is actually the leading cause of death for smokers. Smoking doubles the risk of heart disease and increases the risk of sudden death two to four times. The effect of smoking on risk of heart attack is greater in younger smokers.

Smokers who suffer heart attacks have only a 50 percent chance of recovering. Smokers have a 70 percent higher death rate from heart disease than nonsmokers, and those who smoke heavily have a 200 percent higher death rate.

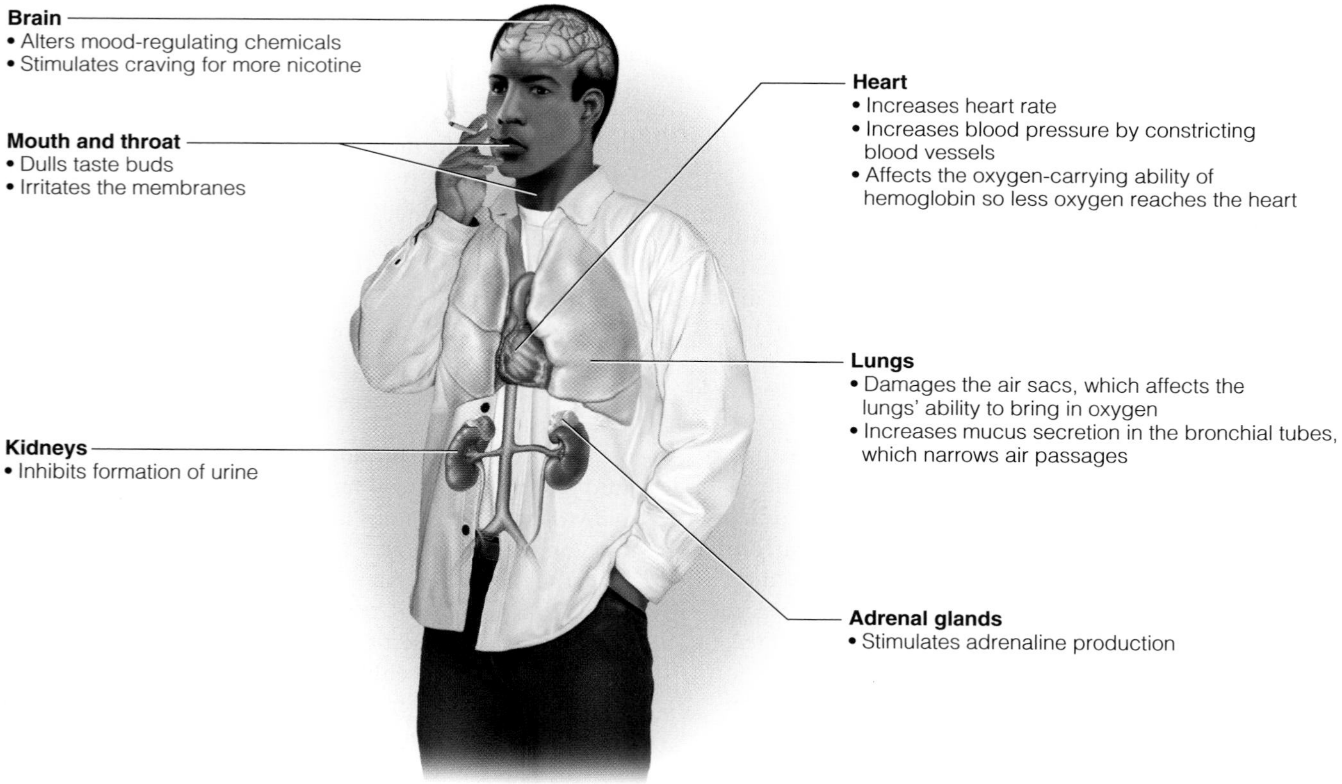

FIGURE 12-9 Some Effects of Smoking on the Body
Smoking harms the respiratory system and the cardiovascular system. The leading cause of death for smokers is heart attack.

The federal Office of the Surgeon General blames cigarettes for one of every ten deaths attributable to heart disease. Smoking is more dangerous than the two most notorious risk factors for heart disease: high blood pressure and high cholesterol. If smoking is combined with one of these, the chances of heart attack are four times greater. Women who smoke and use oral contraceptives have a ten times higher risk of suffering heart attacks than women who do neither.

In addition to contributing to heart attacks, cigarette smoking increases the risk of stroke two to three times in men and women, even after other risk factors are taken into account.

Even people who have smoked for decades can reduce their risk of heart attack if they quit smoking. However, studies indicate some irreversible damage to blood vessels. Progression of atherosclerosis (hardening of the arteries) among former smokers continues at a faster pace than among those who never smoked.

Cancer

Smoking is linked to at least ten different cancers and accounts for 30 percent of all deaths from cancer. It is the cause of more than 80 percent of all cases of lung cancer. The more people smoke, the longer they smoke, and the earlier they start smoking, the more likely they are to develop lung cancer.

Smoking causes about 130,000 lung cancer deaths each year. Smokers of two or more packs a day have lung cancer mortality rates 15 to 25 times greater than nonsmokers. If smokers stop smoking before cancer has started, their lung tissue tends to repair itself, even if there were already precancerous changes.

Chemicals in cigarette smoke and other environmental pollutants switch on a particular gene in the lung cells of some individuals. This gene produces an enzyme that helps manufacture powerful carcinogens, which set the stage for cancer. The gene seems more likely to be activated in some people than others, and people with this gene are at much higher risk of developing lung cancer. However, smokers without the gene still remain at risk, because other chemicals and genes also may be involved in the development of lung cancer.

Smokers who are depressed are more likely to get cancer than nondepressed smokers. Although researchers don't know exactly how smoking and depression may work together to increase the risk of cancer, one possibility is that stress and depression cause biological changes that lower immunity, such as a decline in natural killer cells that fight off tumors.

Respiratory Diseases

Smoking quickly impairs the respiratory system, including the cough reflex, a vital protective response. Even some teenage smokers show signs of respiratory difficulty—breathlessness, chronic cough, excess phlegm production—when compared with nonsmokers of the same age. Cigarette smokers are up to 18 times more likely than nonsmokers to die of noncancerous diseases of the lungs.

Cigarette smoking is the major cause of chronic obstructive lung disease (COLD), which includes emphysema and chronic bronchitis. COLD is characterized by progressive limitation of the flow of air into and out of the lungs. In emphysema, the limitation of air flow is the result of disease changes in the lung tissue, affecting the bronchioles (the smallest air passages) and the walls of the alveoli (the tiny air sacs of the lung). Eventually, many of the air sacs are destroyed, and the lungs become much less able to bring in oxygen and remove carbon dioxide. As a result, the heart has to work harder to deliver oxygen to all organs of the body.

In chronic bronchitis, the bronchial tubes in the lungs become inflamed, thickening the walls of the bronchi, and the production of mucus increases. The result is a narrowing of the air passages. Smoking is more dangerous than any form of air pollution, at least for most Americans, but exposure to both air pollution and cigarettes is particularly harmful.

Other Smoking-Related Problems

Smokers are more likely than nonsmokers to develop gum disease, and they lose significantly more teeth. Even those who quit have worse gum problems than people who never smoked at all. Smoking may also contribute to the loss of teeth and teeth supporting bone, even in individuals with good oral hygiene.

carbon monoxide A colorless, odorless gas produced by the burning of gasoline or tobacco; displaces oxygen in the hemoglobin molecules of red blood cells.

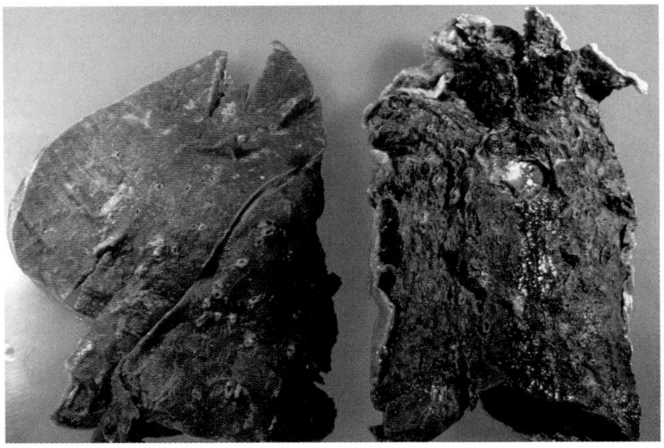

© Arthur Glauberman/PhotoResearchers, Inc.

Healthy nonsmoker's lung (left) and smoker's lung (right). Healthy lungs are pink, with a smooth but porous texture. A smoker's lungs show obvious signs of impairment. Bronchial tubes are inflamed, air passages are constricted, and tar coats the bronchial tubes.

Cigarette smoking is associated with stomach and duodenal ulcers; mouth, throat, and other types of cancer; and cirrhosis of the liver. Smoking may worsen the symptoms or complications of allergies, diabetes, hypertension, peptic ulcers, and disorders of the lungs or blood vessels. Some men who smoke ten cigarettes or more a day may experience erectile dysfunction. Cigarette smokers also tend to miss work one-third more often than nonsmokers, primarily because of respiratory illnesses. In addition, each year cigarette-ignited fires claim thousands of lives.

Smoking is an independent risk factor for high-frequency hearing loss and also adds to the danger of hearing loss for those exposed to noise (Chapter 14). Cigarette smoking also may increase the likelihood of anxiety, panic attacks, and social phobias.

Other Forms of Tobacco

Some 10.7 million Americans smoke cigars; 7.6 million use smokeless tobacco; and 2.1 million smoke pipes. Ingesting tobacco may be less deadly than smoking cigarettes, but it is dangerous. Smoking cigars, clove cigarettes, and pipes and chewing or sucking on smokeless tobacco all put the user at risk of cancer of the lip, tongue, mouth, and throat, as well as other diseases and ailments.

Cigars

Cigar use has declined in the last few years. However, after cigarettes, cigars are the tobacco product most widely used by college students.

Cigar smoking is as dangerous as cigarette smoking even though cigar smokers do not inhale. Cigars can cause cancer of the lung and the digestive tract. The risk of death related to cigars approaches that of cigarettes, depending on the number of cigars smoked and the amount of cigar smoke inhaled. Cigar smoking can lead to nicotine addiction, even if the smoke is not inhaled. The nicotine in the smoke from a single cigar can vary from an amount roughly equivalent to that in a single cigarette to that in a pack or more of cigarettes.

Clove Cigarettes

Sweeteners have long been mixed with tobacco, and clove, a spice, is the latest ingredient to be added to the recipe for cigarettes. Clove cigarettes typically contain two-thirds tobacco and one-third clove. Consumers of these cigarettes are primarily teenagers and young adults.

Many users believe that clove cigarettes are safer because they contain less tobacco, but this isn't necessarily the case. The CDC reports that people who smoke clove cigarettes may be at risk of serious lung injury.

Clove cigarettes deliver twice as much nicotine, tar, and carbon monoxide as moderate-tar American brands. Eugenol, the active ingredient in cloves (which dentists have used as an anesthetic for years), deadens sensation in the throat, allowing smokers to inhale more deeply and hold smoke in their lungs for a longer time. Chemical relatives of eugenol can produce the kind of damage to cells that may lead to cancer.

? FAQ What Are Bidis?

Skinny, sweet-flavored cigarettes called **bidis** (pronounced "beedees") have become a smoking fad among teens and young adults. For centuries, bidis were popular in India, where they are known as the poor man's cigarette and sell for less than five cents a pack. They look strikingly like clove cigarettes or marijuana joints and are available in flavors like grape, strawberry, and mandarin orange. Bidis are legal for adults and even minors in some states and are sold on the Internet as well as in stores.

Although bidis contain less tobacco than regular cigarettes, their unprocessed tobacco is more potent. Smoke from bidis has about three times as much nicotine and carbon monoxide and five times as much tar as smoke from regular filtered cigarettes. Because bidis are wrapped in nonporous brownish leaves, they don't burn as easily as cigarettes, and smokers have to inhale harder and more often to keep them lit. In one study, smoking

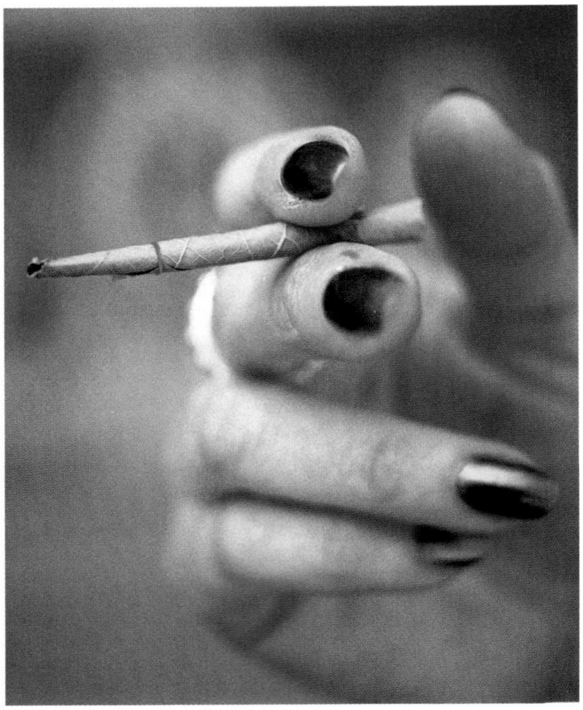

AP Images/John Bazemore

The smoke produced by bidis—skinny, flavored cigarettes—can contain higher concentrations of toxic chemicals than the smoke from regular cigarettes.

SAVVY CONSUMER

Are "Safer" Cigarettes Really Safe?

Tobacco companies are producing "lower-risk" cigarettes that they claim reduce secondhand smoke and have fewer carcinogens and less nicotine. For example, Eclipse cigarettes heat rather than burn tobacco inside a cigarette-like tube to reduce the release of carbon monoxide, a big contributor to heart disease. Users of another product, Accord, insert special cigarettes into a small electronic device about the size of a pager that ignites the cigarette when the smoker puffs and sucks up secondhand smoke. Other brands claim to use genetic engineering or a chemical process to remove major carcinogens.

Are these products truly safer? The answer is no. So-called safer cigarettes may actually lead to increased addiction. In one experiment, smokers puffed on their own brand and then on a so-called safer cigarette brand called Advance. While Advance cigarettes supposedly contain less of a type of cancer-causing substance called nitrosamines, they delivered 25 percent more nicotine, the addictive substance in cigarettes, into the blood than the smokers' own brands.

Accord cigarettes deliver less nicotine and boost smokers' heart rates and carbon monoxide levels less than traditional cigarettes. However, they aren't as satisfying to smokers, who may smoke more of them to reduce withdrawal symptoms such as anxiety, restlessness, and irritability.

Eclipse cigarettes suppress withdrawal symptoms about as well as conventional cigarettes. However, they deliver about 30 percent more carbon monoxide, which has been linked to heart disease, than regular cigarettes.

The bottom line: "Safer" cigarettes may reduce some toxins that are associated with smoking-related diseases, but they may increase levels of other dangerous substances and boost the likelihood of addiction. Don't think that you're protecting your health by switching to a "safe" cigarette. There is no such thing. The only proven way to avoid smoking-related risks of disease and death is to stop smoking.

a single bidi required 28 puffs, compared to 9 puffs for cigarettes.

Pipes

Many cigarette smokers switch to pipes to reduce their risk of health problems. But former cigarette smokers may continue to inhale, even though pipe smoke is more irritating to the respiratory system than cigarette smoke. People who have smoked only pipes and who do not inhale are much less likely to develop lung and heart disease than cigarette smokers. However, they are as likely as cigarette smokers to develop—and die of—cancer of the mouth, larynx, throat, and esophagus.

Smokeless Tobacco

The consumption of smokeless tobacco products (sometimes called "spit") is rising, particularly among young males. However, fewer than 10 percent of college students have ever tried them.[48] These substances include snuff, finely ground tobacco that can be sniffed or placed inside the cheek and sucked, and chewing tobacco, tobacco leaves mixed with flavoring agents such as molasses. With both, nicotine is absorbed through the mucous membranes of the nose or mouth.

Smokeless tobacco causes a user's heart rate, blood pressure, and epinephrine (adrenaline) levels to jump.[49] In addition, it can cause cancer and noncancerous oral conditions and lead to nicotine addiction and dependence. Smokeless tobacco users are more likely than nonusers to become cigarette smokers.

Powerful carcinogens in smokeless tobacco include nitrosamines, polycyclic aromatic hydrocarbons, and radiation-emitting polonium. Its use can lead to

bidis Skinny, sweet-flavored cigarettes.

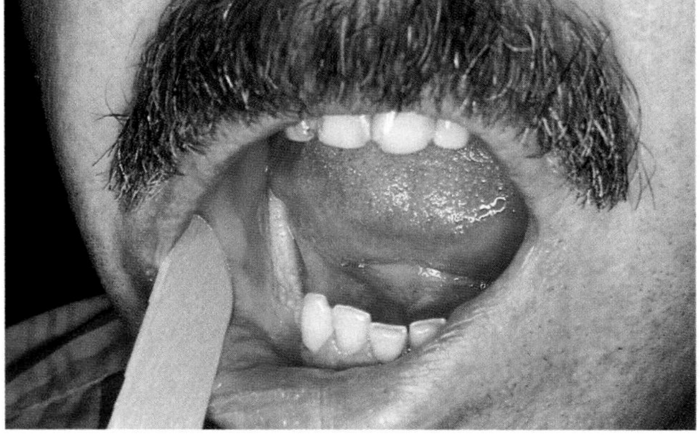

Chewing smokeless tobacco can damage the tissues of the mouth and lead to cancer of the lip, pharynx, larynx, esophagus, kidney, pancreas, and bladder.

the development of white patches on the mucous membranes of the mouth, particularly on the site where the tobacco is placed. Most lesions of the mouth lining that result from the use of smokeless tobacco dissipate six weeks after the use of the tobacco products is stopped, according to a U.S. Air Force study. However, when first found, about 5 percent of these lesions are cancerous or exhibit changes that progress to cancer within ten years if not properly treated. Cancers of the lip, pharynx, larynx, and esophagus have all been linked to smokeless tobacco.

Nicotine replacement with gum or patches (discussed on page 357–358) decreases cravings for smokeless tobacco and helps with short-term abstinence. However, it does not improve long-term abstinence. Behavioral approaches are more effective for long-term quitting.[50]

Quitting

Smoking is a remarkably difficult habit to kick. However, half of all Americans who ever smoked have quit. Half of current smokers try to quit each year, but only 7 percent succeed on their first attempt.[51]

About half of whites who have smoked were able to kick the habit, compared with 45 percent of Asian Americans, 43 percent of Hispanics, and 37 percent of African Americans. Men and women with college and graduate degrees were much more likely to quit successfully than high school dropouts.[52]

Compared with men, women seem to have a higher behavioral dependence on cigarettes. For them, wearing a nicotine patch or chewing nicotine gum does not substitute for the "hand-to-mouth" behaviors associated with smoking, such as lighting a cigarette, inhaling, and handling the cigarette. Some investigators have found that women are more likely to quit successfully when they receive a combination of nicotine replacement and the use of a device like a nicotine inhaler to substitute for smoking behaviors.

Although a large proportion of students have made an attempt to quit, only a minority succeed. Among current smokers, 59 percent report ever making an attempt to quit. Among those who ever smoked daily, 82 percent have tried to quit, while 75 percent are still smokers. The barriers to quitting in college include fears of weight gain, inability to manage stress without nicotine, and denial of nicotine addition.

One campus-based program that employed peer facilitators to help smokers quit and avoid relapse reported a success rate of 88 percent. Being "in the group" was the single most powerful contributor to quitting, and participants said their sense of connectedness helped them quit and stay smoke-free.

Nicotine withdrawal symptoms can behave like characters in a bad horror flick: Just when you think you've killed them, they're back with a vengeance. In recent studies, some people who tried to quit smoking reported a small improvement in withdrawal symptoms over two weeks, but then their symptoms leveled off and persisted. Others found that their symptoms intensified rather than lessened over time. For reasons scientists cannot yet explain, former smokers who start smoking again put their lungs at even greater jeopardy than smokers who never quit.

Once a former smoker takes a single puff, the odds of a relapse are 80 to 85 percent. Smokers are most likely to quit in the third, fourth, or fifth attempt. But thanks to new products and programs, it may be easier now than ever before to become an ex-smoker (Figure 12-10).

Quitting on Your Own

More than 90 percent of former smokers quit on their own—by throwing away all their cigarettes, by gradually cutting down, or by first switching to a less potent brand. One characteristic of successful quitters is that they see themselves as active participants in health maintenance and take personal responsibility for their own health. Often they experiment with a variety of strategies, such as learning relaxation techniques. In women, exercise has proved especially effective for quitting and avoiding weight gain. Making a home a

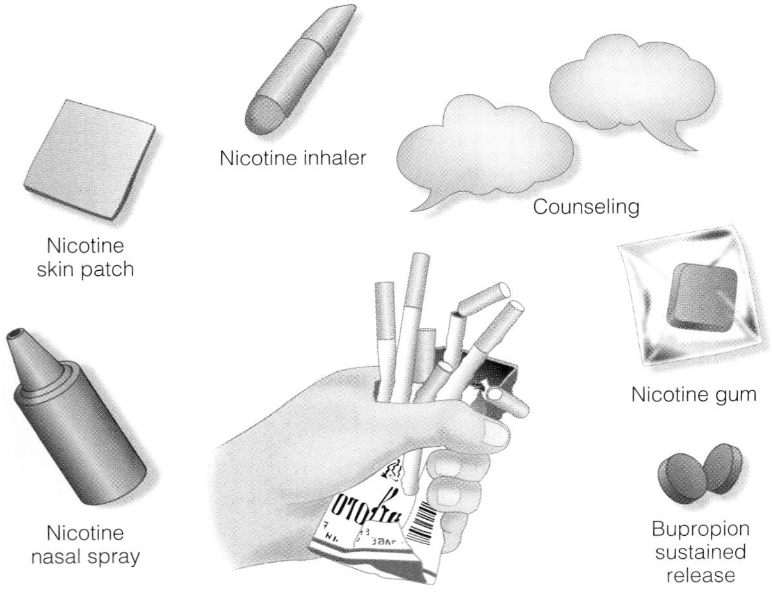

FIGURE 12-10 ▌ How to Quit
Combining one of the four nicotine replacement therapies (or bupropion/Zyban) with counseling is the most effective strategy to quit smoking.

smoke-free zone also increases a smoker's likelihood of successfully quitting.

Stop-Smoking Groups

Joining a support group doubles your chances of quitting for good. The American Cancer Society's FreshStart program runs about 1,500 stop-smoking clinics, each with about 8 to 18 members meeting for eight two-hour sessions over four weeks. Instructors explain the risks of smoking, encourage individuals to think about why they smoke, and suggest ways of unlearning their smoking habit. A quitting day is set for the third or fourth session.

The American Lung Association's Freedom from Smoking program consists of eight one- to two-hour sessions over seven weeks. The approach is similar to the American Cancer Society's, but smokers keep diaries and team up with buddies. Ex-smokers serve as advisers on quitting day. Both groups estimate that 27 or 28 percent of their participants successfully stop smoking.

Stop-smoking classes are also available through science departments and student health services on many college campuses, as well as through community public health departments. The Seventh-Day Adventists sponsor a four-week Breathe Free Plan, in which smokers commit themselves to clean living (no smoking, alcohol, tea, or coffee, along with a balanced diet and regular exercise).

Many businesses sponsor smoking-cessation programs for employees, which generally follow the approaches of professional groups. Motivation may be even higher in these programs than in programs outside the workplace because some companies offer attractive incentives to participants, such as lower rates on their health insurance.

Some smoking-cessation programs rely primarily on **aversion therapy,** which provides a negative experience every time a smoker has a cigarette. This may involve taking drugs that make tobacco smoke taste unpleasant, undergoing electric shocks, having smoke blown at you, or rapid smoking (the inhaling of smoke every six seconds until you're dizzy or nauseated).

Nicotine Anonymous, a nonprofit organization based on the 12 steps to recovery developed by Alcoholics Anonymous (see Chapter 11), acknowledges the power of nicotine and provides support to help smokers, chewers, and dippers live free of nicotine. New members are encouraged to abstain from using nicotine "one day at a time" and to attend meetings regularly. In addition to local meetings, NicA offers online support and networking, which puts people in touch with others in their region who share their desire to quit using nicotine.

Telephone-counseling "quit lines," which advise smokers on how to restructure their lives and deal with urges, are helpful because people can get counseling without leaving their homes. The quality of online smoking cessation websites is not consistent, and information is often hard to find, incomplete, or not based on research.[53]

Nicotine Replacement Therapy (NRT)

This approach uses a variety of products that supply low doses of nicotine in a way that allows smokers to taper off gradually over a period of months. Nicotine replacement therapies include nonprescription products (nicotine gum and nicotine patches) and prescription products (nicotine nasal spray and nicotine inhaler). The nasal spray, dispensed from a pump bottle, delivers nicotine to the nasal membranes and reaches the bloodstream faster than any other nicotine replacement therapy product. The inhaler delivers nicotine into the mouth and enters the bloodstream much more slowly than the nicotine in cigarettes.

Smokers who use NRT are 1.5 to 2 times more likely to quit.[54] Because nicotine is a powerful, addictive substance, using nicotine replacements for a prolonged period is not advised. Pregnant women and individuals with heart disease shouldn't use them.

The most effective approaches combine medication—nicotine patches or Zyban, for instance—with psychological intervention. Each doubles a person's chance of quitting successfully.

Nicotine replacement therapy, which supplies ex-smokers with lower levels of nicotine in the form of a gum or patch, has proved more beneficial for men than women—particularly with higher doses of nicotine. Men who receive more nicotine achieve a higher quit rate than men getting lower doses.

For women, the nicotine "dose" does not have an impact on successful quitting. They are no more likely to stop smoking with high doses than with lower ones, indicating that they may be less dependent on nicotine than men.

Nicotine Gum

Nicotine gum, sold as Nicorette, contains a nicotine resin that's gradually released as the gum is chewed. Absorbed through the mucous membrane of the mouth, the nicotine doesn't produce the same rush as a deeply inhaled drag on a cigarette. However, the gum maintains enough nicotine in the blood to diminish withdrawal symptoms. A month's supply of Nicorette costs roughly $45.

Although this gum is lightly spiced to mask nicotine's bitterness, many users say that it takes several days to become accustomed to its unusual taste. Its side effects include mild

aversion therapy A treatment that attempts to help a person overcome a dependence or bad habit by making the person feel disgusted or repulsed by that habit.

indigestion, sore jaws, nausea, heartburn, and stomachache. Also, because Nicorette is heavier than regular chewing gum, it may loosen fillings or cause problems with dentures. Drinking coffee or other beverages may block absorption of the nicotine in the gum; individuals trying to quit smoking shouldn't ingest any substance immediately before or while chewing nicotine gum. You have to chew nicotine gum until you get a tingling sensation, and then place it between the cheek and gum.

Most people use nicotine gum as a temporary crutch and gradually taper off until they can stop chewing it relatively painlessly. However, 5 to 10 percent of users transfer their dependence from cigarettes to the gum. When they stop using Nicorette, they experience withdrawal symptoms, although the symptoms tend to be milder than those prompted by quitting cigarettes. Intensive counseling to teach smokers coping methods can greatly increase success rates.

Nicotine Patches

Nicotine transdermal delivery system products, or patches, provide nicotine, their only active ingredient, via a patch attached to the skin by an adhesive. Like nicotine gum, the nicotine patch minimizes withdrawal symptoms, such as intense craving for cigarettes. Nicotine patches help nearly 20 percent of smokers quit entirely after six weeks, compared with 7 percent on a placebo patch. Some insurance programs pay for patch therapy. Nicotine patches, which cost between $3.25 and $4 each, are replaced daily during therapy programs that run between 6 and 16 weeks. There is no evidence that continuing their use for more than 8 weeks provides added benefit.

Some patches deliver nicotine around the clock and others for just 16 hours (during waking hours). Those most likely to benefit from nicotine patch therapy are people who smoke more than a pack a day, are highly motivated to quit, and participate in counseling programs. While using the patch, 37 to 77 percent of people are able to abstain from smoking. When combined with counseling, the patch can be about twice as effective as a placebo, enabling 26 percent of smokers to abstain for six months.

Patch wearers who smoke or use more than one patch at a time can experience a nicotine overdose; some users have even suffered heart attacks. Occasional side effects include redness, itching, or swelling at the site of the patch application; insomnia; dry mouth; and nervousness.

Nicotrol Inhaler

Available only by prescription, the Nicotrol Inhaler consists of a mouthpiece and a cartridge containing a nicotine-impregnated plug. The smoker inhales through the mouthpiece, using either shallow or deep puffs. The inhaled air becomes saturated with nicotine, which is absorbed mainly through the tissues of the mouth. The

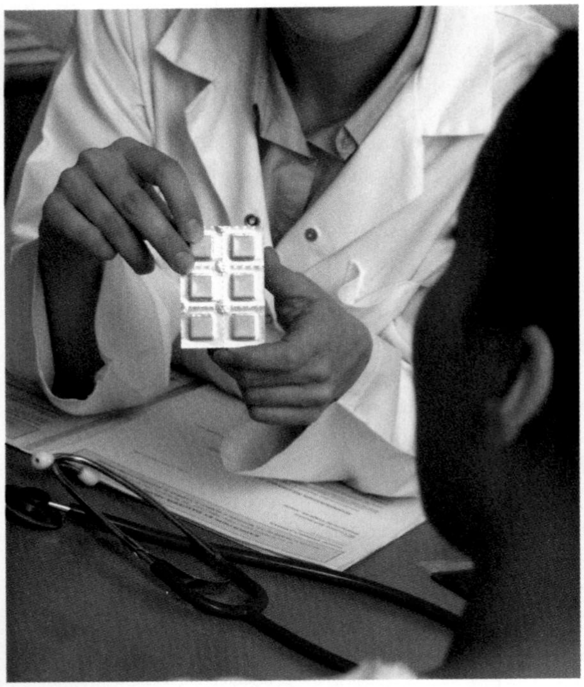

Nicorette gum, when chewed, gradually releases a nicotine resin and helps some smokers break their habit. Nicorette is available without a prescription.

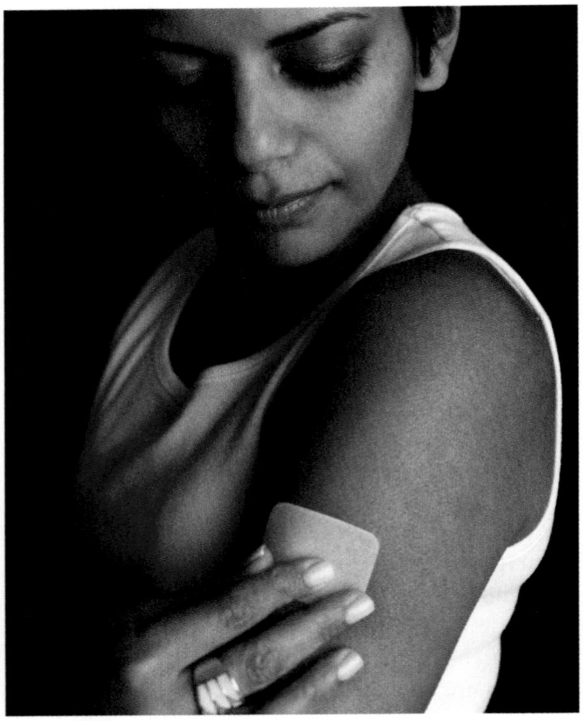

A nicotine patch releases nicotine transdermally (through the skin) in measured amounts, which are gradually decreased over time.

Inhaler releases less nicotine per puff than a cigarette and does not contain a cigarette's harmful tars, carbon monoxide, and smoke. Treatment is recommended for three months with a gradual reduction over the next six to twelve weeks. Total treatment should not exceed six months.[55]

Bupropion (Zyban)

An alternative to the patch is *bupropion,* a drug initially developed to treat depression, that is marketed in a slow-release form for nicotine addiction as Zyban. In studies that have combined Zyban with nicotine replacement and counseling, 40 to 60 percent of those treated have remained smoke-free for at least a year after completing the program. This success rate is much higher than the 10 to 26 percent reported among smokers who try to quit by using nicotine replacement alone. The combination of Zyban and nicotine replacement also prevented the initial weight gain that often accompanies quitting. Other medications used to treat nicotine addiction are clonidine, mecamylamine, and buspirone.

Environmental Tobacco Smoke

Maybe you don't smoke—never have, never will. That doesn't mean you don't have to worry about the dangers of smoking, especially if you live or work with people who smoke. **Environmental tobacco smoke,** or secondhand cigarette smoke, the most hazardous form of indoor air pollution, ranks behind cigarette smoking and alcohol as the third-leading preventable cause of death.

On average, a smoker inhales what is known as **mainstream smoke** eight or nine times with each cigarette, for a total of about 24 seconds. However, the cigarette burns for about 12 minutes, and everyone in the room (including the smoker) breathes in what is known as **sidestream smoke.**

According to the American Lung Association, incomplete combustion from the lower temperatures of a smoldering cigarette makes sidestream smoke dirtier and chemically different from mainstream smoke. It has twice as much tar and nicotine, five times as much carbon monoxide, and 50 times as much ammonia. And because the particles in sidestream smoke are small, this mixture of irritating gases and carcinogenic tar reaches deeper into the lungs. If you're a nonsmoker sitting next to someone smoking seven cigarettes an hour, even in a ventilated room, you'll take in almost twice the maximum amount of carbon monoxide set for air pollution in industry—and it will take hours for the carbon monoxide to leave your body.

Even a little secondhand smoke is dangerous. According to the CDC, every year environmental tobacco smoke causes about 35,000 deaths from heart disease and 3,000 deaths from lung cancer.[56] As a cancer-causing agent, secondhand smoke may be twice as dangerous as radon gas and more than a hundred times more hazardous than outdoor pollutants regulated by federal law. Secondhand smoke also increases sick leave rates among employees.

environmental tobacco smoke Secondhand cigarette smoke; the third-leading preventable cause of death.

mainstream smoke The smoke inhaled directly by smoking a cigarette.

sidestream smoke The smoke emitted by a burning cigarette and breathed by everyone in a closed room, including the smoker; contains more tar and nicotine than mainstream smoke.

LEARN IT / LIVE IT

Taking Charge of Alcohol and Tobacco

As you decide about the role alcohol should play in your life, you might want to follow these guidelines, proposed by BACCHUS, a volunteer college student organization that promotes responsible alcohol-related behavior:

- Set a limit on how many drinks you're going to have ahead of time—and stick to it.
- When you're mixing a drink, measure the alcohol.
- Alternate nonalcoholic and alcoholic drinks.
- Drink slowly; don't guzzle.
- Eat before and while drinking.
- Develop alternatives to drinking so you don't turn to alcohol whenever you're depressed or upset. Exercise is a wonderful release for tension; meditation or relaxation techniques can also help you cope.
- Avoid performing tasks that require skilled reactions during or after drinking.
- Don't encourage or reinforce others' irresponsible behavior.

Above all, keep in mind that drinking should not be the primary focus of any activity. Responsible drinking is a matter of you controlling your drinking rather than the drinking controlling you.

If you smoke—even just a few cigarettes a few times a week—you are at risk of nicotine addiction. Here is how to get back into control:

- Use delaying tactics. Have your first cigarette of the day 15 minutes later than usual, then 15 minutes later than that the next day, and so on.

(Continued)

- Distract yourself. When you feel a craving for a cigarette, talk to someone, drink a glass of water, or get up and move around.
- Establish nonsmoking hours. Instead of lighting up at the end of a meal, for instance, get up immediately, brush your teeth, wash your hands, or take a walk.
- Never smoke two packs of the same brand in a row. Buy cigarettes only by the pack, not by the carton.
- Make it harder to get to your cigarettes. Lock them in a drawer, wrap them in paper, or leave them in your coat or car.
- Change the way you smoke. Smoke with the hand you don't usually use. Smoke only half of each cigarette.
- Stop completely for just one day at a time. Promise yourself 24 hours of freedom from cigarettes; when the day's over, make the same commitment for one more day. At the end of any 24-hour period, you can go back to smoking and not feel guilty.
- Spend more time in places where you can't smoke. Take up bike-riding or swimming. Shower often. Go to movies or other places where smoking isn't allowed.

12 Making This Chapter Work for You

Review Questions

1. Which of these is a standard drink?
   a. A margarita
   b. A 12-oz. regular beer
   c. A double martini
   d. A 16-oz. can of malt liquor
2. An individual's response to alcohol depends on all of the following *except*
   a. the rate at which the drink is absorbed into the body's tissues.
   b. the blood alcohol concentration.
   c. socioeconomic status.
   d. gender and race.
3. Which of the following statements about drinking on college campuses is true?
   a. Students think their peers drink more than they actually do.
   b. The number of women who binge drink has decreased.
   c. Because of peer pressure, students in fraternities and sororities tend to drink less than students in dormitories.
   d. Seniors drink more then freshmen.
4. Which of the following statements about the effects of alcohol on the body systems is true?
   a. In most individuals, alcohol sharpens the responses of the brain and nervous system, enhancing sensation and perception.
   b. Moderate drinking may have a positive effect on the cardiovascular system.
   c. French researchers have found that drinking red wine with meals may have a positive effect on the digestive system.
   d. The leading alcohol-related cause of death is liver damage.
5. Which of the following statements about alcohol abuse and dependence is *false?*
   a. Alcohol dependence involves a persistent craving for and an increased tolerance to alcohol.
   b. An individual may have a genetic predisposition for developing alcoholism.
   c. Alcoholics often abuse other psychoactive drugs.
   d. Alcohol abuse and alcohol dependence are different names for the same problem.
6. Tobacco use on college campuses
   a. is higher among male athletes.
   b. continues to increase despite no-smoking policies by all schools.
   c. is more prevalent among those students who also use marijuana and alcohol.
   d. is most often in the form of smokeless tobacco.
7. Cigarette smokers
   a. are more likely to die of lung cancer than heart disease.
   b. usually develop lung problems after years of tobacco use.
   c. have two to three times the risk of suffering a stroke than nonsmokers.
   d. may completely reverse the damage to their blood vessels if they quit smoking.
8. Quitting smoking
   a. usually results in minor withdrawal symptoms.
   b. will do little to reverse the damage to the lungs and other parts of the body.
   c. can be aided by using nicotine replacement products.
   d. is best done by cutting down on the number of cigarettes you smoke over a period of months.
9. Ways to help yourself quit include all of the following *except*
   a. join a support group.
   b. make your home a smoke-free zone.
   c. try acupuncture.
   d. switch to bidis.
10. Secondhand tobacco smoke is
    a. the smoke inhaled by a smoker.

LACC Extra Credit Assignment

12. Smoking or drinking. Which is better? Discuss.

b. more hazardous than outdoor pollution as a cancer-causing agent.
c. less hazardous than mainstream smoke.
d. less likely to cause serious health problems in children than in adults.

Answers to these questions can be found on page 422.

Critical Thinking

1. Driving home from his high school graduation party, 18-year-old Rick has had too much to drink. As he crosses the dividing line on the two-lane road, the driver of an oncoming car—a young mother with two young children in the backseat—swerves to avoid an accident. She hits a concrete wall and dies instantly, but her children survive. Rick has no record of drunk driving. Should he go to prison? Is he guilty of manslaughter? How would you feel if you were the victim's husband? If you were Rick's friend?
2. Have you ever been around people who have been intoxicated when you have been sober? What did you think of their behavior? Were they fun to be around? Was the experience not particularly enjoyable, boring, or difficult in some way? Have you ever been intoxicated? How do you behave when you are drunk? Do you find the experience enjoyable? What do the people around you think of your actions when you are drunk?
3. Has smoking become unpopular among your friends or family? What social activities continue to be associated with smoking? Can you think of any situation in which smoking might be frowned upon?
4. How would you motivate someone you care about to stop smoking? What reasons would you give for them to stop? Describe your strategy.

Media Menu

ThomsonNOW™ Go to the ThomsonNOW website at **http://www.thomsonedu.com** that will:

- Help you evaluate your knowledge of the material.
- Allow you to take an exam-prep quiz.
- Provide a Personalized Learning Plan targeting resources that address areas you should study.
- Coach you through identifying target goals for behavioral change and creating and monitoring your personal change plan throughout the semester.

INTERNET CONNECTIONS

College Drinking: Changing the Culture
www.collegedrinkingprevention.gov

This website, sponsored by the National Institute of Alcohol Abuse and Alcoholism, focuses on the college alcohol culture with information for students, parents, college health administrators, and more. In addition, the site features information about alcohol prevention, college alcohol policies, research topics, and factual information about the consequences of alcohol abuse and alcoholism.

Al-Anon Family Group Headquarters
www.al-anon.alateen.org

This site provides information and referrals to local Al-Anon and Alateen groups. It also includes a self-quiz to determine if you are affected by someone who has an alcohol problem.

Tobacco Information and Prevention Source (TIPS)
www.cdc.gov/tobacco

This comprehensive feature on the Centers for Disease Control and Prevention (CDC) website provides educational information, research, a report from the U.S. Surgeon General, tips on how to quit, and much more.

Tobacco Facts
www.tobaccofacts.org

This excellent site provides access to many facts and resources regarding tobacco use.

InfoTrac College Edition Activities Log on, insert **alcohol abuse** or **tobacco use** into the Keyword search box, and limit your search to the past year. When you get the results, Mark articles to review, then Select one to read. Summarize three or four key points from the article.

You can find additional readings related to personal health with InfoTrac College Edition, an online library of more than 900 journals and publications. Follow the instructions for accessing InfoTrac College Edition that were packaged with your textbook; then search for articles using a keyword search.

For additional links, resources, and suggested readings on InfoTrac College Edition, visit our Health and Wellness Resource Center at **http://health.wadsworth.com**.

Key Terms

The terms listed are used on the page indicated. Definitions of the terms are in the Glossary at the end of this book.

absorption 330
alcohol abuse 344
alcohol dependence 344
alcoholism 345
aversion therapy 357
bidis 354
binge drinking 332
blood-alcohol concentration (BAC) 328
carbon monoxide 352
environmental tobacco smoke 359
ethyl alcohol 328
fetal alcohol effects (FAE) 342
fetal alcohol syndrome (FAS) 343
mainstream smoke 359
motivational interviewing 339
nicotine 351
proof 328
sidestream smoke 359
tar 351

13 Protecting Yourself, Your Rights, and Your Health

REAL HEALTH

"This can't be happening to me!" This was the phrase that first ran through Parker's mind when the car swerved out of control. He kept repeating it to himself as he felt a terrible crushing pain shoot through his legs.

Later at the hospital, when he woke up after surgery, it was his first thought. And all through his long rehabilitation, on the days when he thought life would never go back to normal, he'd try to tell himself that this too couldn't be happening to him.

At least Parker had been wearing a seat belt. His friend in the back seat wasn't. Thrown from the car, he suffered such severe injuries that the doctors weren't sure he'd survive.

For months after the accident, Parker couldn't get the sounds and sights of that terrible night out of his mind. Why had they let Randy, who'd had just as much to drink as they did, take the wheel? Why didn't they tell him to slow down? Ironically, he walked away from the accident with no more than some scrapes.

"You were lucky too," Parker's mother reminded him. "You'll recover. And maybe you've learned some lessons that may save your life in the future." The biggest lesson, Parker realized, was a wake-up call: Bad things can and do happen, even to him.

Accidents, injuries, assaults, crimes, serious illnesses, chronic medical conditions—all seem like things that happen only to other people, only in other times and places. But no one, regardless of how young, healthy, or strong, is immune from danger.

If you are of traditional college age, the greatest threats to your well-being and your life are intentional and nonintentional injury, for example, an assault or an accident. You may think that the risk of either is simply a matter of chance, of being in the wrong place at the wrong time. That's not the case. Certain behaviors, such as heavy drinking or not buckling your seat belt, greatly increase the risk of harm. Ultimately, you have more control over your personal safety than anyone else.

Regardless of your age, you may suffer chronic pain or other medical symptoms. Although you have many choices in seeking health care, the responsibility for getting the best possible treatment is yours.

Whether you are monitoring your blood pressure, taking medication, or deciding whether to try an alternative therapy, you need to gather information, ask questions, weigh advantages and disadvantages, and take charge of your health. The reason: No one cares more about your health than you do, and no one will do more to promote your well-being than you.

? FAQ **Frequently Asked Questions**

- Is it safe to talk on the phone while driving? *p. 366*
- Is stalking dangerous? *p. 370*
- How can I find good advice online? *p. 374*

After studying the material in this chapter, you should be able to:

- **Describe** key factors in driving safely.
- **Define** hate crimes.
- **Define** sexual victimization, sexual harassment, stalking, and sexual coercion.
- **Describe** recommended actions for preventing rape.
- **List** ways of becoming an informed health-care consumer.
- **Discuss** strategies for self-care, as well as how to get the best possible health care.
- **List** your rights as a medical consumer.
- **Describe** the different types of complementary and alternative therapies and **explain** what research has shown about their effectiveness.
- **Explain** the concept of managed care.

ThomsonNOW™ Log on to ThomsonNOW at **www.thomsonedu.com/thomsonnow** to find your Behavior Change Planner and to explore self-assessments, interactive tutorials, and practice quizzes.

Personal Safety

The major threat to the lives of college students isn't illness but injury. Almost 75 percent of deaths among Americans 15 to 24 years old are caused by "unintentional injuries" (a term public health officials prefer), suicides, and homicides.[1] Accidents, especially motor vehicle crashes, kill more college-age men and women than all other causes combined; the greatest number of lives lost to accidents is among those 25 years of age.

Becoming a Safer Driver

With more drivers and more vehicles on the roads than ever before, accidents kill about 43,000 people a year.[2] Alcohol use is a factor in about 40 percent of these crashes; speeding, in about one-third. Rollovers caused by drivers who lose control of their vehicles kill about 25 people daily. Crashes involving teen drivers result in about 25 fatalities each day. Motor vehicle accidents injure almost three million people, more than any other form of unintentional injury.

College students aren't necessarily safer drivers than others their age. According to national data, full-time college students drink and drive more often than part-time students and other young adults, but they also are more likely to wear seat belts while driving and riding in cars. How can you increase your odds of staying safe on the road? Some key factors are staying sober and alert, using your seat belt, making sure your vehicle has working air bags, and controlling road rage. The number-one culprit in car crashes is distraction—whether by chatting on the phone, fiddling with a radio, or eating.[3]

Stay Sober and Alert

The number of fatalities caused by drunk driving, particularly among young people, has dropped. The National Highway Traffic Safety Administration (NHTSA) attributes this decline to increases in the drinking age, to educational programs aimed at reducing nighttime driving by teens, to the formation of Students Against Destructive Decisions (SADD; originally called Students Against Drunk Driving) and similar groups, and to changes in state laws that lowered the legal blood-alcohol concentration level for drivers under age 21 (some states have zero tolerance blood-alcohol level (BAC) for drivers under 21).

Falling asleep at the wheel is second only to alcohol as a cause of serious motor-vehicle accidents. About half of drivers in the United States drive while drowsy. Nearly 14 million have fallen asleep at the wheel in the past year, according to the National Sleep Foundation.

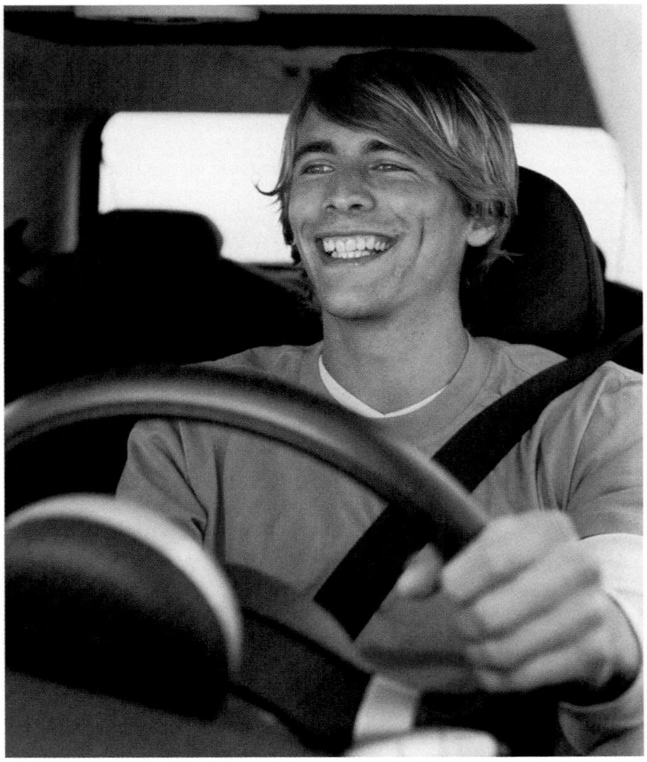

© Nick Clements

Buckling up is one of the simplest and most effective ways of protecting yourself from injury.

Men and young adults between the ages of 18 and 29 are at the highest risk for driving while drowsy or falling asleep at the wheel.

Buckle Up

Seat belt use has reached an all-time high, with three in four Americans buckling up. States with seat belt laws have even higher rates of use: 80 percent. However, young people are less likely to use seat belts. Men between ages 19 and 29 are least likely to wear seat belts while driving or riding in a car. By official estimates, two-thirds of 15- to 20-year-olds killed in motor vehicle accidents were not wearing seat belts. Unbelted crash occupants are three times as likely to die in an emergency department while undergoing treatment.[4]

Seat belts save an estimated 9,500 lives in the United States each year. When lap-shoulder belts are used properly, they reduce the risk of fatal injury to front-seat passengers by 45 percent and the risk of moderate to critical injury by 50 percent. Because an unrestrained passenger can injure others during a crash, the risk of death is lowest when all occupants wear seat belts, according to federal analysts. Seat belt use by everyone in a car may prevent about one in six deaths that might otherwise occur in a crash.

Check for Air Bags

An air bag, either with or without a seat belt, has proved the most effective means of preventing adult death, somewhat more so for women than for men. However, they do not lower the risk of serious injury; seat belts do. Air bags used in conjunction with seat belts do not significantly reduce the risk of injury; without seat belts, they increase the risk of injury, particularly to the head and legs.

Because there is controversy over the potential hazard they pose to children, the American Academy of Pediatrics recommends that children be placed in the backseat, whether or not the car is equipped with a passenger air bag.

Rein in Road Rage

The emotional outbursts known as road rage are a factor in as many as two-thirds of all fatal car crashes and one-third of nonfatal accidents, according to the NHTSA. Psychologist Arnold Nerenberg of Whittier, California, a specialist in motorway mayhem, estimates 1.78 billion episodes of road rage occur each year, resulting in more than 28,000 deaths and 1 million injuries.[5]

Some strategies for reducing road rage include the following:

- **Lower the stress in your life.** Take a few moments to breathe deeply and relax your shoulders before putting the key in the ignition.
- **Consciously decide not to let other drivers get to you.** Decide that whatever happens, it's not going to make your blood pressure go up.
- **Slow down.** If you're going five or ten miles over the speed limit, you won't have the time you need to react to anything that happens.
- **Modify bad driving habits one at a time.** If you tend to tailgate slow drivers, spend a week driving at twice your usual following distance. If you're a habitual horn honker, silence yourself.
- **Be courteous—even if other drivers aren't.** Don't dawdle in the passing lane. Never tailgate or switch lanes without signaling. Don't use your horn or high beams unless absolutely necessary.
- **Never retaliate.** Whatever another driver does, keep your cool. Count to ten. Take a deep breath. If you yell or gesture at someone who's upset with you, the conflict may well escalate.
- **If you do something stupid, show that you're sorry.** On its website, the AAA Foundation for Traffic Safety solicited suggestions for automotive apologies. The most popular: slapping yourself on your forehead or the top of your head to indicate that you know you goofed. Such gestures can soothe a miffed motorist—and make the roads a slightly safer place for all of us.

Strategies for Prevention

What To Do In An Emergency

Life-threatening situations rarely happen more than once or twice in any person's life. When they do, you must think and act quickly to prevent disastrous consequences.

- **Stop, look, and listen.** Your immediate response to an emergency may be overwhelming fear and anxiety. Take several deep breaths. Start by assessing the circumstances. Look for any possible dangers to you or the victim, such as a live electrical wire or a fire. Listen for sounds, such as a cry for help or a siren. Don't attempt rescue techniques, such as cardiopulmonary resuscitation (CPR), unless you're trained.
- **Don't wait for symptoms to go away or get worse.** If you suspect that someone is having a heart attack or stroke, or has ingested something poisonous, *phone for help immediately.* A delay could jeopardize the person's life. Stay on the line long enough to give your name, address, and a brief description of the emergency.
- **Don't move a victim.** The person may have a broken neck or back, and attempting to move him or her could cause extensive damage or even death.
- **Don't drive.** Even if the hospital is just ten minutes away, you're better off waiting for a well-equipped ambulance with trained paramedics who can deliver emergency care on the spot. People rushing to emergency rooms are more likely to get into accidents themselves.
- **Don't do too much.** Often well-intentioned good samaritans make injuries worse by trying to tie tourniquets, wash cuts, or splint broken limbs. Don't give an injured person anything to eat or drink.
- **At home, keep a supply of basic first-aid items in a convenient place.** Beyond the emergency number 911, make sure that telephone numbers for your doctor and neighbors are handy.

FAQ Is It Safe to Talk on the Phone While Driving?

According to the National Highway Traffic Safety Administration, people who use mobile phones while driving are four times more likely to have a serious crash.[6] Most college students with cell phones use them when driving. A third of these have been involved in a serious car accident. In some states, it is now illegal to talk on a cell phone while driving.

Although many believe that hands-free car phones are less hazardous, researchers have shown this is not the case. Talking on a wireless phone while driving a car is just as dangerous with a hands-free or a handheld phone. The reason is that talking while driving distracts the brain as well as the eyes—much more so than talking to another person in the vehicle. Conversation on any type of phone disrupts a driver's attention to the visual environment, leading to what researchers call "inattention blindness," the inability to recognize objects encountered in the driver's visual field. This form of cognitive impairment may distract drivers for up to two minutes after the phone conversation has ended.

On the other hand, mobile phones are helpful in alerting authorities to road hazards, congestion, or problem drivers and in summoning help in case of a breakdown or other emergency.

Car Phone Safety Tips

- Find out if cell phone use while driving is legal in your state.

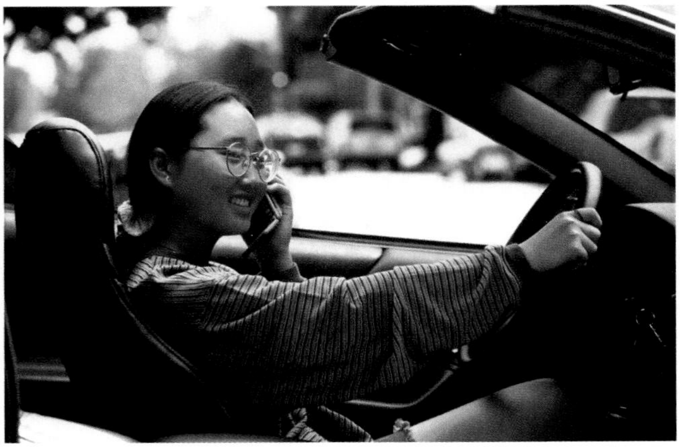

Any form of distraction while driving, including talking on a cell phone, can put you and others at risk.

- Do not dial new calls until you're stopped or in a safe low-traffic environment.
- Keep calls short, less than 1 or 2 minutes.
- When you're on the phone, avoid difficult maneuvers, such as changing lanes, that require a lot of attention.
- Have a passenger send or receive calls.
- Invest in a hands-free model, especially if you use your phone regularly. While the cognitive distraction is the same, it helps to avoid the mechanical distraction.

Safe Cycling

Mile for mile, motorcycling is far more risky than automobile driving. The most common motorcycle injury is head trauma, which can lead to physical disability,

Strategies for Prevention — How to Drive Safely

- Don't drive while under the influence of alcohol or other drugs, including medications that may impair your reflexes, cause drowsiness, or affect your judgment. Never get into a car if you suspect the driver may be intoxicated or affected by a drug.
- Remain calm when dealing with drivers who are reckless or rude. Be alert and anticipate possible hazards. Don't let yourself be distracted by conversations, children's questions, arguments, food or drink, or scenic views.
- Don't get too comfortable. Alertness matters. Use the rearview mirror often. Don't let passengers or packages obstruct your view. Use turn signals when changing lanes or making a turn. If someone cuts you off, back off to a safe distance.
- Watch out for warning signs of fatigue, such as difficulty focusing, frequent blinking or heavy eyelids, trouble keeping one's head up; repeated yawning; trouble remembering the last few miles driven; and drifting from the lane or hitting the shoulder rumble strip.
- Drive more slowly if weather conditions are bad. Avoid driving at all during heavy rain, snow, or other conditions that affect visibility and road conditions. If you must drive in hazardous conditions, make sure that your car has the proper equipment, such as chains or snow tires, and that you know how to respond in case of a skid.
- Maintain your car properly, replacing windshield wipers, tires, and brakes when necessary. Keep flares and a fire extinguisher in your car for use in emergencies.

including paralysis and general weakness, as well as problems reading and thinking. It can also cause personality changes and psychiatric problems, such as depression, anxiety, uncontrollable mood swings, and anger. Complete recovery from head trauma can take four to six years, and the costs can be staggering. Head injury can also result in permanent disability, coma, and death. To prevent head trauma, motorcycle helmets are required in most states.

Approximately 80.6 million people ride bicycles. Each year, bicycle crashes kill about 750 to 1,500 of these individuals and send 450,000 to 587,000 to emergency rooms. Men are more likely to suffer cycling injuries. Head injury is the cause of 70 to 85 percent of bicycle crash deaths.

According to a national survey, 50 percent of all bicycle riders in the United States regularly wear bike helmets—43 percent every time they ride and 7 percent more than half the time. Wearing a helmet can reduce head injuries and deaths by an estimated 29 to 90 percent, depending on the type of helmet.

Living in a Dangerous World

Although the United States remains the most violent country in the Western world, the rate of violent crime is going down. The World Health Organization (WHO) defines violence as "the intentional use of physical force or power, threatened or actual, against oneself, another person, or a group or community, that either results in, or has a high likelihood of resulting in, injury, death, psychological harm, maldevelopment, or deprivation."

Rates of violent crime in the United States have been dropping for more than a decade. Yet more than 300,000 people die each year as a result of violence, suicide, or accidental injury. Interpersonal violence is the third-leading cause of death among people 15 to 44 years old. Some studies show that a third of women age 16 to 49 have, at some point in their lives, been victims of sexual abuse.

Violence in the United States

Gun-related injuries and deaths have declined, but guns remain the second-leading cause of injury-related death in the United States after car accidents. About 260 Americans are injured by firearms every day; one-third die from their wounds.[7] Despite the decline in crime, gun violence annually takes the lives of nearly 30,000 Americans.

Although men commit nine times more violent crimes than women, the rates are getting closer. Individuals with mental illness are somewhat more likely to become violent and to be the victims of violent crimes.

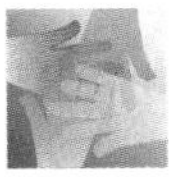

There are ethnic and racial differences in patterns of violence. African Americans are at greater risk of victimization by violent crime than whites or persons of other racial groupings. Hispanics are at greater risk of violent victimization than non-Hispanics. There is little difference between white women and nonwhite women in rape, physical assault, or stalking. Native American and Alaska Native women are significantly more likely than white women or African-American women to report being raped. Mixed-race women also have a significantly higher incidence of rape than white women. Native American and Alaska Native men report significantly more physical assaults than Asian and Pacific Islander men.

Strategies for Prevention — *How to Buy a Bicycle Helmet*

What should you look for when buying a helmet? Here are some basic guidelines:

- A government regulation requires all helmets produced after 1999 to meet the Consumer Product Safety Commission standard; look for a CPSC sticker inside the helmet. The ASTM (American Society for Testing and Materials) standard is comparable to CPSC. The Snell Memorial Foundation's B-90 standard is even better.
- Check the fit. The helmet should sit level on your head, touching all around, comfortably snug but not tight. The helmet should not move more than about an inch in any direction, regardless of how hard you tug at it.
- Pick a bright color for visibility. Avoid dark colors, thin straps, or a rigid visor that could snag in a fall.
- Look for a smooth plastic outer shell, not one with alternating strips of plastic and foam.
- Watch out for excessive vents, which put less protective foam in contact with your head in a crash.
- Mirrors should have a breakaway mount; the wire type mounted on eyeglasses can gouge an eye in a fall.

Hate Crimes

Recent years have seen the emergence of violent crimes motivated by hatred of a particular person's (or group of persons') race, ethnicity, religion, sexual orientation, or political values. These hate crimes have included the dragging death of a young African-American man, the beating death of a young gay man, the shooting of children and teachers at a Jewish community center, and the vandalizing of Muslim-owned businesses after the terrorist attacks of September 11, 2001. Politicians and government leaders have called for an expansion of hate-crime laws that would inflict especially severe sentences on those who commit violence on the basis of racism, sexism, homophobia, anti-Semitism, or other forms of prejudice.

More than half of hate crimes on campus are motivated by race; others by anti-Semitism and sexual orientation. These crimes can take the form of graffiti; verbal slurs; bombings, threatening notes, emails, or phone calls; and physical attacks. They often generate fear and intimidation in large groups of students, undermining health, academic work, and the basic security of a campus.[8]

Crime and Violence on Campus

According to the Bureau of Justice, college students are victims of almost half a million violent crimes a year, including assault, robbery, sexual assault, and rape. While this number may seem high, the overall violent crime rate has dropped by 54 percent since 1995.[9]

College students ages 18 to 24 are less likely to be victims of violent crime, including robbery and assault, than nonstudents of the same age. More than half (58 percent) of crimes against students are committed by strangers. More than nine in ten occur off campus, most often in an open area or street, on public transportation, in a place of business, or at a private home. In about two-thirds of the crimes, no weapon is involved. Most off-campus crimes occur at night, while on-campus crimes are more frequent in the day.[10]

Male college students are twice as likely to be victims of overall violence than female students. White undergraduates have higher rates of violent victimization than students of other races. Simple assault accounts for two-thirds of violent crimes against students; sexual assault or rape account for around 6 percent.[11]

About three in four campus crimes are never reported to the police. The main reasons students give for not reporting crimes are that they are too minor or private or they are not certain that it was a crime. Individuals also may be too ashamed or emotionally overwhelmed to contact authorities.

The Jeanne Clery Disclosure of Campus Security Policy and Campus Crime Statistics Act, originally known as the Student Right-to-Know and Campus Security Act, requires colleges to publish annual crime statistics for their campuses. However, the act excludes certain offenses, such as theft, threats, harassment, and vandalism, so the picture it presents may not be complete. The most recent crime statistics for the nation's 6,269 colleges, universities, and career schools are posted on the Internet at http://ope.ed.gov/security. How safe is your school? Take the Self Survey: "How Safe Is Your School?" in the Self-Assessment Booklet.

Because of concerns about safety on campus, more schools are taking tougher stands on student behavior. Many have established codes of conduct barring the use of alcohol and drugs, fighting, and sexual harassment. Many also have instituted policies requiring suspension or expulsion for students who violate this code.

Some types of violence occur mainly on college campuses. One is hazing, which refers to any activity that humiliates, degrades, or poses a risk of emotional or physical harm for the sake of joining a group or to maintain full status in that group. This behavior may occur in fraternities and sororities, athletic teams, or other campus organizations. Its forms include verbal ridicule and abuse, forced consumption of alcohol or ingestion of vile substances, sexual violation, sleep deprivation, paddling, beating, burning, or branding.

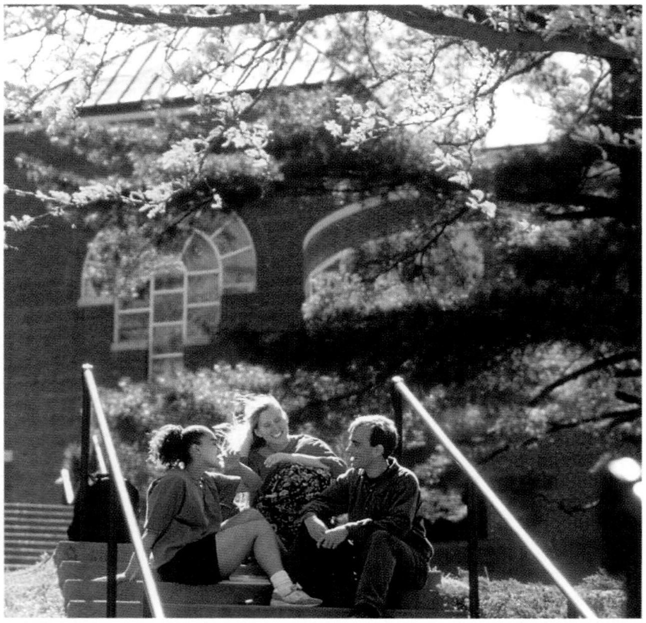

A peaceful scene like this doesn't mean that a campus is safe. Do you know the crime statistics for your college?

Sexual Victimization and Violence

Sexual victimization refers to any situation in which a person is deprived of free choice and forced to comply with sexual acts. This is not only a woman's issue; in fact, men also are victimized. In recent years, researchers have come to view acts of sexual victimization along a continuum, ranging from street hassling, stalking, and obscene telephone calls to rape, battering, and incest.

Sexual Harassment

All forms of **sexual harassment** or unwanted sexual attention—from the display of pornographic photos to the use of sexual obscenities to a demand for sex by anyone in a position of power or authority—are illegal.

Nearly two-thirds of students experience sexual harassment at some point during college, including nearly one-third of first year students, according to a recent research report on campus sexual harassment. Nearly one-third of students say they have experienced physical harassment, such as being touched, grabbed, or pinched in a sexual way. Sexual comments and jokes are the most common form of harassment. More than half of female students and nearly half of male students say they have experienced this type of harassment. Lesbian, gay, bisexual, and transgender (LGBT) students are more likely than heterosexual students to be sexually harassed.[12] (See Student Snapshot: "Sexual Harassment on Campus.")

Sexual harassment takes an especially heavy toll on female students, who often feel upset, self-conscious, embarrassed, or angry. Men are much less likely to admit to being very or somewhat upset. A third of harassed college women say they felt afraid; one-fifth say they were disappointed in their college experience as a result of sexual harassment.

More than a third of students who experience harassment tell no one; about half tell a friend. Only 7 percent of students say they reported sexual harassment to a faculty member or other college employee. More than half of students would like their college or university to offer a Web-based, confidential method for submitting complaints about sexual harassment. Nearly half would like their college or university to designate an office or person to contact about sexual harassment.

About half of college men and a third of women admit that they have sexually harassed someone on campus. Private college students are more likely than their public college peers to have ever done so. Students at large schools (population of 10,000 or more) are more likely than students at small schools with fewer than 5,000 students to say they have experienced sexual harassment. The most common rationale for harassment is "I thought it was funny." Harassment occurs in dorms or student housing as well as outside on campus grounds, in classrooms or lecture halls.[13]

If you encounter sexual harassment as a student, report it to the department chair or dean. If you don't receive an adequate response to your complaint, talk with the campus representatives who handle matters involving affirmative action or civil rights. Federal guidelines prevent any discrimination against you in terms of grades or the loss of a job or scholarship if you report harassment. Schools that do not take measures to remedy harassment could lose federal funds.

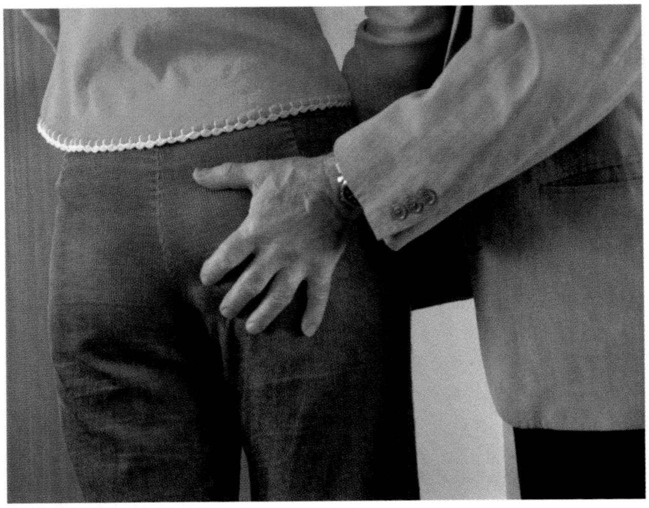

© WoodyStock/Alamy

Sexual harassment can take many forms, ranging from suggestive comments to physical touching, and can occur in classrooms as well as offices and other workplaces.

Student Snapshot
Sexual Harassment on Campus

	Men	Women
Experienced physical harassment	29%	35%
Experienced sexual comments or jokes	48%	57%
Sexually harassed someone on campus	51%	31%
Very or somewhat upset by harassment	68%	35%

Source: Drawing the Line: Sexual Harassment on Campus. Washington, DC: American Association of University Women, January 2006.

© 2006 Jupiter Images

Sexual harassment Unwanted sexual attention.

? FAQ Is Stalking Dangerous?

The "willful, repeated, and malicious following, harassing, or threatening of another person," as stalking is defined, is common on college campuses—perhaps more so than in the general population. In studies, as many as 25 to 30 percent of female students and 11 to 17 percent of male students report having been stalked.

College students may be targeted for several reasons. Simply because they are young and still learning how to manage complex social relationships, some individuals may not recognize their behavior as stalking or even as disturbing. In addition, college students tend to live close to each other and to have flexible schedules and large amounts of unsupervised time.

Stalking is not a benign behavior and can result in emotional or psychological distress, physical harm, or sexual assault. By some estimates, 10 percent of stalking incidents result in forced or attempted sexual contact. The most common consequence is psychological, with victims reporting emotional or psychological distress.

Dating Violence

Actual or threatened physical or sexual violence or psychological and emotional abuse of a current or former dating partner is a form of violence. It can occur between heterosexual, homosexual, or bisexual partners.

Over the course of five years (the national average for a college career), including summers and vacations, one of every four or five female students is raped. In a single academic year, 2.7 percent of coeds are raped—35 rapes for every 1,000 women. According to the Department of Justice, a campus with 6,000 coeds averages one rape a day every day for the entire school year.

In nine surveys of male university students, between 3 and 6 percent had been raped by other men; up to 25 percent had been sexually assaulted. Like female rape victims, male victims suffer long-term psychological problems, physical injuries, and are at risk of contracting a sexually transmitted infection.

Nonvolitional Sex and Sexual Coercion

Nonvolitional sex is sexual behavior that violates a person's right to choose when and with whom to have sex and what sexual behaviors to engage in. The more extreme forms of this behavior include sexual coercion or forced sex, rape, childhood sexual abuse, and violence against people with nonconventional sexual identities. Other forms, such as engaging in sex to keep one's partner or to pass as heterosexual, are so common that many think of them as normal.

Sexual coercion can take many forms, including exerting peer pressure, taking advantage of one's desire for popularity, threatening an end to a relationship, getting someone intoxicated, stimulating a partner against his or her wishes, or insinuating an obligation based on the time or money one has expended. Men may feel that they need to live up to the sexual stereotype of taking advantage of every opportunity for sex. Women are far more likely than men to encounter physical force.

Eight in ten college students report using verbal coercion and two in ten used physical coercion against a dating partner in the last year.[14]

Rape

Rape refers to sexual intercourse with an unconsenting partner under actual or threatened force. Sexual intercourse between a male over the age of 16 and a female under the age of consent (which ranges from 12 to 21 in different states) is called *statutory rape.* In *acquaintance rape,* or *date rape,* the victim knows the rapist. In *stranger rape,* the rapist is an unknown assailant. Both stranger and acquaintance rapes are serious crimes that can have a devastating impact on their victims.

For many years, the victims of rape were blamed for doing something to bring on the attack. However, researchers have shown that women are raped because they encounter sexually aggressive men, not because they look or act a certain way. Although no woman is immune to attack, many rape victims are children or adolescents.

Women who successfully escape rape attempts do so by resisting verbally and physically, usually by yelling and fleeing. Women who use forceful verbal or physical resistance (screaming, hitting, kicking, biting, and running) are more likely to avoid rape than women who try pleading, crying, or offering no resistance.

For every 1,000 college women, 35 will be the victims of rape or attempted rape on campus.[15]

Acquaintance, or Date, Rape

The same factors that lead to other forms of sexual victimization can set the stage for date rape. Socialization into an aggressive role, acceptance of rape myths, and a view that force is justified in certain situations increase the likelihood of a man's committing date rape. Other factors can also play a role, including the following:

- **Personality and early sexual experiences.** Certain factors may predispose individuals to sexual aggression, including first sexual experience at a very young age, earlier and more frequent than usual childhood sexual experiences (both forced and voluntary), hostility toward women, irresponsibility, lack of social consciousness, and a need for dominance over sexual partners.

- **Situational variables (what happens during the date).** Men who initiate a date, pay all expenses, and provide transportation are more likely to be sexually aggressive, perhaps because they feel they can call all the shots.
- **Rape-tolerant attitudes.** As several studies have confirmed, college men hold more rape-tolerant attitudes than do college women. For example, college men are significantly more likely than college women to agree with statements such as, "Some women ask to be raped and may enjoy it" and "If a woman says 'no' to having sex, she means 'maybe' or even 'yes.'"

  Some social groups, such as fraternities and athletic teams, may encourage the use of alcohol; reinforce stereotypes about masculinity; and emphasize violence, force, and competition. The group's shared values, including an acceptance of sexual coercion, may keep individuals from questioning their behavior.
- **Drinking.** Alcohol use is one of the strongest predictors of acquaintance rape. Men who've been drinking may not react to subtle signals, may misinterpret a woman's behavior as a come-on, and may feel more sexually aroused. At the same time, drinking may impair a woman's ability to effectively communicate her wishes and to cope with a man's aggressiveness.
- **Date rape drugs.** Drugs such as Rohypnol (flunitrazepam) and GHB (gamma hydroxybutyrate) have been implicated in cases of acquaintance, or date, rape. Since both drugs are odorless and tasteless, victims have no way of knowing whether their drink has been tampered with. The subsequent loss of memory leaves victims with no explanation for where they've been or what's happened.

  Rohypnol—which can cause impaired motor skills and judgment, lack of inhibitions, dizziness, confusion, lethargy, very low blood pressure, coma, and death—has been outlawed in this country. Deaths also have been attributed to GHB overdoses.
- **Gender differences in interpreting sexual cues.** In research comparing college men and women, the men typically overestimated the woman's sexual availability and interest, seeing friendliness, revealing clothing, and attractiveness as deliberately seductive. In one study of date rape, the men reported feeling "led on," in part because their female partners seemed to be dressed more suggestively than usual.

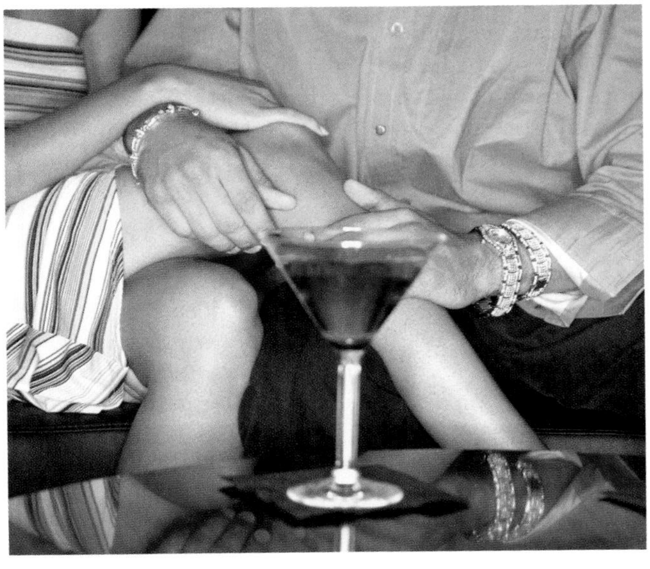

© Master/file

Acquaintance rape and alcohol use are very closely linked. Both men and women may find their judgment impaired or their communications unclear as a result of drinking.

YOUR LIFE COACH

PREVENTING RAPE

Date Rape

According to data from the U.S. Bureau of Justice, nine in ten reported rapes and sexual assaults in the United States involve a single offender with whom the victim had a prior relationship.

Both women and men report having been forced into sexual activity by someone they know. Many college students are in the age group most likely to face this threat: women aged 16 to 25 and men under 25. Women are most vulnerable and men are most likely to commit assaults during their senior year of high school and their first year of college.

Women who describe incidents of sexual coercion that meet the legal definition of rape often don't label it as such. They may have a preconceived notion that true rape consists of a blitzlike attack by a stranger. Or they may blame themselves for getting into a situation in which they couldn't escape. They may feel some genuine concern for others who would be devastated if they knew the truth (for example, if the rapist were the brother of a good friend or the son of a neighbor).

Here are strategies that can lower your risk of being involved in a date rape:

For men:

- Remember that it's okay not to "score" on a date.
- Don't assume that a sexy dress or casual flirting is an invitation to sex.

nonvolitional sex Sexual behavior that violates a person's right to choose when and with whom to have sex and what sexual behaviors to engage in.

sexual coercion Sexual activity forced upon a person by the exertion of psychological pressure by another person.

rape Sexual penetration of a female or a male by means of intimidation, force, or fraud.

- Be aware of your partner's actions. If she pulls away or tries to get up, understand that she's sending you a message—one you should acknowledge and respect.
- Restrict drinking, drug use, or other behaviors (such as hanging out with a group known to be sexually aggressive in certain situations) that could affect your judgment and ability to act responsibly.
- Think of the way you'd want your sister or a close woman friend to be treated by her date. Behave in the same manner.

For women:

- If the man pays for all expenses, he may think he's justified in using force to get "what he paid for." If you cover some of the costs, he may be less aggressive.
- Back away from a man who pressures you into other activities you don't want to engage in on a date, such as chugging beer or drag racing with his friends.
- Avoid misleading messages and avoid behavior that may be interpreted as sexual teasing. Don't tell him to stop touching you, talk for a few minutes, and then resume petting.
- Despite your clearly stated intentions, if your date behaves in a sexually coercive manner, use a strategy of escalating forcefulness—direct refusal, vehement verbal refusal, and if necessary, physical force.
- Avoid using alcohol or other drugs when you definitely do not wish to be sexually intimate with your date.

Stranger Rape

Rape prevention consists primarily of making it as difficult as possible for a rapist to make you his victim:

- Don't advertise that you're a woman living alone. Use initials on your mailbox. Install and use secure locks on doors and windows, changing door locks after losing keys or moving into a new residence.
- Don't open your door to strangers. If a repairman or public official is at your door, ask him to identify himself and call his office to verify that he is a reputable person on legitimate business.
- Lock your car when it is parked, and drive with locked car doors. Should your car break down, attach a white cloth to the antenna and lock yourself in. If someone other than a uniformed officer stops to offer help, ask this person to call the police or a garage but do not open your locked car door.
- Avoid dark and deserted areas, and be aware of the surroundings where you're walking. Should a driver ask for directions when you're a pedestrian, avoid approaching his car. Instead, call out your reply from a safe distance.
- Have house or car keys in hand as you approach the door. Check the back seat before getting into your car.
- Carry a device for making a loud noise, like a whistle or, even better, a small pint-sized compressed air horn available in many sporting goods and boat supply stores. Sound the noise alarm at the first sign of danger.
- Take a self-defense class to learn techniques of physical resistance that can injure the attacker or distract him long enough for you to escape.

Date rape on campus is rarely reported to the police. However, even if a woman decides not to press criminal charges, she can turn to campus authorities. Should colleges establish a zero-tolerance policy and expel students for sexual coercion and assault? Or should colleges leave such matters to law enforcement?

You Decide

Male Nonconsensual Sex and Rape

No one knows how common male rape is because men are less likely to report such assaults than women. Researchers estimate that the victims in about 10 percent of acquaintance rape cases are men. These hidden victims often keep silent because of embarrassment, shame, or humiliation, as well as their own feelings and fears about homosexuality and conforming to conventional sex roles.

Although many people think men who rape other men are always homosexuals, most male rapists consider themselves to be heterosexual. Young boys aren't the only victims. The average age of male rape victims is 24. Rape is a serious problem in prison, where men may experience brutal assaults by men who usually resume sexual relations with women once they're released.

Impact of Rape

Rape-related injuries include unexplained vaginal discharge, bleeding, infections, multiple bruises, and fractured ribs. Victims of sexual violence often develop chronic symptoms, such as headaches, backaches, high blood pressure, sleep disorders, pelvic pain, and sexual fertility problems. But sexual violence has both a physical and a psychological impact. The psychological scars of a sexual assault take a long time to heal. Therapists have linked sexual victimization with hopelessness, low self-esteem, high levels of self-criticism, and self-defeating relationships. An estimated 30 to 50 percent of women develop posttraumatic stress disorder following

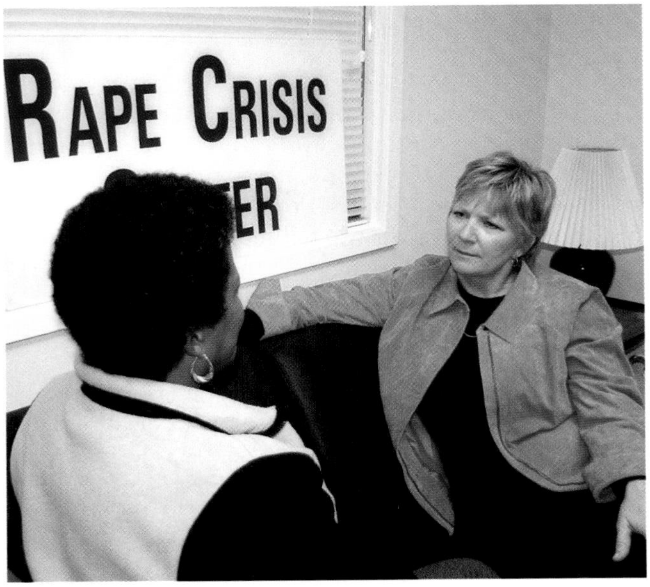

Counseling from a trained professional can help ease the trauma suffered by a rape victim.

a rape. Many do not seek counseling until a year or more after an attack, when their symptoms have become chronic or intensified.

Acquaintance rape may cause fewer physical injuries but greater psychological torment. Often too ashamed to tell anyone what happened, victims may suffer alone, without skilled therapists or sympathetic friends to reassure them. Women raped by acquaintances blame themselves more, see themselves less positively, question their judgment, have greater difficulty trusting others, and have higher levels of psychological distress. Nightmares, anxiety, and flashbacks are common. The women may avoid others, become less capable of protecting themselves, and continue to be haunted by sexual violence for years. A therapist can help these victims begin the slow process of healing.

What to Do in Case of Rape

Fewer than 5 percent of college rapes are reported.[16] Women who are raped should call a friend or a rape crisis center. A rape victim should not bathe or change her clothes before calling. Semen, hair, and material under her fingernails or on her apparel all may be useful in identifying the man who raped her.

A rape victim who chooses to go to a doctor or hospital should remember that she may not necessarily have to talk to police. However, a doctor can collect the necessary evidence, which will then be available if she later decides to report the rape to police. All rape victims should talk with a doctor or health-care worker about testing and treatment for sexually transmitted infections and postintercourse conception.

Even an unsuccessful rape attempt should be reported because the information a woman may provide about the attack—the assaulter's physical characteristics, voice, clothes, car, even an unusual smell—may prevent another woman from being raped.

Halting Sexual Violence

Sexual violence has its roots in social attitudes and beliefs that demean women and condone aggression. According to international research, much sexual violence takes place within families, marriage, and dating relationships. In many settings, rape is a culturally approved strategy to control and discipline women. In these places, laws and policies to improve women's status are critical to ending sexual coercion.

As colleges and universities have become more aware of the different forms of sexual danger, many have taken the lead in setting up primary prevention programs (including newspaper articles; seminars in dormitories, fraternities, and sororities; and lectures) to help students examine their attitudes and values, understand cultural influences, and develop skills for avoiding or escaping from dangerous situations. All men and women should recognize misleading rape myths and develop effective ways of communicating to avoid misinterpretation of sexual cues. Students should also know to whom they can turn to learn more about and seek help for sexual victimization: counselors, campus police, deans of student affairs, fraternity or sorority representatives, and campus ministers.

While most campuses provide self-defense seminars for potential female victims of rape and general campus safety measures, some have tried innovative approaches, such as Men Against Violence, a peer-education program that confronts male students' conceptions of manhood and appropriate gender roles to reduce their likelihood of sexual or physical violence. Such all-male, peer-guided approaches that challenge myths about rape and rape victims also have proved effective with college fraternity men.

Safeguarding Your Health

It's up to you. By learning how to maintain your health, evaluate medical information, and spot early signs of a problem, you're more likely to get the best possible care—and to keep down your medical bills. Self-care means head-to-toe maintenance, including good oral care, appropriate screening tests, knowing your medical rights, and understanding the health-care system.

Chances are that you've tried—or will try—alternative therapies. Many use a "whole-person" approach that addresses all the dimensions of health. You need to be just as savvy a consumer when considering a complementary or alternative treatment as you would with a more mainstream one. You also need to continue your best healthy practices throughout your life so you can function at your best for as long as possible. But your future begins with the healthy choices you make today and every day.

Health Care and the College Student

All of the more than 14 million men and women enrolled in institutions of higher learning need some health-care services, regardless of their age or general health. The Preventive Services Task Force of the U.S. Public Health Service recommends that all have periodic screenings for high blood pressure, obesity, and problem alcohol consumption and that they receive regular counseling concerning the use of drugs, tobacco, and alcohol; sexually transmitted infections; effective contraception; a healthy diet; exercise; oral health; and prevention of motor vehicle injuries and other accidents.

In addition to the medical services available at student health centers, colleges provide health information. According to a CDC survey of approximately 4,600 undergraduates at 136 colleges and universities, about three-quarters of undergraduates have received some form of health information. About half of all students surveyed had been given some information on prevention of alcohol and drug use and HIV infection and AIDS.

Making Smart Health-Care Decisions

Although you may not realize it, you make crucial decisions that affect your health every day. You choose what you eat, whether you exercise, if you smoke or drink, when to fasten your seat belt. You decide when to see health professionals, what to tell them, and whether to follow their advice.

The responsibility for making smart choices about your health lies with you. Never before has so much information about health been available in so many forms and formats. However, not all of it is accurate, objective, or helpful. In order to base your decisions on a solid scientific basis, you have to develop and apply your critical-thinking skills.

The following sections can help.

? FAQ How Can I Find Good Advice Online?

An estimated 85 million Americans—three in four Internet users—are "e-health" consumers who seek information or support, communicate with health-care providers, or buy medical products online. "They use the Internet as an adjunct to physicians, who remain their primary source of health advice," says Mark Bard, president of Manhattan Research, a health-care marketing firm.[17] The American College of Physicians Foundation has launched an "Information Rx" campaign that refers patients to a website (www.medlineplus.gov) operated by the National Library of Medicine. Table 13-1 lists some doctor-endorsed websites.

TABLE 13-1 Doctor-Recommended Websites

National Library of Medicine: MedlinePlus	**www.medlineplus.gov**
MedlinePlus contains links to information on hundreds of health conditions and issues. The site also includes a medical dictionary, an encyclopedia with pictures and diagrams, and links to physician directories.	
FDA Center for Drug Evaluation and Research	**www.fda.gov**
Click on Drugs@FDA for information on approved prescription drugs and some over-the-counter medications.	
WebMD	**www.webmd.com**
WebMD is full of information to help you manage your health. The site's quizzes and calculators are a fun way to test your medical knowledge. Get diet tips, information on drugs and herbs, and check out special sections on men's and women's health.	
MayoClinic	**www.mayoclinic.com**
The renowned Mayo Clinic offers a one-stop health resource website. Use the site's Health Decision Guides to make decisions about prevention and treatment. Learn more about complementary and alternative medicine, sports medicine, and senior health in the Healthy Living Centers.	
Centers for Disease Control and Prevention	**www.cdc.gov**
Stay up to date on the latest public health news and get the CDC's recommendations on travelers' health, vaccines and immunizations, and protecting your health in case of a disaster.	
Medscape	**www.medscape.com**
Medscape delivers news and research specifically tailored to your medical interests. The site requires (free) registration.	

If you go to other websites for medical information, here are some guidelines for evaluating them:

- **Check the creator.** Websites are produced by health agencies, health support groups, school health programs, health-product advertisers, health educators, and health-education organizations. Read site headers and footers carefully to distinguish biased commercial advertisements from unbiased sites created by scientists and health agencies.
- **If you are looking for the most recent research,** check the date the page was created and last updated as well as the links. Several nonworking links signal that the site isn't carefully maintained or updated.
- **Check the references.** As with other health education materials, web documents should provide the reader with references. Unreferenced suggestions may be scientifically unsound and possibly unsafe.
- **Consider the author.** Is he or she recognized in the field of health education or otherwise qualified to publish a health information web document? Does the author list his or her occupation, experience, and education?
- **Look for possible bias.** Websites may be attempting to provide health information to consumers, but they also may be attempting to sell a product. Many sites are merely disguised advertisements.

Evaluating Health News

Cure! Breakthrough! Medical miracle! These words make headlines. Remember that although medical breakthroughs and cures do occur, most scientific progress is made one small step at a time. Rather than putting your faith in the most recent report or the hottest trend, try to gather as much background information and as many opinions as you can. Weigh them carefully—ideally with a trusted physician—and make the decision that seems best for you. (See Savvy Consumer: "Getting Medical Facts Straight.")

Self-Care

Most people do treat themselves. You probably prescribe aspirin for a headache, chicken soup or orange juice for a cold, or a weekend trip to unwind from stress. At the very least, you should know what your **vital signs** are and how they compare against normal readings (Table 13-2).

Once a thermometer was the only self-testing equipment found in most American homes. Now hundreds of home tests are available to help consumers monitor everything from fertility to blood pressure

vital signs Measurements of physiological functioning; specifically, temperature, blood pressure, pulse rate, and respiration rate.

SAVVY CONSUMER

Getting Medical Facts Straight

When reading a newspaper or magazine story or listening to a radio or television report about a medical advance, look for answers to the following questions:

- **Who are the scientists involved?** Are they recognized, legitimate health professionals? What are their credentials? Are they affiliated with respected medical or scientific institutions? Be wary of individuals whose degrees or affiliations are from institutions you've never heard of, and be sure that the person's educational background is in a discipline related to the area of research reported.
- **Where did the scientists report their findings?** The best research is published in peer-reviewed professional journals, such as the *New England Journal of Medicine*. Research developments also may be reported at meetings of professional societies.
- **Is the information based on personal observations?** Does the report include testimonials from cured patients or satisfied customers? If the answer to either question is yes, be wary.
- **Does the article, report, or advertisement include words like *amazing, secret, or quick?*** Does it claim to be something the public has never seen or been offered before? Such sensationalized language is often a tip-off to a dubious treatment.
- **Is someone trying to sell you something?** Manufacturers who cite studies to sell a product have been known to embellish the truth.
- **Does the information defy all common sense?** Be skeptical. If something sounds too good to be true, it probably is.

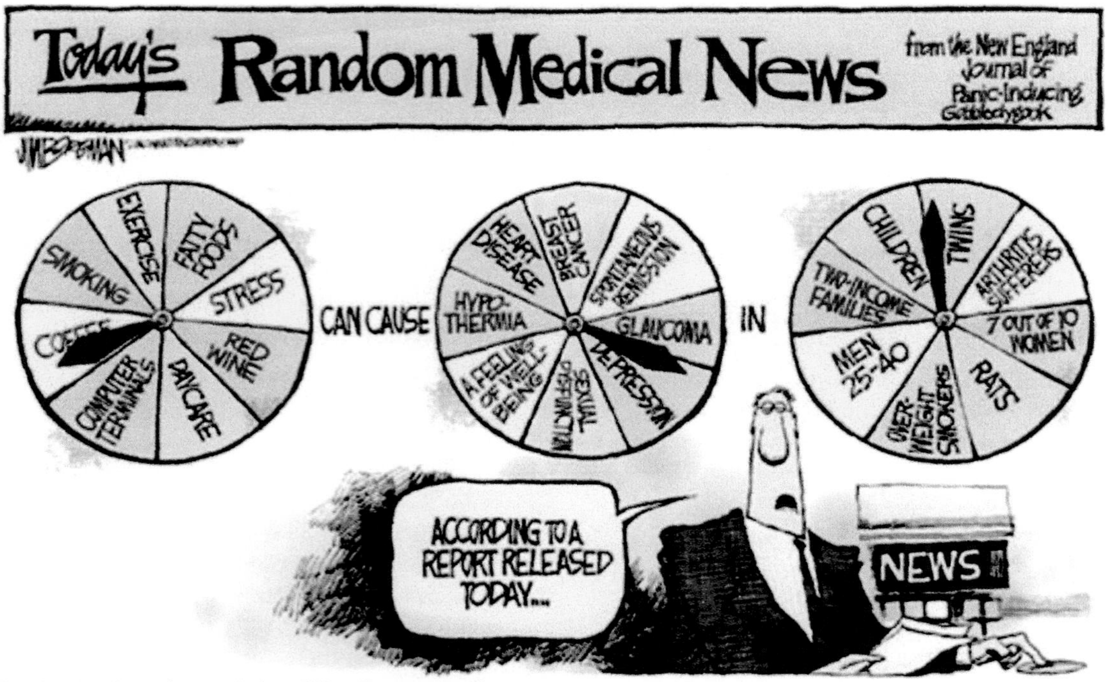

TABLE 13-2 Take Your Own Vital Signs

Vital Sign	Normal Values
Temperature 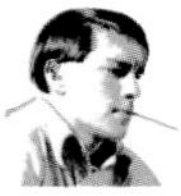	98.9° F in the morning or 99.9° F later in the day is upper limit of the normal oral temperature for people 40 years old or younger. • Women's temperatures are slightly higher than men's. • African Americans' temperatures are slightly higher than white Americans. Measure your temperature with a mercury or digital thermometer.
Blood pressure 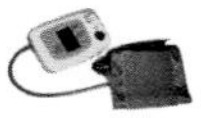	Below 120 (systolic) and below 80 (diastolic) mm Hg. You can measure your own blood pressure if you want to invest in blood pressure equipment. Check your local drugstore to purchase a blood pressure cuff or digital blood pressure monitor.
Pulse 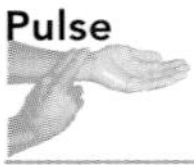	72 beats per minute. Take your pulse rate at your wrist or at the carotid artery in your neck.
Respiration rate 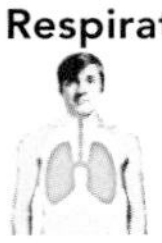	15–20 breaths per minute.

to cholesterol levels (Table 13-3). More convenient and less expensive than a visit to a clinic or doctor's office, the new tests are generally as accurate as those administered by a professional.

Self-care also can mean getting involved in the self-help movement, which has grown into a major national trend. An estimated 20 million people participate in self-help support groups. Many others join virtual support communities online.

Getting the Best Health Care

Once patients simply put their faith in physicians and assumed that they knew best and would make the correct medical decisions. Today health care has become far more complex and impersonal. Increasingly, doctors as well as consumer advocates insist that patients need to take responsibility for their own care. Rather than assuming that health-care providers will do whatever is necessary and appropriate, you must take the initiative to ensure that you get quality care.

The Doctor-Patient Partnership

Once the family doctor was indeed part of the family. The family doctor brought babies into the world, shepherded them through childhood, comforted and counseled them, stood by their bedside in their darkest hours. Patients entrusted the doctor with their cares, their confidences, their very lives. Dramatic breakthroughs in diagnosing and treating illness shifted the focus in medicine from the family physician to the specialist, from

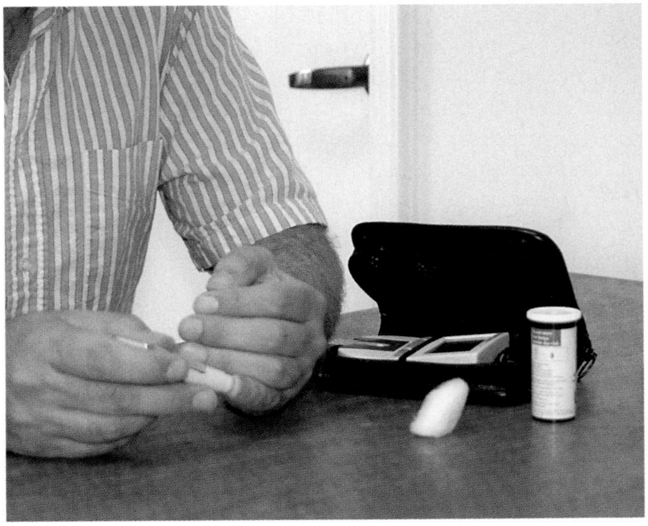

Home health tests can be more convenient and less expensive than a trip to a clinic or doctor's office.

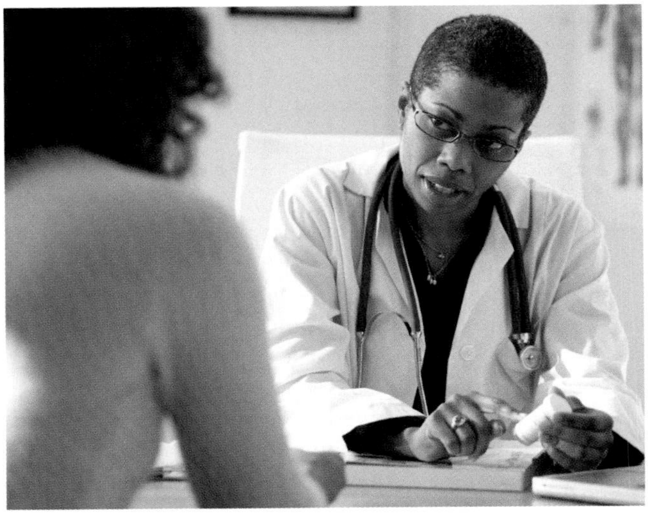

Take charge of your health by educating yourself and asking your doctor questions about your health and treatments.

TABLE 13-3 Home Health Tests: A Consumer's Guide

Type of Test	What It Does
Pregnancy	Determines if a woman is pregnant by detecting the presence of human chorionic gonadotropin in urine. Considered 99 percent accurate.
Fertility	Measures levels of luteinizing hormone (LH), which rise 24 to 36 hours before a woman conceives. Can help women increase their odds of conceiving.
Blood pressure	Measures blood pressure by means of an automatically inflating armband or a cuff for the finger or wrist; helps people taking hypertension medication or suffering from high blood pressure monitor their condition.
Cholesterol	Checks cholesterol in blood from a finger prick; good for anyone concerned about cholesterol.
Colon cancer	Screening test to detect hidden blood in stool; recommended for anyone over 40 or concerned about colorectal disease.
Urinary tract infection	Diagnoses infection by screening for certain white blood cells in urine; advised for women who get frequent UTIs and whose doctors will prescribe antibiotics without a visit.
HIV infection	Detects antibodies to HIV in a blood sample sent anonymously to a lab. Controversial because no face-to-face counseling is available for those who test positive.

basic caring to high-tech medical care. Patients today are more likely to be cured of a vast array of illnesses than were patients a century ago. However, they often complain of insensitive, uncaring physicians who focus on their diseases rather than on them as individuals.

As more physicians have joined managed-care organizations (discussed later in this chapter), which emphasize efficiency, they sometimes feel pressure to see more patients a day, to spend less time with each, and to discourage expensive tests and treatments. Because physicians have less time and less autonomy, patients today must do more. Your first step should be learning more about your body, any medical conditions or problems you develop, and your options for treatment. You can find a great deal of information via computer online services, patient advocacy and support organizations, and libraries.

This information can help you know what questions to ask and how to evaluate what your doctor says. But you have to be willing to speak up. Busy doctors give patients less than a minute on average during a routine visit to say what's bothering them before they interrupt. This doesn't mean your doctor isn't interested, but it does mean that you have to develop good communication skills so you can tell physicians what they need to know to help you.

Complementary and Alternative Medicine

The medical research community uses the term **complementary and alternative medicine (CAM)** to apply to all health-care approaches, practices, and treatments not widely taught in medical schools and not generally used in hospitals. CAM

complementary and alternative medicine (CAM) A term used to apply to all health-care approaches, practices, and treatments not widely taught in medical schools, not generally used in hospitals, and not usually reimbursed by medical insurance companies.

includes many healing philosophies, approaches, and therapies, including preventive techniques designed to delay or prevent serious health problems before they start and **holistic** methods that focus on the whole person and the physical, mental, emotional, and spiritual aspects of well-being. Some approaches are based on the same physiological principles as traditional Western methods; others, such as acupuncture, are based on different healing systems.

According to a recent nationwide government survey of more than 31,000 adults aged 18 and over, 50 percent have used CAM at some time and 46 percent have tried some form of complementary and alternative medicine in the last year. When CAM includes megavitamins and prayer specifically for health, the number reporting they ever used some form of CAM rises to 75 percent; 62 percent did so in the past year.[18]

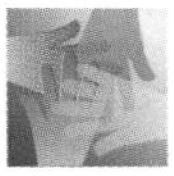

CAM use varies among different groups. Those most likely to use CAM include women, people with higher education, those hospitalized within the past year, and former smokers (compared to current smokers or those who never smoked). African-American adults are more likely than white or Asian adults to use CAM practices, including megavitamin therapy and prayer (Figure 13-1).

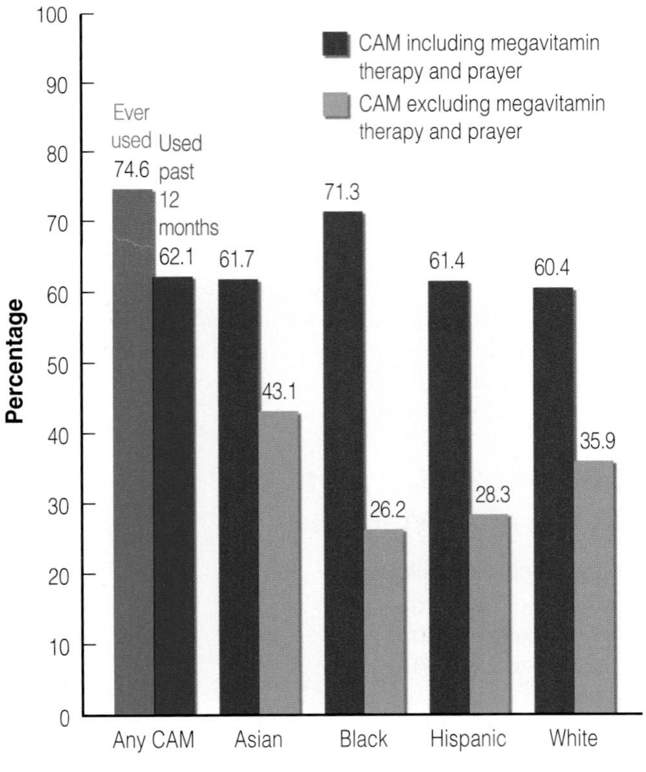

FIGURE 13-1 CAM Use by U.S. Adults and by Race/Ethnicity

Source: NCCAM, http://nccam.nih.gov.

Some states have mandated health insurance coverage for CAM therapies, which also are becoming more common in Canada and Europe. Many medical schools now include training in CAM in their curricula. **Integrative medicine,** which combines selected elements of both conventional and alternative medicine in a comprehensive approach to diagnosis and treatment, has gained greater acceptance within the medical community.

Types of CAM

The National Center for Complementary and Alternative Medicine (NCCAM) has classified CAM therapies into five categories (Figure 13-2).

- **Alternative medical systems**
- **Mind-body medicine**
- **Biologically based therapies**
- **Manipulative and body-based methods**
- **Energy therapies**

Alternative Medical Systems

Systems of theory and practice other than traditional Western medicine are included in this group. They include acupuncture, Eastern medicine, t'ai chi, external and internal qi, Ayurvedic medicine, naturopathy, and unconventional Western systems, such as homeopathy and orthomolecular medicine.

Acupuncture is an ancient Chinese form of medicine, based on the philosophy that a cycle of energy circulating through the body controls health. Pain and

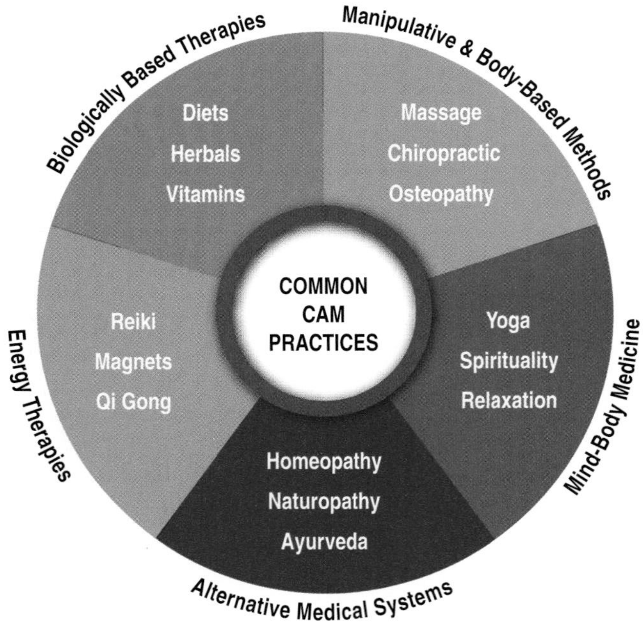

FIGURE 13-2 The Five Categories of CAM

Source: NCCAM, http://nccam.nih.gov.

Strategies for Prevention — What You Should Know Before You Try CAM

You should never decide on any treatment—traditional or CAM—without fully evaluating it. Here are some key questions to ask:

- **Is it safe?** Be particularly wary of unregulated products.
- **Is it effective?** Check the website of the National Center for CAM: http://nccam.nih.gov.
- **Will it interact with other medicines or conventional treatments?** Many widely used alternative remedies can interact with prescription medications in dangerous ways.
- **Is the practitioner qualified?** Find out if your state licenses practitioners who provide acupuncture, chiropractic services, naturopathy, herbal medicine, homeopathy, and other treatments.
- **What has been the experience of others?** Talk to people who have used CAM for a similar problem, both recently and in the past.
- **Can you talk openly and easily with the practitioner?** You should feel comfortable asking questions and confident in the answers you receive. And the practitioner's office should put you at ease.
- **What are the costs?** Many CAM services are not covered by HMOs or health insurers.

disease are the result of a disturbance in the energy flow, which can be corrected by inserting long, thin needles at specific points along longitudinal lines, or *meridians,* throughout the body. Each point controls a different corresponding part of the body. Once inserted, the needles are rotated gently back and forth or charged with a small electric current for a short time. Western scientists aren't sure exactly how acupuncture works, but some believe that the needles alter the functioning of the nervous system.

A National Institute of Health (NIH) consensus development panel that evaluated current research into acupuncture concluded that there is "clear evidence" that acupuncture can control nausea and vomiting in patients after surgery or while undergoing chemotherapy and relieve postoperative dental pain. The panel said that acupuncture is "probably" also effective in the control of nausea in early pregnancy and that there were "reasonable" studies showing satisfactory treatment of addiction to illicit drugs and alcohol (but not to tobacco), stroke rehabilitation, headache, menstrual cramps, tennis elbow, general muscle pain, low back pain, carpal tunnel syndrome, and asthma. Ongoing studies are evaluating its efficacy for chronic headaches and migraines. Acupressure (applying pressure with the thumbs or fingertips to the same points on the body stimulated in acupuncture) seems more effective in reducing low-back pain and providing long-term relief than physical therapy.[19]

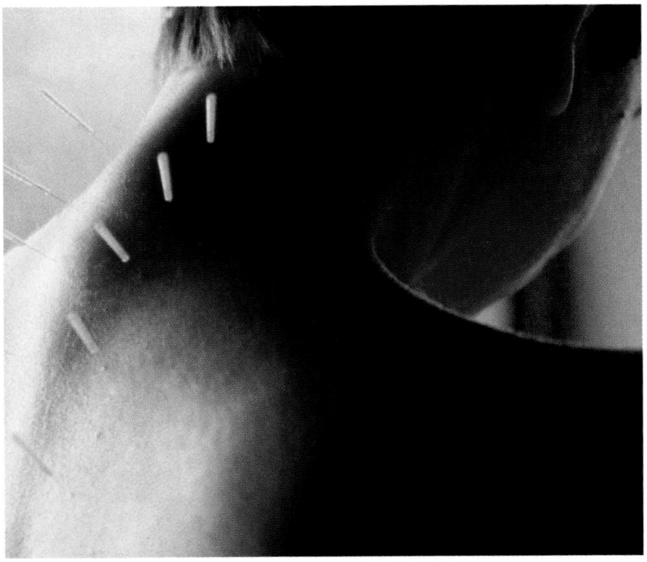

© Jon Feingersh/CORBIS

The ancient Chinese practice of acupuncture produces healing through the insertion and manipulation of needles at specific points throughout the body.

Considered alternative in this country, **Ayurveda** is a traditional form of medical treatment in India, where it has evolved over thousands of years. Its basic premise is that illness stems from incorrect mental attitudes, diet, and posture. Practitioners use a discipline of exercise, meditation, herbal medication, and proper nutrition to cope with such stress-induced conditions as hypertension, the desire to smoke, and obesity.

Homeopathy is based on three fundamental principles: like cures like; treatment must always be indi-

holistic An approach to medicine that takes into account body, mind, emotions, and spirit.

integrative medicine An approach that combines traditional medicine with alternative/complementary therapies.

acupuncture A Chinese medical practice of puncturing the body with needles inserted at specific points to relieve pain or cure disease.

Ayurveda A traditional Indian medical treatment involving meditation, exercise, herbal medications, and nutrition.

homeopathy A system of medical practice that treats a disease by administering dosages of substances that would in healthy persons produce symptoms similar to those of the disease.

vidualized; and less is more—the idea that increasing dilution (and lowering the dosage) can increase efficacy. By administering doses of animal, vegetable, or mineral substances to a large number of healthy people to see if they all develop the same symptoms, homeopaths determine which substances may be given, in small quantities, to alleviate the symptoms. Some of these substances are the same as those used in conventional medicine: nitroglycerin for certain heart conditions, for example, although the dose is minuscule.

Naturopathy emphasizes natural remedies, such as sun, water, heat, and air, as the best treatments for disease. Therapies might include dietary changes (such as more vegetables and no salt or stimulants), steam baths, and exercise. Some naturopathic physicians (who are not MDs) work closely with medical doctors in helping patients.

Mind-Body Medicine

Mind-body medicine uses techniques designed to enhance the mind's capacity to affect bodily function and symptoms. Some techniques that were considered alternative in the past have become mainstream (for example, patient support groups and cognitive-behavioral therapy). Other mind-body approaches are still considered CAM, including meditation, prayer (see Chapter 2), yoga, t'ai chi, visual imagery, mental healing, and therapies that use creative outlets such as art, music, or dance. About 30 percent of Americans report using relaxation techniques and imagery, biofeedback, and hypnosis; 50 percent use prayer.

The physical and emotional risks of using mind-body interventions are minimal. Although we need much more research on how these approaches work and when to apply them most effectively, there is considerable evidence that mind-body interventions have positive effects on psychological functioning and quality of life and may be particularly helpful for patients coping with chronic illnesses.

Mind-body approaches definitely have won some acceptance in modern medical care. Techniques such as hypnosis have proved helpful in reducing discomfort and complications during and after various surgical procedures. With *biofeedback* (discussed in Chapter 2), people can learn to control usually involuntary functions, such as circulation to the hands and feet, tension in the jaws, and heartbeat rates. Biofeedback has been used to treat dozens of ailments, including asthma, epilepsy, pain, and Reynaud's disease (a condition in which the fingers become painful and white when exposed to cold). Many health insurers now cover biofeedback treatments.

Creative *visualization,* (also discussed in Chapter 2) helps patients heal, including some diagnosed as terminally ill with cancer. Other patients use visualization to create a clear idea of what they want to achieve, whether the goal is weight loss or relaxation.

Biologically Based Therapies

Biologically based CAM therapies use substances such as herbs, foods, and vitamins. They include botanical medicine or phytotherapy, the use of individual herbs or combinations; special diet therapies, such as macrobiotics, Ornish, McDougall, and high fiber; Mediterranean orthomolecular medicine (use of nutritional and food supplements for preventive or therapeutic purposes); and use of other products (such as shark cartilage) and procedures applied in an unconventional manner.

Herbal medicine has become an estimated $4 billion-a-year industry, yet questions about the safety and effectiveness of herbal supplements persist. Although more than 1,500 different preparations are on the U.S. market, just a few single-herb preparations account for about half the sales in the United States: echinacea, garlic, ginkgo biloba, ginseng, kava, St. John's wort, and valerian. Unlike medications, herbal products are exempt from the FDA's regulatory scrutiny. The ingredients and the potency of active ingredients can vary from batch to batch.

Rigorous research studies are producing the first scientific evidence on the safety and efficacy of herbal supplements. Their benefits, if any, have proved modest (Table 13-4). Ginkgo biloba, for instance, temporarily boosts memory, but no more so than eating a candy bar. Other agents, such as saw palmetto or garlic, produce slight benefits but far less than available medications.

Most of the herbs tested have proved generally safe, although side effects such as headache and nausea can occur. However, some herbs can cause serious, even fatal dangers. Echinacea, widely used as a cold remedy, may cause liver damage if taken in combination with anabolic steroids. Several widely used herbs, including ginger, garlic, and ginkgo biloba, are dangerous if taken prior to surgery.

The FDA has prohibited the sale of dietary supplements containing ephedra, which was linked with dozens of deaths and more than 1,000 adverse reactions. It has issued warnings on other potentially dangerous herbs, including chaparral, comfrey, yohimbe, lobelia, germander, willow bark, jin bu huan, and products containing magnolia or stephania.

Manipulative and Body-Based Methods

CAM therapies based on manipulation and/or movement of the body are divided into three subcategories:

TABLE 13-4 Evidence-Based Evaluations of Herbal Supplements

Herb	Evidence
Saw Palmetto	Reduces an enlarged prostate, but the effect is small compared with prescription medication
Ginseng	No demonstrated benefits or proven effect on energy
Echinacea	No proven benefits as a cold remedy; can trigger an allergic reaction
Kava	May reduce anxiety, but can cause liver damage
Gingko biloba	No improvement in memory or thinking in the healthy elderly, but a small benefit for patients with dementia
Garlic	Lowers cholesterol when taken in higher doses than you would get with food; much less effective than cholesterol-lowering medications
Black Cohosh	Currently under study as a treatment for hot flashes; long-term effects unknown

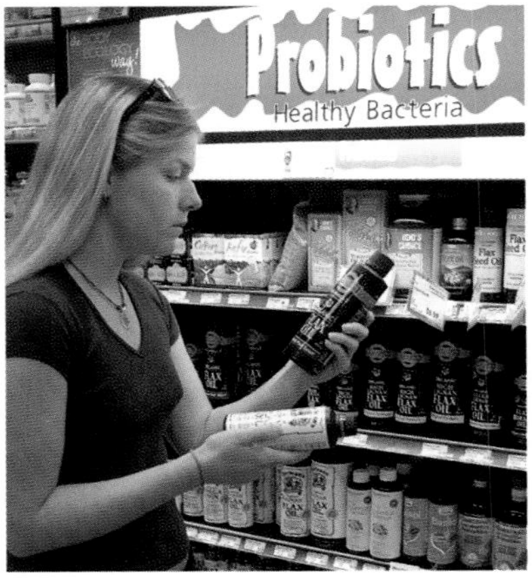

- **Chiropractic medicine.**
- **Massage therapy and body work** (including osteopathic manipulation, Swedish massage, Alexander technique, reflexology, Pilates, acupressure, and rolfing).
- **Unconventional physical therapies** (including colonics, hydrotherapy, and light and color therapies).

Chiropractic is a treatment method based on the theory that many human diseases are caused by misalignment of the bones (subluxation). Chiropractors are licensed in all 50 states, but chiropractic is considered a mainstream therapy by some and a form of CAM by others. Significant research in the last ten years has demonstrated its efficacy for acute lower-back pain. NIH is funding research on other potential benefits, including headaches, asthma, middle ear inflammation, menstrual cramps, and arthritis.

Chiropractors, who emphasize wellness and healing without drugs or surgery, may use X rays and magnetic resonance imaging (MRI) as well as orthopedic, neurological, and manual examinations in making diagnoses. However, chiropractic treatment consists solely of the manipulation of misaligned bones that may be putting pressure on nerve tissue and affecting other parts of the body. Many HMOs offer chiropractic services, which are the most widely used alternative treatment among managed care patients.

Energy Therapies

Various approaches focus on energy fields believed to exist in and around the body. Some use external energy sources, such as electromagnetic fields. Magnets are marketed to relieve pain but there is little scientific evidence of their efficacy. Others, such as therapeutic touch, use a therapist's healing energy to repair imbalances in an individual's biofield.

Becoming a Savvy Health-Care Consumer

By learning about your medical rights, the health-care system, and paying for health care, you can make better, more informed choices.

Your Medical Rights

As a consumer, you have basic rights that help ensure that you know about any potential dangers, receive competent diagnosis and treatment, and retain control and dignity in your interactions with health-care professionals. Many hospitals publish a patient's bill of rights, including your rights to know whether a procedure is experimental; to refuse to undergo a specific treatment; to designate someone else to make decisions about your care if and when you cannot; and to leave the hospital, even against your physician's advice.

You have the right to be treated with respect and dignity, including being called "Mr." or "Ms." or whatever you wish, rather than by your first name. Make clear your preferences. If you feel that health-care pro-

naturopathy An alternative system of treatment of disease that emphasizes the use of natural remedies such as sun, water, heat, and air. Therapies may include dietary changes, steam baths, and exercise.

herbal medicine An ancient form of medical treatment using substances derived from trees, flowers, ferns, seaweeds, and lichens to treat disease.

chiropractic A method of treating disease, primarily through manipulating the bones and joints to restore normal nerve function.

fessionals are being condescending or inconsiderate, say so—in the same tone and manner that you would like others to use with you. If you're hospitalized, find out if there's a patient advocate or representative at your hospital. These individuals can help you communicate with physicians, make any special arrangements, and get answers to questions or complaints.

Your Right to Information

By law, a patient must give consent for hospitalization, surgery, and other major treatments. **Informed consent** is a right, not a privilege. Use this right to its fullest. Ask questions. Seek other opinions. Make sure that your expectations are realistic and that you understand the potential risks, as well as the possible benefits, of a prospective treatment.

Your Right to Privacy and Access to Medical Records

Your medical records are your property. You have the right to see them whenever you choose and to limit who else can see them. Federal standards protecting the privacy of patients' medical information guarantee patients access to their medical records, give them more control over how personal health information is disclosed, and limit the ways that health plans, pharmacies, and hospitals can use personal medical information.

Key provisions include:

- **Access to medical records.** As a patient, you should be able to see and obtain copies of your medical records and request corrections if there are errors. Health-care providers must provide these within 30 days; they may charge for the cost of copying and mailing records.
- **Notice of privacy practices.** Your providers must inform you of how they use personal medical information. Doctors, nurses, and other providers may not disclose information for purposes not related to your health care.
- **Prohibition on marketing.** Pharmacies, health plans, and others must obtain specific authorization before disclosing patient information for marketing.
- **Confidentiality.** Patients can request that doctors take reasonable steps to ensure confidential communications, such as calling a cell phone rather than home or office.

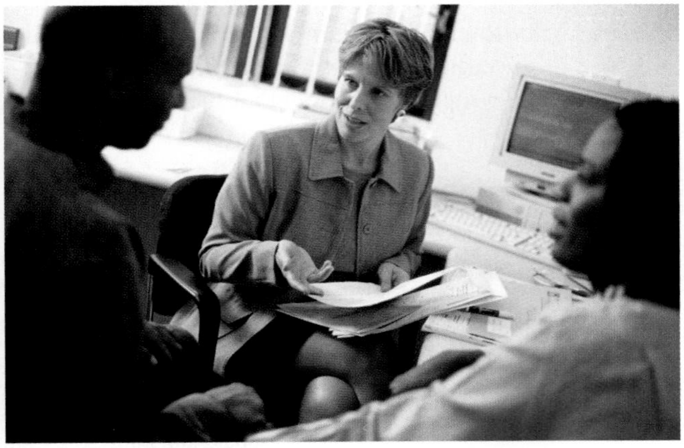

© Mark Thornton/Brand X Pictures/Getty Images

In the hospital, you can discuss the patient's rights and other individual concerns with a patient advocate.

Your Right to Good, Safe Care

According to recent court rulings, patients have the right to sue health insurers that refuse to authorize medically necessary treatment. This enables patients to hold health plans accountable for their role in medical decision making.

Preventing Medical Errors Medical errors, which can occur whenever something goes wrong with a test or treatment, are a leading cause of injury and death. An average of 195,000 people in the United States die due to potentially preventable, hospital medical errors each year, according to a recent study of 37 million patient records.

The risks associated with hospitalization include what health workers call the "terrible I's": infection; inactivity; incorrect actions; and the inherent risks of drugs, X rays, and false lab tests. The simplest method for preventing hospital-acquired infection—handwashing—is often ignored by health-care providers.

Errors, which may involve diagnosis, equipment, lab reports, medications, or surgery, are more likely to occur when doctors and their patients have problems communicating. The single most important thing you can do to prevent errors is take part in every decision about your health care. Make sure you understand what may be wrong with you, as well as which medications you are taking and why:

- **When your doctor writes you a prescription** make sure you can read it and know why and how you are to take the medication.
- **Ask for information about your medicines** in terms you can understand, including explanations of possible interactions with other drugs or dietary supplements and potential side effects.
- **If you must undergo surgery** and you can choose a hospital, select one at which many patients have had the procedure or surgery you need.
- **Consider asking all health-care workers** in direct contact with you whether they have washed their hands. This simple step prevents the spread of infections.

Strategies for Prevention — Protecting Yourself Against Quackery

- Arm yourself with up-to-date information about your condition or disease from appropriate organizations, such as the American Cancer Society or the Arthritis Foundation, which keep track of unproven and ineffective methods of treatment.
- Ask for a written explanation of what a treatment does and why it works, evidence supporting all claims (not just testimonials), and published reports of the studies, including specifics on numbers treated, doses, and side effects. Be skeptical of self-styled "holistic practitioners," treatments supported by crusading groups, and endorsements from self-proclaimed experts or authorities.
- Don't part with your money quickly. Be especially careful because insurance companies won't reimburse for unproven therapies.
- Don't discontinue your current treatment without your physician's approval. Many physicians encourage supportive therapies—such as relaxation exercises, meditation, or visualization—as a supplement to standard treatments.
- To get information on health scams and consumer topics, go to the Federal Trade Commission (FTC) website: www.ftc.gov/bcp/menu-health.htm.

- **Speak up if you have questions or concerns.** Ask a family member or friend to be your advocate and speak up for you if you can't.

Malpractice The essence of a *malpractice* suit is the claim that the physician failed to meet the standard of care required of a reasonably skilled and careful medical doctor. Although physicians don't have to guarantee good results to their patients and aren't held liable for unavoidable errors, they are required to use the same care and judgment in treatment that other physicians in the same specialty would use under similar circumstances. To protect themselves financially, physicians, particularly those in surgical specialties who are most likely to be sued, pay tens of thousands of dollars a year in malpractice insurance premiums. Some of this cost is passed on to patients.

Most lawsuits are based on negligence and assert that a physician failed to render diagnosis and treatment with appropriate professional knowledge and skill. Other cases are brought for failure to provide information, obtain consent, or respect a patient's confidentiality. However, analysis of malpractice cases has shown that, in 70 to 80 percent, a doctor's attitude and inability to communicate effectively—by devaluing patients' views, delivering information poorly, failing to understand patients' perspectives, or displaying an air of superiority—also played a role.

Quackery Every year millions of Americans go searching for medical miracles that never happen. In all, they spend more than $10 billion on medical **quackery,** unproven health products and services. Those who lose only money are the lucky ones. Many also waste precious time, during which their conditions worsen. Some suffer needless pain, along with crushed expectations. Far too many risk their lives on a false hope—and lose.

The Health-Care System

As a college student, you can turn to the student health service if you get sick. There, a nurse, nurse practitioner, physician's assistant, or medical doctor may evaluate your symptoms and provide basic care. However, you may rely on a primary care physician in your hometown to perform regular checkups or manage a chronic condition like asthma. If you're injured in an accident, you probably will be treated at the nearest emergency room. If you become seriously ill and require highly specialized care, you may have to go to a university-affiliated medical center to receive state-of-the-art treatment.

Students can often continue their health-care coverage under their parents' policy until the age of 23. However, if a parent belongs to an HMO with a local network of providers, the student may not be covered for anything outside the plan's service area except emergency care. A more open plan, like a preferred provider organization, may allow students to see doctors near school, but the costs may be high.

Most colleges offer some type of health insurance plan, with the student health center acting as the primary care provider. Many schools require enrollment if the student is not covered under any other plan. Check the plan

informed consent Permission (to undergo or receive a medical procedure or treatment) given voluntarily, with full knowledge and understanding of the procedure or treatment and its possible consequences.

quackery Medical fakery; unproven practices claiming to cure diseases or solve health problems.

carefully. Physicals, gynecological visits, and other preventive care may not be covered. College plans also may not cover preexisting conditions, such as asthma.

Paying for Health Care

In the 1990s, as medical costs spiraled upward, the concept of **managed care,** emerged. Managed-care organizations provide health care or health-care insurance at lower costs to employers. The trade-off for such savings is that a third party makes the final decision on when or if a medical visit or treatment is necessary. This differs from traditional *fee-for-service* medicine, in which patients decide when to seek care and choose which physician to see.

Both fee-for-service and managed-care systems have drawbacks. Fee-for-service medicine errs on the side of doing too much and providing unneeded tests and therapies. Managed-care organizations are more likely to do too little so they can keep costs low.

Managed Care

Managed care has become the predominant form of health care in the United States. Managed-care organizations, which take various forms, deliver care through a network of physicians, hospitals, and other health-care professionals who agree to provide their services at fixed or discounted rates. Nine in ten physicians in the United States have contracted with managed care companies.

Consumers in a managed-care group must follow certain procedures in advance of seeking care (for example, getting prior approval for a test or treatment) and must abide by a limit on reimbursement for certain services. Some procedures may be deemed unnecessary and not be covered at all. Patients who choose to see a physician who is not a participating member of the medical-insurance coverage group may have to pay the entire fee themselves.

Managed-care plans have been criticized for pressuring providers to "undertreat" patients—for example, sending them home from the hospital too soon or denying them costly tests or treatments. Members have complained of long waits, the need to switch primary physicians if their doctor leaves the plan, difficulty getting approval for needed services, and a sense that providers pay more attention to the bottom line than to the health needs of their patients.

As dissatisfaction with managed care has grown, consumers have demanded more choice of physicians, direct access to specialists, and the ability to go "out of network." In response to patients' complaints, many states have approved "patient protection acts" or "comprehensive consumer bills of rights."

According to the National Committee for Quality Assurance, managed-care plans have shown improvement in the delivery of care, but health-care costs continue to rise. As a result, employers are cutting back coverage and asking employees to shoulder more of the burden of their health care in the belief that consumers will seek more efficient care when they are required to pay more out of pocket.

Health Maintenance Organizations (HMOs)

Health maintenance organizations, or **HMOs,** are managed-care plans that emphasize routine care and prevention by providing complete medical services in exchange for a predetermined monthly payment. In a *group-model* HMO, physicians provide care in offices at a clinic run by the HMO. In an *individual practice association (IPA),* or network HMO, independent physicians provide services in their own offices. HMOs generally pay a fixed amount per patient to a physician or hospital, regardless of the type and number of services actually provided. This is called *capitation.*

Members of HMOs pay a regular, preset fee that usually includes diagnostic tests, routine physical exams, and vaccinations as well as treatment of illnesses. HMOs usually do not require a deductible, and copayments for medications or services are small. The primary drawback of standard HMOs is that the consumer is limited to a particular health-care facility and staff.

Preferred Provider Organizations (PPOs)

In a **preferred provider organization (PPO),** a third party—a union, an insurance company, or a self-insured business—contracts with a group of physicians and hospitals to treat members at a discount. PPO members may choose any physician within the network, and usually pay a 10 percent copayment for care within the system and a higher percentage (20 to 30 percent) for care elsewhere. PPOs generally require prior approval for expensive tests or major procedures.

A *point-of-service (POS)* plan is a PPO that permits patients to use physicians outside the network. Consumers pay the difference between the preferred provider's discounted fee and the outside physician's fee. A *gatekeeper* plan requires members to choose a primary physician, as in an HMO, who must approve all referrals to specialists.

Government-Financed Insurance Plans

The government, through programs like Medicare and Medicaid, funds 45 percent of total U.S. health spending. Under Medicare, the federal government pays 80 percent of most medical bills, after a deductible fee, for people over age 65. Medicare also offers options for coverage of prescription medications.

Medicaid, a federal and state insurance plan that protects people with very low or no incomes, is the chief source of coverage for the unemployed. However, many unemployed Americans don't qualify because their family incomes are above the poverty line. Publicly insured patients are more likely than those with private insurance to receive inadequate care and to experience adverse health outcomes.

The Uninsured

The United States is the only industrialized nation that does not have national health insurance. More Americans lack health insurance coverage than a decade ago—a total of more than 43 million. Many more experience temporary lapses in coverage or are underinsured, meaning that they don't have adequate coverage and are less likely to receive preventive care or routine checkups.

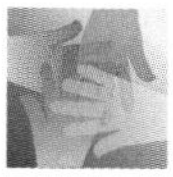

Racial and ethnic minorities are much more likely to be uninsured than white Americans. More than a third of the Hispanic population and over a quarter of Native Americans are uninsured, compared to 12 percent of whites. The uninsured rates among African Americans and Asian Americans are also much higher than among whites. Nearly one-third of the uninsured are Latino, despite the fact that Latinos make up just 13 percent of the population. This disparity results from several factors, including citizenship issues and language barriers.

Young adults, 18 to 24 years of age, are more likely than any other age group to be uninsured. Of Americans between the ages of 18 and 24 years, almost a third are without medical insurance.

A committee of the Institute of Medicine (IOM), after years of exhaustive study, has urged federal leaders to provide health insurance for everyone living in the United States. The consequences of being uninsured, the IOM concluded, include "worse health and earlier death," including 18,000 deaths every year. It proposed that coverage be universal (for all residents, not just citizens), continuous, affordable, sustainable, and provided in such a way as to promote access to high-quality care.

LEARN IT / LIVE IT

Taking Charge of Your Health

You can do more to safeguard and enhance your well-being than any health-care provider. Here are some recommendations to keep in mind:

- **Trust your instincts.** You know your body better than anyone else. If something is bothering you, it deserves medical attention. Don't let your health-care provider—or your health plan administrator—dismiss it without a thorough evaluation.
- **Do your homework.** Go to the library or online and find authoritative articles that describe what you're experiencing. The more you know about possible causes of your symptoms, the more likely you are to be taken seriously.
- **Find a good primary care physician who listens carefully and responds to your concerns.** Look for a family doctor or general internist who takes a careful history, performs a thorough exam, and listens and responds to your concerns.
- **See your doctor regularly.** If you're in your twenties or thirties, you may not need an annual exam, but it's important to get checkups at least every two or three years so you and your doctor can get to know each other and develop a trusting, mutually respectful relationship.
- **Get a second opinion.** If you are uncertain of whether to undergo treatment or which therapy is best, see another physician and listen carefully for any doubts or hesitation about what you're considering.
- **Seek support.** Patient support and advocacy groups can offer emotional support, information on many common problems, and referral to knowledgeable physicians.
- **If your doctor cannot or will not respond to your concerns, get another one.** Regardless of your health coverage, you have the right to replace a physician who is not meeting your health-care needs.
- **Speak up.** If you don't understand, ask. If you feel that you're not being taken seriously or being treated with respect, say so. Sometimes the only difference between being a patient or becoming a victim is making sure your needs and rights are not forgotten or overlooked.
- **Bring your own advocate.** If you become intimidated or anxious talking to physicians, ask a friend to accompany you, to ask questions on your behalf and to take notes.

managed care Health-care services and reimbursement predetermined by third-party insurers.

health maintenance organization (HMO) An organization that provides health services on a fixed-contract basis.

preferred provider organization (PPO) A group of physicians contracted to provide health care to members at a discounted price.

13 Making This Chapter Work for You

Review Questions

1. Safe-driving tips include all of the following *except*:
   a. Avoid driving at night for the first year after getting a license.
   b. Make sure your car has snow tires or chains before driving in hazardous snowy conditions.
   c. If riding with an intoxicated driver, keep talking to him so that he doesn't fall asleep at the wheel.
   d. Don't let packages or people obstruct the rear or side windows.
2. Which statement about violence on college campuses is *false?*
   a. Campus hazing often involves activities that would be called torture if perpetrated elsewhere.
   b. Most crimes against students occur on campus.
   c. Many campuses have codes of conduct on alcohol, drugs, and fighting.
   d. Crime statistics for colleges and universities are posted on the Internet.
3. Sexual victimization
   a. includes sexual harassment, sexual coercion, and rape.
   b. is gender-specific, affecting women who are violated emotionally or physically by men.
   c. is rare in academic environments such as college campuses.
   d. most commonly takes the form of physical assault and stalking.
4. Which of the following statements about rape is true?
   a. When a person is sexually attacked by a stranger, it is referred to as *rape*. When a person is sexually attacked by an acquaintance, it is referred to as *sexual coercion*.
   b. Statutory rape is defined as sexual intercourse initiated by a woman under the age of consent.
   c. Men who rape other men usually consider themselves heterosexuals.
   d. Women who flirt and dress provocatively are typically more willing to participate in aggressive sex than women who dress conservatively and do not flirt.
5. Ways to protect or prevent rape include:
   a. Use alcohol and drugs only in familiar surroundings.
   b. Take a self-defense class.
   c. To avoid angering a sexually aggressive person, become passive and quiet.
   d. Do not discuss your sexual limits on a first or second date, because just talking about sex will encourage your date to think you are interested in a sexual relationship.
6. Which of the following statements about health information is true?
   a. Chat rooms are the most reliable source of accurate medical information.
   b. Physicians who have websites must adhere to a strict set of standards set by the American Medical Association.
   c. Government-sponsored websites such as that of the Centers for Disease Control and Prevention are excellent sources of accurate health-care information.
   d. Testimonials from satisfied users of a health product prove the product's effectiveness.
7. Informed consent means that
   a. the patient has informed the doctor of his or her symptoms and has consented to treatment.
   b. the physician has informed the patient about the treatment to be given and has consented to administer the treatment.
   c. the patient has informed the doctor of his or her symptoms, and the doctor has consented to administer treatment.
   d. the physician has informed the patient about the treatment to be given, and the patient has consented to the treatment.
8. Patients have all the rights below *except* which of the following?
   a. access to their medical records
   b. medical care that meets accepted standards of quality
   c. to donate a body part for compensation
   d. to leave the hospital against their physician's advice
9. Which statement is *false*?
   a. Acupuncture has been shown to control nausea in patients after surgery.
   b. Reflexologists massage points on the foot or hand to relieve stress or pain in corresponding parts of the body.
   c. People can learn to control involuntary functions through biofeedback.
   d. Naturopathy is based on the premise that like cures like.
10. Managed care features all of the following *except*
    a. health maintenance organizations.
    b. a fee-for-service system of insurance.
    c. preferred provider organizations.
    d. limitations on reimbursement for certain health services.

Answers to these questions can be found on page 422.

Critical Thinking

1. A friend of yours, Eric, frequently makes crude or derogatory comments about women. When you finally call him on this, his response is, "I didn't say anything wrong. I like women." What might you say to him?
2. At one college, women raped by acquaintances on dates scrawled the names of their assailants on the walls of women's restrooms on campus. Several young men

LACC Extra Credit Assignment

13. You live alone. What precautionary measures should you consider? List at least 10 and discuss.

whose names appeared on the list objected, protesting that they were innocent and were being unfairly accused. How do you feel about this method of fighting back against date rape? Do you think it violates the rights of men? How do you feel about naming women who've been raped in news reports? Are there circumstances in which a woman's identity should be revealed? Would fewer women report a rape if not assured of privacy?

3. Have you used any complementary or alternative approaches to health care? If so, were you satisfied with the results? How did your experience with the CAM therapist compare with your most recent experience with a traditional medical practitioner? Do you feel confident that you know the difference between alternative care and quackery?
4. If you're young and healthy, you'll have little problem getting health insurance. However, if you develop a chronic illness, sustain serious injuries in an accident, or simply get older, you may find insurance harder to get and more expensive to keep. What is your insurance coverage? Do you believe insurance companies have the right to turn down applicants with preexisting conditions, such as high blood pressure? Do they have the right to require screening for potentially serious health problems, such as HIV infection, or to cancel the policies of individuals who have run up high medical bills in the past?

Media Menu

ThomsonNOW™ Go to the ThomsonNOW website at **http://www.thomsonedu.com** that will:

- Help you evaluate your knowledge of the material.
- Allow you to take an exam-prep quiz.
- Provide a Personalized Learning Plan targeting resources that address areas you should study.
- Coach you through identifying target goals for behavioral change and creating and monitoring your personal change plan throughout the semester.

INTERNET CONNECTIONS

National Safety Council (NSC)

www.nsc.org

The mission of the NSC is to educate and influence society to adopt safety, health, and environmental policies, practices, and procedures that prevent human suffering and economic losses arising from preventable causes.

RAINN-Rape Assault Incest National Network

www.rainn.org

This site provides great information from an organization fighting against rape, assault, and incest.

National Center for Complementary and Alternative Medicine

http://nccam.nih.gov

This National Institutes of Health site features a variety of fact sheets on alternative therapies and dietary supplements, research, current news, and databases for the public as well as for practitioners.

MedicineNet

www.medicinenet.com

This comprehensive site is written for the consumer by board-certified physicians and contains medical news, a directory of procedures, a medical dictionary, a pharmacy, and first aid information. You can use the information at medicinenet.com to prepare for a doctor visit, learn about a diagnosis, or understand a prescribed treatment or procedure.

InfoTrac College Edition Activities Log on, insert **seat belts** or **complementary alternative medicine** into the Keyword search box, and limit your search to the past year. When you get the results, Mark articles to review, then Select one to read. Summarize three or four key points from the article.

You can find additional readings related to personal health with InfoTrac College Edition, an online library of more than 900 journals and publications. Follow the instructions for accessing InfoTrac College Edition that were packaged with your textbook; then search for articles using a keyword search.

For additional links, resources, and suggested readings on the InfoTrac College Edition, visit our Health and Wellness Resource Center at **http://health.wadsworth.com.**

Key Terms

The terms listed are on the page indicated. Definitions of the terms are in the Glossary at the end of this book.

acupuncture 378
Ayurveda 379
chiropractic 381
complementary and alternative medicine (CAM) 377
health maintenance organizations (HMO) 384
herbal medicine 380
holistic 378
homeopathy 379
informed consent 382
integrative medicine 378
managed care 384
naturopathy 380
nonvolitional sex 370
preferred provider organization (ppo) 384
quackery 383
rape 370
sexual coercion 370
sexual harassment 369
vital signs 375

14 *Working Toward a Healthy Environment*

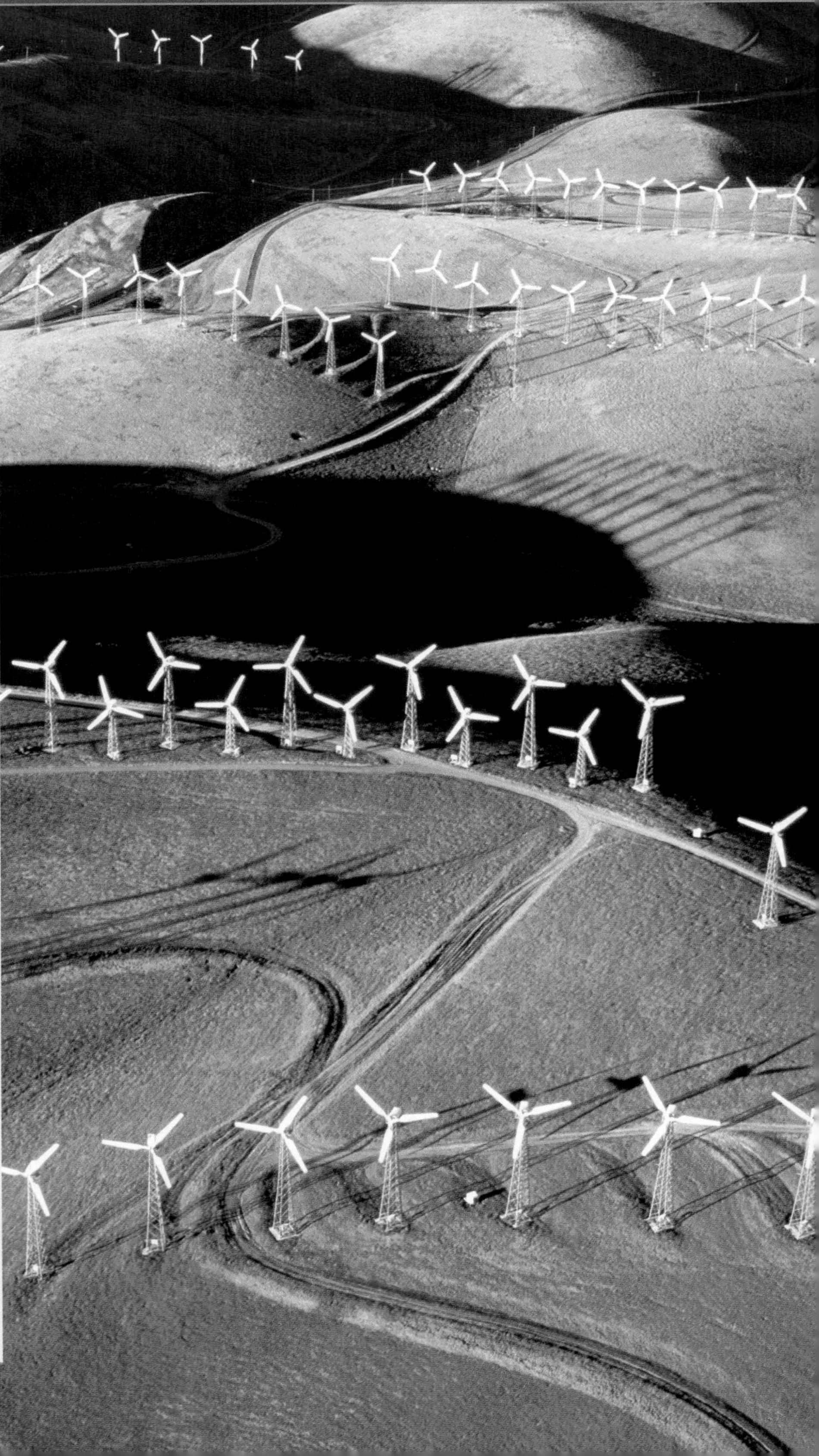

REAL HEALTH

Jeremy never thought twice about the setting of the thermostat or whether he left the lights on at home. But when his university announced the opening of a new "green" dorm, he was intrigued. In engineering and ecology courses, he studied "sustainability" and liked the idea of taking as little as possible from resources that cannot be renewed.

Jeremy's dorm used highly energy-efficient heating, water, and air circulation systems. The architectural design let in so much natural light that artificial illumination was unnecessary during the day.

Jeremy couldn't explain exactly why, but his new residence hall "felt" different. The air was cleaner. The rooms were brighter. At times the water pressure fell while he was showering, but he learned to accept it as a minor irritant. A kiosk in the lobby recorded the daily energy use of the building and its residents and compared it with previous days. Jeremy took pride in seeing how low his dormmates could go.

In his classes Jeremy became involved in sustainability projects, such as designing rooftops of plants, grass, and gravel. Before college he had thought that being green meant recycling and lead-free gasoline. Now Jeremy sees it as a way of life—and as the career he hopes to pursue.

© Owaki-Kulla/CORBIS

Ours is a planet in peril. Sea levels are rising. Forests are being destroyed. Droughts in Asia and Africa have become more frequent and more intense. Heat waves have killed tens of thousands. Hurricanes and floods have ravaged cities. Millions of people have died from the effects of air pollution and contaminated water.

No one has more stake in the future of the planet than the young. Environmental concerns may seem so enormous that nothing any individual can do will have an effect. This is not the case. All of us, as citizens of the world, can help find solutions to the challenges confronting our planet. The first step is realizing that you have a personal responsibility for safeguarding the health of your environment and, thereby, your own well-being.

This chapter explores the complex interrelationships between your world and your well-being. It discusses major threats to the environment—including atmospheric changes; air, water, and noise pollution; chemical risks; and radiation—and provides specific guidance on what you can do about them.

? FAQ Frequently Asked Questions

- What is global warming? *p. 391*
- Is mold dangerous? *p. 394*
- Is listening to music through earbuds hazardous to my hearing? *p. 396*
- Is bottled water better? *p. 396*
- What health risks are caused by pesticides? *p. 397*

After studying the material in this chapter, you should be able to:

- **Discuss** the health effects of depletion of the ozone layer and of global warming.
- **List** the health effects of air pollution.
- **Describe** actions that individuals can take to protect the environment.
- Name ways to protect your ears from noise-induced hearing loss.
- **List** the key sources and health risks of electromagnetic fields.

ThomsonNOW™ Log on to ThomsonNOW at **www.thomsonedu.com/thomsonnow** to find your Behavior Change Planner and to explore self-assessments, interactive tutorials, and practice quizzes.

The Environment and Your Health

The planet Earth—once taken for granted as a ball of rock and water that existed for our use for all time—now is seen as a single, fragile **ecosystem** (a community of organisms that share a physical and chemical environment). Our environment is a closed ecosystem, powered by the sun. The materials needed for the survival of this planet must be recycled over and over again. Increasingly, we're realizing just how important the health of this ecosystem is to our own well-being and survival.

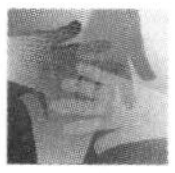

As shown in Student Snapshot: "Do Students Care About the Environment?" the majority of undergraduates do not share this concern, but higher numbers of students express concern than in the past. Students at all-black colleges are much more likely to express environmental concerns.[1]

Our environment affects our well-being both directly and indirectly. Changes in temperature and rainfall patterns disturb ecological processes in ways that can be hazardous to health. The environment may account for 25 to 40 percent of diseases worldwide. Children are the most vulnerable because of their greater sensitivity to toxic threats. In response to this trend, Congress has approved funding to create a nationwide system to track environmental links to chronic diseases.

No individual is immune to environmental health threats. Depletion of the ozone layer has already been implicated in the increase in skin cancers and cataracts. Global warming, according to some theorists, might lead to changes in one-third to one-half of the world's vegetation types and to the extinction of many plant and animal species. A warmer world is expected to produce more severe flooding in some places and more severe droughts in others, jeopardizing natural resources and the safety of our water supply. Warmer weather—a consequence of changes in atmospheric gases and climate—worsens urban-industrial air pollution and, if the air also is moist, increases concentrations of allergenic pollens and fungal spores. These are truly problems without borders.

For good or for ill, we cannot separate our individual health from that of the environment in which we live. The air we breathe, the water we drink, the chemicals we use all have an impact on the quality of our lives. At the same time, the lifestyle choices we make, the products we use, the efforts we undertake to clean up a beach or save wetlands affect the quality of our environment.

Student Snapshot

Do Students Care About the Environment?

Freshmen who say that "becoming involved in programs to clean up the environment" is essential or very important

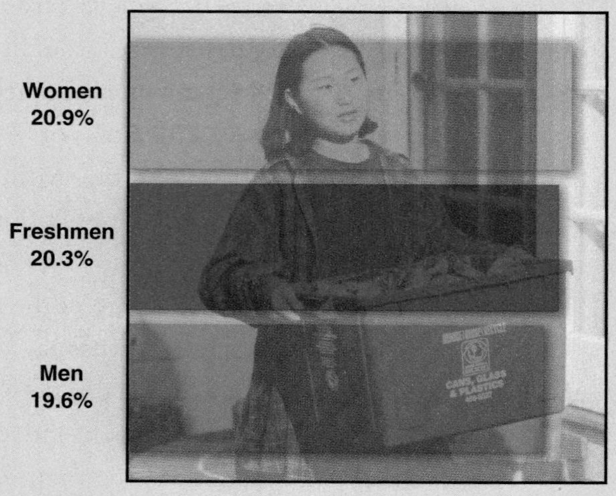

David Young-Wolff/Getty Images

Source: The American Freshman: National Norms for Fall 2005. Los Angeles, CA: Higher Education Research Institute, UCLA, 2005

The Impact of Pollution

Any change in the air, water, or soil that could reduce its ability to support life is a form of *pollution.* Natural events, such as smoke from fires triggered by lightning, can cause pollution. The effects of pollution depend on the concentration (amount per unit of air, water, or soil) of the **pollutant,** how long it remains in the environment, and its chemical nature. An *acute effect* is a severe, immediate reaction, usually after a single, large exposure. For example, pesticide poisoning can cause nausea and dizziness, even death. A *chronic effect* may take years to develop or may be a recurrent or continuous reaction, usually after repeated exposure. The development of cancer after repeated exposure to a pollutant such as asbestos is an example of a chronic effect.

Environmental agents that trigger changes, or *mutations,* in the genetic material (the DNA) of living cells are called **mutagens.** The changes that result can lead to the development of cancer. A substance or agent that causes cancer is a *carcinogen:* All carcinogens are mutagens; most mutagens are carcinogens. Furthermore, when a mutagen affects an egg or a sperm cell, its effects can be passed on to future generations. Mutagens that can cross the placenta of a pregnant woman and cause a spontaneous abortion or birth defects in the fetus are called **teratogens.**

Pollution is a hazard to all who breathe. Deaths caused by air pollution exceed those from motor vehicle injuries. Those with respiratory illnesses are at greatest risk during days when smog or allergen counts are high. However, even healthy joggers are affected; carbon monoxide has been shown to impair their exercise performance. The effects of carbon monoxide are much worse in smokers, who already have higher levels of the gas in their blood.

Toxic substances in polluted air can enter the human body in three ways: through the skin, through the digestive system, and through the lungs. The combined interaction of two or more hazards can produce an effect greater than that of either one alone. Pollutants can affect an organ or organ system directly or indirectly.

Among the health problems that have been linked with pollution are the following:

- Headaches and dizziness.
- Eye irritation and impaired vision.
- Nasal discharge.
- Cough, shortness of breath, and sore throat.
- Constricted airways.
- Constriction of blood vessels and increased risk of heart disease.
- Chest pains and aggravation of the symptoms of colds, pneumonia, bronchial asthma, emphysema, chronic bronchitis, lung cancer, and other respiratory problems.
- Birth defects and reproductive problems.
- Nausea, vomiting, and stomach cancer.
- Allergy and asthma from diesel fumes in polluted air.

? FAQ What Is Global Warming?

The Earth's average temperature increased about 1 degree in the twentieth century to approximately 59 degrees, but the rate of warming in the last three decades has been three times the average rate since 1900. Seas have risen about six to eight feet globally over the last century and are rising at a higher rate. By 2010, sea levels could be several feet higher than they are now.[2]

Why is our planet getting warmer? Figure 14-1 shows the normal greenhouse effect: Certain gases in Earth's atmosphere trap energy from the sun and retain heat somewhat like the glass panels of a greenhouse. These "greenhouse" gases include carbon dioxide, methane, and nitrous oxide. Human activities have increased the greenhouse gases in our atmosphere. We burn fossil fuels (oil, natural gas, coal) and wood products, which release carbon dioxide into the atmosphere. We produce coal, natural gas, and oil, which emit methane. Livestock and the decomposition of organic wastes also produce methane. Agricultural and industrial processes emit nitrous oxide. These emissions enhance the normal greenhouse effect, trapping more heat and raising the temperature of the atmosphere and

ecosystem A community of organisms sharing a physical and chemical environment and interacting with each other.

pollutant A substance or agent in the environment, usually the by-product of human industry or activity, that is injurious to human, animal, or plant life.

mutagen An agent that causes alterations in the genetic material of living cells.

teratogen Any agent that causes spontaneous abortion, defects, or malformations in a fetus.

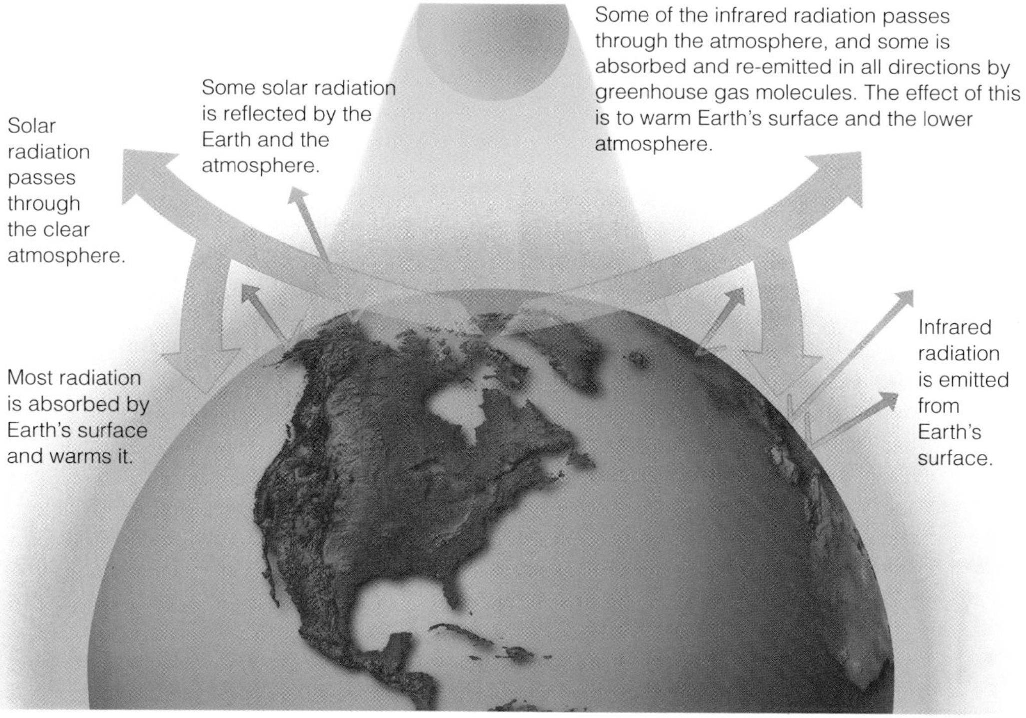

Some of the infrared radiation passes through the atmosphere, and some is absorbed and re-emitted in all directions by greenhouse gas molecules. The effect of this is to warm Earth's surface and the lower atmosphere.
Some solar radiation is reflected by the Earth and the atmosphere.
Solar radiation passes through the clear atmosphere.
Most radiation is absorbed by Earth's surface and warms it.
Infrared radiation is emitted from Earth's surface.

FIGURE 14-1 The Greenhouse Effect
The normal greenhouse effect warms the Earth to a hospitable temperature. An increase in greenhouse gases intensifies the greenhouse effect, trapping more heat and raising the Earth's temperature.

Earth's surface. This is **global warming.** Some 163 countries—not including the United States—have signed the first international treaty to fight global warming by implementing the rules known as the Kyoto Protocol. The treaty calls on industrialized nations to limit carbon emissions or reduce them to levels below those of 1990. The United States, which is responsible for 23 percent of greenhouse-gas emissions, rejected the accord as harmful to the U.S. economy and unfair because it excused heavily polluting nations, such as India and China, from any obligation.

YOUR LIFE COACH

Going Green

More universities are developing programs to achieve **sustainability,** the use of as little as possible of resources that cannot be renewed. Innovative programs include "green" dorms and campaigns to reduce energy waste.[3] (See "You Decide.")

By the choices you make and the actions you take, you can improve the state of the world. No one expects you to sacrifice every comfort or spend great amounts of money. However, for almost everyone, there's plenty of room for improvement. If enough people make small individual changes, they can have an enormous impact.

One basic environmental action is **precycling:** buying products packaged in recycled materials. According to Earthworks, a consumer group, packaging makes up a third of what people in the United States throw away. When you precycle, you consider how you're going to dispose of a product and the packaging materials before purchasing it. For example, you might choose eggs in recyclable cardboard packages, rather than in plastic cartons, and look for juice and milk in refillable bottles.

Recycling—collecting, reprocessing, marketing, and reusing materials once considered trash—serves several important functions, including:

- **Preserving natural resources.** Reprocessing used materials to make new products and packaging reduces the consumption of natural resources. Recycling steel saves iron ore, coal, and limestone. Recycling newsprint, office paper, and mixed paper saves trees.
- **Saving energy.** Recycling used aluminum cans, for instance, requires only about 5 percent of the energy needed to produce aluminum. Recycling just one can save enough electricity to light a 100-watt bulb for 3½ hours.
- **Reducing greenhouse gas emissions.** Recycling cuts these gases by decreasing the amount of energy used to produce and transport new products.
- **Decreasing the need for landfill storage or incineration.** Both are more costly and can contribute to air pollution.

Different communities take different approaches to recycling. Many provide regular curbside pickup of recyclables, and others have drop-off centers. Buyback centers pay for recyclables. In some places, reverse vending machines accept returned beverage containers and provide deposit refunds.

Discarded computers, other electronic devices, and printer cartridges also should be recycled, by donating them to schools or charitable organizations. "Tech trash" buried in landfills is creating a new hazard because trace amounts of potentially hazardous agents, such as lead and mercury, can leak into the ground and water.

With *composting*—which some people describe as nature's way of recycling—the benefits can be seen as close as your backyard. Organic products, such as leftover food and vegetable peels, are mixed with straw or other dry material and kept damp. Bacteria eat the organic material and turn it into a rich soil. Some people keep a compost pile (which should be stirred every few days) in their backyard; others take their organic garbage (including mowed grass and dead leaves) to community gardens or municipal composting sites.

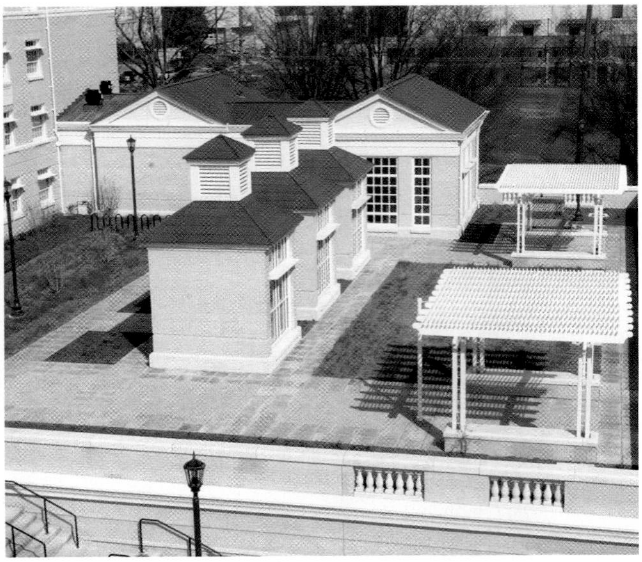

Courtesy of University of South Carolina Publications

Many colleges are conserving energy, designing environmentally friendly buildings, restricting traffic, and limiting use of hazardous materials. Does your campus have a "green" program?

A growing number of colleges and universities are designing innovative buildings and programs to increase energy efficiency and conserve natural resources. Some argue that such efforts are too little too late or that they are not part of the mission of educating young people. Should students support and participate in the search for innovative solutions to environmental problems? Or should that be a mission for scientists and national policy makers?

You Decide

Air Pollution

In most places in the United States, you can breathe easier today than you would have a quarter century ago. Smog has declined by about a third, although there are now 85 percent more vehicles being driven 105 percent more miles a year. Current model automobiles emit an average of 80 percent less pollution per mile than was emitted by new cars in 1970. However, tailpipe emissions from cars and trucks still account for almost a third of the air pollution in the United States. Even a small shift of support away from fossil fuels toward clean renewable energy could save millions of lives and help slow global warming.

According to the Harvard School of Public Health, living in a city with even moderately sooty air may shorten your lifespan by about a year. In fact, air pollution can be as harmful to breathing capacity as smoking. Residents of polluted cities are exposed to some of the same toxic gases, such as nitrogen oxide and carbon monoxide, found in cigarettes.

Air pollution of any sort can cause numerous ill effects. As pollutants destroy the hairlike cilia that remove irritants from the lungs, individuals may suffer chronic bronchitis, characterized by excessive mucus flow and continuous coughing. Emphysema may develop or worsen, as pollutants constrict the bronchial tubes and destroy the air sacs in the lungs, making breathing more difficult.

When air pollution levels are high, heart attacks, strokes, heart failure flare-ups, and lung troubles increase. Air contamination also has enduring effects on heart health and increases atherosclerosis and deaths due to heart disease. For the elderly and people with asthma or heart disease, polluted air can be life-threatening. Even healthy individuals can be affected, particularly if they exercise outdoors during high-pollution periods.

A combination of smoke and fog, **smog** is made up of chemical vapors from auto exhaust, industrial and commercial pollutants (volatile organic compounds, carbon monoxide, nitrogen oxides, sulfur oxides, particulates), and ozone. The most obvious sources of these pollutants are motor vehicles, industrial factories, electric utility plants, and wood-burning stoves.

Gray-air, or *sulfur-dioxide,* smog, often seen in Europe and much of the eastern United States, is produced by burning oil of high sulfur content. Among the cities that must deal with gray-air smog are Chicago, Baltimore, Detroit, and Philadelphia. Like cigarette smoke, gray-air smog affects the cilia in the respiratory passages; the lungs are unable to expel particulates, such as soot, ash, and dust, which remain and irritate the tissues. This condition is hazardous to people with chronic respiratory problems.

Brown-air, or *photochemical,* smog is found in large traffic centers such as Los Angeles, Salt Lake City, Denver, Mexico City, and Tokyo. This type of smog results principally from nitric oxide in car exhaust reacting with oxygen in the air, forming nitrogen dioxide, which produces a brownish haze and, when exposed to sunlight, other pollutants.

One of these, *ozone,* the most widespread pollutant, can impair the body's immune system and cause long-term lung damage. (Ozone in the upper atmosphere protects us by repelling harmful ultraviolet radiation from the sun, but ozone in the lower atmosphere is a harmful component of air pollution.) Automobiles also produce carbon monoxide, a colorless and odorless gas that diminishes the ability of red blood cells to carry oxygen. The resulting oxygen deficiency can affect breathing, hearing, and vision in humans and stunt the growth of plants and trees.

Indoor Pollutants

Because people in industrialized nations spend more than 90 percent of their time in buildings, the quality of the air they breathe inside can have an even greater impact on their well-being than outdoor pollution.

The most hazardous form of indoor air pollution is cigarette smoke. Nearly half of all nonsmoking Americans are regularly exposed to secondhand smoke, which contains more than 50 cancer-causing chemicals. According to a major 2006 scientific report from the U.S. Surgeon General, secondhand smoke exposure can cause heart disease and lung cancer in nonsmoking adults and sudden infant death syndrome (SIDS), respiratory problems, ear infections, and asthma attacks in babies and children. Even brief exposure to secondhand smoke has immediate adverse effects on the cardiovascular system and increases risk for heart disease and lung cancer.[4]

Other threats include formaldehyde, asbestos, and lead—indoor pollutants that come from the very materials the buildings are made of and from the appliances inside them. Most manufacturers have voluntarily quit

global warming Increase in Earth's surface and atmospheric temperature due to increased levels of greenhouse gases (carbon dioxide, methane, and nitrous oxide) that trap heat in the atmosphere.

sustainability A method of using a resource so that the resource is not depleted or permanently damaged.

precycling The use of products that are packaged in recycled or recyclable material.

recycling The processing or reuse of manufactured materials to reduce consumption of raw materials.

smog A grayish or brownish fog caused by the presence of smoke and/or chemical pollutants in the air.

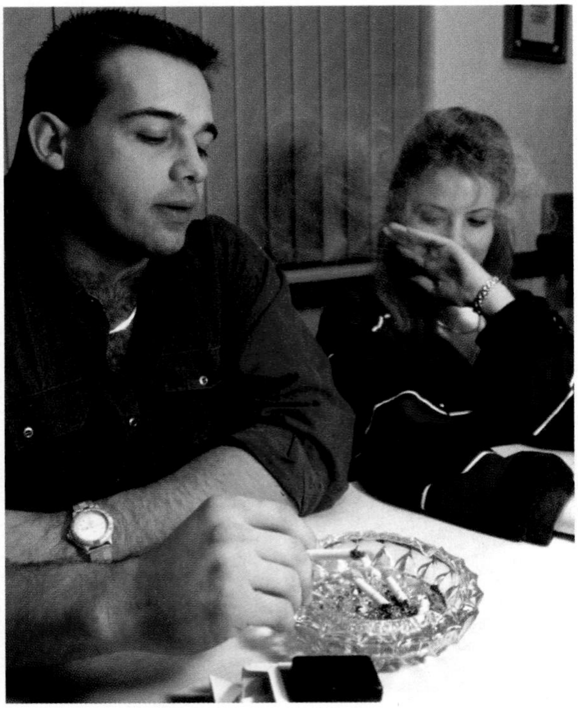

Nonsmokers exposed to secondhand smoke, at home or at work, increase their risk of developing lung cancer by 20 percent to 30 percent and their risk of developing heart disease by 25 to 30 percent.

using formaldehyde, but many homes already contain materials made with urea-formaldehyde, which can seep into the air. To avoid formaldehyde exposure, buy solid wood or nonwood products whenever possible, and ask about the formaldehyde content of building products, cabinets, and furniture before purchasing them.

Asbestos exposure can cause serious lung problems and cancer. Exposure usually occurs by breathing contaminated air in workplaces that make or use asbestos. Asbestos is also found in the air of buildings containing asbestos that are being torn down or renovated.

Lead lurks in some 57 million American homes, most built before 1960, with walls, windows, doors, and banisters coated with more than 3 million metric tons of lead-based paint. Fetuses and children under age 7 are particularly vulnerable to lead because their nervous systems are still developing and because their body mass is so small that they ingest and absorb more lead per pound than adults. Adults exposed to low levels of lead (which once were thought to be safe) may develop headaches, high blood pressure, irritability, tremors, and insomnia. Health effects increase with exposure to higher levels.

? FAQ Is Mold Dangerous?

One of the oldest and most widespread substances on earth, mold—a type of fungus that decomposes organic matter and provides plants with nutrients—has emerged as a major health concern. Common molds include *Aspergillus, Penicillium,* and *Stachybotrys,* a slimy, dark green mold that has been blamed for infant deaths and various illnesses, from Alzheimer's disease to cancer, in adults that breathe in its spores. Faulty ventilation systems and airtight buildings have been implicated as contributing to the increased mold problem.

Experts agree that mold may trigger or worsen a number of health problems, including dizziness, breathing problems, nausea, and asthma attacks. However, mold usually is harmful only to allergic or sensitive individuals.[5] In the last decade, high-profile lawsuits have resulted in multimillion dollar judgments, despite a lack of scientific evidence linking mold exposure and cancer or brain damage.

Mold problems can range from small patches to large infestations of entire rooms or even a whole building. The first step to reduce mold exposure is moisture control, which may require new methods of keeping rainwater and ground water away from the interior and maintaining the heating ventilation and air conditioning systems appropriately. Bleach or soap and water can clean up small infestations. Larger ones may require appropriate protective respiratory equipment or professionally trained, licensed, and experienced contractors.

Your Hearing Health

Hearing loss is the third-most common chronic health problem, after high blood pressure and arthritis, among older Americans. Loud noises cause hearing loss in an estimated 10 million Americans every year. Only about one-fifth of the 28 million Americans suffering from hearing loss have sought professional help.[6]

How Loud Is That Noise?

Loudness, or the intensity of a sound, is measured in **decibels (dB).** A whisper is 20 decibels; a conversation in a living room is about 50 decibels. On this scale, 50 isn't two and a half times louder than 20, but 1,000 times louder: Each 10-dB rise in the scale represents a tenfold increase in the intensity of the sound. Very loud but short bursts of sounds (such as gunshots and fireworks) and quieter but longer-lasting sounds (such as power tools) can induce hearing loss.

Sounds under 75 dB don't seem harmful. However, prolonged exposure to any sound over 85 dB (the equivalent of a power mower or food blender) or brief exposure to louder sounds can harm hearing. The noise level at rock concerts can reach 110 to 140 dB, about as loud as an air raid siren. Personal sound systems (boom boxes) can blast sounds of up to 115 dB. Cars with extremely loud music systems, known as boom cars, can

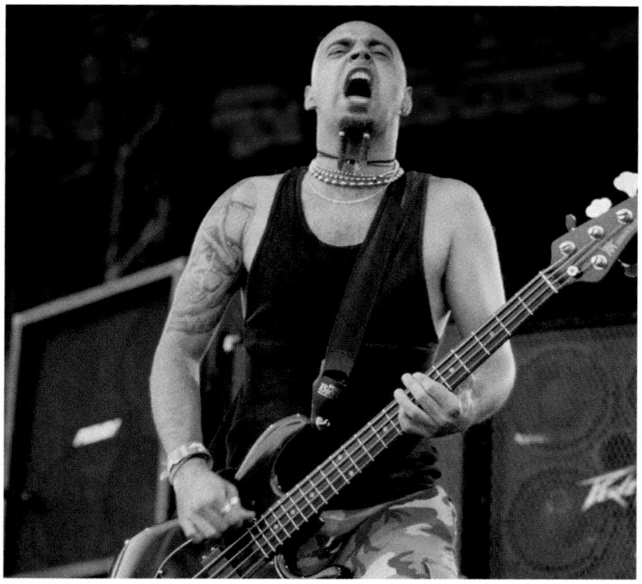

© Rune Hellestad/CORBIS

Besides listening to the music at your next concert, tune in to the noise level and how your ears are feeling.

produce an earsplitting 145 dB—louder than a jet engine or thunderclap (Figure 14-2).

Common "sound offenders" are nightclubs (with sustained levels of well over 100 decibels), restaurants (with levels of 80 to 96 decibels), and street traffic (80 decibels or more). However, even low-level office noise can undermine well-being and increase health risks.

Effects of Noise

Noise-induced hearing loss is 100 percent preventable—and irreversible. Hearing aids are the only treatment, but they do not correct the problem; they just amplify sound to compensate for hearing loss.

The healthy human ear can hear sounds within a wide range of frequencies (measured in hertz), from the low-frequency rumble of thunder at 50 hertz to the high-frequency overtones of a piccolo at nearly 20,000 hertz. High-frequency noise damages the delicate hair cells that serve as sound receptors in the inner ear. Damage first begins as a diminished sensitivity to frequencies around 4,000 hertz, the highest notes of a piano.

Early symptoms of hearing loss include difficulty understanding speech and *tinnitus* (ringing in the ears). Brief, very loud sounds, such as an explosion or gunfire, can produce immediate, severe, and permanent hearing loss. Longer exposure to less intense but still hazardous sounds, such as those common at work or in public places, can gradually impair hearing, often without the individual's awareness.

Conductive hearing loss, often caused by ear infections, cuts down on perception of low-pitched sounds.

Decibels	Example	Zone
0	The softest sound a typical ear can hear	Safe
10dB	Just audible	
20dB	Watch ticking; leaves rustling	
30dB	Soft whisper at 16 feet	
40dB	Quiet office; suburban street (no traffic)	
50dB	Interior of typical urban home; rushing stream	1,000 times louder than 20dB
60dB	Normal conversation; busy office	
70dB	Vacuum cleaner at 10 feet; hair dryer	
80dB	Alarm clock at 2 feet; loud music; average daily traffic	1,000 times louder than 50dB
90dB*	Motorcycle at 25 feet; jet 4 miles after takeoff	Risk of injury
100dB*	Video arcade; loud factory; subway train	
110dB*	Car horn at 3 feet; symphony orchestra; chain saw	1,000 times louder than 80dB
120dB	Jackhammer at 3 feet; boom box; nearby thunderclap	Injury
130dB	Rock concert; jet engine at 100 feet	
140dB	Jet engine nearby; amplified car stereo; firearms	1,000 times louder than 110dB

FIGURE 14-2 Loud and Louder

The human ear perceives a 10-decibel increase as a doubling of loudness. Thus, the 100 decibels of a subway train sound much more than twice as loud as the 50 decibels of a rushing stream.

*Note: The maximum exposure allowed on the job by federal law, in hours per day: 90 decibels, 8 hours; 100 decibels, 2 hours; 110 decibels, ½ hour.

Sensorineural loss involves damage or destruction of the sensory cells in the inner ear that convert sound waves to nerve signals.

Noise can harm more than our ears: High-volume sound has been linked to high blood pressure and other stress-related problems that can lead to heart disease, insomnia, anxiety, headaches, colitis, and ulcers. Noise frays the nerves; people tend to be more anxious, irritable, and angry when their ears are constantly barraged with sound.

decibel (dB) A unit for measuring the intensity of sounds.

? FAQ Is Listening to Music Through Earbuds Hazardous to My Hearing?

Although there is limited research, audiologists (who specialize in hearing problems) report seeing greater noise-induced hearing loss in young people. One probable culprit is extended use of earbuds, tiny earphones used with portable music players that deliver sound extremely close to the eardrum. Hearing loss can be temporary or permanent.

The dangers to your hearing depend on how loud the music is and how long you listen. Because personal music players have long-lasting rechargeable batteries, people—especially young ones—both listen for long periods and turn up the volume. As long as the sound level is within safety levels (see Figure 14-2), you can listen as long as you'd like. If you listen to music so loud that someone else can hear it two or three feet away, it's too loud.[7]

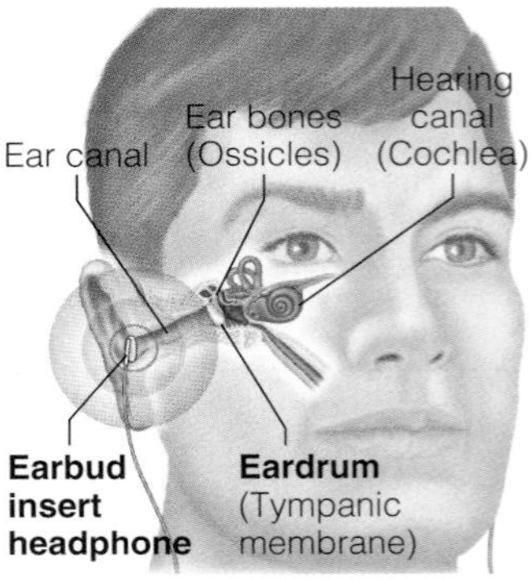

For safe listening, limit listening to a portable music player with earphones at 60 percent of its potential volume to one hour a day. At the very least, take a five-minute break after an hour of listening and keep the volume low.

Ask yourself the following questions to determine if you should have your hearing checked:

- Do you frequently have to ask people to repeat themselves?
- Do you have difficulty hearing when someone speaks in a whisper?
- Do people complain that you turn up the volume too much when watching television or listening to music?
- Do you have difficulty following conversation in a noisy environment?
- Do you avoid groups of people because of hearing difficulty?
- Have your friends or family suggested you might have hearing loss?

The Quality of Your Drinking Water

Fears about the public water supply have led many Americans to turn off their taps. About two-thirds take steps to drink purer water, either by using filtration and distillation methods or by drinking bottled water. However, Consumer Union, a nonprofit advocacy group, maintains that the United States has the safest water supply in the world. The Environmental Protection Agency has set standards for some 80 contaminants. These include many toxic chemicals and heavy metals—including lead, mercury, cadmium, and chromium—that can cause kidney and nervous system damage and birth defects.

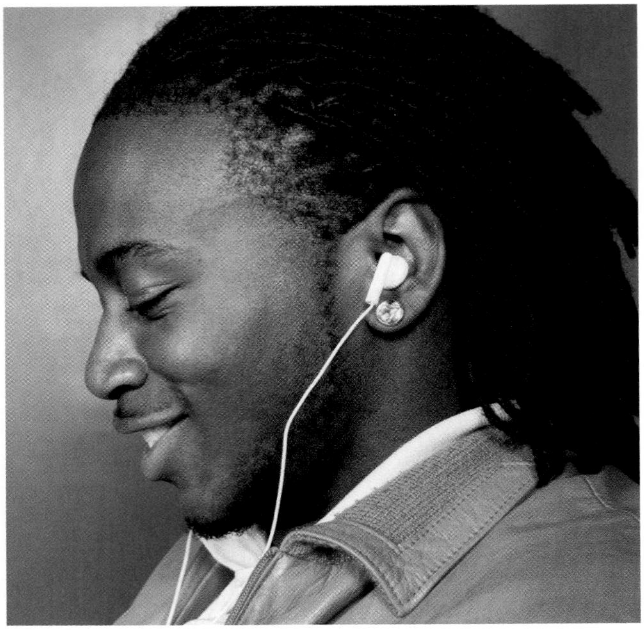

How loudly do you play your favorite music? How long do you use earbuds?

Each year the CDC reports an average of 7,400 cases of illness related to the water people drink. The most common culprits include parasites, bacteria, viruses, chemicals, and lead. Health officials suggest having your water tested if you live near a hazardous waste dump or industrial park, if the pipes in your house are made of lead or joined together with lead solder, if your water comes from a well, or if you purchase water from a private company. Check to see if your state health department or local water supplier will provide free testing. If not, use a state-certified laboratory that tests water in accordance with EPA standards.

? FAQ Is Bottled Water Better?

Is bottled water better? That's what consumers have often assumed. Bottled water sales have tripled in the past ten years. Women and college-age Americans make up the majority of bottled-water drinkers. Yet in the past, the Food and Drug Administration (FDA) simply defined bottled water as "sealed in bottles or other con-

Strategies for Change — Protecting Your Ears

- If you must live or work in a noisy area, wear hearing protectors to prevent exposure to blasts of very loud noise. Don't think cotton or facial tissue stuck in your ears can protect you; foam or soft plastic earplugs are more effective. Wear them when operating lawn mowers, weed trimmers, or power tools.
- Give your ears some quiet time. Rather than turning up the volume on your personal music player to blot out noise, look for truly quiet environments, such as the library, where you can rest your ears and focus your mind.
- Soundproof your home by using draperies, carpets, and bulky furniture. Put rubber mats under washing machines, blenders, and other noisy appliances. Seal cracks around windows and doors.
- Beware of large doses of aspirin. Researchers have found that eight aspirin tablets a day can aggravate the damage caused by loud noise; twelve a day can cause ringing in the ears (tinnitus).
- Don't drink in noisy environments. Alcohol intensifies the impact of noise and increases the risk of lifelong hearing damage.
- When you hear a sudden loud noise, press your fingers against your ears. Limit your exposure to loud noise. Several brief periods of noise seem less damaging than one long exposure.

tainers and intended for human consumption." Bottled water wasn't required to be "pure" or even to be tested for toxic chemicals. One survey found chemical contaminants associated with cancer in 22 of 100 brands tested.

The FDA has called for federal monitoring of the purity of bottled water. Some states, including California and New York, have their own bottled-water safety standards to ensure that bottled water is at least as safe as drinking water.

Chemical Risks

Various chemicals, including benzene, asbestos, and arsenic, have been shown to cause cancer in humans. Probable carcinogens include DDT and PCB. Risks can be greatly increased with simultaneous exposures to more than one carcinogen, for example, tobacco smoke and asbestos.[8]

According to the CDC, the levels of potentially harmful chemicals, including pesticides and lead, in Americans' blood have declined. Still, an estimated 50,000 to 70,000 U.S. workers die each year of chronic diseases related to past exposure to toxic substances, including lung cancer, bladder cancer, leukemia, lymphoma, chronic bronchitis, and disorders of the nervous system. **Endocrine disruptors,** chemicals that act as or interfere with human hormones, particularly estrogen, may pose a different threat. Scientists are investigating their impact on fertility, falling sperm counts, and cancers of the reproductive organs. Exposure to toxic chemicals causes about 3 percent of developmental defects.

? FAQ What Health Risks Are Caused by Pesticides?

High quantities of toxic chemical waste from unused or obsolete pesticides are posing a continuing and worsening threat to people and the environment in Eastern Europe, Africa, Asia, the Middle East, and Latin America. In the United States, the FDA estimates that 33 to 39 percent of our food supply contains residues of pesticides that may pose a long-term danger to our health. Scientists have detected traces of pesticides in groundwater in both urban and rural areas.

No relationship has been found between fertility, as measured by time to pregnancy (that is, the time taken for a couple to conceive once they decide they want to), and male exposure to pesticides. Exposure to pesticides may, however, pose a risk to pregnant women and their unborn children. Men whose jobs routinely expose them to pesticides may be at increased risk of prostate cancer. Parental exposure does not increase the likelihood of childhood brain cancer.

Chlorinated hydrocarbons include several high-risk substances—such as DDT, kepone, and chlordane—that have been restricted or banned because they may cause cancer, birth defects, neurological disorders, and damage to wildlife and the environment. They are extremely resistant to breakdown.

endocrine disruptors Synthetic chemicals that interfere with the ways that hormones work in humans and wildlife.

chlorinated hydrocarbons Highly toxic pesticides, such as DDT and chlordane, that are extremely resistant to breakdown; may cause cancer, birth defects, neurological disorders, and damage to wildlife and the environment.

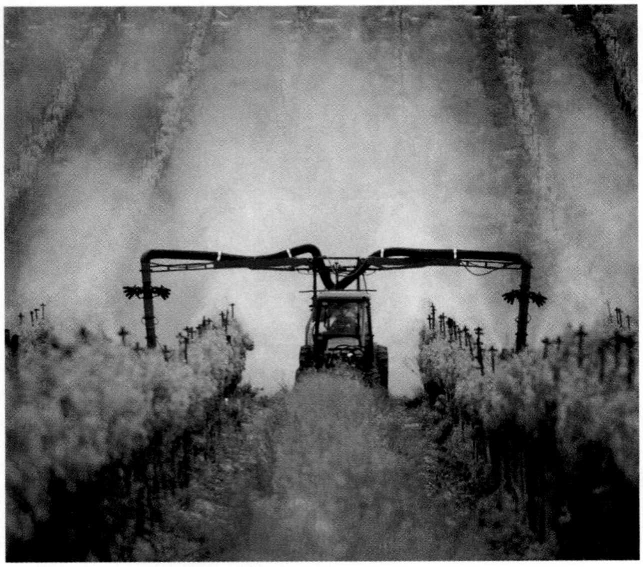

© Spencer Grant/PhotoEdit, Inc.

Pesticides protect crops from harmful insects, plants, and fungi but may endanger human health.

Organic phosphates, including chemicals such as malathion, break down more rapidly than the chlorinated hydrocarbons. Most are highly toxic, causing cramps, confusion, diarrhea, vomiting, headaches, and breathing difficulties. Higher levels in the blood can lead to convulsions, paralysis, coma, and death.

Farmworkers and those in the communities surrounding agricultural land are at greatest risk for pesticide exposure. However, even city dwellers aren't out of range. About half (52 percent) of the nation uses insect repellents, including some made with potent insecticides.

Invisible Threats

Among the unseen threats to health are various forms of *radiation,* energy radiated in the form of waves or particles.

Electromagnetic Fields

Any electrically charged conductor generates two kinds of invisible fields: electric and magnetic. Together they're called **electromagnetic fields (EMFs).** For years, these fields, produced by household appliances, home wiring, lighting fixtures, electric blankets, and overhead power lines, were considered harmless. However, epidemiological studies have revealed a link between exposure to high-voltage lines and cancer (especially leukemia, a blood cancer) in electrical workers and children.

Laboratory studies on animals have shown that alternating current, which changes strength and direction 60 times a second (and electrifies most of North America), emits EMFs that may interfere with the normal functioning of human cell membranes, which have their own electromagnetic fields. The result may be mood disorders, changes in circadian rhythms (our inner sense of time), miscarriage, developmental problems, or cancer. Researchers have documented increases in breast cancer deaths in women who worked as electrical engineers, electricians, or in other high-exposure jobs, and a link between EMF exposure and increased risk of leukemia and possibly brain cancer.

After six years of congressionally mandated research, the National Institute of Environmental Health Sciences concluded that the evidence of a risk of cancer and other human disease from the electric and magnetic fields around power lines is "weak." This finding applies to the extremely low frequency electric and magnetic fields surrounding both the big power lines that distribute power and the smaller but closer electric lines in homes and appliances. However, the researchers also noted that EMF exposure "cannot be recognized as entirely safe."

Expectant mothers who often use electric blankets or heated water beds during winter have a higher miscarriage rate than nonusers. Babies conceived in the winter by electric blanket-users grow more slowly in the womb and tend to have a lower birthweight than others. Federal officials urge "prudent avoidance" of electric blankets for women who are pregnant or hoping to conceive.

Cell phones emit low levels of electromagnetic energy (see Savvy Consumer: "Are Cell Phones Safe to Use?").

Microwaves

Microwaves (extremely high frequency electromagnetic waves) increase the rate at which molecules vibrate; this vibration generates heat. There's no evidence that existing levels of microwave radiation encountered in the environment pose a health risk to people, and all home microwave ovens must meet safety standards for leakage.

Another concern about the safety of microwave ovens stems from the chemicals in plastic wrapping and plastic containers used in microwave ovens. Chemicals may leak into food. In high concentrations, some of the chemicals (such as DEHA, which makes plastic more pliable) can cause cancer in mice. Consumers should be cautious about using clingy plastic wrap when reheating leftovers, and plastic-encased metal "heat susceptors" included in convenience foods such as popcorn and pizza. Although these materials seem safe when tested in conventional ovens at temperatures of 300° to 350° Fahrenheit, microwave ovens can boost temperatures to 500° Fahrenheit.

SAVVY CONSUMER

Are Cell Phones Safe to Use?

Since cellular phone service was introduced in the United States in 1984, mobile and handheld phones have become ubiquitous. More than 86 million people use cell phones, and concern has grown about their possible health risks. The federal government sets upper exposure limits to electromagnetic energy from cell phones known as the specific absorption rate, or SAR. A phone emits the most radiation during a call, but it also emits small amounts periodically whenever it's turned on.

Can exposure to low levels of electromagnetic energy that the body absorbs from a cell phone be harmful? More than 70 research papers on the potentially harmful effects of cell phone use have raised concerns about cancer, neurological disorders, sleep problems, or headaches; others have shown no association or were inconclusive. The Food and Drug Administration (FDA) and Federal Communications Commission (FCC) have stated that "the available scientific evidence does not show that any health problems are associated with using wireless phones. There is no proof, however, that wireless phones are absolutely safe." Additional studies are underway.

Swedish and Finnish researchers have found no "consistent evidence" of increased risk of cancer from use for up to five years, but they did document protein changes in human cells exposed to cell phone radiation and an increased rate of benign brain tumors. Health experts in Britain, France, and Germany have discouraged children from using cell phones largely because of concerns that their developing nervous systems may be especially vulnerable.

A headset can keep the phone's antenna away from your head and body. Shields that claim to reduce exposure generally don't work as advertised, say the FDA and FCC.

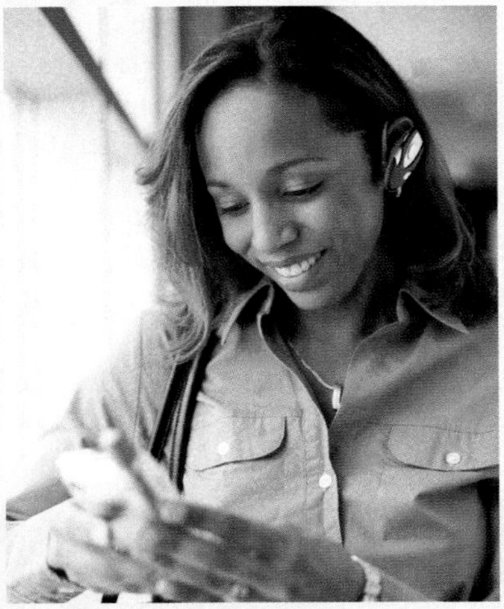

© Jim Craigmyle/ CORBIS

LEARN IT / LIVE IT

Taking Care of Mother Earth

Environmental problems can seem so complex that you may think there's little you can do about them. That's not the case. This world can be made better instead of worse. The job isn't easy, and all of us have to do our part. Just as many diseases of the previous century have been eradicated, so in time we may be able to remove or reduce many environmental threats. Your future—and our planet's future—may depend on it.

- **Plant a tree.** Even a single tree helps absorb carbon dioxide and produces cooling that can reduce the need for air-conditioning.
- **Look for simply packaged items.** Whenever possible, choose items packed in recycled materials or something recyclable.
- **Bring your own bag.** Whenever possible, avoid using plastic or paper bags for items you could carry in a cloth or string carryall.
- **Hit the switch.** Turn off all electrical appliances (TVs, CD players, radios, lights, computers, printers) when you're not in the room or paying attention to them.
- **Avoid disposables.** Use a mug instead of a paper or Styrofoam cup, a sponge instead of a paper towel, a cloth napkin instead of a paper one.
- **Be water wise.** Turn off the tap while you shave or brush your teeth. Install water-efficient faucets, toilets, and shower heads. Wash clothes in cold water.
- **Cancel junk mail.** It consumes 100 million trees a year. To get off mailing lists, write: Di-

(Continued)

organic phosphates Toxic pesticides that may cause cancer, birth defects, neurological disorders, and damage to wildlife and the environment.

electromagnetic fields (EMFs) The invisible electric and magnetic fields generated by an electrically charged conductor.

microwaves Extremely high frequency electromagnetic waves that increase the rate at which molecules vibrate, thereby generating heat.

rect Mail Association, Mail Preference Service, P.O. Box 9008, Farmingdale, NY 11735-9008

- **Spare the seas.** If you live near the coast or are picnicking or hiking near the ocean, don't use plastic bags (which are often blown into the water) or plastic six-pack holders (which can get caught around the necks of sea birds).
- **Don't buy products made of endangered substances.** Examples include coral, ivory, tortoise shell, or wood from endangered forests (teak, mahogany, ebony, rosewood).
- **Speak out.** E-mail your senators and congressional representatives, who vote on pollution controls, budgets for the enforcement of safety regulations, and the preservation of forests and wildlife. Identify the particular bill or issue you're addressing. Be as specific, brief, and to the point as possible. Go to www.senate.gov and click on "Senators" to find the e-mail addresses. To find your congressional representative, go to www.house.gov and click on "Write Your Representative."

14 Making This Chapter Work for You

Review Questions

1. Threats to the environment include
   a. an open ecosystem.
   b. depletion of the oxygen layer.
   c. ecological processes.
   d. global warming.
2. Mutagens
   a. are caused by birth defects.
   b. result in changes to the DNA of body cells.
   c. are agents that trigger changes in the DNA of body cells.
   d. are caused by repeated exposure to pollutants.
3. Which of the following statements about global warming is true?
   a. In 2001, the United States signed the first international treaty to fight global warming.
   b. Global warming may result in severe drought and a rise in ocean levels.
   c. Increasing tree cover and agricultural lands will contribute to global warming.
   d. Increasing carbon dioxide production will slow the progress of global warming.
4. One of the most important things you can do to help protect the environment is
   a. recycle paper, bottles, cans, and unwanted food.
   b. use as much water as possible to help lower the ocean water levels.
   c. avoid energy-depleting fluorescent bulbs.
   d. use plastic storage containers and plastic wrap to save trees from being cut down.
5. Which of the following statements about air pollution is *false?*
   a. Current model automobiles emit much less pollution per mile than new cars in 1970.
   b. The three types of smog include sulfur-dioxide smog, produced by burning oil; photochemical smog, resulting from car exhaust; and carbon-monoxide smog, caused by fossil fuels.
   c. Ozone in the upper atmosphere protects us from harmful ultraviolet radiation from the sun, but in the lower atmosphere, it is a harmful air pollutant.
   d. Air pollution can cause the same types of respiratory health problems as smoking.
6. An example of the concept of sustainability is
   a. getting enough to eat at every meal.
   b. lowering the price of gas to 1990 levels.
   c. using wind power to generate electricity.
   d. maintaining our current levels of energy usage.
7. You can protect your hearing by
   a. avoiding prolonged exposure to sounds under 75 decibels.
   b. using foam earplugs when operating noisy tools or attending rock concerts.
   c. limiting noise exposure to short bursts of loud sounds such as fireworks.
   d. drinking alcohol in noisy environments to mute the sounds.
8. Drinking water safety
   a. may be compromised if your water comes from a well.
   b. is low in the United States because of chemical treatment.
   c. can be guaranteed by using bottled water, which is completely free of chemical contaminants.
   d. is measured by the cases of illness reported each year.
9. Pesticide risks to health include:
   a. reduced male fertility.
   b. higher incidence of childhood brain cancer if parents have been exposed.
   c. higher incidence of cancer and birth defects from chlorinated hydrocarbons such as DDT.
   d. higher incidence of diabetes.
10. Which statement about radiation is *false?*
    a. Evidence indicates a weak link between electromagnetic fields around power lines and cancer and other diseases.
    b. Radio frequency signals from cell phones cause brain cancer.

LACC Extra Credit Assignment

14. What in your estimation is the greatest problem that our environment faces? Discuss.

c. Women who are pregnant should not use electric blankets.
d. Chemicals in plastic wrap may leak into foods heated in microwave ovens.

Answers to these questions can be found on page 422.

Critical Thinking

1. How do you contribute to environmental pollution? How might you change your habits to protect the environment?
2. An excerpt from a recent newspaper article stated, "Children living in a public housing project near a local refinery suffer from a high rate of asthma and allergies, and an environmental group says the plant may be to blame." The refinery has met all the local air quality standards, employs hundreds in the community, and pays substantial city taxes, which support police, fire, and social services. If you were a city council member, how would you balance health and environmental concerns with the need for industry in your community? What actions would you recommend in this particular situation?
3. In one Harris poll, 84 percent of Americans said that, given a choice between a high standard of living (but with hazardous air and water pollution and the depletion of natural resources) and a lower standard of living (but with clean air and drinking water), they would prefer clean air and drinking water and a lower standard of living. What about you? What exactly would you be willing to give up: air conditioning, convenience packaging and products, driving your own car rather than using public transportation? Do you think most people are willing to change their lifestyles to preserve the environment?

Media Menu

ThomsonNOW™ Go to the ThomsonNOW website at **http://www.thomsonedu.com** that will:

- Help you evaluate your knowledge of the material.
- Allow you to take an exam-prep quiz.
- Provide a Personalized Learning Plan targeting resources that address areas you should study.
- Coach you through identifying target goals for behavioral change and creating and monitoring your personal change plan throughout the semester.

INTERNET CONNECTIONS

Envirolink
www.envirolink.org

Envirolink is a nonprofit organization that brings together individuals and groups concerned about the environment and provides access to a wealth of online environmental resources.

Student Environmental Action Coalition
www.seac.org

Since 1988, the Student Environmental Action Coalition has been empowering students and youth to fight for environmental and social justice in our schools and communities.

Environmental Protection Agency
www.epa.gov

This comprehensive government site features environmental topics, including ecosystems, global warming, air and water pollution, compliance and enforcement, pesticides and toxins, accident prevention, and treatment.

National Center for Environmental Health (NCEH)
www.cdc.gov/nceh/

This site, sponsored by the U.S. Centers for Disease Control and Prevention, features a searchable database as well as fact sheets and brochures on a variety of environmental topics, from emergency preparedness and public health tracking to environmental hazards and lead poisoning prevention.

InfoTrac College Edition Activities Log on, insert **hearing** into the Keyword search box, and limit your search to the past year. When you get the results, Mark articles to review, then Select one to read. Summarize three or four key points from the article.

You can find additional readings related to personal health with InfoTrac College Edition, an online library of more than 900 journals and publications. Follow the instructions for accessing InfoTrac College Edition that were packaged with your textbook; then search for articles using a keyword search.

For additional links, resources, and suggested readings on the InfoTrac College Edition, visit our Health and Wellness Resource Center at **http://health.wadsworth.com.**

Key Terms

The terms listed are used on the page indicated. Definitions of the terms are in the Glossary at the end of this book.

chlorinated hydrocarbons 397
decibel (dB) 394
ecosystem 390
electromagnetic fields (EMFs) 398
endocrine disruptors 397
global warming 392
microwaves 398
mutagen 390
organic phosphates 398
pollutant 390
precycling 392
recycling 392
smog 393
sustainability 392
teratogen 390

15 A Lifetime of Health

REAL HEALTH

Rina didn't feel old until she enrolled in a college personal health course. Formal at first, the other students—some young enough to be her children—started calling her "Mom." When the professor announced that the next week's topic would be aging, Rina beamed, "I'll be the expert!"

Rina soon discovered that a lot of what she believed about aging wasn't true. In her mind it seemed inevitable that people would slow down, lose their zest for living, and give up the activities they once loved. In her health class she learned this isn't the case.

Just being back in college energized Rina. Always curious, she told her husband she could almost feel her brain tingle with the stimulation of new ideas and information. Intrigued by the notion that exercise is the best anti-aging pill in existence, Rina began working out at the campus gym. She applied her new knowledge about nutrition as she prepared healthy meals at home.

By the end of her first year as a "nontraditional" student, Rina stopped thinking of the age gap between her and most of her classmates. Although she didn't set out to turn back the clock, she proudly announced to her family that she was feeling younger than she had in years.

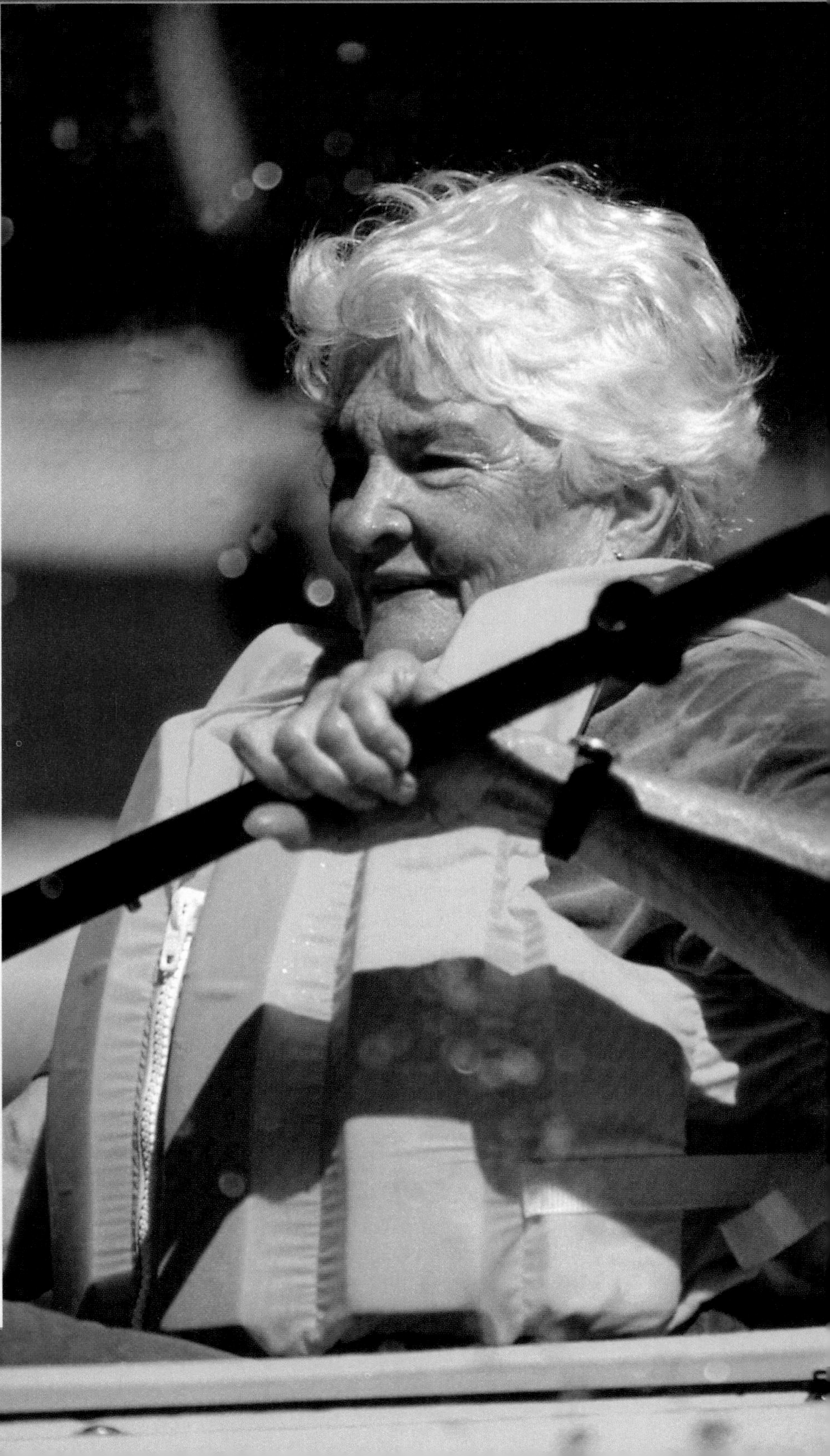

Although **aging**—the characteristic pattern of normal life changes that occurs as humans, plants, and animals grow older—remains inevitable, you can do a great deal to influence the impact that the passage of time has on you. Whether you're in your teens, twenties, thirties, or older, now is the time to start taking the steps that will add healthy, active, productive years to your life.

This chapter provides a preview of the changes age brings, the steps you can take to age healthfully, and the ways you can make the most of all the years of your life.

Invariably, though, no one gets out of this life alive. Death is the natural completion of things, as much a part of the real world as life itself. In time we all lose people we cherish: grandparents, aunts and uncles, parents, friends, neighbors, coworkers, siblings. With each loss, part of us may seem to die, yet each loss also reaffirms how precious life is.

This chapter explores the meaning of death, describes the process of dying, provides information on end-of-life issues, and offers advice on comforting the dying and helping their survivors.

? FAQ Frequently Asked Questions

- How long can I expect to live? *p. 404*
- What are advance directives? *p. 413*
- What do we know about near-death experiences? *p. 416*

After studying the material in this chapter, you should be able to:

- **List** the benefits that older Americans can gain from physical activity.
- **Discuss** hormone therapy for menopause symptoms.
- **Identify** some of the challenges of aging and **discuss** their risk factors and possible ways of preventing them.
- **Explain** the purposes of advanced directives and a holographic will.
- **Define** death and **explain** the stages of emotional reaction experienced in facing death.
- **Name** some of grief's effects on health.

aging The characteristic pattern of normal life changes that occur as humans grow older.

ThomsonNOW™ Log on to ThomsonNOW at **www.thomsonedu.com/thomsonnow** to find your Behavior Change Planner and to explore self-assessments, interactive tutorials, and practice quizzes.

Living in an Aging Society

America is turning gray. People age 65 and older make up 13 percent of the U.S. population. By the year 2014, this group will grow to 15 percent. By the midpoint of the twenty-first century, 80 million Americans—one in five—will be seniors (65 or older).[1] (See Figure 15-1)

Throughout your life, you will confront a variety of issues related not just to your age, but also to that of the aging American population. These include:

- **Retirement costs.** Unless changes are made to decrease the demand on the Social Security system, Social Security taxes on workers may be increased.
- **Health costs.** Health-care costs for those over 65 years are three to five times greater than for younger men and women.
- **Gray-power politics.** Senior citizens go to the polls in larger numbers than younger voters. With such voting power, programs for the elderly may make up a larger share of future federal budgets.
- **Anti-aging gimmicks.** As the population ages, health hucksters push an ever-growing number of unproven anti-aging treatments, such as melatonin or the hormone DHEA. Because some preparations have the potential to harm, consumers must be wary of all claims to turn back or slow down the biological clock.

? FAQ How Long Can I Expect to Live?

The answer depends on you. Statistically, you're likely to live longer than your parents or grandparents. Life expectancy has been increasing steadily over the last century, reaching an all-time high in the United States of 77.6 years. The longevity gender gap also has been shrinking since 1990. According to the National Center for Health Statistics, life expectancy for American women now stands at 80.1 years; for men, it is a record high of 74.8 years.

Contrary to common belief, heredity doesn't determine how long you'll live or how well you'll age. Genes, as studies of identical twins have revealed, influence only about 30 percent of the rate and ways in which we age.

When does a person become old? That answer may depend on your gender. In a survey of 441 undergraduates at a large southeastern university, men said that a person becomes "old" at

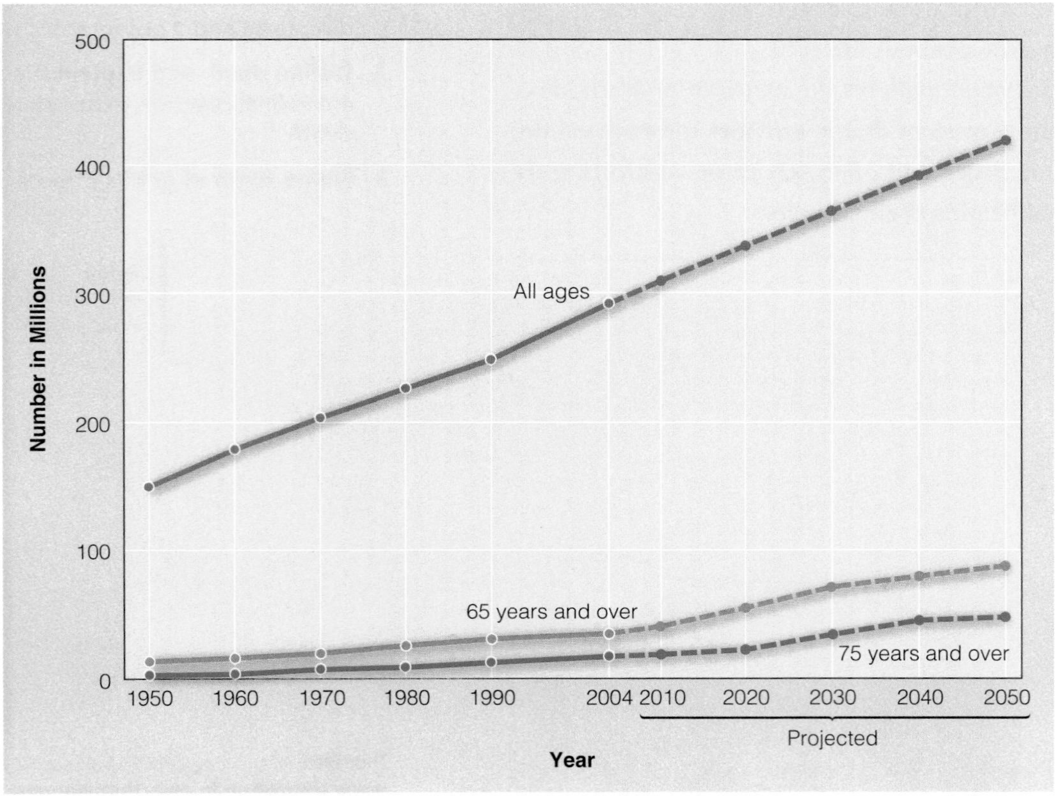

FIGURE 15-1 Total Population and Older Population

Source: U.S. Census Bureau.

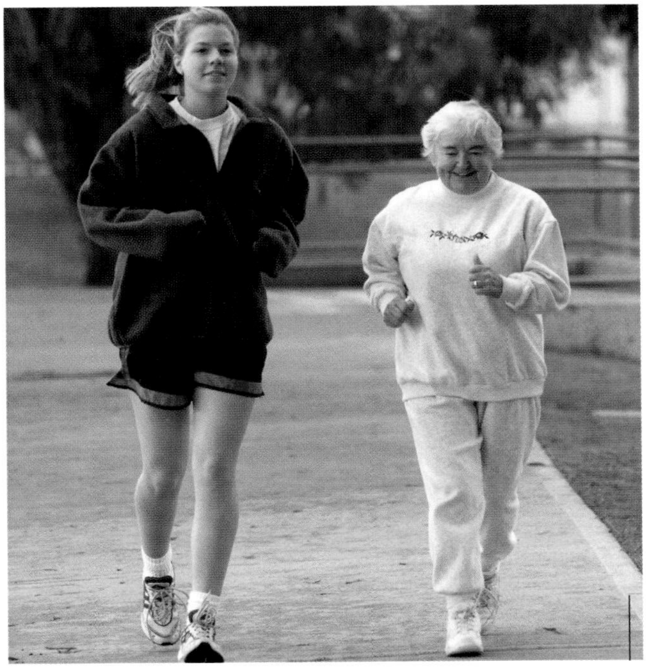

© David Young Wolf/PhotoEdit

Why do you think this student would probably say "old" is about 60, while the older person would likely say 70?

age 58. Women viewed a person becoming "old" at age 62. But "old," like beauty, may be in the eye of the beholder. In other studies individuals between the ages of 65 and 74 identified 70 as the age at which a person becomes "old."[2]

Women's lifespans average 5 to 10 percent longer than men's. No one knows exactly why. But the gender gap in longevity narrows over time. At birth a baby boy has a life expectancy about five years shorter than a girl's. By age 65, a man can expect to live an additional 15.1 years, just 3.8 years less than a woman. By age 85, the difference in projected life expectancies is down to 1.2 years.

YOUR LIFE COACH

Staying Healthy Longer

If you want to feel young when you're older, the time to start taking care of yourself is now—whether you're 25, 45, or 65. The healthier you become now, the longer you're likely to stay healthy in the future.

Since genes influence only about 30 percent of the aging process, "the rest is up to us," says Michael Roizen, M.D., coauthor of *You: The Owner's Manual,* who notes that it's possible to turn back the biological clock. "With relatively simple changes, someone whose chronological age is 69 can have a physiological age of 45. And the most amazing thing is that it's never too late to live younger—until one foot is six feet under."[3]

Keep Your Arteries Young

"You are as young—or as old—as your arteries," says Roizen. Problems like high blood pressure, high cholesterol, and buildup of atherosclerotic plaque increase the likelihood of stroke, heart disease, kidney problems, even memory impairment. If your arteries are healthy, you're much more likely to have a healthy heart and a healthy brain. People with "young" arteries tend to retain a higher level of cognitive functioning.

Premature aging of the arteries is largely self-inflicted; common culprits are a high-fat diet, lack of exercise, obesity, and a high-stress lifestyle. At any age, the unexercised body—though free of the symptoms of illness—will rust out long before it could ever wear out.

Avoid Illness

In studies of centenarians, most have had no serious chronic illnesses. Among the most important strategies: not smoking, avoiding weight gain in middle age, and recognizing and treating conditions like elevated cholesterol and high blood pressure.

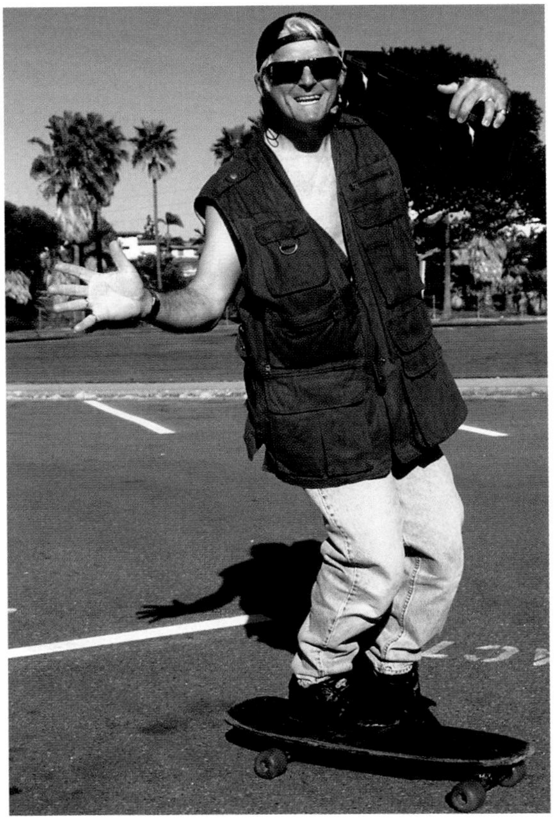

© Photo Network/PictureQuest

Age is partly a matter of attitude.

Also important is keeping up with immunizations against diseases, such as influenza and pneumococcal pneumonia, that take a greater toll on the elderly. For women at risk of osteoporosis, new options, including "designer estrogens" like raloxifene, can preserve their bones' health. A healthy diet, chockful of fruits and vegetables, also can contribute to a healthy old age, in part because they contain antioxidants that may ward off many age-related problems.

Maintain Your Zest for Living

Attitude matters. The healthiest seniors are "engaged" in life, resilient, optimistic, productive, and socially involved. While they are not immune to life's slings and arrows, successful agers bounce back after a setback and have a "can-do" attitude about the challenges they face. They also tend to be lifelong learners who may take up entirely new hobbies late in life—pursuits that stimulate production of more connections between neurons and may slow aging within the brain. Social interactions, such as entertaining friends and getting involved with religious activities, lead to greater life satisfaction as people get older.

Just as with muscles, the best advice to keep your brain healthy as you age is "use it or lose it." Some memory losses among healthy older people are normal—but reversible with training in simple methods, such as word associations, that improve recall.

Stay Strong

For years, experts assumed that older meant weaker. Landmark research with frail nursing home residents in their eighties and nineties showed this isn't so. After just eight to ten weeks of strength training, even the oldest seniors increased muscle and bone, sped up their metabolic rate, improved sleep and mobility, boosted their spirits, and gained in self-confidence. Other studies have found that exercise programs can increase lung capacity, double leg strength, and decrease the risk of disability and premature death.

Successful Aging

Although the proportion of people who live beyond 100 years is still very small, the worldwide number is rapidly growing. The United Nations estimates that in 2050, there will be 3.2 million centenarians, an increase of about eighteen times. The number of Americans living long enough to blow out 100 birthday candles has increased 35 percent from a decade ago.

Americans are living better as well as longer. Disability decreased steadily through the 1980s and 1990s, and the rate of improvement is accelerating. Nursing home use has fallen. Senior citizens are healthier and more independent. Among the factors contributing to a longer healthspan are improved medical care, diet, exercise, and public health advances.

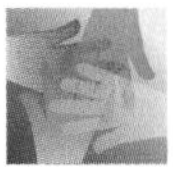

When surveyed, about half of Americans aged 65 to 69 say, "These are the best years of my life." Many people in their seventies and eighties agree. Sixty percent of older black and 57 percent of older Hispanic respondents say these are their best years. When asked about the keys to a meaningful and vital life, older adults rate having family and friends and taking care of their health as most important, followed by spiritual life.[4]

Physical Activity: It's Never Too Late

The effects of ongoing activity are so profound that gerontologists sometimes refer to exercise as "the closest thing to an antiaging pill." Exercise slows many changes associated with advancing age, such as loss of lean muscle tissue, increase in body fat, and decreased work capacity. The bottom line: What you *don't* do may matter more than what you do do.

No one is ever too old to get in shape. The American College of Sports Medicine encourages seniors to engage in the full range of physical activities, including aerobic conditioning. With regular conditioning, 60-year-olds can regain the fitness they had at age 40 to 45. Adults over the age of 72 who exercise more and smoke less than their peers are most likely to enjoy long, healthy, and happy lives, according to a study that followed 1,000 seniors for nine years.

Exercise lowers the risk of heart disease and stroke in the elderly—and greatly improves general health. Male and female runners over age 50 have much lower rates of disability and much lower health-care expenses than less active seniors. Even less intense activities, such as gardening, dancing, and brisk walking, can delay chronic physical disability and cognitive decline.

According to the U.S. surgeon general, physical activity offers older Americans additional benefits, including the following:

- **Greater ability to live independently.**
- **Reduced risk of falling and fracturing bones.**
- **Lower risk of dying from coronary heart disease** and of developing high blood pressure, colon cancer, and diabetes.
- **Reduced blood pressure** in some people with hypertension.
- **Fewer symptoms of anxiety** and depression.
- **Improvements in mood** and feelings of well-being.

Despite these potential benefits, many seniors are not active. By age 75, about one in three men and one in two women engage in no physical activity. Yet even sedentary individuals in their eighties and nineties can participate in an exercise program—and gain significant benefits.

Nutrition and Obesity

The most common nutritional disorder in older persons is obesity. Among Americans between 65 to 74 years old, approximately 34 percent of women and 44 percent of men are overweight; an additional 27 percent of women and 24 percent of men are obese. They face higher risk of diabetes, heart disease, stroke, and other health problems, including arthritis.[5]

As many as 40 percent of elderly people who live independently do not get adequate amounts of one or more essential nutrients. The reasons are many: limited income, difficulty getting to stores, chronic illness, medications that interfere with the metabolism of nu trients, problems chewing or digesting, poor appetite, inactivity, illness, depression. Nutritionists urge the elderly, like other Americans, to concentrate on eating healthful foods; many also recommend daily nutritional supplements, which may provide the added benefit of improving cognitive function in healthy people over 65.

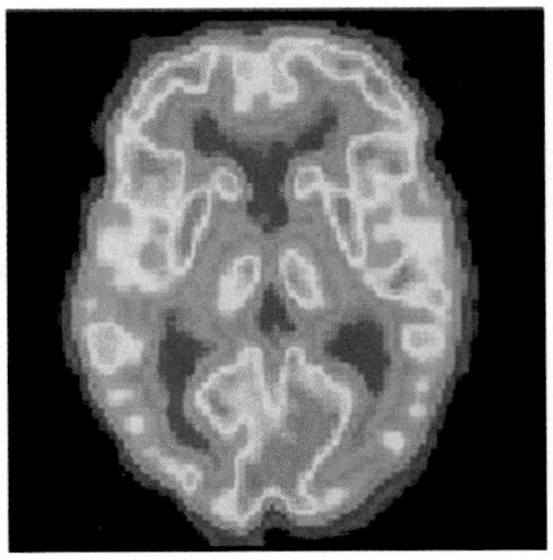

PET scan of a 20-year-old brain

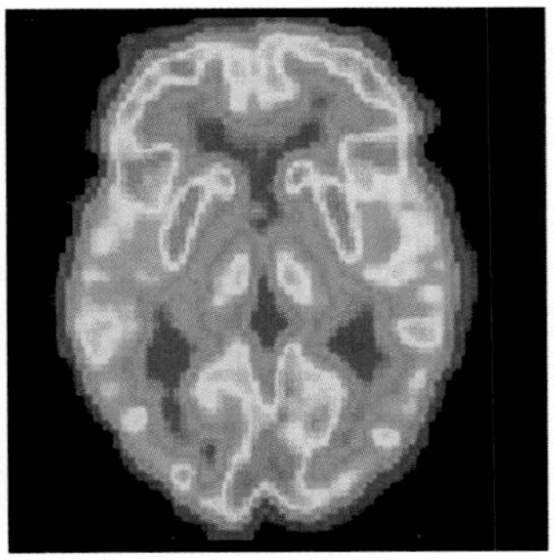

PET scan of an 80-year-old brain

Alzheimer's Disease Education & Referral Center (both)

In these PET scans, the red and yellow show greater neuron activity in the young adult. The brain of the older person shows less activity and more dark areas, indicating that the fluid-filled ventricles have grown larger.

The Aging Brain

Scientists used to think that the aging brain, once worn out, could never be fixed. Now they know that the brain can and does repair itself. When neurons (brain cells) die, the surrounding cells develop "fingers" to fill the gaps and establish new connections, or synapses, between surviving neurons. Although self-repair occurs more quickly in young brains, the process continues in older brains. Even victims of Alzheimer's disease, the most devastating form of senility, have enough healthy cells in the diseased brain to regrow synapses. Scientists hope to develop drugs that someday may help the brain repair itself.

Mental ability does not decline along with physical vigor. Researchers have been able to reverse the supposedly normal intellectual declines of 60- to 80-year-olds by tutoring them in problem solving. Reaction time, intellectual speed and efficiency, nonverbal intelligence, and maximum work rate for short periods may diminish by age 75. However, understanding, vocabulary, ability to remember key information, and verbal intelligence remain about the same.

Memory

Between the ages of 30 and 90, the brain loses about 10 percent of its volume. Forgetfulness isn't an automatic result, however. Crossword puzzles, practicing the piano, and playing chess exercise the brain and can counteract natural changes in memory. Exercise also helps cognitive function.

Some memory skills, particularly the ability to retrieve names and quickly process information, inevitably diminish over time. What normal changes should you expect? Here is a preview:

- **Recalling information takes longer.** As individuals reach their mid- to late sixties, the brain slows down, but usually just by a matter of milliseconds. As long as they're not rushed, older adults eventually adapt and perform just as well as younger ones.
- **Distractions become more disruptive.** College students can study and listen to the stereo at the same time. Thirty-something moms can soothe the baby, field questions about homework, and prepare dinner all at once. But older individuals find it much more difficult to divide their attention or to remember details after having switched their attention to something else. Inability to ignore background information while focusing on a task may underlie the memory problems associated with aging.
- **"Accessing" names gets harder.** The ability to remember names, especially those you don't use frequently, diminishes by as much as 50 percent between ages 25 and 65. Preventive strategies can help, such as repeating a person's name when introduced, writing down the name as soon as possible, and making obvious associations (the Golden Gate for a man named Bridges).
- **Learning new information is harder.** The quality of memory doesn't change, just the speed at which we receive, absorb, and react to information. That's why strategies like taking notes or outlining material become critical for older students, especially when learning new skills. However, adding to existing knowledge remains as easy as ever.
- **Wisdom matters.** In any memory test involving knowledge of the world, vocabulary, or judgment, older people outperform their younger counterparts.

Women at Midlife

In the next two decades some 40 million American women will end their reproductive years. "The primary misconception is that this is a terrible time when all women suffer horrible symptoms," says Sherry Sherman, M.D., project officer for the National Institute of Aging's Study of Women Across the Nation, which has followed 3,300 women through midlife since 1996. "When you look at healthy women in the community in terms of what actually affects their lives, their periods stop. That's it."[6]

Perimenopause

While the average age of **menopause**—defined as the complete cessation of menstrual periods for 12 consecutive months—is 51.5, a woman's reproductive system begins changing more than a decade earlier. "The change of life starts in our thirties with irregular menstrual cycles and then heats up in our forties with hot flashes and night sweats"[7] says psychiatrist Marsha Speller, M.D., author of *The Menopause Answer Book.*

For many women, **perimenopause**—the four-to-ten-year span before a woman's last period—is more baffling and bothersome than the years after. During this time the egg cells, or oocytes, in a woman's ovaries start to *senesce* or die off at a faster rate. Eventually, the number of egg cells drops to a tiny fraction of the estimated 2 million packed into her ovaries at birth. Trying to coax some of the remaining oocytes to ripen, the pituitary gland churns out extra follicle-stimulating hormone (FSH). This surge is the earliest harbinger of menopause, occurring six to ten years before a woman's final periods. Eventually, the other menstrual messenger, luteinizing hormone (LH), also increases, but at a slower rate.

These hormonal shifts can trigger an array of symptoms. The most common are night sweats (a *subdromal hot flash,* in medical terms), which can be just intense enough to disrupt sleep. The drop in estrogen levels also may cause hot flashes (bursts of perspiration that last from a few seconds to 15 minutes).

A woman's habits and health history also have an impact. Women with a lifelong history of depression are more likely to experience early perimenopause. Smokers experience more symptoms at an earlier age than nonsmokers. Heavier women also have more severe symptoms.

Menopause

About 10 to 15 percent of women breeze through this transition with only trivial symptoms. Another 10 to 15 percent are virtually disabled. The majority fall somewhere in between these extremes. Women who undergo surgical or medical menopause (the result of removal of their ovaries or chemotherapy) often experience abrupt symptoms, including flushing, sweating, sleeplessness, early morning awakenings, involuntary urination, changes in libido, mood swings, perception of memory loss, and changes in cognitive function.

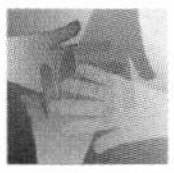

Race and ethnicity profoundly affect women's experience. African-American women report more hot flashes and night sweats but have more positive attitudes toward menopause. Japanese and Chinese women experience more muscle stiffness and fewer hot flashes but view menopause more negatively. Hispanic women reach menopause a year or two earlier than Caucasian women; Asian women, a year or two later.

Dwindling levels of estrogen subtly affect many aspects of a woman's health, from her mouth (where dryness, unusual tastes, burning, and gum problems can develop) to her skin (which may become drier, itchier, and overly sensitive to touch). With less estrogen to block them, a woman's androgens, or male hormones, may have a greater impact, causing acne, hair loss, and according to some anecdotal reports, surges in sexual appetite. (Other women, however, report a drop in sexual desire.)

At the same time, a woman's clitoris, vulva, and vaginal lining begin to shrivel, sometimes resulting in pain or bleeding during intercourse. Since the thinner genital tissues are less effective in keeping out bacteria and other pathogens, urinary tract infections may become more common. Some women develop breast or ovarian cysts, which usually go away on their own. Eventually, a woman's ovaries don't respond at all to her pituitary hormones. After the last ovulatory cycle, progesterone is no longer secreted, and estrogen levels decrease rapidly. A woman's testosterone level also falls.

In the United States, the average woman who reaches menopause has a life expectancy of about 30 more years. However, she faces risks of various diseases, including an increased risk of obesity, metabolic syndrome, heart disease, stroke, and breast cancer. Women can reduce these risks by exercise, good nutrition, and controlling weight both before and after menopause.

"Exercise is the best thing a woman can do for herself at midlife," says JoAnn Pinkerton, M.D., of the National Women's Health Resource Center. "It improves your heart function so you have less chance of heart disease. It improves your cognition so you think better. It decreases your risk of breast cancer. It helps your mood. It lessens the likelihood of depression. It increases energy and protects your bones."[8]

Hormone Therapy

Hormone therapy (HT) was long believed to prevent heart disease and strokes and help women live longer. But medical thinking on HT, particularly a combination of estrogen and progestin, has changed completely in recent years. HT is no longer recommended for reasons other than short-term relief of symptoms such as hot flashes and night sweats.

The Women's Health Initiative (WHI)—a series of clinical trials begun in 1991 on postmenopausal women—halted its study of combination estrogen/progestin therapy in July 2002 and its study of estrogen-only therapy in 2004 because of safety concerns. Combination therapy slightly increased the risk of breast cancer, heart disease, blood clots, and stroke. Women taking only estrogen for shorter periods did not have an elevated rate of breast cancer, but their risk increased significantly after 15 years of use.[9] In African-American women, estrogen use has been linked to higher breast cancer risk, particularly in leaner women.[10]

The Food and Drug Administration recommends hormone therapy for women with *acute* menopausal symptoms—but in the lowest possible dose and for the shortest possible time. For alternatives to HT, see Savvy Consumer: "Alternative Treatments for Menopausal Symptoms."

Researchers now think that many symptoms that had been linked with menopause, such as joint pain and stiffness, low backaches, and tiredness, are in fact related to aging or other conditions.

Men at Midlife

Although men don't experience the dramatic hormonal upheaval that women do, they do experience a decline by as much as 30 to 40 percent in their primary sex hormone, testosterone, between the ages of 48 and 70. This change, sometimes called *andropause,* may cause a range of symptoms, including decreased muscle mass, greater body fat, loss of bone density, flagging energy, lowered fertility, and impaired virility. Some researchers are experimenting with testosterone supplements, which in tests with young men have been shown to increase lean body mass and decrease body fat—at least temporarily. However, other researchers warn that, particularly in older men, excess testosterone might raise the risk of prostate cancer and heart disease.

After age 40, the prostate gland, which surrounds the urethra at the base of the bladder, enlarges. This condition, called *benign prostatic hypertrophy,* occurs in every man. By age 50, half of all men have some enlargement of the gland; after 70, three-quarters do. As it expands, the prostate tends to pinch the urethra, decreasing urinary flow and creating a sense of urinary urgency, particularly at night. Other warning signs of prostate problems include difficult urination, blood in the urine, painful ejaculation, or constant lower-back pain.

The drug Proscar (generic name, finasteride), which shrinks an

menopause The complete cessation of ovulation and menstruation for twelve consecutive months.

perimenopause The period from a woman's first irregular cycles to her last menstruation.

hormone therapy (HT) The use of supplemental hormones during and after menopause.

SAVVY CONSUMER

Alternative Treatments for Menopausal Symptoms

For Hot flashes

- **Lifestyle changes.** These include dressing and eating to avoid being too warm, sleeping in a cool room, and reducing stress. Avoid spicy foods and caffeine. Try deep breathing and stress reduction techniques, including meditation and other relaxation methods.
- **Antidepressants,** such as Effexor, Paxil, and Prozac. These medications have proved moderately effective in clinical trials.

For Vaginal Dryness

- **Vaginal lubricants** and moisturizers (available over the counter).
- **Products that release estrogen** locally (such as vaginal creams, a vaginal suppository, called Vagifem, and a plastic ring, called an Estring) are used for more severe dryness.

For Mood Swings

- **Lifestyle behaviors,** including getting enough sleep and being physically active.
- **Relaxation exercises.**
- **Antidepressant** or antianxiety drugs.

For Insomnia

- **Over-the-counter sleep aids.**
- **Milk products,** such as a glass of milk or cup of yogurt—choose low-fat or fat-free varieties—consumed at bedtime.
- **Do physical activity** in the morning or early afternoon—exercising later in the day may increase wakefulness.
- **Hot shower or bath** immediately before going to bed.

For Memory Problems

- **Mental exercises.**
- **Lifestyle behaviors,** especially getting enough sleep and being physically active.

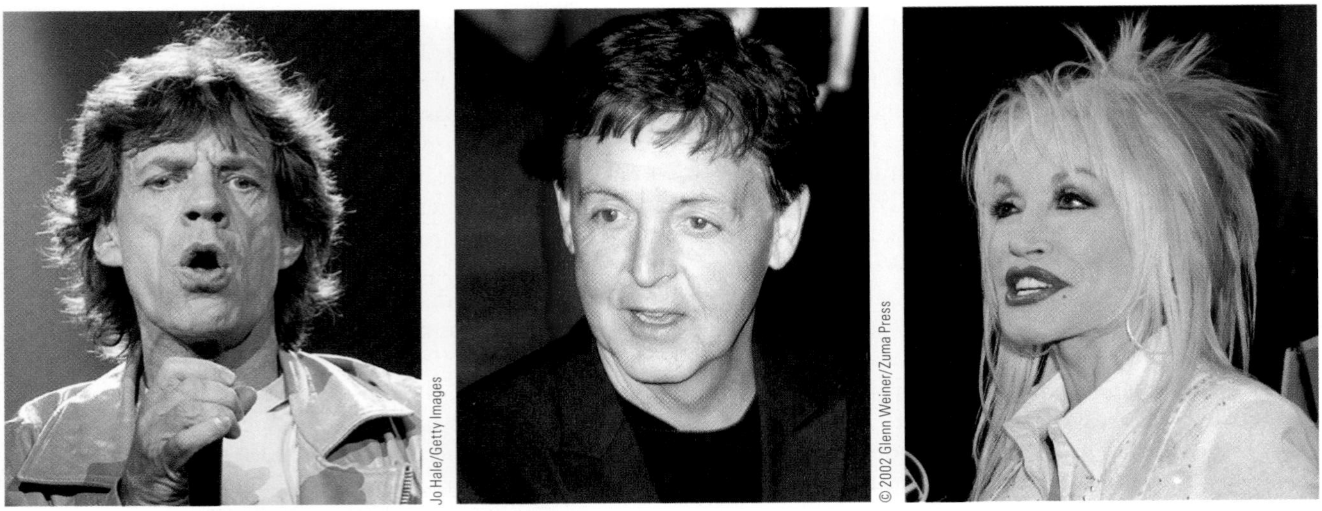

Jo Hale/Getty Images

© 2002 Glenn Weiner/Zuma Press

© Fred Prouser/Reuters/Corbis

What life after 60 can look like.

enlarged prostate, has provided an alternative to corrective surgery for many men. Other drugs are being tried experimentally. The older a man gets, the more likely he is to develop prostate cancer.

Sexuality and Aging

Health and sexuality interact in various ways as we age. When they are healthy and have a willing partner, a substantial number of older men remain sexually active. The fittest men and women report more frequent sexual activity.

Other research has found a relationship between sex and longevity. A Swedish study found that men, but not women, who had discontinued intercourse had higher death rates. A study of the entire male population of a small Welsh town found that the sexually active men had half the mortality of the inactive group. In a Duke University study, longevity in women correlated with enjoyment of sexual intercourse, rather than with its frequency.

Aging does cause some changes in sexual response: Women produce less vaginal lubrication. An older man needs more time to achieve an erection or orgasm and to attain another erection after ejaculating. Both men and women experience fewer contractions during orgasm. However, none of these changes reduces sexual pleasure or desire.

In a poll of more than 4,000 people between the ages of 40 and 80 in the United States, Canada, Australia, and New Zealand, around 30 percent of men aged 70 to 80 reported having sex five times in the past month, although only 8 percent of women reported doing so. Most women said the lack of sex was due to the absence of a partner. Some 40 percent of men reported problems such as erectile dysfunction.

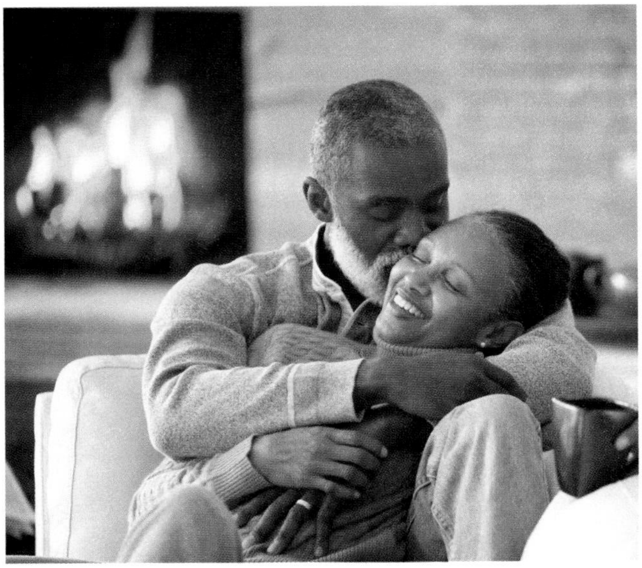

© Blend Images/Alamy

For older couples, sexual desire and pleasure can be enhanced by years of intimacy and affection.

The Challenges of Age

No matter how well we eat, exercise, and take care of ourselves, some physical changes are inevitable as we age. Figure 15-2 shows some of these changes, but most of them are not debilitating, and people can remain active and vital into extreme old age. Aging brains and bodies do become vulnerable to diseases like Alzheimer's and osteoporosis. Other common life problems, such as depression, substance misuse, and safe driving, become more challenging as we age.

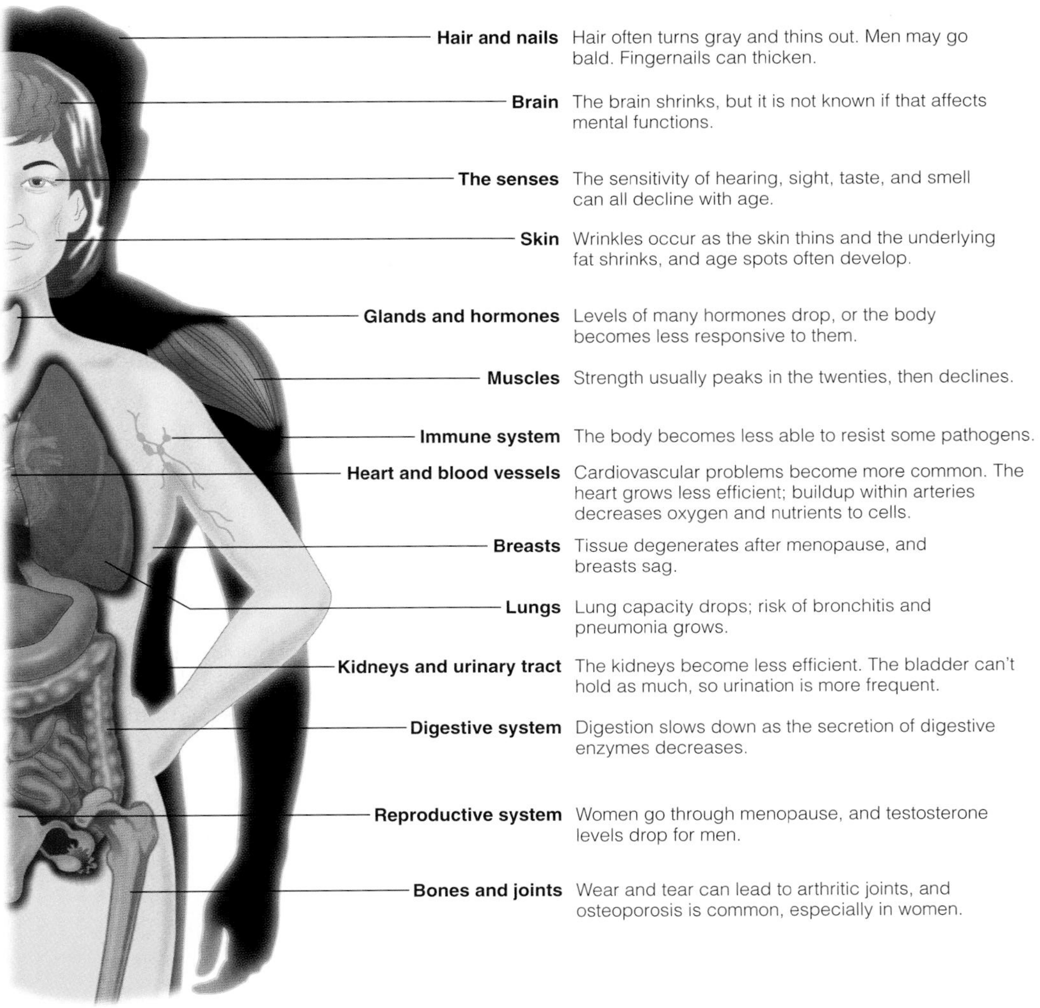

Hair and nails
Hair often turns gray and thins out. Men may go bald. Fingernails can thicken.
Brain
The brain shrinks, but it is not known if that affects mental functions.
The senses
The sensitivity of hearing, sight, taste, and smell can all decline with age.
Skin
Wrinkles occur as the skin thins and the underlying fat shrinks, and age spots often develop.
Glands and hormones
Levels of many hormones drop, or the body becomes less responsive to them.
Muscles
Strength usually peaks in the twenties, then declines.
Immune system
The body becomes less able to resist some pathogens.
Heart and blood vessels
Cardiovascular problems become more common. The heart grows less efficient; buildup within arteries decreases oxygen and nutrients to cells.
Breasts
Tissue degenerates after menopause, and breasts sag.
Lungs
Lung capacity drops; risk of bronchitis and pneumonia grows.
Kidneys and urinary tract
The kidneys become less efficient. The bladder can't hold as much, so urination is more frequent.
Digestive system
Digestion slows down as the secretion of digestive enzymes decreases.
Reproductive system
Women go through menopause, and testosterone levels drop for men.
Bones and joints
Wear and tear can lead to arthritic joints, and osteoporosis is common, especially in women.

FIGURE 15-2 The Effects of Aging on the Body

Alzheimer's Disease

About 15 percent of older Americans lose previous mental capabilities, a brain disorder called **dementia.** Sixty percent of these—a total of 4.5 million men and women over age 65—suffer from the type of dementia called **Alzheimer's disease,** a progressive deterioration of brain cells and mental capacity.

The percentage of people with Alzheimer's doubles for every five-year age group beyond 65. By age 85, nearly half of men and women have Alzheimer's. A person with the disease typically lives eight years after the onset of symptoms, but some live as long as 20 years. Some 13.2 million older Americans will develop Alzheimer's disease by 2050. The greatest increase will be among people age 85 and older.

Women are more likely to develop Alzheimer's than men, and women with Alzheimer's perform significantly worse than men in various visual, spatial, and memory tests. Initiating hormone therapy after age 60 increases the risk of Alzheimer's disease, but earlier use may reduce a woman's risk of this devastating illness.

African Americans have higher rates of Alzheimer's disease than Africans living in Africa, according to the first study to find differences in the incidence of this illness in an industrial and a nonindustrial country.

The early signs of dementia—insomnia, irritability, increased sensitivity to alcohol and other drugs, and decreased energy and tolerance of frustration—are usually subtle and insidious. Diagnosis requires a comprehensive assessment of an individual's medical history, physical health, and mental status, often involving brain scans and a variety of other tests.

dementia Deterioration of mental capability.

Alzheimer's disease A progressive deterioration of intellectual powers due to physiological changes within the brain; symptoms include diminishing ability to concentrate and reason, disorientation, depression, apathy, and paranoia.

Strategies for Prevention | Lowering Your Risk of Osteoporosis

Regardless of your age and gender, you can prevent future bone problems by taking some protective steps now. The most important guidelines are as follows:

- Get adequate calcium. Increased calcium intake, particularly during childhood and the growth spurt of adolescence, may produce a heavier, denser skeleton and reduce the risk of the complications of bone loss later in life. College-age women also can strengthen their bones and reduce their risk of osteoporosis by increasing their calcium intake and physical activity.
- If you do not get enough calcium in your diet, take daily supplements.
- Drink alcohol only moderately. More than two or three alcoholic beverages a day impairs intestinal calcium absorption.
- Don't smoke. Smokers tend to be thin and enter menopause earlier, thus extending the period of jeopardy from estrogen loss.
- Let the sunshine in (but don't forget your sunscreen). Vitamin D, a vitamin produced in the skin in reaction to sunlight, boosts calcium absorption.
- Exercise regularly. Both aerobic exercise and weight training can help preserve bone density.

Even though medical science cannot restore a brain that is in the process of being destroyed by an organic brain disease like Alzheimer's, medications can control difficult behavioral symptoms and enhance or partially restore cognitive ability. Often physicians find other medical or psychiatric problems, such as depression, in these patients; recognizing and treating these conditions can have a dramatic impact.

The FDA has approved several prescription drugs for people with mild to moderate dementia, including Cognex, Aricept, Exelon, and Reminyl. They all increase the level of the brain chemical acetylcholine. Researchers are studying other medications that might delay Alzheimer's or stop its progression.

Osteoporosis

Another age-related disease is *osteoporosis,* a condition in which losses in bone density become so severe that a bone will break after even slight trauma or injury (see photos). A chronic disease, osteoporosis is silent for years or decades before a fracture occurs.

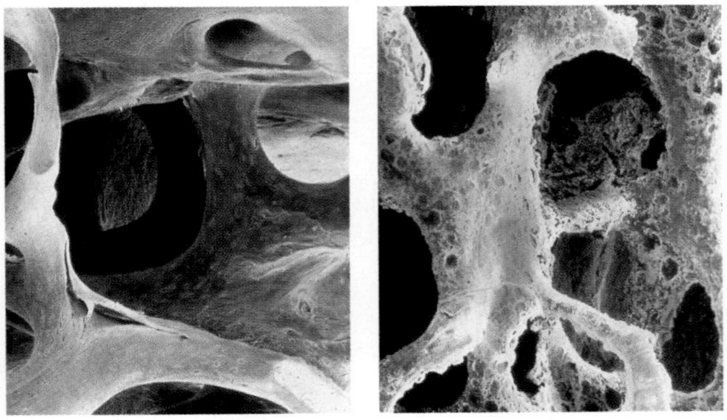

The effect of osteoporosis on bone density (a) Normal bone tissue. (b) After the onset of osteoporosis, bones lose density and become hollow and brittle.

Source: © Dr. P. Motta, Department of Anatomy, University "La Sapienza," Rome/Science Photo Library/Photo Researchers, Inc.

Women, who have smaller skeletons, are more vulnerable than men; in extreme cases, their spines may become so fragile that just bending causes severe pain. But although commonly seen as an illness of women, osteoporosis occurs frequently in men. One in every two women and one in four men over 50 will have an osteoporosis-related fracture in their lifetimes.

Calcium and vitamin D supplements in healthy postmenopausal women provide a modest benefit in preserving bone mass and preventing hip fractures but do not prevent other types of fractures, according to the results of a major clinical trial, part of the Women's Health Initiative (WHI), which studied more than 36,000 women over age 50.[11]

Preparing for Medical Crises and the End of Life

Throughout this book, we have stressed the ways in which you can determine how well and how long you live. You can also make decisions about the end of your life.

Various racial and ethnic groups have different preferences for their end-of-life wishes. Many Arab Americans prefer not to go to nursing homes as they near the end of their lives, while many African Americans are comfortable with nursing homes and hospitals. Hispanic individuals express strong concerns about dying with dignity. Many white people don't want their families to take care of them, although they—like members of other racial and ethnic groups—want their families nearby as they live out their last days.[12]

? FAQ What Are Advance Directives?

Every state and the District of Columbia has laws authorizing the use of **advance directives** to specify the kind of medical treatment individuals want in case of a medical crisis. These documents are important because, without clear indications of a person's preferences, hospitals and other institutions often make decisions on an individual's behalf, particularly if family members are not available or disagree.

The two most common advance directives are health-care proxies and living wills. Each state has different legal requirements for these forms. You can find state-specific forms at www.caringinfo.org. Once the forms are completed, make copies of your advance directives and give them to anyone who might have input in decisions on your behalf. Also give copies to your physician or health-care organization and ask that they be made part of your medical record.

Health-Care Proxy

A *health-care proxy* is an advance directive that gives someone else the power to make health decisions on your behalf. This advance directive is also called Medical Power of Attorney or Health-Care Power of Attorney. People typically name a relative or close friend as their agent. Let family and friends know that you have completed a health care-proxy. Tell your primary physician, but you should not designate your doctor as your agent. Many states prohibit this. Even when allowed, it is not a good idea because your doctor's primary responsibility is to administer care.

Living Will

Individuals can use a **living will** (also called health-care directive or physician's directive) to indicate whether they want or don't want all possible medical treatments and technology used to prolong their lives. Figure 15-3 shows a physician's directive for Texas and notes where state laws may differ.

The Five Wishes

An innovative document called "Five Wishes" helps the aged, the seriously ill, their loved ones, and caregivers prepare for medical crises. Written with the help of the American Bar Association's Commission on the Legal Problems of the Elderly, the Five Wishes document has a health-care proxy, a health-care directive, and three other "wishes":

- Which person they want to make health-care decisions for them when they are no longer able to do so.
- Which kinds of medical treatments they do or don't want.
- How comfortable they want to be made.
- How they want people to treat them.
- What they want loved ones to know.

The Five Wishes document (at www.agingwithdignity.org) is legally valid in 38 states. Churches, synagogues, hospices, hospitals, physicians, social service agencies, and employers also are distributing the document to help people plan for their own care or that of aging parents.

DNR Order

You can also sign an advance directive specifying that you want to be allowed to die naturally—you do not want to be resuscitated in case your heart stops beating. **Do-not-resuscitate (DNR)** orders apply mainly to hospitalized, terminally ill patients and must be signed by a physician. However, in some states, it is possible to complete a *nonhospital DNR* form that specifies an individual's wish not to be resuscitated at home. Patients in the final stages of advanced cancer or AIDS may choose to use such forms to protect their rights in case paramedics are called to their home.

Even healthy young people may suffer injuries or illnesses that leave them capable of surviving only with artificial assistance. Some individuals would rather not face the possibility of making end-of-life decisions. Others argue that the surviving family should do what they feel is right. Is it better to make your preferences clear in an advance directive? Or can such difficult decisions be left until old age?

You Decide

Holographic Wills

Perhaps you think that only wealthy or older people need to write wills. However, if you're married, have children, or own property, you should either hire a lawyer to draw up a will, use software to generate a will, or at least write a **holographic will** yourself, specifying who you wish to raise your children and who should have your property. If you die *intestate* (without a will), the state will make these decisions for you. Even a modest estate can be tied up in court for a long period

advance directives Documents that specify an individual's preferences regarding treatment in a medical crisis.

living will An advance directive providing instructions for the use of life-sustaining procedures in the event of terminal illness or injury.

do-not-resuscitate (DNR) An advance directive expressing an individual's preference that resuscitation efforts not be made during a medical crisis.

holographic will A will wholly in the handwriting of its author.

Directives are effective until they're revoked. Still, it's considered a good idea to initial and date your directive every few years to show that it still expresses your wishes.

DIRECTIVE TO PHYSICIANS
For Persons 18 Years of Age and Over

I, ______________, recognize that the best health care is based upon a partnership of trust and communication with my physician. My physician and I will make health care decisions together as long as I am of sound mind and able to make my wishes known. If there comes a time that I am unable to make medical decisions about myself because of illness or injury, I direct that the following treatment preferences be honored:

If, in the judgment of my physician, I am suffering with a terminal condition from which I am expected to die within six months, even with available life-sustaining treatment provided in accordance with prevailing standards of medical care:

____ I request that all treatments other than those needed to keep me comfortable be discontinued or withheld and my physician allow me to die as gently as possible; OR

____ I request that I be kept alive in this terminal condition using available life-sustaining treatment (THIS SELECTION DOES NOT APPLY TO HOSPICE CARE).

If, in the judgment of my physician, I am suffering with an irreversible condition so that I cannot care for myself or make decisions for myself and am expected to die without life-sustaining treatment provided in accordance with prevailing standards of care:

____ I request that all treatments other than those needed to keep me comfortable be discontinued or withheld and my physician allow me to die as gently as possible; OR

____ I request that I be kept alive in this irreversible condition using available life-sustaining treatment (THIS SELECTION DOES NOT APPLY TO HOSPICE CARE).

Additional requests: (After discussion with your physician, you may wish to consider listing particular treatments in this space that you do or do not want in specific circumstances, such as artificial nutrition and fluids, intravenous antibiotics, etc. Be sure to state whether you do or do not want the particular treatment).

In most states, directives will have a space to specify treatment you do or don't want. Ask your physician what to include here. You can:

- Ask for or prohibit use of artificial feeding tubes, cardiopulmonary resuscitation, antibiotics, dialysis, and respirators.
- Ask for pain medication to keep you comfortable.
- State whether you would prefer to die in the hospital or at home.
- Designate a proxy—someone to make decisions about your treatment when you're unable.
- Donate organs or other body parts.

After signing this DIRECTIVE, if my representative or I elect hospice care, I understand and agree that only those treatments needed to keep me comfortable would be provided and I would not be given available life-sustaining treatments.

If I do not have a Medical Power of Attorney and I am unable to make my wishes known, I designate the following person(s) to make treatment decisions with my physician compatible with my personal values.

Name ______________________________

Address ______________________________

Name ______________________________

Address ______________________________

(If a Medical Power of Attorney has been executed, then an agent already has been named and you should not list additional names in this document.)

If the above persons are not available, or if I have not designated a spokesperson, I understand that a spokesperson will be chosen for me following standards specified in the laws of Texas. If, in the judgment of my physician, my death is imminent within minutes to hours, even with the use of all available medical treatment provided within the prevailing standard of care, I acknowledge that all treatments may be withheld or removed except those needed to maintain my comfort.

In some states the directive is valid for pregnant women. Others exclude women during all or part of their pregnancy, although that has been challenged on the grounds that a woman's right to privacy doesn't end when she becomes pregnant.

I understand that under Texas law this Directive has no effect if I have been diagnosed as pregnant. This DIRECTIVE will remain in effect until I revoke it. No other person may do so. I understand that I may revoke this DIRECTIVE at any time.

You can revoke or amend your directive at any time simply by making a statement to a physician, nurse, or other health-care worker.

I understand the full import of this DIRECTIVE and I am emotionally and mentally competent to make this DIRECTIVE.

Signed ______________________________

City, County, and State of Residence ______________________________

Date ______________________________

Two competent witnesses must sign below, acknowledging your signature. The witness designated as "Witness 1" may not be a person designated to make a treatment decision for the patient and may not be related to the patient by blood or marriage. The witness may not be entitled to any part of the estate and may not have a claim against the estate of the patient. The witness may not be the attending physician or an employee of the attending physician. If this witness is an employee of the health care facility in which the patient is being cared for, this witness may not be involved in providing direct patient care to the patient. This witness may not be an officer, director, partner, or business office employee of the health care facility in which the patient is being cared for or of any parent organization of the health care facility.

Witness 1 ______________________________

Witness 2 ______________________________

TEXAS LAW DOES NOT REQUIRE THIS DIRECTIVE TO BE NOTARIZED.

In some states your signature must be notarized. Elsewhere, the signature of the witnesses is adequate, although if you're in a hospital or nursing home, in some states you may need as an additional witness the chief of staff or medical director.

FIGURE 15-3 Preparing a Physician's Directive

Source: Texas Medical Association.

of time, depriving family members of money when they need it most.

A holographic will is a handwritten (not typed) statement that some states will recognize. You can:

- **Name a family member** or friend as the executor, the person who sees that your wishes are carried out.
- **List the things you own** and to whom you want them to go; include addresses and telephone numbers, if possible.
- **Select a guardian for your children** (if any), presumably someone whose ideas about raising children are similar to your own. Be sure that any named guardians are willing and able to accept this responsibility before writing them into your will.
- **Specify any funeral arrangements.**

Be sure to keep the will in a safe place, where your executor, family members, or closest beneficiary can find it quickly and easily; tell them where it is.

Death and Dying

Some 2.4 million people die in the United States each year. Although most are older, death occurs in all age groups. The causes of death vary with both age and gender. Among those under age 35, intentional and nonintentional injury are the primary causes of death. Among older Americans, cancer and heart disease are the top killers. Men typically die at a younger age than women. College-age individuals are most likely to die as a result of accidents or assaults. (See Student Snapshot: "Dying Young.")

Student Snapshot

Dying Young

The Five Leading Causes of Death for College-Age Americans

1. Unintentional injury (accidents)
2. Homicide/Assault
3. For men } Suicide
4. For women } Suicide
3. For women } Cancer
4. For men } Cancer
5. Heart disease

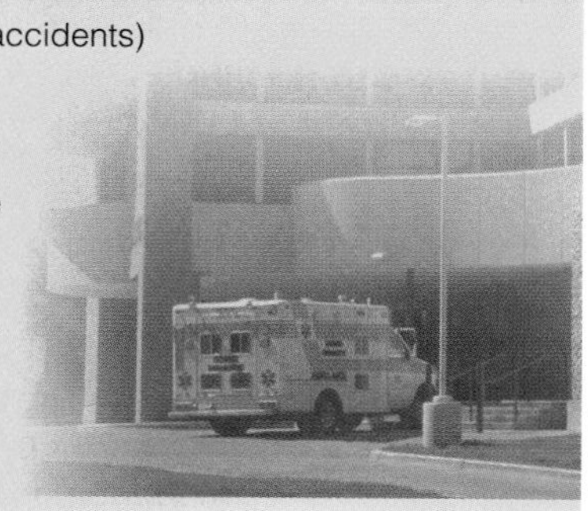

© 2006 Jupiter Images

Source: National Center for Injury Prevention and Control.

Defining Death

In our society, death isn't a part of everyday life, as it once was. Because machines can now keep alive people who, in the past, would have died, the definition of death has become more complex. Death has been broken down into the following categories:

- **Functional death.** The end of all vital functions, such as heartbeat and respiration.
- **Cellular death.** The gradual death of body cells after the heart stops beating. If placed in a tissue culture or, as is the case with various organs, transplanted to another body, some cells can remain alive indefinitely.
- **Death.** The moment when the heart stops beating.
- **Brain death.** The end of all brain activity, indicated by an absence of electrical activity (confirmed by an electroencephalogram, or EEG) and a lack of reflexes. The notion of brain death is bound up with what we consider to be the actual person, or self. The destruction of a person's brain means that his or her personality no longer exists; the lower brain centers controlling respiration and circulation no longer function.
- **Spiritual death.** The moment when the soul, as defined by many religions, leaves the body.

When does a person actually die? The traditional legal definition of death is failure of the lungs or heart to function. However, because respiration and circulation can be maintained by artificial means, most states have declared that an individual is considered dead only when the brain, including the brain stem, completely stops functioning. Brain-death laws prohibit a medical staff from "pulling the plug" if there is any hope of sustaining life.

Denying Death

Most of us don't quite believe that we're going to die. A reasonable amount of denial helps us focus on the day-to-day realities of living. However, excessive denial can be life-threatening. Some drivers, for instance, refuse to buckle their seat belts because they refuse to acknowledge that a drunk driver might collide with them. Similarly, cigarette smokers deny that lung cancer will ever strike them, and people who eat high-fat meals deny that they'll ever suffer a heart attack.

One important factor in denial is the nature of the threat. It's easy to believe that death is at hand when someone's pointing a gun at you; it's much harder to think that cigarette smoking might cause your death 20 or 30 years down the road. The late Elisabeth Kübler-Ross, a psychiatrist who extensively studied the process of dying, described the downside of denying death in *Death: The Final Stage of Growth.*

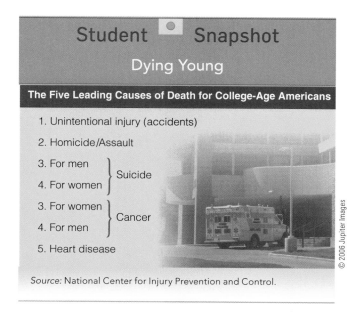

> It is the denial of death that is partially responsible for people living empty, purposeless lives; for when you live as if you'll live forever, it becomes too easy to postpone the things you know that you must do. You live your life in preparation for tomorrow or in the remembrance of yesterday—and meanwhile, each today is lost. In contrast, when you fully understand that each day you awaken could be the last you have, you take the time that day to grow, to become more of who you really are, to reach out to other human beings.[13]

Emotional Responses to Dying

Kübler-Ross identified five typical stages of reaction that a person goes through when facing death (Figure 15-4).

1. **Denial ("No, not me").** At first knowledge that death is coming, a terminally ill patient rejects the news. The denial overcomes the initial shock and allows the person to begin to gather together his or her resources. Denial, at this point, is a healthy defense mechanism. It can become distressful, however, if it's reinforced by the relatives and friends of the dying patient.
2. **Anger ("Why me?").** In the second stage, the dying person begins to feel resentment and rage regarding imminent death. The anger may be directed at God or at the patient's family and caregivers, who can do little but try to endure any expressions of anger, provide comfort, and help the patient on to the next stage.
3. **Bargaining ("Yes, me, but . . .").** In this stage, a patient may try to bargain, usually with God, for a way to reverse or at least postpone dying. The patient may promise, in exchange for recovery, to do good works or to see family members more often. Alternatively, the patient may say, "Let me live long enough to see my grandchild born" or "to see the spring again."
4. **Depression ("Yes, it's me").** In the fourth stage, the patient gradually realizes the full consequences of his or her condition. This may begin as grieving for health that has been lost and then become anticipatory grieving for the loss that is to come of friends, loved ones, and life itself. This stage is perhaps the most difficult: The dying person should not be left alone during this period. Neither should loved ones try to cheer up the patient, who must be allowed to grieve.
5. **Acceptance ("Yes, me; and I'm ready").** In this last stage, the person has accepted the reality of death: The moment looms as neither frightening nor painful, neither sad nor happy—only inevitable. The person who waits for the end of life may ask to see fewer visitors, to separate from other people, or perhaps to turn to just one person for support.

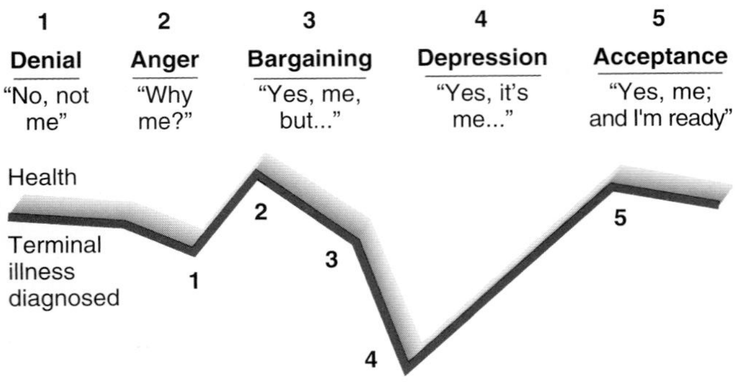

FIGURE 15-4 ▮ Kübler-Ross's Five Stages of Adjustment to Facing Death

Several stages may occur at the same time and some may happen out of sequence. Each stage may take days or only hours or minutes. Throughout, denial may come back to assert itself unexpectedly, and hope for a medical breakthrough or a miraculous recovery is forever present.

Some experts dispute Kübler-Ross's basic five-stage theory as too simplistic and argue that not all people go through such well-defined stages in the dying process. The way a person faces death is often a mirror of the way he or she has faced other major stresses in life: Those who have had the most trouble adjusting to other crises will have the most trouble adjusting to the news of their impending death.

An individual's will to live can postpone death for a while. In a study of elderly Chinese women, researchers found that their death rate decreased before and during a holiday during which the senior women in a household play a central role; it increased after the celebration. A similar temporary drop occurs among Jews at the time of Passover. However, different events may have different effects. The prospect of an upcoming birthday postpones death in women but hastens it in men. The will to live typically fluctuates in terminal patients, varying along with depression, anxiety, shortness of breath, and a sense of well-being.

The family of a dying person experiences a spectrum of often wrenching emotions. Family members, too, may deny the verdict of death, rage at the doctors and nurses who can't do more to save their loved one, bargain with God to give up their own health if necessary, sink into helplessness and depression, and finally accept the reality of their anticipated loss.

? FAQ What Do We Know About Near-Death Experiences?

Reports of near-death experiences have grown, thanks largely to advances in emergency medical care. Most are remarkably similar, whether they occur in children or adults, whether they're the result of accidents or illnesses, even whether the individuals actually are near death or only think they are. Some individuals who have survived a close brush with death report **autoscopy** (watching, from several feet in the air, resuscitation attempts on their own bodies) or **transcendence** (the sense of passing into a foreign region or dimension). Some see light, often at the end of a tunnel. Their vision seems clearer; their hearing, sharper. Some recall scenes from their lives or feel the presence of loved ones who have died. Many report profound feelings of joy, calm, and peace. Fewer than 1 percent of those who've reported near-death experiences described them as frightening or distressing, although a larger number recall transitory feelings of fear or confusion.

Many near-death experiences occur in individuals who've been sedated or given other medications; however, many others do not. Several studies have shown that individuals who received medication or anesthesia were actually less likely to remember near-death experiences than those who hadn't had any drugs. Some scientists have speculated that lack of oxygen, changes in blood gases, altered brain functioning, or the release of neurotransmitters (messenger chemicals in the brain) may play a role in near-death experiences. However, there's little solid evidence that physiological events are responsible. There's also no proof that wishful thinking, cultural conditioning, posttraumatic stress, or other psychological mechanisms may be at work. For now, the most that scientists can say for sure about this medical mystery is that it needs further study.

Suicide

Suicide increases with age and is most common in persons aged 65 years and older. This age group accounts for 18 percent of all suicides in the United States.[14] For every completed suicide, there are 10 to 40 unsuccessful attempts. (Chapter 2 presents a detailed discussion of the risk factors and warning signs of suicide.)

One of the main factors leading to suicide is illness, especially terminal illness. A great deal of debate centers on quality of life, yet there is no reliable or consistent way to measure this. Patients who are dying may feel some quality of life, even when others do not recognize it, or their evaluations of the quality of their lives may fluctuate. Dying patients who say their lives are not worth living may be suffering from depression; hopelessness is one of its characteristic symptoms.

"Rational" Suicide

An elderly widow suffering from advanced cancer takes a lethal overdose of sleeping pills. A young man with several AIDS-related illnesses shoots himself. A woman in her fifties, diagnosed as having Alzheimer's disease, asks a doctor to help her end her life. Are these suicides "rational" because these individuals used logical reasoning in deciding to end their lives?

The question is intensely controversial. Advocates of the right to "self-deliverance" argue that individuals in great pain or faced with the prospect of a debilitating, hopeless battle against an incurable disease can and should be able to decide to end their lives. As legislatures and the legal system tackle the thorny questions of an individual's right to die, mental health professionals worry that, even in those with fatal diseases, suicidal wishes often stem from undiagnosed depression.

Numerous studies have indicated that most patients with painful, progressive, or terminal illnesses do not want to kill themselves. The percentage of those who report thinking about suicide ranges from 5 to 20 percent; most of these have major depressions. Many mental health professionals argue that what makes patients with severe illnesses suicidal is depression, not their physical condition. Cognitive therapy (discussed in Chapter 2) has proved effective in reducing the risk of suicide in even extremely suicidal patients, many of whom were already taking drugs for depression.[15]

Because depression may indeed warp the ability to make a rational decision about suicide, mental health professionals urge physicians and family members to make sure individuals with chronic or fatal illnesses are evaluated for depression and given medication, psychotherapy, or both. It is also important for everyone to allow enough time—an average of three to eight weeks—to see if treatment for depression will make a difference in their desire to keep living.

The Practicalities of Death

At a time of great emotional pain, grieving family members must cope with medical, legal, and practical concerns, including obtaining a medical certificate of the cause of death, registering the death, and making funeral arrangements. They also may want to arrange for organ donations and, in some circumstances, an autopsy.

Funeral Arrangements

A body can be either buried or cremated. Burial requires the purchase of a cemetery plot, which many families do decades before death. A burial is typically the third most expensive purchase of a lifetime, behind the cost of a house and car. The average national costs range as high as $6,000, although they vary consider-

autoscopy The sensation of one's self being outside the body, often experienced by individuals in near-death medical crises.

transcendence The sense of passing into a foreign region or dimension, often experienced by a person near death.

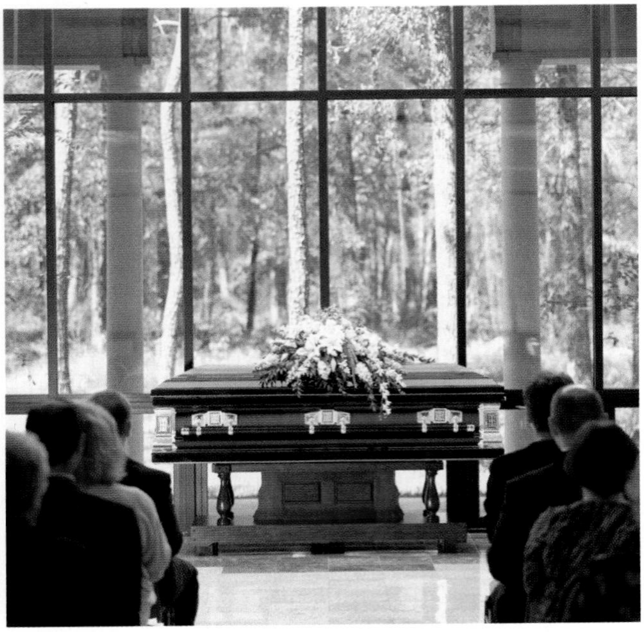

© Terry Vine/Stone/Getty Images

Funerals and memorial services help those in mourning to honor the deceased and to come to terms with their loss.

ably. Memorial societies are voluntary groups that help people plan in advance for death. They obtain services at moderate cost, keep the arrangements simple and dignified, and—most important, perhaps—ease the emotional and financial burden on the rest of the family when death finally does come.

If the body is to be cremated, you must comply with some additional formalities, with which the funeral director can help you. After a *cremation* (incineration of the remains), you can either collect the ashes to keep, bury, or scatter yourself, or ask the crematorium to dispose of them.

The tradition of a funeral may help survivors come to terms with the death, enabling them to mourn their loss and to celebrate the dead person's life. Funerals are usually held two to four days after the death. Many have two parts: a religious ceremony at a church or funeral home, and a burial ceremony at the grave site.

Alternatively, the body may be disposed of immediately, through burial, cremation, or bequeathal to a medical school, and a memorial service held later. In a memorial service, the body is not present, which may change the focus of the service from the person's death to his or her life.

Grief

An estimated 8 million Americans lose a member of their immediate family each year. Each death leaves an average of five people bereaved. Such loss may be the single most upsetting and feared event in a person's life. It produces a wide range of reactions, including anxiety, guilt, anger, and financial concern. Many may see the death of an old person as less tragic than the death of a child or young person. A sudden death is more of a shock than one following a long illness. A suicide can be particularly devastating, because family members may wonder whether they could have done anything to prevent it. The cause of death also can affect the reactions of friends and acquaintances. Some people express less sympathy and support when individuals are murdered or take their own lives.

Encountering death can make us feel alone and vulnerable. The most common and one of the most painful experiences is the death of a parent. When both parents die, individuals may feel like orphaned children. They mourn not just for the father and mother who are gone, but also for their lost role of being someone's child.

The death of a child can be even more devastating. Eventually parents may be able to resolve their grief and accept the death as "God's will" or as "something that happens." Time erases their pain and they feel a desire to get on with their lives, consciously putting the loss behind them. Others deal with their grief by keeping busy or by substituting other problems or situations to take their minds off their loss. Yet many parents who lose a child continue to grieve for many years. Although the pain of their loss diminishes with time, they view it as part of themselves and describe an emptiness inside—even though most have rich, meaningful, and happy daily lives.

The loss of a mate can also have a profound impact, although men's and women's responses to the death—and their subsequent health risks—may depend on how their spouses died. Men whose wives die suddenly face a much greater risk of dying themselves than those whose wives die after a long illness. On the other hand, women whose husbands die after a long illness face greater risk of dying than other widows. The reason may be that men whose wives were chronically ill learned how to cope with the loss of their nurturers, while women who spend a long time caring for an ill husband may be at greater risk because of the combined burdens of caregiving and loss of financial support.

Bereavement is not a rare occurrence on college campuses, but it is largely an ignored problem. Counselors have called upon universities to help students who have lost a loved one through initiatives such as training nonbereaved students to provide peer support and raising consciousness about bereavement.

Grief's Effects on Health

Men and women who lose partners, parents, or children endure so much stress that they're at increased risk of serious physical and mental illness, and even of prema-

Strategies for Change: Coping with Grief

- **Accept your feelings**—sorrow, fear, emptiness, whatever—as normal. Don't try to deny emotions such as anger, guilt, despair, or relief.
- **Let others help you**—by bringing you food, by taking care of daily necessities, by providing companionship and comfort. (It will make them feel better, too.)
- **Face each day as it comes.** Let yourself live in the here-and-now until you're ready to face the future. Give yourself time—perhaps more than you ever imagined—for the pain to ebb, the scars to heal, and your life to move on.
- **Don't think there's a right or wrong way to grieve.** Mourning takes many forms, and there's no set timetable for working through the various stages of grief.
- **Seek professional counseling** if you remain intensely distressed for more than six months or your grief does not ease over time. Therapy can help prevent potentially serious physical and psychological problems.

ture death. Studies of the health effects of grief have found the following:

- Grief produces changes in the respiratory, hormonal, and central nervous systems and may affect functions of the heart, blood, and immune systems.
- Grieving adults may experience mood swings between sadness and anger, guilt and anxiety.
- They may feel physically sick, lose their appetite, sleep poorly, or fear that they're going crazy because they "see" the deceased person in different places.
- Friendships and remarriage offer the greatest protection against health problems.
- Some widows may have increased rates of depression, suicide, and death from cirrhosis of the liver. The greatest risk factors are poor previous mental and physical health and a lack of social support.
- Grieving parents, partners, and adult children are at increased risk of serious physical and mental illness, suicide, and premature death.

Sometimes grief progresses from an emotionally painful but normal experience to a more persistent problem, called *complicated grief*.[16] Individuals who experience very long-lasting or severe symptoms, including inability to accept a loved one's death, persistent thoughts about the death, and preoccupation with the lost loved one, can benefit from professional treatment.

LEARN IT / LIVE IT

Living Long and Well

"Every man desires to live long," wrote Jonathan Swift, "but no man would be old." We all wish for long lives, yet we want to avoid the disease and disability that can tarnish our golden years. Here are the best ways to do so.

- **Exercise regularly.** By improving blood flow, staving off depression, warding off heart disease, and enhancing well-being, regular workouts help keep mind and body in top form.
- **Don't smoke.** Every cigarette you puff can snuff out seven minutes of your life, according to the Centers for Disease Control and Prevention.
- **Watch your weight and blood pressure.** Increases in these vital statistics can increase your risk of hypertension, cardiovascular disease, and other health problems.
- **Eat more fruits and vegetables.** These foods, rich in vitamins and protective antioxidants, can reduce your risk of cancer and damage from destructive free radicals.
- **Cut down on fat.** Fatty foods can clog the arteries and contribute to various cancers.
- **Limit drinking.** Alcohol can undermine physical health and sabotage mental acuity.
- **Cultivate stimulating interests.** Elderly individuals with complex and interesting lifestyles are most likely to retain sharp minds and memories beyond age 70.
- **Don't worry; be happy.** At any age, emotional turmoil can undermine well-being. Relaxation techniques, such as meditation, help by reducing stress.
- **Reach out.** Try to keep in contact with other people of all ages and experiences. Make the effort to invite them to your home or go out with them. On a regular basis, do something to help another person.
- **Make the most of your time.** Greet each day with a specific goal—to take a walk, write letters, visit a friend.

15 Making This Chapter Work for You

Review Questions

1. Factors that contribute to staying healthy longer include all of the following *except*
   a. avoiding illness.
   b. moderate smoking.
   c. regular exercise.
   d. lifelong learning.
2. Physically fit people over age 60
   a. have lower risk of dying from chronic heart disease.
   b. can regain the fitness level of a 25-year-old.
   c. show no difference in levels of anxiety and depression.
   d. have higher health-care expenses.
3. Which statement about the aging brain is *false?*
   a. When brain cells die, surrounding cells can fill the gaps to maintain cognitive function.
   b. Remembering names and recalling information may take longer.
   c. "Use it or lose it."
   d. Mental ability and physical ability both decline with age.
4. Which statement about aging is *false?*
   a. The most common nutritional disorder in the elderly is obesity.
   b. In men, sexual activity and longevity are linked.
   c. Hormone therapy reduces the risk of heart disease in menopausal women.
   d. Seniors who take up new hobbies late in life may slow aging within the brain.
5. Which statement about age-related problems is correct?
   a. Osteoporosis affects only women.
   b. Alzheimer's disease is a form of dementia.
   c. Osteoporosis treatment includes surgery.
   d. Drug interactions do not occur in the elderly.
6. When should concern change to intervention?
   a. Uncle Charlie is 85 and continues to drive himself to the grocery store and to the Senior Center during the daytime.
   b. Nana takes pills at breakfast, lunch, and dinner but sometimes mixes them up.
   c. Mom's hot flashes have become a family joke.
   d. Your older brother can never remember where he put his car keys.
7. According to Elisabeth Kübler-Ross, an individual facing death goes through all of the following emotional stages *except*
   a. bargaining.
   b. acceptance.
   c. denial.
   d. repression.
8. The gender gap related to longevity
   a. is due to deficiencies in the Y chromosome.
   b. results from the presence of a mutant gene.
   c. may be due to the X chromosome and its hormonal influences on the immune system.
   d. is about 13 years in the United States.
9. An advance directive
   a. indicates who should have your property in the event you die.
   b. may authorize which individuals may not participate in your health care if you are unable to care for yourself.
   c. can specify your desires related to the use of medical treatments and technology to prolong your life.
   d. should specify which physician you designate to be your health-care proxy.
10. You can best help a friend who is bereaved by
    a. encouraging him to have a few drinks to forget his pain.
    b. simply spending time with her.
    c. avoiding talking about his loss because it is awkward.
    d. reminding her about all she still has in her life.

Answers to these questions can be found on page 422.

Critical Thinking

1. How are your parents or other mentors staying fit and alert as they age? Do you think you might use similar strategies?
2. Do you think that coming to terms with mortality allows an individual to live each day to its fullest, rather than putting off what he or she would like to do until tomorrow? How does this concept affect your own life? Explain. Do you believe in a next life? How does this affect your view of life and death?
3. Have your living parents and grandparents written advanced directives or a living will? Have you discussed with them their preferences regarding treatment in the event of a medical crisis? If you haven't had this discussion with your family, how can you begin the process of helping your parents or grandparents communicate their wishes?
4. As many as 10,000 people in this country are chronically unconscious, kept alive by artificial respirators and feeding tubes. If you were in an accident that left you in a vegetative state, would you want doctors to do everything possible to fight for your life? Would you want to spend months or even years totally unaware of your surroundings? Should health-care professionals have the right to declare that anyone is too old, too ill, or too frail to try to save? Should they have the right to insist that someone live on even if that person isn't experiencing much of a life?

LACC Extra Credit Assignment

15. Given that you will not be as active as a 20 year old when you are 65 or older. Draft an exercise prescription for a 65 year old if:

   A. He/she is in poor shape
   B. He/she is in moderate shape
   C. He/she is in good shape

Media Menu

ThomsonNOW™ Go to the ThomsonNOW website at **http://www.thomsonedu.com** that will:

- Help you evaluate your knowledge of the material.
- Allow you to take an exam-prep quiz.
- Provide a Personalized Learning Plan targeting resources that address areas you should study.
- Coach you through identifying target goals for behavioral change and creating and monitoring your personal change plan throughout the semester.

INTERNET CONNECTIONS

National Institute on Aging
www.nia.nih.gov

This government site features a comprehensive array of resources on aging, including publications on a variety of geriatric health topics, current news events, and a resource directory for older people.

RealAge
www.realage.com

This site features diet and exercise assessment tools—such as a BMI calculator, exercise estimator, and RealAge assessment quizzes on a variety of health topics—to help you determine your risk of disease and what you can do to reduce this risk. The main feature is an interactive, online personal lifestyle assessment that also gives you options for "growing younger."

U.S. Administration on Aging
http://aoa.gov

This site, part of the Department of Health and Human Services, has information for seniors and their families on promoting healthy lifestyles and general aging topics.

The End of Life: Exploring Death in America
www.npr.org/programs/death/

This site, sponsored by National Public Radio, contains transcripts and resources from an *All Things Considered* series focusing on how Americans deal with death and dying. Features include personal stories, a place where you can tell your own story, and a comprehensive list of organizations that can help families who are coping with death, dying, and the diseases of old age.

InfoTrac College Edition Activities Log on, insert **advance directives** into the Keyword search box, and limit your search to the past year. When you get the results, Mark articles to review, then Select one to read. Summarize three or four key points from the article.

You can find additional readings related to personal health with InfoTrac College Edition, an online library of more than 900 journals and publications. Follow the instructions for accessing InfoTrac College Edition that were packaged with your textbook; then search for articles using a keyword search.

For additional links, resources, and suggested readings on the InfoTrac College Edition, visit our Health and Wellness Resource Center at **http://health.wadsworth.com.**

Key Terms

The terms listed are used on the page indicated. Definitions of the terms are in the Glossary at the end of this book.

advance directives 413
aging 403
Alzheimer's disease 411
autoscopy 417
dementia 411
do-not-resuscitate (DNR) 413
holographic will 413
hormone therapy (HT) 408
living will 413
menopause 408
perimenopause 408
transcendence 417

Making This Chapter Work for You

Answers to multiple choice questions

Chapter 1
1. d; 2. c; 3. b; 4. c; 5. a; 6. b; 7. c; 8. d; 9. c; 10. c

Chapter 2
1. b; 2. d; 3. a; 4. c; 5. c; 6. c; 7. a; 8. b; 9. d; 10. b

Chapter 3
1. b; 2. d; 3. a; 4. a; 5. c; 6. b; 7. a; 8. c; 9. d; 10. b

Chapter 4
1. c; 2. b; 3. c; 4. b; 5. c; 6. d; 7. b; 8. b; 9. b; 10. d

Chapter 5
1. c; 2. a; 3. d; 4. a; 5. d; 6. c; 7. a; 8. a; 9. a; 10. b

Chapter 6
1. c; 2. b; 3. c; 4. c; 5. d; 6. a; 7. c; 8. c; 9. a; 10. c

Chapter 7
1. d; 2. a; 3. b; 4. a; 5. d; 6. c; 7. d; 8. d; 9. b; 10. d

Chapter 8
1. c; 2. d; 3. a; 4. c; 5. c; 6. b; 7. c; 8. a; 9. b; 10. d

Chapter 9
1. a; 2. c; 3. a; 4. b; 5. c; 6. a; 7. d; 8. b; 9. b; 10. c

Chapter 10
1. b; 2. a; 3. b; 4. b; 5. d; 6. a; 7. d; 8. a; 9. d; 10. b

Chapter 11
1. a; 2. c; 3. d; 4. b; 5. c; 6. c; 7. d; 8. a; 9. b; 10. d

Chapter 12
1. b; 2. c; 3. a; 4. b; 5. d; 6. c; 7. c; 8. c; 9. d; 10. b

Chapter 13
1. c; 2. b; 3. a; 4. c; 5. b; 6. c; 7. d; 8. c; 9. d; 10. b

Chapter 14
1. d; 2. c; 3. b; 4. a; 5. b; 6. c; 7. b; 8. a; 9. c; 10. b

Chapter 15
1. b; 2. a; 3. d; 4. c; 5. b; 6. b; 7. d; 8. c; 9. c; 10. b

Glossary

abscess A localized accumulation of pus and disintegrating tissue.

absorption The passage of substances into or across membranes or tissues.

abstinence Voluntary refrainment from sexual intercourse.

acquired immune deficiency syndrome (AIDS) The final stages of HIV infection, characterized by a variety of severe illnesses and decreased levels of certain immune cells.

active stretching A technique that involves stretching a muscle by contracting the opposing muscle.

acupuncture A Chinese medical practice of puncturing the body with needles inserted at specific points to relieve pain or cure disease.

acute injuries Physical injuries, such as sprains, bruises, and pulled muscles, which result from sudden traumas, such as falls or collisions.

adaptive response The body's attempt to reestablish homeostasis or stability.

addiction A behavioral pattern characterized by compulsion, loss of control, and continued repetition of a behavior or activity in spite of adverse consequences.

adoption The legal process for becoming the parent to a child of other biological parents.

advance directives Documents that specify individual's preferences regarding treatment in a medical crisis.

aerobic exercise Physical activity in which sufficient or excess oxygen is continually supplied to the body.

affirmation A single positive sentence used as a tool for behavior change.

aging The characteristic pattern of normal life changes that occur as humans grow older.

alcohol abuse Continued use of alcohol despite awareness of social, occupational, psychological, or physical problems related to its use, or use of alcohol in dangerous ways or situations, such as before driving.

alcohol dependence Development of a strong craving for alcohol due to the pleasurable feelings or relief of stress or anxiety produced by drinking.

alcoholism A chronic, progressive, potentially fatal disease characterized by impaired control of drinking, a preoccupation with alcohol, continued use of alcohol despite adverse consequences, and distorted thinking, most notably denial.

allergy A hypersensitivity to a particular substance in one's environment or diet.

altruism Acts of helping or giving to others without thought of self-benefit.

Alzheimer's disease A progressive deterioration of intellectual powers due to physiological changes within the brain; symptoms include diminishing ability to concentrate and reason, disorientation, depression, apathy, and paranoia.

amenorrhea The absence or suppression of menstruation.

amino acids Organic compounds containing nitrogen, carbon, hydrogen, and oxygen; the essential building blocks of proteins.

amnion The innermost membrane of the sac enclosing the embryo or fetus.

amphetamine Any of a class of stimulants that trigger the release of epinephrine, which stimulates the central nervous system; users experience a state of hyper-alertness and energy, followed by a crash as the drug wears off.

anabolic steroids Drugs derived from testosterone and approved for medical use, but often used by athletes to increase their musculature and weight.

anaerobic exercise Physical activity in which the body develops an oxygen deficit.

angioplasty Surgical repair of an obstructed artery by passing a balloon catheter through the blood vessel to the area of disease and then inflating the catheter to compress the plaque against the vessel wall.

anorexia nervosa A psychological disorder in which refusal to eat and/or an extreme loss of appetite leads to malnutrition, severe weight loss, and possibly death.

antibiotics Substances produced by microorganisms, or synthetic agents, that are toxic to other types of microorganisms; in dilute solutions, used to treat infectious diseases.

antidepressant A drug used primarily to treat symptoms of depression.

antioxidants Substances that prevent the damaging effects of oxidation in cells.

antiviral drug A substance that decreases the severity and duration of a viral infection if taken prior to or soon after onset of the infection.

anxiety A feeling of apprehension and dread, with or without a known cause; may range from mild to severe and may be accompanied by physical symptoms.

anxiety disorders A group of psychological disorders involving episodes of apprehension, tension, or uneasiness, stemming from the anticipation of danger and sometimes accompanied by physical symptoms, which cause significant distress and impairment to an individual.

aorta The main artery of the body, arising from the left ventricle of the heart.

appetite A desire for food, stimulated by anticipated hunger, physiological changes within the brain and body, the availability of food, and other environmental and psychological factors.

artificial insemination The introduction of viable sperm into the vagina by artificial means for the purpose of inducing conception.

assertive Behaving in a confident manner to make your needs and desires clear to others in a nonhostile way.

atrium (plural **atria**) Either of the two upper chambers of the heart, which receive blood from the veins.

attention deficit/hyperactivity disorder (ADHD) A spectrum of difficulties in controlling motion and sustaining attention, including hyperactivity, impulsivity, and distractibility.

autonomy The ability to draw on internal resources; independence from familial and societal influences.

autoscopy The sensation of one's self being outside the body, often experienced by individuals in near-death medical crises.

aversion therapy A treatment that attempts to help a person overcome a dependence or bad habit by making the person feel disgusted or repulsed by that habit.

Ayurveda A traditional Indian medical treatment involving meditation, exercise, herbal medications, and nutrition.

bacteria (singular, **bacterium**) One-celled microscopic organisms; the most plentiful pathogens.

bacterial vaginosis A vaginal infection caused by overgrowth and depletion of various microorganisms living in the vagina, resulting in a malodorous white or gray vaginal discharge.

ballistic stretching Rapid bouncing movements.

barbiturates Antianxiety drugs that depress the central nervous system, reduce activity, and induce relaxation, drowsiness, or sleep;

often prescribed to relieve tension and treat epileptic seizures or as a general anesthetic.

barrier contraceptives Birth-control devices that block the meeting of egg and sperm, either by physical barriers, such as condoms, diaphragms, or cervical caps, or by chemical barriers, such as spermicide, or both.

basal metabolic rate (BMR) The number of calories required to sustain the body at rest.

behavioral therapy Psychotherapy that emphasizes application of the principles of learning to substitute desirable responses and behavior patterns for undesirable ones.

benzodiazepines Antianxiety drugs that depress the central nervous system, reduce activity, and induce relaxation, drowsiness, or sleep; often prescribed to relieve tension, muscular strain, sleep problems, anxiety, and panic attacks; also used as an anesthetic and in the treatment of alcohol withdrawal.

bidis Skinny, sweet-flavored cigarettes.

binge drinking For a man, having five or more alcoholic drinks at a single sitting; for a woman, having four drinks or more at a single sitting.

binge eating The rapid consumption of an abnormally large amount of food in a relatively short time.

biofeedback A technique of becoming aware, with the aid of external monitoring devices, of internal physiological activities in order to develop the capability of altering them.

bipolar disorder Severe depression alternating with periods of manic activity and elation.

bisexual Sexually oriented toward both sexes.

blood-alcohol concentration (BAC) The amount of alcohol in the blood, expressed as a percentage.

body composition The relative amounts of fat and lean tissue (bone, muscle, organs, water) in the body.

body mass index (BMI) A mathematical formula that correlates with body fat; the ratio of weight to height squared.

botulism Possibly fatal food poisoning caused by a type of bacterium that grows and produces its toxin in the absence of air and is found in improperly canned food.

bulimia nervosa Episodic binge eating, often followed by forced vomiting or laxative abuse, and accompanied by a persistent preoccupation with body shape and weight.

caesarean delivery The surgical procedure in which an infant is delivered through an incision made in the abdominal wall and uterus.

calorie The amount of energy required to raise the temperature of 1 gram of water by 1 degree Celsius. In everyday usage related to the energy content of foods and the energy expended in activities, a calorie is actually the equivalent of a thousand such calories, or a kilocalorie.

candidiasis An infection of the yeast *Candida albicans,* commonly occurring in the vagina, vulva, penis, and mouth and causing burning, itching, and a whitish discharge.

capillary A minute blood vessel that connects an artery to a vein.

carbohydrates Organic compounds, such as starches, sugars, and glycogen, that are composed of carbon, hydrogen, and oxygen, and are sources of bodily energy.

carbon monoxide A colorless, odorless gas produced by the burning of gasoline or tobacco; displaces oxygen in the hemoglobin molecules of red blood cells.

carcinogen A substance that produces cancerous cells or enhances their development and growth.

cardiorespiratory fitness The ability of the heart and blood vessels to circulate blood through the body efficiently.

celibacy Abstention from sexual activity; can be partial or complete, permanent or temporary.

cervical cap A thimble-sized rubber or plastic cap that is inserted into the vagina to fit over the cervix and prevent the passage of sperm into the uterus during sexual intercourse; used with a spermicidal foam or jelly, it serves as both a chemical and a physical barrier to sperm.

cervix The narrow, lower end of the uterus that opens into the vagina.

chanchroid A soft, painful sore or localized infection usually acquired through sexual contact.

chiropractic A method of treating disease, primarily through manipulating the bones and joints to restore normal nerve function.

chlamydia A sexually transmitted disease caused by the bacterium *Chlamydia trachomatis,* often asymptomatic in women, but sometimes characterized by urinary pain; if undetected and untreated, may result in pelvic inflammatory disease (PID).

chlorinated hydrocarbons Highly toxic pesticides, such as DDT and chlordane, that are extremely resistant to breakdown; may cause cancer, birth defects, neurological disorders, and damage to wildlife and the environment.

cholesterol An organic substance found in animal fats; linked to cardiovascular disease, particularly atherosclerosis.

chronic fatigue syndrome (CFS) A cluster of symptoms whose cause is not yet known; a primary symptom is debilitating fatigue.

circumcision The surgical removal of the foreskin of the penis.

clitoris A small erectile structure on the female, corresponding to the penis on the male.

club drugs Illegally manufactured psychoactive drugs that have dangerous physical and psychological effects.

cocaine A white crystalline powder extracted from the leaves of the coca plant that stimulates the central nervous system and produces a brief period of euphoria followed by a depression.

cognitive therapy A technique used to identify an individual's beliefs and attitudes, recognize negative thought patterns, and educate in alternative ways of thinking.

cohabitation Two people living together as a couple, without official ties such as marriage.

coitus interruptus The removal of the penis from the vagina before ejaculation.

complementary and alternative medicine (CAM) A term used to apply to all health-care approaches, practices, and treatments not widely taught in medical schools, not generally used in hospitals, and not usually reimbursed by medical insurance companies.

complementary proteins Incomplete proteins that, when combined, provide all the amino acids essential for protein synthesis.

complete proteins Proteins that contain all the amino acids needed by the body for growth and maintenance.

complex carbohydrates Starches, including cereals, fruits, and vegetables.

conception The merging of a sperm and an ovum.

condom A latex sheath worn over the penis during sexual acts to prevent conception and/or the transmission of disease; the female condom lines the walls of the vagina.

contraception The prevention of conception; birth control.

corpus luteum A yellowish mass of tissue that is formed, immediately after ovulation, from the remaining cells of the follicle; it secretes estrogen and progesterone for the remainder of the menstrual cycle.

Cowper's glands Two small glands that discharge into the male urethra; also called bulbourethral glands.

culture The set of shared attitudes, values, goals, and practices of a group that are internalized by an individual within the group.

cunnilingus Sexual stimulation of a woman's genitals by means of oral manipulation.

cystitis Inflammation of the urinary bladder.

decibel (dB) A unit for measuring the intensity of sounds.

decisional balance Weighing the positive and negative consequences of change to yourself and to others.

defense mechanism A psychological process that alleviates anxiety and eliminates mental conflict; includes denial, displacement, projection, rationalization, reaction formation, and repression.

dementia Deterioration of mental capability.

depression In general, feelings of unhappiness and despair; as a mental illness, also characterized by an inability to function normally.

diabetes mellitus A disease in which the inadequate production of insulin leads to failure of the body tissues to break down carbohydrates at a normal rate.

diaphragm A bowl-like rubber cup with a flexible rim that is inserted into the vagina to cover the cervix and prevent the passage of sperm into the uterus during sexual intercourse; used with a spermicidal foam or jelly, it serves as both a chemical and a physical barrier to sperm.

diastole The period between contractions in the cardiac cycle, during which the heart relaxes and dilates as it fills with blood.

diastolic blood pressure Lowest blood pressure between contractions of the heart.

dietary fiber The nondigestible form of carbohydrates found in plant foods, such as leaves, stems, skins, seeds, and hulls.

dilation and evacuation (D and E) A medical procedure in which the contents of the uterus are removed through the use of instruments.

distress A negative stress that may result in illness.

do-not-resuscitate (DNR) An advance directive expressing an individual's preference that resuscitation efforts not be made during a medical crisis.

drug Any substance, other than food, that affects bodily functions and structures when taken into the body.

drug abuse The excessive use of a drug in a manner inconsistent with accepted medical practice.

drug misuse The use of a drug for a purpose (or person) other than that for which it was medically intended.

dynamic flexibility The ability to move a joint quickly and fluidly through its entire range of motion with little resistance.

dysfunctional Characterized by negative and destructive patterns of behavior between partners or between parents and children.

dysmenorrhea Painful menstruation.

eating disorders Bizarre, often dangerous patterns of food consumption, including anorexia nervosa and bulimia nervosa.

ecosystem A community of organisms sharing a physical and chemical environment and interacting with each other.

ecstasy (MDMA) A synthetic compound, also known as methylenedioxymethamphetamine, that is similar in structure to methamphetamine and has both stimulant and hallucinogenic effects.

ectopic pregnancy A pregnancy in which the fertilized egg has implanted itself outside the uterine cavity, usually in the fallopian tube.

ejaculatory duct The canal connecting the seminal vesicles and vas deferens.

electromagnetic fields (EMFs) The invisible electric and magnetic fields generated by an electrically charged conductor.

embryo An organism in its early stage of development; in humans, the embryonic period lasts from the second to the eighth week of pregnancy.

emergency contraception Types of oral contraceptive pills, usually taken within 72 hours after intercourse, that can prevent pregnancy.

emotional health The ability to express and acknowledge one's feelings and moods and exhibit adaptability and compassion for others.

emotional intelligence A term used by some psychologists to evaluate the capacity of people to understand themselves and relate well with others.

enabling factors The skills, resources, and physical and mental capabilities that shape our behavior.

endocrine disruptors Synthetic chemicals that interfere with the ways that hormones work in humans and wildlife.

endometrium The mucous membrane lining the uterus.

endorphins Mood-elevating, pain-killing chemicals produced by the brain.

environmental tobacco smoke Secondhand cigarette smoke; the third-leading preventable cause of death.

epididymis That portion of the male duct system in which sperm mature.

erogenous Sexually sensitive.

essential nutrients Nutrients that the body cannot manufacture for itself and must obtain from food.

ethyl alcohol The intoxicating agent in alcoholic beverages; also called ethanol.

eustress Positive stress, which stimulates a person to function properly.

failure rate The number of pregnancies that occur per year for every 100 women using a particular method of birth control.

fallopian tubes The pair of channels that transport ova from the ovaries to the uterus; the usual site of fertilization.

family A group of people united by marriage, blood, or adoption; residing in the same household; maintaining a common culture; and interacting with one another on the basis of their roles within the group.

fellatio Sexual stimulation of a man's genitals by means of oral manipulation.

fertilization The fusion of sperm and egg nucleus.

fetal alcohol effects (FAE) Milder forms of FAS, including low birthweight, irritability as newborns, and permanent mental impairment as a result of the mother's alcohol consumption during pregnancy.

fetal alcohol syndrome (FAS) A cluster of physical and mental defects in the newborn, including low birthweight, smaller-than-normal head circumference, intrauterine growth retardation, and permanent mental impairment caused by the mother's alcohol consumption during pregnancy.

fetus The human organism developing in the uterus from the ninth week until birth.

FITT A formula that describes the frequency, intensity, type, and length of time for physical activity.

flexibility The range of motion allowed by one's joints; determined by the length of muscles, tendons, and ligaments attached to the joints.

folic acid A form of folate used in vitamin supplements and fortified foods.

functional fiber Isolated, nondigestible carbohydrates with beneficial effects in humans.

fungi (singular, **fungus**) Organisms that reproduce by means of spores.

gamma globulin The antibody-containing portion of the blood fluid (plasma).

GBL (gamma butyrolactone) The main ingredient in gamma hydroxybutyrate (GHB), also known as the "date rape drug"; once ingested, GBL converts to GHB and can cause the ingestor to lose consciousness.

general adaptation syndrome (GAS) The sequenced physiological response to a stressful situation; consists of three stages: alarm, resistance, and exhaustion.

generalized anxiety disorder (GAD) An anxiety disorder characterized by chronic distress.

GHB (gamma hydroxybutyrate) A brain messenger chemical that stimulates the release of human growth hormone; commonly abused for its high and its alleged ability to trim fat and build muscles. Also known as "blue nitro" or the "date rape drug."

global warming Increase in Earth's surface and atmospheric temperature due to increase levels of greenhouse gases (carbon dioxide, methane, and nitrous oxide) that trap heat in the atmosphere.

gonorrhea A sexually transmitted disease caused by the bacterium *Neisseria gonorrhoeae;* symptoms include discharge from the penis; women are generally asymptomatic.

guided imagery An approach to stress control, self-healing, or motivating life changes by means of visualizing oneself in the state of calmness, wellness, or change.

hallucinogen A drug that causes hallucinations.

hashish A concentrated form of a drug, derived from the cannabis plant, containing the psychoactive ingredient TCH, which causes a sense of euphoria when inhaled or eaten.

health A state of complete well-being, including physical, psychological, spiritual, social, intellectual, and environmental dimensions.

health belief model (HBM) A model of behavioral change that focuses on the individual's attitudes and beliefs.

health maintenance organization (HMO) An organization that provides health services on a fixed-contract basis.

health promotion An educational and informational process in which people are helped to change attitudes and behaviors in an effort to improve their health.

helminth A parasitic roundworm or flatworm.

hepatitis An inflammation and/or infection of the liver caused by a virus, often accompanied by jaundice.

herbal medicine An ancient form of medical treatment using substances derived from trees, flowers, ferns, seaweeds, and lichens to treat disease.

herpes simplex A condition caused by one of the herpes viruses and characterized by lesions of the skin or mucous membranes; herpes virus type 2 is sexually transmitted and causes genital blisters or sores.

heterosexual Primary sexual orientation toward members of the other sex.

holistic An approach to medicine that takes into account body, mind, emotions, and spirit.

holographic will A will wholly in the handwriting of its author.

homeopathy A system of medical practice that treats a disease by administering dosages of substances that would in healthy persons produce symptoms similar to those of the disease.

homeostasis The body's natural state of balance or stability.

homosexual Primary sexual orientation toward members of the same sex.

hormone therapy (HT) The use of supplemental hormones during and after menopause.

host A person or population that contracts one or more pathogenic agents in an environment.

human immunodeficiency virus (HIV) A type of virus that causes a spectrum of health problems, ranging from a symptomless infection to changes in the immune system, to the development of life-threatening diseases because of impaired immunity.

human papilloma virus (HPV) A pathogen that causes genital warts and increases the risk of cervical cancer.

hunger The physiological drive to consume food.

hypertension High blood pressure occurring when the blood exerts excessive pressure against the arterial walls.

hypothermia An abnormally low body temperature; if not treated appropriately, coma or death could result.

immune deficiency Partial or complete inability of the immune system to respond to pathogens.

immunity Protection from infectious diseases.

immunotherapy A series of injections of small but increasing doses of an allergen, used to treat allergies.

implantation The embedding of the fertilized ovum in the uterine lining.

incomplete proteins Proteins that lack one or more of the amino acids essential for protein synthesis.

incubation period The time between a pathogen's entrance into the body and the first symptom.

infertility The inability to conceive a child.

infiltration A gradual penetration or invasion.

inflammation A localized response by the body to tissue injury, characterized by swelling and the dilation of the blood vessels.

influenza Any of a type of fairly common, highly contagious viral diseases.

informed consent Permission (to undergo or receive a medical procedure or treatment) given voluntarily, with full knowledge and understanding of the procedure or treatment and its possible consequences.

inhalants Substances that produce vapors having psychoactive effects when sniffed.

integrative medicine An approach that combines traditional medicine with alternative/complementary therapies.

intercourse Sexual stimulation by means of entry of the penis into the vagina; coitus.

interpersonal therapy (IPT) A technique used to develop communication skills and relationships.

intimacy A state of closeness between two people, characterized by the desire and ability to share one's innermost thoughts and feelings with each other either verbally or nonverbally.

intoxication Maladaptive behavioral, psychological, and physiologic changes that occur as a result of substance abuse.

intramuscular Into or within a muscle.

intrauterine device (IUD) A device inserted into the uterus through the cervix to prevent pregnancy by interfering with implantation.

intravenous Into a vein.

ionizing radiation A form of energy emitted from atoms as they undergo internal change.

isokinetic Having the same force; exercise with specialized equipment that provides resistance equal to the force applied by the user throughout the entire range of motion.

isometric Of the same length; exercise in which muscles increase their tension without shortening in length, such as when pushing an immovable object.

isotonic Having the same tension or tone; exercise requiring the repetition of an action that creates tension, such as weight lifting or calisthenics.

labia majora The fleshy outer folds that border the female genital area.

labia minora The fleshy inner folds that border the female genital area.

labor The process leading up to birth: effacement and dilation of the cervix; the movement of the baby into and through the birth canal, accompanied by strong contractions; and contraction of the uterus and expulsion of the placenta after the birth.

lacto-vegetarians People who eat dairy products as well as fruits and vegetables (but not meat, poultry, or fish).

Lamaze method A method of childbirth preparation taught to expectant parents to help the woman cope with the discomfort of labor; combines breathing and psychological techniques.

laparoscopy A surgical sterilization procedure in which the fallopian tubes are observed, with a laparoscope inserted through a small incision, and then cut or blocked.

lipoprotein A compound in blood that is made up of proteins and fat; a high-density lipoprotein (HDL) picks up excess cholesterol in the blood; a low-density lipoprotein (LDL) carries more cholesterol and deposits it on the walls of arteries.

listeria A bacterium commonly found in deli meats, hot dogs, and soft cheeses that can cause an infection called listeriosis.

living will An advance directive providing instructions for the use of life-sustaining procedures in the event of terminal illness or injury.

locus of control An individual's belief about the source of power and influence over his or her life.

lumpectomy The surgical removal of a breast tumor and its surrounding tissue.

Lyme disease A disease caused by a bacterium carried by a tick; it may cause heart arrhythmias, neurological problems, and arthritis symptoms.

lymph nodes Small tissue masses in which some immune cells are stored.

macronutrients Nutrients required by the human body in the greatest amounts, including water, carbohydrates, proteins, and fats.

mainstream smoke The smoke inhaled directly by smoking a cigarette.

major depression Sadness that does not end; ongoing feelings of utter hopelessness.

male pattern baldness The loss of hair at the vertex, or top, of the head.

mammography A diagnostic X-ray exam used to detect breast cancer.

managed care Health-care services and reimbursement predetermined by third-party insurers.

marijuana The drug derived from the cannabis plant, containing the psychoactive ingredient THC, which causes a mild sense of euphoria when inhaled or eaten.

mastectomy The surgical removal of an entire breast.

medical abortion Method of ending a pregnancy within nine weeks of conception using hormonal medications that cause expulsion of the fertilized egg.

meditation A group of approaches that use quiet sitting, breathing techniques, and/or chanting to relax, improve concentration, and become attuned to one's inner self.

meningitis An extremely serious, potentially fatal illness that attacks the membranes around the brain and spinal cord; caused by the bacterium *Neisseria meningitis*.

menopause The complete cessation of ovulation and menstruation for twelve consecutive months.

menstruation Discharge of blood from the vagina as a result of the shedding of the uterine lining at the end of the menstrual cycle.

mental disorder Behavioral or psychological syndrome associated with distress or disability or with a significantly increased risk of suffering death, pain, disability, or loss of freedom.

mental health The ability to perceive reality as it is, respond to its challenges, and develop rational strategies for living.

metabolic syndrome A cluster of disorders of the body's metabolism that make diabetes, heart disease, or stroke more likely.

metastasize To spread to other parts of the body via the bloodstream or lymphatic system.

micronutrients Vitamins and minerals needed by the body in very small amounts.

microwaves Extremely high frequency electromagnetic waves that increase the rate at which molecules vibrate, thereby generating heat.

mindfulness A method of stress reduction that involves experiencing the physical and mental sensations of the present moment.

minerals Naturally occurring inorganic substances, small amounts of some being essential in metabolism and nutrition.

minipill An oral contraceptive containing a small amount of progestin and no estrogen, which prevents contraception by making the mucus in the cervix so thick that sperm cannot enter the uterus.

miscarriage A pregnancy that terminates before the twentieth week of gestation; also called spontaneous abortion.

mononucleosis An infectious viral disease characterized by an excess of white blood cells in the blood, fever, bodily discomfort, a sore throat, and kidney and liver complications.

monophasic pill An oral contraceptive that releases synthetic estrogen and progestin at constant levels throughout the menstrual cycle.

mons pubis The rounded, fleshy area over the junction of the female pubic bones.

mood A sustained emotional state that colors one's view of the world for hours or days.

motivational interviewing A nonjudgmental but directive method for supporting motivation to change.

multiphasic pill An oral contraceptive that releases different levels of estrogen and progestin to mimic the hormonal fluctuations of the natural menstrual cycle.

muscular endurance The ability to withstand the stress of continued physical exertion.

muscular strength Physical power; the maximum weight one can lift, push, or press in one effort.

mutagen An agent that causes alterations in the genetic material of living cells.

myocardial infarction (MI) A condition characterized by the dying of tissue areas in the myocardium, caused by interruption of the blood supply to those areas; the medical name for a heart attack.

naturopathy An alternative system of treatment of disease that emphasizes the use of natural remedies such as sun, water, heat, and air. Therapies may include dietary changes, steam baths, and exercise.

nicotine The addictive substance in tobacco; one of the most toxic of all poisons.

nonexercise activity thermogenesis (NEAT) Nonvolitional movement that can be an effective way of burning calories.

nongonococcal urethritis (NGU) Inflammation of the urethra caused by organisms other than the gonococcus bacterium.

nonvolitional sex Sexual behavior that violates a person's right to choose when and with whom to have sex and what sexual behaviors to engage in.

norms The unwritten rules regarding behavior and conduct expected or accepted by a group.

nutrition The science devoted to the study of dietary needs for food and the effects of food on organisms.

obesity The excessive accumulation of fat in the body; class 1 obesity is defined by a BMI between 30.0 and 34.9; class 2 obesity by a BMI between 35.0 and 39.9; class 3 or severe obesity by a BMI of 40 or higher.

obsessive-compulsive disorder (OCD) An anxiety disorder characterized by obsessions and/or compulsions that impair one's ability to function and form relationships.

opioids Drugs that have sleep-inducing and pain-relieving properties, including opium and its derivatives and nonopioid, synthetic drugs.

oral contraceptives Preparations of synthetic hormones that inhibit ovulation; also referred to as birth control pills or simply the pill.

organic Term designating food produced with, or production based on the use of, fertilizers originating from plants or animals, without the use of pesticides or chemically formulated fertilizers.

organic phosphates Toxic pesticides that may cause cancer, birth defects, neurological disorders, and damage to wildlife and the environment.

osteoporosis A condition common in older people in which the bones become increasingly soft and porous, making them susceptible to injury.

ovary The female sex organ that produces egg cells, estrogen, and progesterone.

overload principle Providing a greater stress or demand on the body than it is normally accustomed to handling.

overloading Method of physical training involving increasing the number of repetitions or the amount of resistance gradually to work the muscle to temporary fatigue.

over-the-counter (OTC) drugs Medications that can be obtained legally without a prescription from a medical professional.

overtrain Working muscles too intensely or too frequently, resulting in persistent muscle soreness, injuries, unintended weight loss, nervousness, and an inability to relax.

overuse injuries Physical injuries to joints or muscles, such as strains, fractures, and tendinitis, which result from overdoing a repetitive activity.

overweight A condition of having a BMI between 25.0 and 29.9.

ovo-lacto-vegetarians People who eat eggs, dairy products, and fruits and vegetables (but not meat, poultry, or fish).

ovulation The release of a mature ovum from an ovary approximately 14 days prior to the onset of menstruation.

ovum (plural, **ova**) The female gamete (egg cell).

panic attack A short episode characterized by physical sensations of light-headedness, dizziness, hyperventilation, and numbness of extremities, accompanied by an inexplicable terror, usually of a physical disaster such as death.

panic disorder An anxiety disorder in which the apprehension or experience of recurring panic attacks is so intense that normal functioning is impaired.

passive stretching A stretching technique in which an external force or resistance (your body, a partner, gravity, or a weight) helps the joints move through their range of motion.

pathogen A microorganism that produces disease.

PCP (phencyclidine) A synthetic psychoactive substance that produces effects similar to other psychoactive drugs when swallowed, smoked, sniffed, or injected, but also may trigger unpredictable behavioral changes.

pelvic inflammatory disease (PID) An inflammation of the internal female genital tract, characterized by abdominal pain, fever, and tenderness of the cervix.

penis The male organ of sex and urination.

perimenopause The period from a woman's first irregular cycles to her last menstruation.

perineum The area between the anus and vagina in the female and between the anus and scrotum in the male.

phobia An anxiety disorder marked by an inordinate fear of an object, a class of objects, or a situation, resulting in extreme avoidance behaviors.

physical dependence The physiological attachment to, and need for, a drug.

physical fitness The ability to respond to routine physical demands, with enough reserve energy to cope with a sudden challenge.

phytochemicals Chemicals such as indoles, coumarins, and capsaicin, which exist naturally in plants and have disease-fighting properties.

placenta An organ that develops after implantation and to which the embryo attaches, via the umbilical cord, for nourishment and waste removal.

plaque The sludgelike substance that builds up on the inner walls of arteries; the sticky film of bacteria that forms on teeth.

pollutant A substance or agent in the environment, usually the by-product of human industry or activity, that is injurious to human, animal, or plant life.

polyabuse The misuse or abuse of more than one drug.

posttraumatic stress disorder (PTSD) The repeated reliving of a trauma through nightmares or recollection.

preconception care Health care to prepare for pregnancy.

precycling The use of products that are packaged in recycled or recyclable material.

predisposing factors The beliefs, values, attitudes, knowledge, and perceptions that influence our behavior.

preferred provider organization (PPO) A group of physicians contracted to provide health care to members at a discounted price.

prehypertension A condition of slightly elevated blood pressure, which is likely to worsen in time.

premature labor Labor that occurs after the twentieth week but before the thirty- seventh week of pregnancy.

premenstrual dysphoric disorder (PMDD) A disorder that causes symptoms of psychological depression during the last week of the menstrual cycle.

premenstrual syndrome (PMS) A disorder that causes physical discomfort and psychological distress prior to a woman's menstrual period.

prevention Information and support offered to help healthy people identify their health risks, reduce stressors, prevent potential medical problems, and enhance their well-being.

progestin-only pill *See* minipill.

progressive overloading Gradually increasing physical challenges once the body adapts to the stress placed upon it to produce maximum benefits.

progressive relaxation A method of reducing muscle tension by contracting, then relaxing, certain areas of the body.

proof The alcoholic strength of a distilled spirit, expressed as twice the percentage of alcohol present.

prostate gland A structure surrounding the male urethra that produces a secretion that helps liquefy the semen from the testes.

protection Measures that an individual can take when participating in risky behavior to prevent injury or unwanted risks.

proteins Organic compounds composed of amino acids; one of the essential nutrients.

protozoa Microscopic animals made up of one cell or a group of similar cells.

psychiatric drugs Medications that regulate a person's mental, emotional, and physical functions to facilitate normal functioning.

psychoactive Mind-affecting.

psychodynamic Interpreting behaviors in terms of early experiences and unconscious influences.

psychological dependence The emotional or mental attachment to the use of a drug.

psychotherapy Treatment designed to produce a response by psychological rather than physical means, such as suggestion, persuasion, reassurance, and support.

quackery Medical fakery; unproven practices claiming to cure diseases or solve health problems.

range of motion The fullest extent of possible movement in a particular joint.

rape Sexual penetration of a female or a male by means of intimidation, force, or fraud.

recycling The processing or reuse of manufactured materials to reduce consumption of raw materials.

reinforcement Reward or punishment for a behavior that will increase or decrease one's likelihood of repeating the behavior.

reinforcing factors Rewards, encouragement, and recognition that influence our behavior in the short run.

relative risk The risk of developing cancer in persons with a certain exposure or trait compared to the risk in persons who do not have the same exposure or trait.

rep (or **repetition**) In weight training, a single performance of a movement or exercise.

resting heart rate The number of heartbeats per minute during inactivity.

reversibility principle The physical benefits of exercise are lost through disuse or inactivity.

rhythm method A birth-control method in which sexual intercourse is avoided during those days of the menstrual cycle in which fertilization is most likely to occur.

rubella An infectious disease that may cause birth defects if contracted by a pregnant woman; also called German measles.

satiety A feeling of fullness after eating.

saturated fat A chemical term indicating that a fat molecule contains as many hydrogen atoms as its carbon skeleton can hold. These fats are normally solid at room temperature.

scrotum The external sac or pouch that holds the testes.

self-actualization A state of wellness and fulfillment that can be achieved once certain human needs are satisfied; living to one's full potential.

self-efficacy Belief in one's ability to accomplish a goal or change a behavior.

self-esteem Confidence and satisfaction in oneself.

self-talk Repetition of positive messages about one's self-worth to learn more optimistic patterns of thought, feeling, and behavior.

semen The viscous, whitish fluid that is the complete male ejaculate; a combination of sperm and secretions from the prostate gland, seminal vesicles, and other glands.

seminal vesicles Glands in the male reproductive system that produce the major portion of the fluid of semen.

sets In weight training, the number of repetitions of the same movement or exercise.

sex Maleness or femaleness, resulting from genetic, structural, and functional factors.

sexual coercion Sexual activity forced upon a person by the exertion of psychological pressure by another person.

sexual harassment Unwanted sexual attention.

sexual health The integration of the physical, emotional, intellectual, and social aspects of sexual being in ways that are positively enriching and that enhance personality, communication, and love.

sexual orientation The direction of an individual's sexual interest, either to members of the opposite sex or to members of the same sex.

sexually transmitted infections (STIs) Any of a number of diseases that are acquired through sexual contact.

sidestream smoke The smoke emitted by a burning cigarette and breathed by everyone in a closed room, including the smoker; contains more tar and nicotine than mainstream smoke.

simple carbohydrates Sugars; like all carbohydrates, they provide the body with glucose.

smog A grayish or brownish fog caused by the presence of smoke and/or chemical pollutants in the air.

social isolation A feeling of unconnectedness with others caused by and reinforced by infrequency of social contacts.

social phobia A severe form of social anxiety marked by extreme fears and avoidance of social situations.

specificity principle Each part of the body adapts to a particular type and amount of stress placed upon it.

sperm The male gamete produced by the testes and transported outside the body through ejaculation.

spermatogenesis The process by which sperm cells are produced.

spiritual health The ability to identify one's basic purpose in life and achieve one's full potential; the sense of connectedness to a greater power.

spiritual intelligence The capacity to sense, understand, and tap into ourselves, others, and the world around us.

static flexibility The ability to assume and maintain an extended position at one end point in a joint's range of motion.

static stretching A gradual stretch held for a short time of 10 to 30 seconds.

sterilization A surgical procedure to end a person's reproductive capability.

stimulant An agent, such as a drug, that temporarily relieves drowsiness, helps in the performance of repetitive tasks, and improves capacity for work.

stress The nonspecific response of the body to any demands made upon it; may be characterized by muscle tension and acute anxiety, or may be a positive force for action.

stressor Specific or nonspecific agents or situations that cause the stress response in a body.

stroke A cerebrovascular event in which the blood supply to a portion of the brain is blocked.

subcutaneous Under the skin.

suction curettage A procedure in which the contents of the uterus are removed by means of suction and scraping.

sustainability A method of using a resource so that the resource is not depleted or permanently damaged.

syphilis A sexually transmitted disease caused by the bacterium *Treponema pallidum* and characterized by early sores, a latent period, and; a final period of life-threatening symptoms, including brain damage and heart failure.

systemic disease A pathologic condition that spreads throughout the body.

systole The contraction phase of the cardiac cycle.

systolic blood pressure Highest blood pressure when the heart contracts.

tar A thick, sticky dark fluid produced by the burning of tobacco, made up of several hundred different chemicals, many of them poisonous, some of them carcinogenic.

target heart rate Sixty to eighty-five percent of the maximum heart rate; the heart rate at which one derives maximum cardiovascular benefit from aerobic exercise.

teratogen Any agent that causes spontaneous abortion, defects, or malformations in a fetus.

testes (singular, **testis**) The male sex organs that produce sperm and testosterone.

toxic shock syndrome (TSS) A disease characterized by fever, vomiting, diarrhea, and often shock, caused by a bacterium that releases toxic waste products into the bloodstream.

toxicity Poisonousness; the dosage level at which a drug becomes poisonous to the body, causing either temporary or permanent damage.

transcendence The sense of passing into a foreign region or dimension, often experienced by a person near death.

trans-fat Fat formed when liquid vegetable oils are processed to make table spreads or cooking fats; also found in dairy and beef products; considered to be especially dangerous dietary fats.

transgender Having a gender identity opposite one's biological sex.

transtheoretical model of change A model of behavioral change that focuses on the individual's decision making; it states that an individual progresses through a sequence of six stages as he or she makes a change in behavior.

trichomoniasis An infection of the protozoan *Trichomonas vaginalis;* females experience vaginal burning, itching, and discharge, but male carriers may be asymptomatic.

triglyceride A blood fat that flows through the blood after meals and is linked to increased risk of coronary artery disease.

tubal ligation The suturing or tying shut of the fallopian tubes to prevent pregnancy.

tubal occlusion The blocking of the fallopian tubes to prevent pregnancy.

tuberculosis A highly infectious bacterial disease that primarily affects the lungs and is often fatal.

twelve-step programs Self-help group programs based on the principles of Alcoholics Anonymous.

unsaturated fat A chemical term indicating that a fat molecule contains fewer hydrogen atoms than its carbon skeleton can hold. These fats are normally liquid at room temperature.

urethra The canal through which urine from the bladder leaves the body; in the male, also serves as the channel for seminal fluid.

urethral opening The outer opening of the thin tube that carries urine from the bladder.

urethritis Infection of the urethra.

uterus The female organ that houses the developing fetus until birth.

vagina The canal leading from the exterior opening in the female genital area to the uterus.

vaginal contraceptive film (VCF) A small dissolvable sheet saturated with spermicide that can be inserted into the vagina and placed over the cervix.

vaginal spermicide A substance that kills or neutralizes sperm, inserted into the vagina in the form of a foam, cream, jelly, or suppository.

values The criteria by which one makes choices about one's thoughts and actions and goals and ideals.

vas deferens Two tubes that carry sperm from the epididymis into the urethra.

vasectomy A surgical sterilization procedure in which each vas deferens is cut and tied shut to stop the passage of sperm to the urethra for ejaculation.

vector A biological or physical vehicle that carries the agent of infection to the host.

vegans People who eat only plant foods.

ventricle Either of the two lower chambers of the heart, which pump blood out of the heart and into the arteries.

virus A submicroscopic infectious agent; the most primitive form of life.

visualization An approach to stress control, self-healing, or motivating life changes by means of guided, or directed, imagery.

vital signs Measurements of physiological functioning; specifically, temperature, blood pressure, pulse rate, and respiration rate.

vitamins Organic substances that are needed in very small amounts by the body and carry out a variety of functions in metabolism and nutrition.

waist-to-hip ratio (WHR) The proportion of one's waist circumference to one's hip circumference.

wellness A deliberate lifestyle choice characterized by personal responsibility and optimal enhancement of physical, mental, and spiritual health.

withdrawal Development of symptoms that cause significant psychological and physical distress when an individual reduces or stops drug use.

zygote A fertilized egg.

References

Chapter 1

1. "Constitution of the World Health Organization." *Chronicle of the World Health Organization,* Geneva, Switzerland: WHO, 1947.
2. Travis, John, and Regina Sara Ryan. *The Wellness Workbook,* 3rd ed. Berkeley, CA: Celestial Arts, 2004.
3. Travis, John. Personal interview.
4. Travis and Ryan, *The Wellness Workbook.*
5. Benson, Herbert, et al. "Study of the Therapeutic Effects of Intercessory Prayer (STEP) in Cardiac Bypass Patients: A Multicenter Randomized Trial of Uncertainty and Certainty of Receiving Intercessory Prayer." *American Heart Journal,* Vol. 151, No. 4, April 2006, pp. 934–942.
6. Krucoff, Mitchell, et al. "From Efficacy to Safety Concerns: A STEP Forward or a Step Back for Clinical Research and Intercessory Prayer? The Study of Therapeutic Effects of Intercessory Prayer (STEP)." *American Heart Journal,* Vol. 151, No. 4, April 2006, p. 762.
7. Miniño, Arladi, et al. *Deaths: Preliminary Data for 2004.* National Center for Health Statistics, April 2006, www.cdc.gov.
8. Barford, Anna, et al. "Life Expectancy: Women Now on Top Everywhere." *British Medical Journal,* Vol. 332, April 8, 2006, www.bmj.com.
9. *Health, United States, 2005.* Washington, DC: U.S. Department of Health and Human Services, November 2005.
10. Harris, Kathleen Mullan, et al. "Longitudinal Trends in Race/Ethnic Disparities in Leading Health Indicators from Adolescence to Young Adulthood." *Archives of Pediatric and Adolescent Medicine,* Vol. 160, No. 1, January 2006, p. 74.
11. *Healthy People 2010,* www.healthypeople.gov.
12. *Healthy Campus 2010,* University of Southern California, Health Promotion and Prevention Services, www.usc.edu/student-affairs/Health_Center/hpps.hp2010.shtml.
13. Harris, et al., "Longitudinal Trends in Race/Ethnic Disparities in Leading Health Indicators from Adolescence to Young Adulthood."
14. American College Health Association. "American College Health Association-National College Health Assessment (ACHA-NCHA) Spring 2004 Reference Group Data Report (abridged)." *Journal of American College Health,* Vol. 54, No. 4, January–February 2006, p. 201.
15. American College Health Association. American College Health Association-National College Health Assessment (ACHA-NCHA) Web Summary, April 2006, www.acha.org/projects_programs/ncha_sampledata.cfm.
16. Bylund, Carma, et al. "Accuracy of Parents' Perceptions of Their College Student Children's Health and Health Risk Behaviors." *Journal of American College Health,* Vol. 54, No. 1, July–August 2005, p. 31.
17. American College Health Association. ACHA-NCHA Web Summary.
18. Escoffery, Cam, et al. "Internet Use for Health Information Among College Students." *Journal of American College Health,* Vol. 53, No. 4, January–February 2005, p. 183.
19. "Health Disparities Experienced by Black or African Americans—United States." *Morbidity and Mortality Weekly Report,* Vol. 54, No. 1, January 14, 2005, p. 1(3).
20. Tashiro, Cathy. "The Meaning of Race in Health Care and Research—Part 1: The Impact of History." *Pediatric Nursing,* Vol. 31, No. 3, May–June 2005, p. 208(3).
21. Brawley, Otis. "Lung Cancer and Race: Equal Treatment Yields Equal Outcome Among Equal Patients, But There Is No Equal Treatment." *Journal of Clinical Oncology,* Vol. 24, No. 3, January 2006, p. 332.
22. Ibid.
23. Blackstock, A. William, et al. "Similar Outcomes Between African American and Non-African American Patients with Extensive-Stage Small-Cell Lung Carcinoma: Report from the Cancer and Leukemia Group B." *Journal of Clinical Oncology,* Vol. 24, No. 3, January 2006, p. 407.
24. Tashiro, "The Meaning of Race in Health Care and Research."
25. National Eye Institute, Press release, *U.S. Latinos Have High Rates of Eye Disease and Visual Impairment,* www.nei.nih.gov/latinoeyestudy/.
26. "Cancer Facts for Minorities in the United States." National Center for Chronic Disease Prevention and Health Promotion, www.cdc.gov/cancer/minorityawareness.htm.
27. Asch, Steven, et al. "Who Is at Greatest Risk for Receiving Poor-Quality Health Care?" *New England Journal of Medicine,* Vol. 354, No. 11, March 16, 2006, p. 1147.
28. Prochaska, James, et al. *Changing for Good.* New York: Quill, 1994.
29. Steinman, K. J. "College Students' Early Cessation from Episodic Heavy Drinking: Prevalence and Correlates." *Journal of American College Health,* Vol. 51, No. 5, March 2003, p. 197.
30. Martens, Matthew, et al. "Differences Between Actual and Perceived Student Norms: An Examination of Alcohol Use, Drug Use, and Sexual Behavior." *Journal of American College Health,* Vol. 54, No. 5, March–April 2006, p. 205.
31. Seligman, Martin. Personal interview.
32. Christian, Kenneth W. Personal interview.

Chapter 2

1. Kessler, Ronald, et al. "Lifetime Prevalence and Age-of-Onset Distributions of *DSM-IV* Disorders in the National Comorbidity Survey Replication." *Archives of General Psychiatry,* Vol. 62, No. 6, June 2005, p. 593.
2. Wang, Philip, et al. "Failure and Delay in Initial Treatment Contact After First Onset of Mental Disorders in the National Comorbidity Survey Replication." *Archives of General Psychiatry,* Vol. 62, No. 6, June 2005, p. 603.
3. Edwards, Paul. Personal interview.
4. Seligman, Martin. *Authentic Happiness.* New York: Free Press, 2002.
5. Ricard, Mathieu. *Happiness: A Guide to Developing Life's Most Important Skill.* New York: Little Brown, April 2006.
6. Seligman, *Authentic Happiness.*
7. Flora, Carlin. "Happy Hour." *Psychology Today,* Vol. 38, No. 1, January–February 2005, p. 40.
8. Larsen, Randy. Personal interview.
9. Storch, Eric, et al. "Religiosity and Depression in Intercollegiate Athletes." *College Student Journal,* Vol. 36, No. 4, December 2002, p. 526.
10. Pryor, John, et al. *The American Freshman: National Norms for Fall 2005.* Los Angeles: Higher Education Research Institute, UCLA, December 2005.

11. Koenig, Harold. Personal interview.
12. Aaronson, Lauren. "Make a Gratitude Adjustment: Feeling Thankful Is One Key to Happiness." *Psychology Today,* March–April 2006, Vol. 39, No. 2, p. 60(2).
13. McCullough, Michael. Personal interview.
14. Hale, Cara, et al. "Social Support and Physical Health: The Importance of Belonging." *Journal of American College Health,* Vol. 53, No. 6, May–June 2005, p. 276.
15. Hermann, Karen, and Nancy Betz. "Path Models of the Relationships of Instrumentality and Expressiveness to Social Self-Efficacy, Shyness, and Depressive Symptoms." *Sex Roles: A Journal of Research,* Vol. 51, No. 1–2, July 2004, pp. 55(12).
16. Colten, Harvey, and Altevogt, Bruce (eds.), Committee on Sleep Medicine and Research of the Institute of Medicine. *Sleep Disorders and Sleep Deprivation: An Unmet Public Health Problem.* Washington, DC: National Academies Press, 2006.
17. National Sleep Foundation. *2006 Sleep In America Poll,* www.sleepfoundation.org.
18. Brown, Franklin, et al. "Development and Evaluation of the Sleep Treatment and Education Program for Students (STEPS)." *Journal of American College Health,* Vol. 54, No. 4, January–February 2006, p. 201.
19. Ibid.
20. Vorona, R. D., et al. "Overweight and Obese Patients in a Primary Care Population Report Less Sleep than Patients with a Normal Body Mass Index." *Archives of Internal Medicine,* Vol. 165, No. 1, January 10, 2005, p. 25.
21. Egan, Brent. "Sleep and Hypertension: Burning the Candle at Both Ends Really Is Hazardous to Your Health." *Hypertension,* Vol. 47, No. 5, May 2006, p. 816.
22. Brown et al. "Development and Evaluation of the Sleep Treatment Education Program for Students."
23. Millman, Richard. "Excessive Sleepiness in Adolescents and Young Adults: Causes, Consequences, and Treatment Strategies." *Pediatrics,* Vol. 115, No. 6, June 2005, p. 774.
24. Kobau, R., et al. "Sad, Blue, or Depressed Days, Health Behaviors and Health-Related Quality of Life, Behavioral Risk Factor Surveillance System, 1995–2000." *Health Quality of Life Outcomes.* Vol. 2, No. 1, July 30, 2004, p. 40.
25. *Diagnostic & Statistical Manual IV TR*(electronic). Washington, DC: American Psychiatric Publishing, 2003.
26. Schwartz, Allan. "Are College Students More Disturbed Today? Stability in the Acuity and Qualitative Character of Psychopathology of College Counseling Center Clients: 1992–1993 through 2001–2002." *American Journal of College Health,* Vol. 54, No. 6, May–June 2006, p. 327–337.
27. Ibid.
28. American College Health Association. American College Health Association-National College Health Assessment (ACHA-NCHA) Web Summary, April 2006, www.acha.org/projects_programs/ncha_sampledata.cfm.
29. American College Health Association. "American College Health Association-National College Health Assessment (ACHA-NCHA) Spring 2004 Reference Group Data Report (abridged)." *Journal of American College Health,* Vol. 54, No. 4, January–February 2006, p. 201.
30. Voelker, Rebecca. "Stress, Sleep Loss, and Substance Abuse Create Potent Recipe for College Depression." *Journal of the American Medical Association,* Vol. 291, No. 18, May 12, 2004, p. 2177.
31. Wart, Paula. "Why Be Happy?" *Health Plus,* Vanderbilt University, January 3, 2005.
32. Johns Hopkins University Evidence-Based Practice Center. *Post-Myocardial Infarction Depression.* Rockville, MD: Agency for Healthcare Research and Quality, May 2005.
33. Miller, Michael Craig. "Is Exercise a Good Treatment for Depression?" HEALTHBeat, July 6, 2005, www.health.harvard.edu/mental.
34. Turner, R. J., and D. A. Lloyd. "Stress Burden and the Lifetime Incidence of Psychiatric Disorder in Young Adults: Racial and Ethnic Contrasts." *Archives of General Psychiatry,* Vol. 61, No. 5, May 2004, p. 481.
35. "Depression Is Up for College Students." *Getting Paid in Behavioral Healthcare,* Vol. 10, No. 5, May 2005, p. 7.
36. Tija, Jennifer, et al. "Factors Associated with Undertreatment of Medical Student Depression." *Journal of American College Health,* Vol. 53, No. 5, March–April 2005, p. 219.
37. Franko, Debra, et al. "Self-Reported Symptoms of Depression in Late Adolescence to Early Adulthood: A Comparison of African-American and Caucasian Females." *Journal of Adolescent Health,* Vol. 37, No. 6, December 2005, pp. 526–529.
38. Jensen, Peter. Personal interview.
39. Lenz, Brenda. "Tobacco, Depression, and Lifestyle Choices in the Pivotal Early College Years." *Journal of American College Health,* Vol. 52, No. 5, March–April 2004, p. 213.
40. Kuehn, Bridget. "Link Between Smoking and Mental Illness May Lead to Treatments." *Journal of American Medical Association,* Vol. 295, No. 5, February 1, 2006, p. 483.
41. Cohen, Lee, et al. "Relapse of Major Depression During Pregnancy in Women Who Maintain or Discontinue Antidepressant Treatment." *Journal of American Medical Association,* Vol. 295, No. 5, February 1, 2006, p. 499.
42. Hampton, Tracy. "Antidepressants and Pregnancy." *Journal of American Medical Association,* Vol. 295, No. 14, April 12, 2006, p. 1631.
43. Kendler, Kenneth, et al. "Sex Differences in the Relationship between Social Support and Risk for Major Depression: A Longitudinal Study of Opposite-Sex Twin Pairs." *American Journal of Psychiatry,* Vol. 162, No. 2, February 2005, p. 250.
44. Trivedi, M. H., et al. "Medication Augmentation After the Failure of SSRIs for Depression." *New England Journal of Medicine,* Vol. 354, No. 12, March 23, 2006, pp. 1243–1252.
45. Schatzberg, Alan, et al. "Medication (Nefazodone) or Psychotherapy (CBASP) Is Effective When the Other Is Not." *Archives of General Psychiatry,* Vol. 62, No. 6, June 2005, p. 513.
46. Fitzgerald, Paul, et al. "A Randomized, Controlled Trial of Sequential Bilateral Repetitive Transcranial Magnetic Stimulation for Treatment-Resistant Depression." *American Journal of Psychiatry,* January 2006, Vol. 163, No. 1, p. 5.
47. Greden, John. Personal interview.
48. Hammad, T. A., et al. "Suicidality in Pediatric Patients Treated with Antidepressant Drugs." *Archives of General Psychiatry,* Vol. 63, No. 3, March 2006, pp. 332–339.
49. Simon, Gregory, et al. "Suicide Risk During Anti-Depressant Treatment." *American Journal of Psychiatry,* Vol. 163, No. 1, January 2006, p. 5.
50. Swann, Alan. "What Is Bipolar Disorder?" *American Journal of Psychiatry,* Vol. 163, No. 1, February 2006, p. 177.
51. Kennedy, Noel, et al. "Gender Differences in Incidence and Age at Onset of Mania and Bipolar Disorder over a 35-Year Period in Camberwell, England." *American Journal of Psychiatry,* Vol. 162, No. 2, February 2005, p. 257.
52. Teter, Christian, et al. "Prevalence and Motives for Illicit Use of Prescription Stimulants in an Undergraduate Student Sample." *Journal of American College Health,* Vol. 53, No. 6, May–June 2005, p. 253.
53. Gold, Lisa. "Suicide and Gender." *Textbook of Suicide Assessment and Management,* Simon, Robert and Robert Hales, (eds.). Washington, DC: American Psychiatric Publishing, 2006, p. 77.
54. Ash, Peter. "Children and Adolescents." *Textbook of Suicide Assessment and Management,* Simon, Robert and Robert Hales, (eds.). Washington, DC: American Psychiatric Publishing, 2006, p. 35.
55. Schwartz, Allan. "College Student Suicide in the United States: 1990–1991 through 2003–2004." *American Journal of College Health,* Vol. 54, No. 6, May–June 2006, pp. 341–352.

56. Schwartz, Allan. "Four Eras of Study of College Student Suicide in the United States: 1920–2004." *American Journal of College Health,* Vol. 54, No. 6, May–June 2006, pp. 353–366.
57. Gould, Madelyn. Personal interview.
58. Horton, Leslie. "Social, Cultural, and Demograpic Factors in Suicide." *Textbook of Suicide Assessment and Management,* Simon, Robert and Robert Hales, (eds.). Washington, DC: American Psychiatric Publishing, 2006, p. 107.
59. Ash, "Children and Adolescents."
60. Hammad et al. "Suicidality in Pediatric Patients Treated with Antidepressant Drugs."
61. Simon et al. "Suicide Risk During Anti-Depressant Treatment."
62. Frankenberger, Kristi, et al. "Effects of Information on College Students' Perceptions of Antidepressant Medication." *Journal of American College Health,* Vol. 53, No. 1, July–August 2004, p. 35.

Chapter 3

1. Lazarus, R., and R. Launier. "Stress-Related Transactions Between Person and Environment." *Perspectives in Interactional Psychology.* New York: Plenum, 1978.
2. Schmeelk-Cone, K. H., et al. "The Buffering Effects of Active Coping on the Relationship Between SES and Cortisol Among African American Young Adults." *Behavioral Medicine,* Vol. 29, No. 2, Summer 2003, p. 85.
3. Jones, M. P. "The Role of Psychosocial Factors in Peptic Ulcer Disease: Beyond *Helicobacter pylori* and NSAIDs." *Journal of Psychosomatic Research.* Vol. 60, No. 4, April 2006, pp. 407–412.
4. Freeman, L. M., and K. M. Gil. "Daily Stress, Coping, and Dietary Restraint in Binge Eating." *International Journal of Eating Disorders,* Vol. 36, No. 2, September 2004, p. 204.
5. Uhart, M., et al. "Hormonal Responses to Psychological Stress and Family History of Alcoholism." *Neuropsychopharmacology.* March 22, 2006 (Epub ahead of print).
6. Pryor, John, et al. *The American Freshman: National Norms for Fall 2006.* Los Angeles, University of California, Los Angeles Higher Education Research Institute, December 2006
7. Uhart, M., et al. "Gender Differences in Hypothalamic-Pituitary-Adrenal (HPA) Axis Reactivity." *Psychoneuroendocrinology,* Vol. 60, No. 4, April 2006, pp. 407–412.
8. Evans, Sybil. Personal interview.
9. Green, B. L., et al. "Effects of Adolescent Trauma Exposure on Risky Behavior in College Women." *Psychiatry.* Vol. 68, No. 4, Winter 2005, pp. 363–378.
10. "Americans Engage in Unhealthy Behaviors to Manage Stress; New Survey Findings Show Gender Differences, Effects on Mind/Body Health." *US Newswire,* February 23, 2006.
11. Utay, Joe, and Miller, Megan. "Guided Imagery as an Effective Therapeutic Technique: A Brief Review of Its History and Efficacy Research." *Journal of Instructional Psychology,* Vol. 33, No. 1, March 2006, p. 40.
12. Archer, Shirley. "Tangible Proof of Brain Changes Associated with Meditation." *IDEA Fitness Journal,* Vol. 3, No. 3, March 2006, p. 88(1).
13. Archer, Shirley. "More College Students Turn to Meditation." *IDEA Fitness Journal,* Vol. 3, No. 4, April 2006, p. 86(1).
14. Foley, Kevin. "PTSD in African Americans." *Clinical Psychiatry News,* Vol. 33, No. 4, April 2005, p. 20.
15. Schafer, I., et al. "Posttraumatic Syndromes in Children and Adolescents after Road Traffic Accidents—A Prospective Cohort Study." *Psychopathology,* Vol. 39, No. 4, April 11, 2006, pp. 159–164.
16. Foa, E. B. "Psychosocial Therapy for Posttraumatic Stress Disorder." *Journal of Clinical Psychiatry,* Vol. 67, Suppl. 2, 2006, pp. 40–45.
17. Rosenbaum, Jerrold, and Covino, Jennifer. "Stress and Resilience: Implications for Depression and Anxiety." *Medscape Psychiatry & Mental Health,* Vol. 2, No. 10, 2005.

Chapter 4

1. American College Health Association. "American College Health Association-National College Health Assessment (ACHA-NCHA) Spring 2004 Reference Group Data Report (abridged)." *Journal of American College Health,* Vol. 54, No. 4, January–February 2006, p. 201.
2. Carnethon, M. R., et al. "Prevalence and Cardiovascular Disease Correlates of Low Cardiorespiratory Fitness in Adolescents and Adults." *Journal of American Medical Association,* Vol. 294, No. 23, December 21, 2005, pp. 2981–2988.
3. American College Health Association. American College Health Association-National College Health Assessment (ACHA-NCHA) Web Summary, April 2006, www.acha.org/projects_programs/ncha_sampledata.cfm.
4. Buckworth, Janet, and Claudio Nigg. "Physical Activity, Exercise, and Sedentary Behavior in College Students." *Journal of American College Health,* Vol. 53, No. 1, July–August 2004, p. 28.
5. Whang, William, et al. "Physical Exertion, Exercise, and Sudden Cardiac Death in Women." *Journal of American Medical Association,* Vol. 295, No. 12, March 22/29, 2006, p. 1399.
6. Mora, Samia, et al. "Association of Physical Activity and Body Mass Index with Novel and Traditional Cardiovascular Biomarkers in Women." *Journal of American Medical Association,* Vol. 295, No. 12, March 22/29, 2006, p. 1412.
7. Orakzai, R. H., et al. "Association of Increased Cardiorespiratory Fitness with Low Risk for Clustering of Metabolic Syndrome Components in Asymptomatic Men." *Archives of Medicine Research,* Vol. 37, No. 4, May 2006, pp. 522–528.
8. Patel, Alpa, et al. "Recreational Physical Activity and Sedentary Behavior in Relation to Ovarian Cancer Risk in a Large Cohort of US Women." *American Journal of Epidemiology,* Vol. 163, 2006, pp. 709–716.
9. Bauer, Jeff. "Regular Exercise May Help Ward Off Dementia." *RN,* Vol. 69, No. 3, March 2006, p. 20.
10. Miller, Michael Craig. "Is Exercise A Good Treatment for Depression?" HEALTHBeat, July 6, 2005, www.health.harvard.edu/mental.
11. "Keys to Healthy Bones: A New Surgeon General's Report Warns of a Coming Osteoporosis Crisis." *Tufts University Health & Nutrition Letter,* Vol. 22, No. 11, January 2005, p. 4.
12. "Step Up to Denser Bones." *Science News,* Vol. 167, No. 17, April 23, 2005, p. 270.
13. "Physical Activity for Lifelong Bone Health: The American College of Sports Medicine Promotes Osteoporosis Prevention." *Journal of Musculoskeletal Medicine,* Vol. 22, No. 1, January 2005, p. 6.
14. Penhollow, Tina, and Michael Young. "Sexual Desirability and Sexual Performance: Does Exercise and Fitness Really Matter?" *Electronic Journal of Human Sexuality,* Vol. 7, October 5, 2004, www.ejhs.org.
15. *Dietary Guidelines for Americans 2005,* U.S. Department of Health and Human Services (USDHHS), U.S. Department of Agriculture (USDA), www.healthierus.gov/dietaryguidelines.
16. Zizzi, Sam, et al. "The Interaction of Goal Orientation and Stage of Change on Exercise Behavior in College Students." *Journal of Sport Behavior,* Vol. 29, No. 1, March 2006, p. 96(15).
17. Keating, Xiaofen Deng, et al. "A Meta-Analysis of College Students' Physical Activity Behaviors." *Journal of American College Health,* Vol. 54, No. 2, September–October 2005, p. 116.
18. Reed, Julian, and Dawn Wilson. "Awareness and Use of a University Recreational Trail." *Journal of American College Health,* Vol. 54, No. 4, January–February 2006, p. 227.
19. Suminski, Richard, and Petosa, Rick. "Web-Assisted Instruction for Changing Social Cognitive Variables Related to Physical Activity." *Journal of American College Health,* Vol. 54, No. 4, January–February 2006, p. 219.
20. Kilpatrick, Marcus, et al. "College Students' Motivation for Physical Activity: Differentiating Men's and Women's

Motives for Sports Participation and Exercise." *Journal of American College Health,* Vol. 54, No. 2, September–October 2005, p. 87.
21. *Dietary Guidelines for Americans 2005,* USDHHS, USDA.
22. Hampton, Tracy. "Researchers Address Use of Performance-Enhancing Drugs in Nonelite Athletes." *Journal of American Medical Association,* Vol. 295, No. 6, February 8, 2006, p. 607.
23. Mosca, Lorie, et al. "Waist Circumference Predicts Cardiometabolic and Global Framingham Risk among Women Screened during National Women's Heart Day." *Journal of Women's Health,* Vol. 15, No. 1, January 2006, pp. 24–34.

Chapter 5

1. *Dietary Guidelines for Americans 2005,* U.S. Department of Health and Human Services (USDHHS), U.S. Department of Agriculture (USDA), www.healthierus.gov/dietaryguidelines.
2. Bell, John. "Jury Out on Value of Low-Carb Diets." *Family Practice News,* Vol. 36, No.6, March 15, 2006, p. 20(1).
3. University of Sydney, Australia, Glycemic Index Testing Service, Human Nutrition Unit, www.glycemicindex.com.
4. Hooper, Lee, et al. "Risks and Benefits of Omega 3 Fats for Mortality, Cardiovascular Disease, and Cancer: Systematic Review." *British Medical Journal,* Vol. 332, No. 7544, April 1, 2006, pp. 752–760.
5. Brunner, Eric. "Oily Fish and Omega 3 Fat Supplements." *British Medical Journal,* Vol. 332, No. 7544, April 1, 2006, pp. 739–740.
6. Prentice, Ross, et al. "Low-Fat Dietary Pattern and Risk of Invasive Breast Cancer." *Journal of the American Medical Association,* Vol. 295, No. 6, February 8, 2006, p. 629.
7. Beresford, Shirley, et al. "Low-Fat Dietary Pattern and Risk of Colorectal Cancer." *Journal of the American Medical Association,* Vol. 295, No. 6, February 8, 2006, p. 643.
8. Howard, Barbara, et al. "Low-Fat Dietary Pattern and Risk of Cardiovascular Disease." *Journal of the American Medical Association,* Vol. 295, No. 6, February 8, 2006, p. 655.
9. Ornish, Dean. "Set the Record Straight on Low-Fat Diets." *Family Practice News,* Vol. 36, No. 7, April 1, 2006, p. 7(1).
10. Buzdar, Aman. "Dietary Modification and Risk of Breast Cancer." *Journal of the American Medical Association,* Vol. 295, No. 6, February 8, 2006, p. 691.
11. Anderson, Cheryl, and Lawrence Appel. "Dietary Modification and CVD Prevention." *Journal of the American Medical Association,* Vol. 295, No. 6, February 8, 2006, p. 693.
12. *Dietary Guidelines for Americans 2005,* USDHHS, USDA.
13. Jackson, R. D., et al. "Calcium Plus Vitamin D Supplementation and the Risk of Fractures." *New England Journal of Medicine,* Vol. 354, February 16, 2006, pp. 669–683.
14. "Calcium and Vitamin D May Offer Modest Bone Benefits." *Association of Operating Room Nurses Journal,* Vol. 83, No. 4, April 2006, p. 846.
15. *Dietary Guidelines for Americans 2005,* USDHHS, USDA.
16. I-Min, Lee, et al. "Vitamin E in the Primary Prevention of Cardiovascular Disease and Cancer." *Journal of the American Medical Association,* Vol. 294, No. 1, July 6, 2005, p. 56.
17. Neff, Matthew. "Antioxidant Vitamin Supplements and Cardiovascular Disease Risk Reduction." *American Family Physician,* Vol. 71, No. 7, April 1, 2005, p. 1433.
18. "Vitamin E Gets an F." *Harvard Health Letter,* June 2005.
19. Jacobs, Eric, and Michael Thun. "Low-Dose Aspirin and Vitamin E: Challenges and Opportunities in Cancer Prevention." *Journal of the American Medical Association,* Vol. 294, No. 1, July 6, 2005, p. 105.
20. "The Riddle of MyPyramid." *Harvard Heart Letter,* April 2006.
21. "One Year Later: Lessons from New Guidelines and Pyramid." *Tufts University Health & Nutrition Letter,* Vol. 23, No. 12, February 2006, p. 4(2).
22. "Rebuilding the Pyramid: The Government's New Food Pyramid Replaces 'One Size Fits All' with a Customizable Eating and Exercise Plan." *Tufts University Health & Nutrition Letter,* Vol. 23, No. 4, June 2005, p. 1.
23. Forshee R. A., et al. "Changes in Calcium Intake and Association with Beverage Consumption and Demographics: Comparing Data from CSFII 1994–1996, 1998 and NHANES 1999–2002." *Journal of American Colllege Nutrition,* Vol. 25, No. 2, April 2006, pp. 108–116.
24. Racette, Susan, et al. "Weight Changes, Exercise, and Dietary Patterns During Freshman and Sophomore Years of College." *Journal of American College Health,* Vol. 53, No. 6, 2005, p. 245.
25. Gray, L. E., et al. "Assessment of Dietary Fiber Intake Among University Students." *Journal of the American Dietetic Association,* Vol. 104, No. 8, August 2004, p. A26.
26. *Dietary Guidelines for Americans 2005,* USDHHS, USDA.
27. *Dietary Guidelines for Americans 2005,* USDHHS, USDA.
28. Conklin, Martha, et al. "Nutrition Information at Point of Selection Could Benefit College Students." *Topics in Clinical Nutrition,* Vol. 20, No. 2, April–June 2005, p. 90(7).
29. Lofshult, Diane. "More Natural Snacks." *IDEA Fitness Journal,* Vol. 2, No. 5, May 2005, p. 77.
30. Partnership for Food Safety, www.fightbac.org.
31. Chapman, Jean, et al. "Food Allergy: A Practice Parameter." *Annals of Allergy, Asthma and Immunology,* Vol. 96, No. 3, Supp. 2, March 2006, pp. 1–68.

Chapter 6

1. American Obesity Association, www.obesity.org.
2. Ogden, Cynthia, et al. "Prevalence of Overweight and Obesity in the United States, 1999–2004." *Journal of the American Medical Association,* Vol. 295, No. 13, April 5, 2006, pp. 1549.
3. "Global Strategy on Diet, Physical Activity and Health." World Health Organization, www.who.int/dietphysicalactivity/publications/facts/obesity/en/.
4. Ogden et al. "Prevalence of Overweight and Obesity in the United States, 1999–2004."
5. Ibid.
6. Pereira, M. A., et al. "Fast-food Habits, Weight Gain, and Insulin Resistance (The CARDIA Study): 15-year Prospective Analysis." *Lancet,* Vol. 365, No. 9453, January 1, 2005, pp. 36–42.
7. Davison, Tany, and Marita McCabe. "Relationships Between Men's and Women's Body Image and Their Psychological, Social, and Sexual Functioning." *Sex Roles: A Journal of Research,* Vol. 52, No. 7–8, April 2005, p. 463.
8. American College Health Association. American College Health Association-National College Health Assessment (ACHA-NCHA) Web Summary. Updated April 2006. Available at www.acha.org/projects_programs/ncha_sampledata.cfm.
9. American Obesity Association.
10. Long, D., et al. "The Cost of Lifestyle Health Risks: Obesity." *Journal of Occupational & Environmental Medicine.* Vol. 48, No. 3, March 2006, pp. 244–251.
11. Simons-Morton, Denise, et al. "Obesity Research—Limitations of Methods, Measurements, and Medications." *Journal of the American Medical Association,* Vol. 295, No. 7, February 15, 2006, p. 826.
12. Yan, Lijing, et al. "Excessive Adiposity, Calorie Restriction, and Aging." *Journal of the American Medical Association,* Vol. 295, No. 13, April 5, 2006, p. 1577.
13. Eisenberg, Marla, et al. "Weight-Related Issues and High-Risk Sexual Behaviors among College Students." *Journal of American College Health,* Vol. 54, No. 2, September–October 2005, p. 95.
14. American College Health Association. ACHA-NCHA Web Summary.

15. Slawson, David. "Popular Diets Equally Effective for Losing Weight." *American Family Physician,* Vol. 71, No. 9, May 1, 2005, p. 1783.
16. Dansinger, Michael, et al. "Comparison of the Atkins, Ornish, Weight Watchers, and Zone Diets for Weight Loss and Heart Disease Risk Reduction: A Randomized Trial." *Journal of the American Medical Association,* Vol. 293, No. 1, January 5, 2005, p. 43.
17. Tsai, Adam, and Wadden, Thomas. "Systematic Review: An Evaluation of Major Commercial Weight Loss Programs in the United States." *Annals of Internal Medicine,* Vol. 142, No. 1, January 4, 2005, p. 56.
18. Prentice, Ross, et al. "Low-Fat Dietary Pattern and Risk of Invasive Breast Cancer." *Journal of the American Medical Association,* Vol. 295, No. 6, February 8, 2006, p. 629.
19. Beresford, Shirley, et al. "Low-Fat Dietary Pattern and Risk of Colorectal Cancer." *Journal of the American Medical Association,* Vol. 295, No. 6, February 8, 2006, p. 643.
20. Howard, Barbara, et al. "Low-Fat Dietary Pattern and Risk of Cardiovascular Disease." *Journal of the American Medical Association,* Vol. 295, No. 6, February 8, 2006, p. 655.
21. Anderson, Cheryl, and Lawrence Appel. "Dietary Modification and CVD Prevention." *Journal of the American Medical Association,* Vol. 295, No. 6, February 8, 2006, p. 693.
22. Levine, James, et al. "Interindividual Variation in Posture Allocation: Possible Role in Human Obesity." *Science,* Vol. 307, No. 5709, January 28, 2005, p. 584.
23. Ibid.
24. Helmering, Doris, and Dianne Hales. *Think Thin, Be Thin.* New York: Broadway Books, 2005.
25. National Weight Control Registry, www.lifespan.org/services/bmed/wt_loss/nwcr/.
26. Simons-Morton et al. "Obesity Research—Limitations of Methods, Measurements, and Medications."
27. Encinosa, W. E., et al. "Use and Costs of Bariatric Surgery and Prescription Weight-Loss Medications." *Health Affairs,* Vol. 24, No. 4, July–August 2005, p. 1039.
28. American Obesity Association. www.obesity.org.
29. National Eating Disorders Center, www.nationaleatingdisorders.org.
30. Kirn, Timothy. "Four Factors Useful in Identifying Eating Disorders in Girls." *Clinical Psychiatry News,* Vol. 33, No. 1, January 2005, p. 42.
31. Hinton, Pamela, et al. "Psychosocial Correlates of Disordered Eating in Female Collegeiate Athletes: Validation of the ATHLETE Questionnaire." *Journal of American College Health,* Vol. 54, No. 3, November–December 2005, p. 149.

Chapter 7

1. American College Health Association. "American College Health Association-National College Health Assessment (ACHA-NCHA) Spring 2004 Reference Group Data Report (abridged)." *Journal of American College Health,* Vol. 54, No. 4, January–February 2006, p. 201.
2. Laumann, Edward. Personal interview.
3. Buss, David. *The Evolution of Desire.* New York: Basic Books, 1994.
4. U.S. Census Bureau, Washington, DC, www.census.gov.
5. Poponoe, David, and Barbara Dafoe Whitehead. *The State of Our Unions 2005.* Rutgers, NJ: National Marriage Project, 2005, http://marriage.rutgers.edu.
6. Sternberg, Robert. Personal interview.
7. National Center for Health Statistics, www.nchs.gov.
8. American College Health Association. "ACHA-NCHA Spring 2004 Reference Group Data Report."
9. "Just the Facts . . . Circumcision." American Adademy of Pediatrics, www.aap.org/mrt/factscir.htm.
10. American College Health Association. American College Health Association-National College Health Assessment (ACHA-NCHA) Web Summary, www.acha.org/projects_programs/ncha_sampledata.cfm.
11. Martens, Matthew, et al. "Differences between Actual and Perceived Student Norms: An Examination of Alcohol Use, Drug Use, and Sexual Behavior." *Journal of American College Health,* Vol. 54, No. 5, March–April 2006, p. 295.
12. Raffaelli, Marccela, et al. "Acculturation Status and Sexuality among Female Cuban American College Students." *Journal of American College Health,* Vol. 54, No. 1, July–August 2005, p. 7
13. Ibid.
14. Eisenberg, Marla, et al. "Weight-Related Issues and High-Risk Sexual Behaviors among College Students." *Journal of American College Health,* Vol. 54, No. 2, September–October 2005, p. 95.
15. "Abstinence-Only Education Policies and Programs: A Position Paper of the Society for Adolescent Medicine." *Journal of Adolescent Health,* January 2006, Vol. 38, p. 83.

Chapter 8

1. Guttmacher Institute, www.guttmacher.org.
2. American College Health Association. "American College Health Association National College Health Assessment (ACHA-NCHA) Spring 2005 Reference Group Data Report (abridged)." *Journal of American College Health,* Vol. 55, No. 1, 2006, pp. 5–16.
3. Fennell, Reginald. "The Emperor Has No Clothes": Emergency Contraception Should Be Available Over-the-Counter." *Journal of American College Health,* Vol. 54, No. 5, March–April 2006, p. 257(3).
4. "Birth Control Patch-Wearers at Higher Risk of Blood Clots." *Contemporary OB/GYN,* Vol. 5, No. 1, January 2006, p. 17.
5. Ibid.
6. "Birth Control and Weight Gain." *Family Practice News,* Vol. 36, No. 5, March 1, 2006, p. 21(1).
7. American College Health Association. "ACHA-NCHA Spring 2005 Reference Group Data Report (abridged)."
8. American College Health Association. American College Health Association-National College Health Assessment (ACHA-NCHA) Web Summary, www.acha.org/projects_programs/ncha_sampledata.cfm.
9. Crosby, Richard, et al. "Condom Discomfort and Associated Problems with their Use among University Students." *Journal of American College Health,* Vol. 54, No. 3, November–December 2005, p. 143.
10. James, Chris. "Prevalence of Erectile Dysfunction and Use of ED Medications Among Teens, Young Men." News Release, Children's Memorial Hospital and Northwestern University, April 24, 2006.
11. Fennell, "The Emperor Has No Clothes."
12. Miller, Laura McKeller, and Robin Sawyer. "Emergency Contraceptive Pills: A 10-Year Follow-Up Survey of Use and Experiences at College Health Centers in the Mid-Atlantic United States." *Journal of American College Health,* Vol. 54, No. 5, March–April 2006, p. 257(3).
13. Conard, Lee, and Melanie Gold. "What You Need to Know About Providing Emergency Contraception: This Update Answers Key Questions About Emergency Contraception and Will Help Increase Your Patients' Access to This Form of Pregnancy Prevention." *Contemporary Pediatrics,* Vol. 23, No. 2, February 2006, p. 49.
14. Miller and Sawyer, "Emergency Contraceptive Pills."
15. "Plan B Emergency Contraception Information Sheet." *Journal of the American Academy of Child and Adolescent Psychiatry,* Vol. 45, No. 3, March 2006, p. 313(1).
16. American College Health Association. "ACHA-NCHA Spring 2004 Reference Group Data Report."
17. Miller and Sawyer, "Emergency Contraceptive Pills."
18. Ibid.
19. "Emergency Contraception." *State Policies in Brief,* Guttmacher Institute, www.guttmacher.org.
20. American Cancer Society, www.cancer.org/docroot/cri/content/cri_2

_6x_can_having_an_abortion_cause_or_contribute_to_breast_cancer.asp?sitearea=cri.

21. Schneider, Mary Ellen. "South Dakota Enacts Far-Reaching Abortion Ban." *Internal Medicine News,* Vol. 39, No. 8, April 15, 2006, p. 76(1).

Chapter 9

1. Kuehn, Bridget. "Animal-Human Diseases Targeted to Stop Pandemics Before They Start." *Journal of the American Medical Association,* Vol. 295, No. 17, May 3, 2006, p. 1987.
2. American College Health Association. American College Health Association-National College Health Assessment (ACHA-NCHA) Web Summary, April 2006, www.acha.org/projects_programs/ncha_sampledata.cfm.
3. Robinson, June. "Anatomical and Hormonal Influences on Women's Dermatologic Health." *Journal of the American Medical Association,* Vol. 295, No. 12, March 22/29, 2006, p. 1443.
4. Mitka, Mike. "Age Range Widens for Pertussis Vaccine." *Journal of the American Medical Association,* Vol. 295, No. 8, February 22, 2006, p. 871.
5. Hampton, Tracy. "New Guidelines Released for Managing Cough." *Journal of the American Medical Association,* Vol. 295, No. 7, February 15, 2006, p. 746.
6. Bright, Rick, et al. "Adamantane Resistance among Influenza A Viruses Isolated Early During the 2005–2006 Influenza Season in the United States." *Journal of the American Medical Association,* Vol. 295, No. 8, February 22, 2006, p. 891.
7. Nichol, Kristin, et al. "Colds and Influenza-Like Illnesses in University Students: Impact on Health, Academic and Work Performance, and Health Care Use." *Clinical Infectious Diseases,* Vol. 40, No. 9, May 1, 2005, p. 1263(8).
8. U.S. Department of Health and Human Services, Washington, DC, www.pandemicflu.gov.
9. Shinya, K., et al. "Avian Flu: Influenza Virus Receptors in the Human Airway." *Nature.* Vol. 440, No. 7083, March 23, 2006, pp. 435–436.
10. Tully, Joanna, et al. "Risk and Protective Factors for Meningococcal Disease in Adolescents: Matched Cohort Study." *British Medical Journal,* Vol. 332, No. 7539, February 15, 2006, pp. 445–450.
11. Chang, T. T., et al. "A Comparison of Entecavir and Lamivudine for HBeAg-Positive Chronic Hepatitis B." *New England Journal of Medicine,* Vol. 354, No. 10, March 9, 2006, pp. 1001–1010.
12. "Hepatitis C Fact Sheet." CDC, Washington, DC, www.cdc.gov/hepatitis.
13. "Bird Flu Expands Range." *Journal of the American Medical Association,* Vol. 295, No. 11, March 15, 2006, p. 1239.
14. Komaroff, Anthony (ed.). *Bird Flu.* Boston, MA: Harvard Health Publications, 2006.
15. Hampton, Tracy. "Avian Flu Risk to Humans Probed." *Journal of the American Medical Association,* Vol. 295, No. 16, April 26, 2006, p. 1885.
16. Shinya et al., "Avian Flu."
17. Hampton, Tracy. "Avian Flu Researchers Make Strides." *Journal of the American Medical Association,* Vol. 295, No. 10, March 8, 2006, p. 1107.
18. National Library of Medicine and National Institutes of Health, Medline Plus, Bethesda, MD, www.nlm.nih.gov/medlineplus/birdflu.html.
19. American College Health Association. "American College Health Association-National College Health Assessment (ACHA-NCHA) Spring 2004 Reference Group Data Report (abridged)." *Journal of American College Health,* Vol. 54, No. 4, January–February 2006, p. 201.
20. Ibid.
21. Preidt, Robert. "College Freshmen at High Chlamydia Risk." *HealthDay,* May 9, 2006, www.nlm.nih.gov/medlineplus.
22. Fox, Maggie. "Younger Women Often Reinfected With Chlamydia." *HealthDay,* May 9, 2006, www.nlm.nih.gov/medlineplus.
23. McPartland, Tara, et al. "Men's Perceptions and Knowledge of Human Papillomavirus (HPV) Infection and Cervical Cancer." *Journal of American College Health,* Vol. 53, No. 5, March–April 2005, p. 225.
24. Cuzick, Jack, et al. "Overview of the European and North American Studies on HPV Testing in Primary Cervical Cancer Screening." *International Journal of Cancer,* April 3, 2006 (epub).
25. "African Americans and HIV/AIDS." *Kaiser Family Foundation HIV/AIDS* Fact Sheet, February 2006, www.kff.org.
26. "Women and HIV/AIDS in the United States." *Kaiser Family Foundation HIV/AIDS Fact Sheet,* February 2006, www.kff.org.

Chapter 10

1. Gulati, Martha, et al. "The Prognostic Value of a Nomogram for Exercise Capacity in Women." *New England Journal of Medicine,* Vol. 353, No. 5, August 4, 2005, pp. 517–519.
2. Hooper, Lee, et al. "Risks and Benefits of Omega 3 Fats for Mortality, Cardiovascular Disease, and Cancer: Systematic Review." *British Medical Journal,* Vol. 332, No. 7544, April 1, 2006, pp. 752–760.
3. Brunner, Eric. "Oily Fish and Omega 3 Fat Supplements." *British Medical Journal,* Vol. 332, No. 7544, April 1, 2006, pp. 739–740.
4. Torpy, Janet. "The Metabolic Syndrome." *Journal of the American Medical Association,* Vol. 295, No. 7, February 15, 2006, p. 850.
5. "Type D Personality and Cardiovascular Risk." *Harvard Health Letter,* August 2005.
6. Schiffter, A., et al. "The Distressed (Type D) Personality Is Independently Associated with Impaired Health Status and Increased Depressive Symptoms in Chronic Heart Failure." *European Journal of Cardiovascular Prevention and Rehabilitation,* Vol. 12, No. 4, August 2005, p. 341.
7. "Type D for Distressed." *Harvard Health Letter,* August 2005.
8. Berger, Jeffrey, et al. "Aspirin for the Primary Prevention of Cardiovascular Events in Women and Men." *Journal of the American Medical Association,* Vol. 295, No. 3, January 18, 2006, p. 306.
9. Hsia, Judith, et al. "Conjugated Equine Estrogens and Coronary Heart Disease: The Women's Health Initiative." *Archives of Internal Medicine,* Vol. 166, No. 3, February 13, 2006, pp. 357-365.
10. Robertson, Rose Marie. Personal interview.
11. Thom, T., N. Haas, and R. Wayne. "Heart Disease and Stroke Statistics—2006 Update: A Report from the American Heart Association Statistics Committee and Stroke Statistics Subcommittee." *Circulation,* Vol. 113, No. 6, Feb 14, 2006, pp. 85–151.
12. Quyyumi, A. A. "Women and Ischemic Heart Disease: Pathophysiologic Implications from the Women's Ischemia Syndrome Evaluation (WISE) Study and Future Research Steps." *Journal of the American College of Cardiology,* Vol. 47, Suppl. 3, February 7, 2006, pp. 566–571.
13. Mitka, Mike. "Studies Explore Stroke's Gender Gap." *Journal of the American Medical Association,* Vol. 295, No. 15, April 19, 2006, p. 1755.
14. Deng, Y. Z., et al. "IV Tissue Plasminogen Activator Use in Acute Stroke: Experience from a Statewide Registry." *Neurology,* Vol. 63, No. 3, February 14, 2006, 66(3):306-312.
15. Berger et al., "Aspirin for the Primary Prevention of Cardiovascular Events in Women and Men."
16. *Cancer Facts and Figures 2006.* Atlanta, GA: American Cancer Society.
17. Ibid.
18. Prentice, Ross, et al. "Low-Fat Dietary Pattern and Risk of Invasive Breast Cancer." *Journal of the American Medical Association,* Vol. 295, No. 6, February 8, 2006, p. 629.
19. Beresford, Shirley, et al. "Low-Fat Dietary Pattern and Risk of Colorectal Cancer." *Journal of the American Medical Association,* Vol. 295, No. 6, February 8, 2006, p. 643.
20. "Indoor Tanning Contributes to Increased Incidence of Skin Cancer." News Release, American Academy of Dermatology, January 12, 2006.

21. Warthan, M. M., et al. "UV Light Tanning as a Type of Substance-Related Disorder." *Archives of Dermatology,* Vol. 141, No. 8, August 2005, pp. 963–966.
22. Chen, W. Y., et al. "Unopposed Estrogen Therapy and the Risk of Invasive Breast Cancer." *Archives of Internal Medicine,* Vol. 166, No. 9, May 8, 2006, pp. 1027–1032.
23. Rosenberg, Lynn, et al. "A Prospective Study of Female Hormone Use and Breast Cancer Among Black Women." *Archives of Internal Medicine,* Vol. 166, No. 7, April 10, 2006, pp. 760–765.
24. "Diagnosing Ovarian Cancer." *Journal of the American Medical Association,* Vol. 295, No. 16, April 26, 2006, p. 1889.
25. Beresford et al. "Low-Fat Dietary Pattern and Risk of Colorectal Cancer."
26. Torpy, Janet. "Colon Cancer Screening." *Journal of the American Medical Association,* Vol. 295, No. 10, March 8, 2006, p. 1208.
27. American Cancer Society. *Cancer Facts and Figures,* 2006, www.cancer.org.
28. American Diabetes Association, www.diabetes.org.
29. Parmet, Sharon. "Weight and Diabetes." *Journal of the American Medical Association,* Vol. 295, No. 11, March 15, 2006, p. 1330.

Chapter 11

1. Kuehn, Bridget. "Shift Seen in Patterns of Drug Use Among Teens." *Journal of the American Medical Association,* Vol. 295, No. 6, February 8, 2006, p. 612.
2. American College Health Association. "American College Health Association-National College Health Assessment (ACHA-NCHA) Spring 2004 Reference Group Data Report (abridged)." *Journal of American College Health,* Vol. 54, No. 4, January–February 2006, p. 201.
3. McCabe, Sean, et al. "Medical Use, Illicit Use, and Diversion of Abusable Prescription Drugs." *Journal of American College Health,* Vol. 54, No. 5, March–April, 2006, p. 269.
4. American College Health Association. ACHA-NCHA Spring 2004 Reference Group Data Report.
5. Martens, Matthew, et al. "Differences Between Actual and Perceived Student Norms: An Examination of Alcohol Use, Drug Use, and Sexual Behavior." *Journal of American College Health,* Vol. 54, No. 5, March–April, 2006, p. 295.
6. Kilmer, Jason, et al. "Misperceptions of College Student Marijuana Use: Implications for Prevention." *Journal of Studies on Alcohol,* Vol. 67, No. 2, March 2006, p. 277(5).
7. Hirschfeld, Lindsay, et al. "A Systematic Analysis of College Substance Use Policies." *Journal of American College Health,* Vol. 54, No. 3, November–December 2005, p. 169.
8. West, Steven, and Carolyn Graham. "A Survey of Substance Abuse Prevention Efforts at Virginia's Colleges and Universities." *Journal of American College Health,* Vol. 54, No. 3, November–December 2005, p. 185.
9. Platz, Laurie, et al. "Gambling by Underage College Students: Preferences and Pathology." *College Student Journal,* Vol. 39, No. 1, March 2005, p. 3.
10. Black, D. W., et al. "A Family Study of Pathological Gambling." *Psychiatry Research,* Vol. 141, No. 3, March 30, 2006, pp. 295–303.
11. Tamminga, Carol, and Eric Nestler. "Pathological Gambling: Focusing on the Addiction, Not the Activity." *American Journal of Psychiatry,* Vol. 163, No. 2, February 2006, p. 1815.
12. Institute for Safe Medication Practices, www.ismp.org.
13. Radley, D. C., et al. "Off-Label Prescribing Among Office-Based Physicians." *Archives of Internal Medicine,* Vol. 166, No. 9, May 8, 2006, pp. 1021–1026.
14. "Expert Warns of Overdose of Over-the-Counter Pain Medication." News release, University of Michigan Health System, March 6, 2006.
15. "National Institutes of Health State-of-the-Science Conference Statement: Manifestations and Management of Chronic Insomnia in Adults." Bethesda, MD: National Institutes of Health, 2005.
16. McCabe et al. "Medical Use, Illicit Use, and Diversion of Abusable Prescription Drugs."
17. Bongartz, Tim, et al. "Anti-TNF Antibody Therapy in Rheumatoid Arthritis and the Risk of Serious Infections and Malignancies: Systematic Review and Meta-analysis of Rare Harmful Effects in Randomized Controlled Trials." *Journal of the American Medical Association,* Vol. 295, No. 19, May 17, 2006, pp. 2275–2285.
18. McCabe et al. "Medical Use, Illicit Use, and Diversion of Abusable Prescription Drugs."
19. Ibid.
20. Labig, Chalmer, et al. *Journal of American College Health,* Vol. 54, No. 3, November–December 2005, p. 177.
21. Cornelis, Marilyn, et al. "Coffee, CYP1A2 Genotype, and Risk of Myocardial Infarction." *Journal of the American Medical Association,* Vol. 295, No. 10, March 8, 2006, p. 1135.
22. Duncan, Greg, et al. "Peer Effects in Drug Use and Sex Among College Students." *Journal of Abnormal College Psychology,* Vol. 33, No. 3, June 2005, p. 375.
23. "Marijuana and Mental Health Problems." *Drug Detection Report,* Vol. 15, No. 13, June 30, 2005, p. 104.
24. FDA Press Office. "U.S. Food and Drug Agency Inter-Agency Advisory Regarding Claims That Smoked Marijuana Is a Medicine." April 20, 2006.
25. Messinis, L., et al. "Neuropsychological Deficits in Long-Term Frequent Cannabis Users." *Neurology,* Vol. 66, No. 5, March 14, 2006, pp. 737–739.
26. Ricuarte, George, and Una McCann. "Recognition and Management of Complications of New Recreational Drug Use." *The Lancet,* Vol. 365, No. 9477, June 18, 2005, p. 2137(9).
27. White, Barbara, et al. "Stimulant Medication Use, Misuse, and Abuse in an Undergraduate and Graduate Student Sample." *Journal of American College Health,* Vol. 54, No. 5, March–April 2006, p. 261.
28. Ibid.
29. "Prescription Narcotics: Methamphetamine Tops List of Treatment Admissions." *Alcoholism & Drug Abuse Weekly,* Vol. 17, No. 28, July 25, 2005, p. 1(2).
30. Colyar, Margaret, and Tracy Call-Schmidt. "Methamphetamine Abuse in the Primary Care Patient." *Clinician Reviews,* Vol. 16, No. 3, March 2006, p. 55.
31. Curtis, E. K. "Meth Mouth: A Review of Methamphetamine Abuse and Its Oral Manifestations." *General Dentistry,* Vol. 54, No. 2, March–April, 2006, pp. 125–129.
32. McCabe, S. E., et al. "Nonmedical Use of Prescription Opioids Among U.S. College Students: Prevalence and Correlates from a National Survey." *Addiction Behavior,* May 2005, Vol. 30, No. 4, pp. 789–805.
33. National Institute on Drug Abuse, www.nida.nih.gov.
34. White, Helene, et al. "Evaluating Two Brief Substance-Use Interventions for Mandated College Students." *Journal of Studies on Alcohol,* Vol. 67, No. 2, March 2006, p. 309(9).

Chapter 12

1. National Institute on Alcohol Abuse and Alcoholism, www.collegedrinkingprevention.gov.
2. American College Health Association. "American College Health Association-National College Health Assessment (ACHA-NCHA) Spring 2004 Reference Group Data Report (abridged)." *Journal of American College Health,* Vol. 54, No. 4, January–February 2006, p. 201.
3. White, A. M., et al. "College Students Lack Knowledge of Standard Drink Volumes: Implications for Definitions of Risky Drinking Based on Survey Data." *Alcoholism, Clinical and Experimental Research,* Vol. 29, No. 4, April 2005, pp. 631–63.
4. Nelson, T. F., et al. "'Binge' Drinking and Blood Alcohol Concentration." *Journal of Studies on Alcohol,* Vol. 66, No. 3, May 2005, pp. 438–439.
5. Wilsnack, Richard, et al. "Are U.S. Women Drinking Less (or More)? His-

torical and Aging Trends, 1981–2001." *Journal of Studies on Alcohol*, Vol. 67, No. 3, May 2006, p. 341(8).
6. Schiller, J. S., et al. "Early Release of Selected Estimates Based on Data from the January–September 2005 National Health Interview Survey." National Center for Health Statistics, March 2006, www.cdc.gov/nchs/nhis.htm.
7. American College Health Association. American College Health Association-National College Health Assessment (ACHA-NCHA) Web Summary, www.acha.org/projects_programs/ncha_sampledata.cfm.
8. Shinew, Kimberly, and Diana Parry. "Examining College Students' Participation in the Leisure Pursuits of Drinking and Illegal Drug Use." *Journal of Leisure Research,* Vol. 37, No. 3, Summer 2005 p. 364.
9. Brewer, Robert, and Monica Swahn. "Binge Drinking and Violence." *Journal of the American Medical Association,* Vol. 294, No. 5, August 3, 2005, p. 616.
10. Schiller et al. "Early Release of Selected Estimates Based on Data from the January–September 2005 National Health Interview Survey."
11. Hingson, Ralph, et al. "Magnitude of Alcohol-Related Mortality and Morbidity among U.S. College Students Ages 18–24." *Annual Review of Public Health,* Vol. 26, April 2005, pp. 259–279.
12. Wechsler, Henry, et al. "Drinking and Driving Among College Students: The Influence of Alcohol-Control Policies." *Journal of American College Health,* Vol. 53, No. 14, January–February 2005, p. 192.
13. National Institute on Alcohol Abuse and Alcoholism, www.collegedrinking prevention.gov.
14. Shinew and Parry, "Examining College Students' Participation in the Leisure Pursuits of Drinking and Illegal Drug Use."
15. American College Health Association. "ACHA-NCHA Spring 2004 Reference Group Data Report."
16. Ibid.
17. Martens, Matthew, et al. "Differences between Actual and Perceived Student Norms: An Examination of Alcohol Use, Drug Use, and Sexual Behavior." *Journal of American College Health*, Vol. 54, No. 5, March–April, 2006, p. 295.
18. Rice, Richard. "College Drinking: Norms vs. Perceptions." *The Scientist*, Vol. 20, No. 2, February 2006, p. 54(2).
19. Neighbors, Clayton, et al. "Normative Misperceptions and Temporal Precedence of Perceived Norms and Drinking." *Journal of Studies on Alcohol*, Vol. 67, No. 2, March 2006, p. 290(10).
20. Neighbors, Clayton, et al. "Event- and Context-Specific Normative Misperceptions and High-Risk Drinking: 21st Birthday Celebrations and Football Tailgating." *Journal of Studies on Alcohol*, Vol. 67, No. 2, March 2006, p. 282(8).
21. Mallet, Kimberley, et al. "Do We Learn From our Mistakes? An Examination of the Impact of Negative Alcohol-Related Consequences on College Students' Drinking Patterns and Perceptions." *Journal of Studies on Alcohol*, Vol. 67, No. 2, March 2006, p. 269(8).
22. Cho, Hyunyi, et al. "Readiness to Change, Norms, and Self-Efficacy Among Heavy-Drinking College Students." *Journal of Studies on Alcohol*, Vol. 67, No. 1, January 2006, p. 131(8).
23. Shinew and Parry, "Examining College Students' Participation in the Leisure Pursuits of Drinking and Illegal Drug Use."
24. Neal, Dan, et al. "It's All Fun and Games . . . or Is It? Collegiate Sporting Events and Celebratory Drinking." *Journal of Studies on Alcohol,* March 2005, Vol. 66, No. 2, p. 291.
25. Boyle, Jennifer, et al. "Perceived Parental Approval of Drinking and Its Impact on Problem Drinking Behaviors among First Year College Students." *Journal of American College Health*, Vol. 54, No. 4, January–February 2006, p. 238.
26. Sheffield, Felicia, et al. "Binge-Drinking and Alcohol-Related Problems among Community College Students: Implications for Prevention Policy." *Journal of American College Health*, Vol. 54, No. 3, November–December 2005, p. 137.
27. Lewis, Melissa, and Clayton Neighors. "Social Norms Approaches Using Descriptive Drinking Norms Education: A Review of the Research on Personalized Normative Feedback." *Journal of American College Health*, Vol. 54, No. 4, January–February 2006, p. 213.
28. Bozell, L. Brent. "Spring Break: Hazardous to Your Health?" *The Washington Post*, March 20, 2006 (online).
29. National Institute on Alcohol Abuse and Alcoholism, www.collegedrinking prevention.gov.
30. American College Health Association. "ACHA-NCHA Spring 2004 Reference Group Data Report."
31. Boyle et al. "Perceived Parental Approval of Drinking and Its Impact on Problem Drinking Behaviors Among First-Year College Students."
32. American College Health Association. "ACHA-NCHA Spring 2004 Reference Group Data Report."
33. LaBrie, Joseph, et al. "Heads UP! A Nested Intervention with Freshman Male College Students and the Broader Campus Community to Promote Responsible Drinking." *Journal of American College Health*, Vol. 54, No. 5, March–April 2006, p. 301.
34. White, Helene, et al. "Evaluating Two Brief Substance-Use Interventions for Mandated College Students." *Journal of Studies on Alcohol*, Vol. 67, No. 2, March 2006, p. 309(9).
35. Ehrlich, Peter, et al. "Screening and Brief Intervention for Alcohol Problems in a University Student Health Clinic." *Journal of American College Health*, Vol. 54, No. 5, March–April 2006, p. 301.
36. Ibid.
37. West, Steven, and Carolyn Graham. "A Survey of Substance Abuse Prevention Efforts at Virginia's Colleges and Universities." *Journal of American College Health*, Vol. 54, No. 3, November–December 2005, p. 185.
38. Hirschfeld, Lindsay, et al. "A Systematic Analysis of College Substance Use Policies." *Journal of American College Health*, Vol. 54, No. 3, November–December 2005, p. 169.
39. Ringold, Sarah. "Alcohol Abuse and Alcoholism." *Journal of the American Medical Association*, Vol. 295, No. 17, May 3, 2006, p. 2100.
40. Anton, Raymond, et al. "Combined Pharmacotherapies and Behavioral Interventions for Alcohol Dependence." *Journal of the American Medical Association*, Vol. 295, No. 17, May 3, 2006, p. 2003.
41. Krantzler, Henry. "Evidence-Based Treatments for Alcohol Dependence." *Journal of the American Medical Association*, Vol. 295, No. 17, May 3, 2006, p. 2075.
42. "Cigarette Smoking among Adults—United States, 2004." *Journal of the American Medical Association*, Vol. 295, No. 7, January 15, 2006, p. 749.
43. Kuehn, Bridget. "Shift Seen in Patterns of Drug Use among Teens." *Journal of the American Medical Association*, Vol. 295, No. 6, February 8, 2006, p. 612.
44. American College Health Association. "ACHA-NCHA Spring 2004 Reference Group Data Report."
45. Morrell, Holley, et al. "Predictors of Smoking and Smokeless Tobacco Use in College Students: A Preliminary Study Using Web-Based Survey Methodology." *Journal of American College Health*, Vol. 54, No. 2, September–October 2005, p. 108.
46. Morrison, Sharon, and Lara Talbott. "TRUCE for Advocacy and Peer Education in Tobacco Prevention." *Journal of American College Health*, Vol. 54, No. 3, November–December 2005, p. 193.
47. Gerson, Megan, et al. "Impact of Smoke-Free Residence Hall Policies: The Views of Administrators at Three Universities." *Journal of American College Health*, Vol. 54, No. 3, November–December 2005, p. 157.
48. American College Health Association. "ACHA-NCHA Spring 2004 Reference Group Data Report."
49. "Smokeless Tobacco Threatens Heart Health." *Medical Update,* Vol. 30, No. 111–112, May–June 2005, p. 6(1).
50. Smith, Kenesha, et al. "What Interventions Can Help Patients Stop Using

Chewing Tobacco?" *Journal of Family Practice,* Vol. 54, No. 4, April 2005, p. 368(2).
51. Mitchell, Amy, and Thomas Parish. "Using Combination Therapy for Smoking Cessation." *Clinician Reviews,* Vol. 15, No. 5, May 2005, p. 39(8).
52. Centers for Disease Control and Prevention, www.cdc.gov.
53. "Study Finds Online Smoking Cessation Treatments Fall Short." *The Brown University Digest of Addiction Theory and Application,* Vol. 24, No. 5, May 2005, p. 5(1).
54. "Nicotine Replacement Use on the Rise." *Alcoholism & Drug Abuse Weekly,* Vol. 17, No. 31, August 15, 2005, p. 7(1).
55. Nicotrol, www.nicotrol.com.
56. Chriqui, J., et al. "State Smoking Restrictions for Private-Sector Worksites, Restaurants, and Bars—United States, 1998 and 2004." *Morbidity and Mortality Weekly Report,* Vol. 54, No. 26, July 8, 2005, p. 649(5).

Chapter 13

1. National Safety Council, www.nsc.org.
2. National Highway Traffic Safety Administration, www.nhtsa.dot.gov.
3. Ibid.
4. Allen, Shane, et al. "A Comprehensive Statewide Analysis of Seatbelt Non-use with Injury and Hospital Admissions: New Data, Old Problem." *Academic Emergency Medicine,* Vol. 13, 2006, pp. 427–434.
5. Nerenberg, Arnold. Personal interview.
6. McEvoy, Suzanne, et al. "Role of Mobile Phones in Motor Vehicle Crashes Resulting in Hospital Attendance: A Case-Crossover Study." *British Medical Journal,* Vol. 331, No. 7514, August 20, 2005, p. 428.
7. Centers for Disease Control and Prevention (CDC), www.cdc.com.
8. Carr, Joetta. *Campus Violence White Paper.* Baltimore, MD: American College Health Association, February 5, 2005.
9. Baum, Katrina, and Patsy Klaus. "Violent Victimization of College Students, 1995–2002." *Bureau of Justice Statistics Special Report,* January 2005.
10. Ibid.
11. Carr, *Campus Violence White Paper.*
12. *Drawing the Line: Sexual Harassment on Campus.* Washington, DC: American Association of University Women, January 2006.
13. Ibid.
14. Oswald, Debra, and Brenda Russell. "Perceptions of Sexual Coercion in Heterosexual Dating Relationships: The Role of Aggressor Gender and Tactics." *The Journal of Sex Research,* Vol. 43, No. 1, February 2006, p. 87(9).
15. Gips, Michael. "Campus Rape Still Not Well Reported." *Security Management,* Vol. 50, No. 3, March 2006, p. 22(1).
16. Ibid.
17. Bard, Mark. Personal interview.
18. National Center for Complementary and Alternative Medicine, http://nccam.nih.gov.
19. Hsieh, Lisa Li-Chen, et al. "Treatment of Low Back Pain by Acupressure and Physical Therapy: Randomized Controlled Trial." *British Medical Journal,* Vol. 332, No. 7543, March 25, 2006, pp. 696-700.

Chapter 14

1. Pryor, John, et al. *The American Freshman: National Norms for Fall 2005.* Los Angeles: Cooperative Institutional Research Program, Higher Education Research Institute, UCLA, December 2005.
2. Revkin, Andrew. "Yelling 'Fire' on a Hot Planet." *New York Times,* April 23, 2006.
3. Egan, Timothy. "The Greening of America's Campuses." *New York Times,* January 8, 2006.
4. U.S. Office of Health and Human Services. *The Health Consequences of Involuntary Exposure to Tobacco Smoke.* Washington, DC: Office of the Surgeon General, 2006.
5. Portnoy, Jay, et al. "Health Effects of Indoor Fungi." *Annals of Allergy, Asthma & Immunology,* Vol. 94, No. 3, March 2005, p. 313.
6. Hales, Dianne. "New Help for Hearing Loss." *Parade,* May 14, 2006, p. 16.
7. "Cranked Up Music on Headphones Can Lead to Hearing Loss." University of Michigan Health System, January 3, 2006.
8. "Environmental Cancer Risks." *Cancer Facts & Figures 2006,* American Cancer Society, 2006.

Chapter 15

1. U.S. Census Bureau.
2. Knox, David, et al. "College Student Views of the Elderly: Some Gender Differences." *College Student Journal,* Vol. 39, No. 1, March 2005, p. 14(3).
3. Roizen, Michael. Personal interview.
4. "Facts About Older Americans." National Council on Aging, www.aoa.gov.
5. Leveille, Susan, et al. "Trends in Obesity and Arthritis Among Baby Boomers and Their Predecessors, 1971–2002." *American Journal of Public Health,* Vol. 95, No. 9, September 2005, p. 1607–1613.
6. Sherman, Sherry. Personal interview.
7. Speller, Marsha. Personal interview.
8. Pinkerton, JoAnn. Personal interview.
9. Chen, W. Y., et al. "Unopposed Estrogen Therapy and the Risk of Invasive Breast Cancer." *Archives of Internal Medicine,* Vol. 166, No. 9, May 8, 2006, pp. 1027–1032.
10. Rosenberg, Lynn, et al. "A Prospective Study of Female Hormone Use and Breast Cancer Among Black Women." *Archives of Internal Medicine,* Vol. 166, No. 7, April 10, 2006, pp. 760–765.
11. Prentice, Ross, et al. "Low-Fat Dietary Pattern and Risk of Invasive Breast Cancer." *Journal of the American Medical Association,* Vol. 295, No. 6, February 8, 2006, p. 629.
12. Duffy, S. A., et al. "Racial/Ethnic Preferences, Sex Preferences, and Perceived Discrimination Related to End-of-Life Care." *Journal of the American Geriatrics Society,* Vol. 54, No. 1, January 2006, pp. 150–157.
13. Kübler-Ross, Elisabeth. *Death: The Final Stage of Growth.* Englewood Cliffs, NJ: Prentice-Hall, 1975.
14. Simon, Robert, and Robert Hales (eds.). *Textbook of Suicide Assessment and Management.* Washington, DC: American Psychiatric Publishing, 2006.
15. Ibid.
16. Ringold, Sarah. "Grief." *Journal of the American Medical Association,* Vol. 293, No. 21, June 1, 2005, p. 2686.

Index